MEDICAL SECRETS

MEDICAL SECRETS

Anthony J. Zollo, Jr., M.D.
Assistant Professor
Department of Internal Medicine
Baylor College of Medicine
Ambulatory Care Service
Houston VA Medical Center
Houston, Texas

HANLEY & BELFUS, INC./Philadelphia
MOSBY – YEAR BOOK, INC./St. Louis • Baltimore • Boston • Chicago • London
Philadelphia • Sydney • Toronto

Publisher: HANLEY & BELFUS, INC.
                  210 S. 13th Street
                  Philadelphia, PA 19107
                  (215) 546-7293

North American and worldwide sales and distribution:

                  MOSBY-YEAR BOOK, INC.
                  11830 Westline Industrial Drive
                  St. Louis, MO 63146

In Canada: THE C.V. MOSBY COMPANY, LTD.
                  5240 Finch Avenue East
                  Unit 1
                  Scarborough, Ontario M1S 5A2
                  Canada

Library of Congress Cataloging-in-Publication Data

Medical secrets / |edited by| Anthony J. Zollo, Jr.
      p.   cm.
      Includes bibliographical references and index.
      ISBN 1-56053-011-1 (paper)
      1. Internal medicine—Examinations, questions, etc.   I. Zollo, Anthony J., 1954-
      |DNLM: 1. Internal Medicine—examination questions.   WB 18 M4885| RC58.M43   1991
      616'.0076—dc20
      DNLM/DLC
      for Library of Congress   91-7092
                                                                                     CIP

MEDICAL SECRETS   ISBN 1-56053-011-1

Library of Congress catalog card number   91-71526

Last digit is the print number: 9   8   7   6   5   4   3   2

CONTENTS

CONTRIBUTORS

Carol M. Ashton, M.D., M.P.H.
Assistant Professor of Medicine, Department of Internal Medicine, Baylor College of
Medicine; Director, General Medicine Consultation Service, Houston Veterans Affairs
Medical Center, Houston, Texas

Robert L. Atmar, M.D.
Assistant Professor of Medicine, Department of Internal Medicine, Baylor College of
Medicine, Houston, Texas

Douglas W. Axelrod, M.D., Ph.D.
Medical Director, Bone and Mineral Research, Norwich Eaton Pharmaceuticals, Inc.,
Norwich, New York

J. Todd Bagwell, M.D.
Fellow in Infectious Diseases, Section of Infectious Diseases, Department of Internal
Medicine, Baylor College of Medicine, Houston, Texas

Robert Bressler, M.D.
Assistant Professor of Medicine, Section of Allergy & Immunology, Department of
Internal Medicine, and Assistant Professor, Department of Microbiology & Immunology,
Baylor College of Medicine, Houston, Texas

Rhonda A. Cole, M.D.
Assistant Professor, Department of Internal Medicine, Baylor College of Medicine;
Assistant Chief, Admissions & Evaluations Unit, Houston Veterans Affairs Medical
Center, Houston, Texas

Sheila Goodnight White, M.D.
Assistant Professor of Medicine, Section of Pulmonary Medicine, Department of Internal
Medicine, Baylor College of Medicine; Director of Pulmonary Function, Pulmonary
Section, Houston Veterans Affairs Medical Center, Houston, Texas

Gabriel B. Habib, M.D.
Assistant Professor of Medicine, Section of Cardiology, Department of Internal
Medicine, Baylor College of Medicine; Director, Coronary Care Unit, Houston Veterans
Affairs Medical Center, Houston, Texas

Richard J. Hamill, M.D.
Assistant Professor of Medicine & Microbiology/Immunology, Departments of Internal
Medicine and Microbiology & Immunology, Baylor College of Medicine; Associate Chief,
Medical Service, Houston Veterans Affairs Medical Center, Houston, Texas

Mary P. Harward, M.D.
Assistant Professor of Medicine, Department of Internal Medicine, University of Florida
Health Sciences Center, Gainesville, Florida

Christopher J. Lahart, M.D.
Assistant Professor of Medicine, Department of Internal Medicine, Baylor College of
Medicine; Chief, AIDS Unit, Houston Veterans Affairs Medical Center, Houston, Texas

Patrice A. Michaletz, M.D.
Clinical Assistant Professor, Section of Gastroenterology, Department of Internal Medicine, University of Washington College of Medicine; Gastroenterologist, The Polyclinic, Seattle, Washington

Sangubhotla Prabhakar, M.D.
Assistant Professor of Medicine, Mount Sinai School of Medicine, New York, New York

Loren A. Rolak, M.D.
Associate Professor of Clinical Neurology, Department of Neurology, Baylor College of Medicine; Assistant Chief, Section of Neurology, Houston Veterans Affairs Medical Center, Houston, Texas

Richard A. Rubin, M.D.
Clinical Instructor in Medicine, Section of Rheumatology, Department of Internal Medicine, Baylor College of Medicine, Houston, Texas

George E. Taffet, M.D.
Assistant Professor of Medicine, Department of Internal Medicine, Baylor College of Medicine; Staff Physician, Huffington Center on Aging, Houston, Texas

Mark M. Udden, M.D.
Assistant Professor of Medicine, Section of Hematology, Department of Internal Medicine, Baylor College of Medicine, Houston, Texas

Donald E. Wesson, M.D.
Assistant Professor of Medicine, Department of Internal Medicine, Baylor College of Medicine; Assistant Chief, Renal Section, Houston Veterans Affairs Medical Center, Houston, Texas

Karen L. Woods, M.D.
Assistant Professor of Medicine, Section of Gastroenterology, Department of Internal Medicine, Baylor College of Medicine; Chief, Therapeutic Endoscopy, Harris County Hospital District, Houston, Texas

Nelda P. Wray, M.D., M.P.H.
Associate Professor of Clinical Medicine, Department of Internal Medicine; Clinical Associate Professor of Medical Ethics, Center for Ethics, Medicine & Public Issues, Baylor College of Medicine; Director, Houston Center for Quality of Care and Utilization Studies, Houston Veterans Affairs Medical Center, Houston, Texas

Anthony J. Zollo, Jr., M.D.
Assistant Professor of Medicine, Department of Internal Medicine, Baylor College of Medicine; Ambulatory Care Service, Houston Veterans Affairs Medical Center, Houston, Texas

Mary Anne Zubler, M.D.
Assistant Professor of Medicine, Section of Oncology, Department of Internal Medicine, Baylor College of Medicine; Chief, Oncology Service, Houston Veterans Affairs Medical Center, Houston, Texas

DEDICATION

To my wife, Mary, without whose help and support
this book, and many other things, would not have been
possible.

PREFACE

The art of Internal Medicine involves questions. It involves questions asked when taking a medical history, when forming a differential diagnosis, or when planning a diagnostic and therapeutic plan. Students of Internal Medicine, regardless of their level of training, are constantly confronted with questions posed from patients, from mentors, and from within themselves. The time-honored, question-based, Socratic approach to teaching is alive and well in the academic and clinical world of Internal Medicine. This book is intended to provide the reader with many of the questions (and answers) commonly encountered in training.

The knowledge base of Internal Medicine is substantial, probably more than any other specialty. Its acquisition is the goal of medical students, house officers, and all others who endeavor to learn and practice the discipline. There are many formal textbooks of internal medicine that provide complete coverage of all topics within the field. This work is not meant to replace the use of those texts. Rather, it is intended to focus on the lead-in questions and topics commonly encountered on teaching rounds, in clinical situations, and in examinations.

In preparing this text, we have attempted to take a middle ground between over-simplification and over-complication. We have included questions on common subjects and on "zebras," which, owing to their academic interest, are frequently discussed. We are grateful to our patients, our teachers, and our students for these questions and answers. As editor, I am indebted to my contributors on the faculty of Baylor College of Medicine for their assistance in this enjoyable and educational undertaking.

Anthony J. Zollo, Jr., M.D.
Baylor College of Medicine

Dear Reader:

If you would like to contribute question/answer sets for the next edition of *Medical Secrets*, please do so. The questions should be those that medical students and interns commonly encounter on rounds, in clinics, and in departmental or "Board"-type examinations. They may be in any area or subspecialty of internal medicine. Credit will be given if your contributions are used. Please remove this page, or photocopy it as many times as needed, and submit your question/answer sets to:

> Anthony J. Zollo, Jr., MD
> c/o Hanley & Belfus, Inc.
> 210 South 13th Street
> Philadelphia, PA 19107

Question:

Answer:

Reference (optional):

FROM: Name: _____

Address: _____

_____

THE FAR SIDE

By GARY LARSON

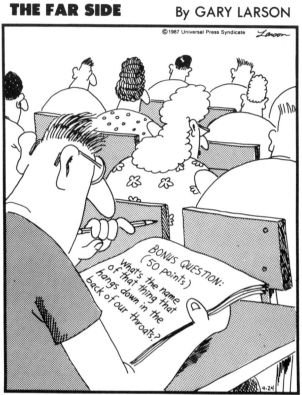

Final page of the Medical Boards

1. GENERAL MEDICINE SECRETS

Rhonda A. Cole, M.D. and Anthony J. Zollo, Jr., M.D.

> *The extraordinary development of modern science may be her undoing. Specialism, now a necessity, has fragmented the specialties themselves in a way that makes the outlook hazardous. The workers lose all sense of proportion in a maze of minutiae.*
>
> Sir William Osler (1849–1919)
> *Address, Classical Association, Oxford, May 16, 1910*

> *Choose your specialist and you choose your disease.*
>
> Anonymous
> *The Westminster Review, May 18, 1906*

1. What are Loeb's Laws of Medicine?
1. If what you're doing is working, keep doing it.
2. If what you're doing is not working, stop doing it.
3. If you don't know what to do, don't do anything.
4. Above all, never let a surgeon get your patient.

(From Matz R: Principles of medicine. NY State J Med 77:99–101, 1977, with permission.)

2. What are the predominant organisms constituting the normal flora of the various areas of the healthy human body?

Predominant Microorganisms Inhabiting Various Surfaces of the Healthy Human Body*

Oropharynx	**Lower genitourinary tract**	**Skin**
Viridans (alpha-hemolytic) streptococci	Staphylococci	Staphylococci (including *Staph. aureus)*
Staphylococci	Streptococci (including enterococcus)	Corynebacteria
Str. pyogenes	Lactobacilli (vaginal)	Propionibacteria
Str. pneumoniae	Corynebacteria	Candida sp.
Branhamella catarrhalis	Neisseria sp.	*Malassezia furfur*
Neisseria sp.	Obligate anaerobes	Dermatophytic fungi
Lactobacilli	Aerobic gram-negative bacilli	
Corynebacteria	*C. albicans*	**Large intestine and feces**
Haemophilus sp.	*Trichomonas vaginalis*	Obligate anaerobes (including *B. fragilis*)
Obligate anaerobes (not *Bacteroides fragilis*)	**Conjunctiva**	Aerobic gram-negative bacilli
Candida albicans	Staphylococci	Streptococci (including enterococcus)
Various protozoa	Corynebacteria	*C. albicans*
	Haemophilus sp.	Various protozoa
Upper intestine		
Streptococci	**Nasopharynx**	
Lactobacilli	Staphylococci (including *Staph. aureus)*	
Candida sp.	Streptococci (including *Str. pneumoniae)*	
	B. catarrhalis	
	Neisseria sp.	
	Haemophilus sp.	

*Adapted from Rosebury T: Microorganisms Indigenous to Man. New York, McGraw-Hill, 1962, pp 310–384.
(From Mackowiak PA: The normal microbial flora. N Engl J Med 307(2):83–93, 1982, Table 1, p 84, with permission.)

3. What are the principles of "diagnostic roundsmanship"?

1. Common things occur commonly.
2. The race may not always be to the swift nor the battle to the strong, but it's a good idea to bet that way.
3. When you hear hoofbeats think of horses, not zebras.
4. Place your bets on uncommon manifestations of common conditions rather than common manifestations of uncommon conditions.

(From Matz R: Principles of medicine. NY State J Med 77:99–101, 1977, with permission.)

4. What are the risk factors for thromboembolism?

Risk Factors for Thromboembolism

1. Heart disease, especially:	8. Fractures, especially of the hip
a. Myocardial infarction (MI)	9. Obesity
b. Atrial fibrillation	10. Varicose veins
c. Cardiomyopathy	11. Prior history of thromboembolic disease
d. Congestive heart failure (CHF)	12. Drugs, especially oral contraceptives and
2. Postoperative states, especially following	estrogens
operations on the abdomen or pelvis,	13. Following cerebrovascular accidents
splenectomy, and orthopedic procedures	14. Abnormal blood flow
on the lower extremities.	15. Myeloproliferative disorders with
3. Pregnancy and parturition	thrombocytosis
4. Neoplastic disease	16. Antithrombin III deficiency
5. Polycythemia	17. Protein C deficiency, protein S deficiency
6. Prolonged immobilization	18. Abnormal fibrinolysis
7. Hemorrhage	

(From Greenberger NF, et al: The Medical Book of Lists, 3rd ed. Chicago, Year Book Medical Publishers, 1990, Table I-36, p 28, with permission.)

5. What are the sensitivity, specificity, benefits, and shortcomings of the various tests used in the diagnosis of deep venous thrombosis?

Tests for Venous Thrombosis

TEST	LOCATION	SENSITIVITY (%)	SPECIFICITY (%)	COMMENTS
[125]I-fibrinogen scan	Distal	90	90	Contraindicated in pregnant or lactating women; insensitive for pelvic vein thrombi; unreliable in upper thigh
Impedance plethysmography	Proximal	>90	>90	Insensitive to calf thrombi; false-positives with incorrect patient position, low arterial flow, increased venous pressure
Doppler ultrasound	Proximal	>90	>90	Insensitive to calf thrombi; interpretation subjective; requires expert technician
Contrast venography	Proximal, distal	95	95	Expensive; technically difficult; increased side-effects; interpretation can be difficult
Fibrinogen scan and plethysmography	Proximal, distal	90	90	Noninvasive alternative to venography

(From Becker DM: Venous thromboembolism: Epidemiology, diagnosis, prevention. J Gen Intern Med 1:402–411, 1986, Table 3, with permission.)

6. What is a Baker's cyst and what condition can its rupture simulate?

A Baker's cyst is caused by posterior herniation of the knee capsule or leakage of synovial fluid into the popliteal fossa. It is also called popliteal bursitis and is most common in males 15–30 years of age. Its symptoms are limitation of knee extension, and pain. It can be felt as a swelling in the popliteal space. Rupture of a Baker's cyst, usually with trauma, can cause acute inflammation, pain, and swelling that can extend down into the posterior calf. This presentation can be confused with venous thrombophlebitis.

7. What is Munchausen's syndrome?

This syndrome, named after Baron von Munchausen, an 18th century German soldier/storyteller reputed to have been prone to wild exaggeration, describes a patient with a history of repeated factitious symptoms, illnesses, and accidents, usually of a dramatic or emergency nature. It is seen in women more frequently than men. The patients often have a history of multiple invasive procedures with negative findings. It is considered to be a psychiatric condition and must be separated from malingering, which is characterized by conscious intent to deceive.

8. What are the risk factors for anticoagulation?

Risk Factors for Anticoagulation

1. Recent central nervous system hemorrhage, stroke, or surgery	6. Salicylate therapy
2. Active gastrointestinal (GI) ulcerative disease (gastric, duodenal, ulcerative colitis, etc.)	7. Pregnancy
	8. Bacterial endocarditis
3. Chronic alcoholism, alcoholic liver disease	9. Old age
4. Bleeding diathesis	10. Blindness (unless supervised)
5. Malignant hypertension	11. Poor patient compliance

9. What factors indicate a poor prognosis in hypertension?

Factors Indicating an Adverse Prognosis in Hypertension

1. Black race	9. Evidence of end-organ damage
2. Youth	a. Cardiac (cardiac enlargement, electro-cardiographic [ECG] changes of ischemia or left ventricular strain, MI, CHF)
3. Male	
4. Persistent diastolic pressure >115 mmHg	
5. Smoking	b. Eyes (retinal exudates and hemorrhages, papilledema)
6. Diabetes mellitus	
7. Hypercholesterolemia	c. Renal (impaired renal function)
8. Obesity	d. Nervous system (cerebrovascular accident)

(From Wilson JD, et al (eds): Harrison's Principles of Internal Medicine, 12th ed. New York, McGraw Hill, 1991, Table 196-3, p 1004, with permission.)

10. What are the cerebrospinal fluid (CSF) findings in bacterial, tuberculous, fungal, and aseptic meningitis?

CSF Findings

	APPEARANCE	WBC COUNT (cells/μl)	WBC (diff.*)	GLUCOSE (mg/dl)	PROTEIN (mg/dl)
Normal	Clear	0–4	100% L* (<2 PMN)*	50–100	10–45
Bacterial	Hazy	200–10,000	75–100% PMN	0–45	100–1,000
Tuberculous	Hazy	50–300	50–90% L	5–45	75–300
Fungal	Clear/hazy	20–300	50–90% L	5–45	40–300
Aseptic	Clear	10–200	Mixed	50–100	25–100

* Diff. = differential count; L = lymphocytes; PMN = polymorphonuclear leukocytes.

11. Which organisms are implicated in meningitis of the adult?

Organisms Implicated in Adult Meningitis

Bacterial
H. influenzae
N. meningitidis
S. pneumoniae
Group A streptococci
S. aureus
Enterobacteriaceae
Klebsiella sp.
Pseudomonas sp.
Proteus sp.
Listeria monocytogenes
N. gonorrhoeae
Clostridium sp.

Spirochetal
Syphilis
Lyme disease

Viral
Nonparalytic poliomyelitis
Mumps
Enterovirus
Echovirus
Coxsackievirus
Adenovirus
Lymphocytic choriomeningitis

Other considerations
Neoplastic disease
Leptospirosis
Tuberculosis
Toxoplasmosis
Cryptococcus

Bensan CA, et al: Acute neurological infection. Med Clin North Am 70:987, 1986.

12. Which cranial nerves (CN) are commonly affected in tuberculous meningitis?

CN VI (abducens—usually bilateral)
CN III (oculomotor)
CN VII (facial)
CN VIII (acoustic)

Meyers B: Tuberculous meningitis. Med Clin North Am 66:733–762, 1982.

13. What criteria should be used to evaluate any preventative health care intervention?

Frame proposed the following six criteria:

1. The condition must have a significant effect on the quantity or quality of life.
2. Acceptable methods of treatment must be available.
3. The condition must have an asymptomatic period during which detection and treatment could significantly reduce the morbidity or mortality.
4. Treatment during the early asymptomatic period must yield a therapeutic result superior to that obtained if treatment is delayed until symptoms appear.
5. Tests to detect the condition in the asymptomatic period must be acceptable to patients and available at a reasonable cost.
6. The incidence of the condition must be sufficient to justify the cost of a screening program.

Frame PS: A critical review of adult health maintenance (Parts 1–4). J Fam Pract 22:341, 417, 511; 23:29, 1986.

14. What is meant by sensitivity, specificity, and predictive value of a test and how are they calculated?

The terms sensitivity, specificity, and positive or negative predictive values are frequently used in the assessment of a test and its ability to rule in or rule out a given condition (also called the **accuracy** of the test). To be able to use these values it is necessary to understand how they are derived.

Since a test can be positive or negative (if we disregard inconclusive results) and a patient either had or does not have a condition, there are four possible outcomes in any test situation. These are reflected in the following matrix:

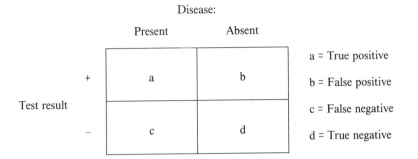

Disease:

	Present	Absent	
+	a	b	a = True positive
			b = False positive
Test result			c = False negative
−	c	d	d = True negative

The terms in question are derived from this matrix. Their definitions and derivations are as follows:

Definitions

Sensitivity $= \dfrac{a}{a+c} =$ The percentage of patients with the disease in whom the test is positive ("% positive in disease").

Specificity $= \dfrac{d}{b+d} =$ The percentage of persons without the disease in whom the test is negative ("% negative in health").

Positive predictive value $= \dfrac{a}{a+b} =$ The percentage of patients with a positive test result who actually do have the disease.

Negative predictive value $= \dfrac{d}{c+d} =$ The percentage of patients with a negative test result who really do not have the disease.

15. What is the pneumococcal polysaccharide vaccine (Pneumovax 23, Pnu-Imune 23) and to whom should it be administered?

This vaccine is composed of 25 micrograms of purified capsular polysaccharide antigens from 23 types of *Streptococcus pneumoniae*. In 1983, when introduced, it replaced the older 14-valent vaccine (released in 1977). These 23-capsular types represent 88% of the bacteremic pneumococcal disease in the U.S. Cross reactivity with other capsular types may increase this coverage another 8%. In healthy adults, antibody levels remain elevated for at least 5 years but then may fall to prevaccination levels within 10 years in some patients. Revaccination is recommended if more than 5 years have elapsed since the previous dose. The overall protective efficacy of the vaccine against pneumococcal bacteremia has been shown to be approximately 60%.

The Public Health Service's Immunization Practices Advisory Committee recommends that the pneumococcal polysaccharide vaccine be administered to the following groups:

1. Adults 65 years of age or older.

2. Adults with chronic illnesses who are at increased risk for pneumococcal disease or its complications (e.g., cardiovascular disease, pulmonary disease, diabetes mellitus, alcoholism, cirrhosis, cerebrospinal fluid leaks).

3. Immunocompromised adults at increased risk for pneumococcal disease or its complications (e.g., persons with splenic dysfunction or anatomic asplenia, Hodgkin's disease, lymphoma, multiple myeloma, chronic renal failure, nephrotic syndrome, organ transplantation).

4. Adults or children (age 2 or greater) with asymptomatic or symptomatic HIV infection.

5. Children (age 2 or greater) with chronic illnesses associated with increased risk for pneumococcal disease or its complications (e.g., anatomic or functional asplenia [including sickle cell disease], nephrotic syndrome, cerebrospinal fluid leaks and conditions associated with immunosuppression).

6. Persons living in special environments or social settings associated with an increased risk for pneumococcal disease or its complications (e.g., certain Native American populations).

Note: The vaccine is *not* recommended for patients with only recurrent upper respiratory tract disease, including otitis media and sinusitis.

CDC: Pneumococcal polysaccharide vaccine. MMWR 38(5):64–68, 73–76, 1989.

16. Are routine, periodic chest x-rays recommended as screening for lung cancer?

Routine screening chest x-rays are not recommended for lung cancer screening. Most lung cancers are already systemic diseases at the time of earliest possible detection by chest x-rays and the outcome as a result of screening by routine chest x-rays is not changed.

17. What is the Hemoccult Slide Test and what can lead to false positive or false negative test results?

The Hemoccult Slide Test (Smith-Kline Diagnostics, Sunnyvale, CA) tests for the presence of hemoglobin in feces. The slides use the peroxidase ability of hemoglobin to oxidize the guaiac-impregnated paper and produce a blue color. False negative results are obtained in patients with colonic neoplasms that are not bleeding (lesions < 1–2 cm, nonulcerated lesions), bleed intermittently, or are not producing the estimated 20 ml of blood per day that are required for a reliably positive result. Stool that is stored prior to testing and large doses of ascorbic acid may also lead to false negative results.

False positive results can be produced by the dietary intake of rare beef or fruits and vegetables that contain peroxidases. This effect is mainly seen in tests performed on rehydrated stool specimens. Oral iron preparations have been implicated in some studies and not in others. The mechanism by which iron preparations could cause false positive results is unclear, but it would be prudent to have patients avoid them during testing. False positive results can occur due to blood from sources other than colorectal carcinoma, such as the increased gastric blood loss caused by the use of nonsteroidal anti-inflammatory drugs (NSAIDs).

Fleischer DE, et al: Detection and surveillance of colorectal cancer. JAMA 261:580–586, 1989.

18. What screening program for colorectal cancer is recommended for patients who are asymptomatic and not members of a high risk group?

Annual digital rectal examination beginning at age 40, followed by annual fecal occult blood testing and initial flexible sigmoidoscopy beginning at age 50 are recommended. Positive screening tests require further evaluation

For maximum sensitivity in detecting colorectal cancer, follow-up evaluations should be performed even if only one out of a series of fecal occult blood tests is positive. The preferred method of evaluation is full colonoscopy. If this is not available, a flexible sigmoidoscopy and double-contrast barium enema examination should be performed. Positive flexible sigmoidoscopy requires total removal of all polyps.

Fleischer DE, et al: Detection and surveillance of colorectal cancer. JAMA 261:580–586, 1989.

19. What screening programs for colorectal cancer are recommended for patients in various high risk groups?

*Patient Groups at High Risk for Colorectal Cancer and Recommended Surveillance Program**

PATIENT GROUP AND RISK	SURVEILLANCE PROGRAM[†]
Markedly increased risk	
Familial polyposis coli and associated syndromes	FS every 6–12 mo from teens to age 40 yr; colectomy if multiple polyps found
Cancer family syndrome	Annual FOBT and colonoscopy every 2–3 yr, beginning at age 20 yr
Universal ulcerative colitis for 8–10 yr	Annual colonoscopy with multiple biopsies; colectomy if severe dysplasia is found and confirmed
Moderately increased risk	
Previous colon cancer or previous adenoma(s)	Colonoscopy 1 yr after resection and then every 3 yr if findings are normal; annual FOBT
Left-sided ulcerative colitis for 15–20 yr	Colonoscopy every 1–2 yr with multiple biopsies; colectomy if severe dysplasia found and confirmed
First-degree relative(s) with history of colon cancer	Annual FOBT and FS every 3–5 yr beginning at age 35–40 yr; if ≥ 2 relatives, colonoscopy every 3–5 yr
Woman undergoing irradiation for gynecologic cancer	Annual FOBT and FS every 3 yr after diagnosis and radiation therapy
Probable increased risk	
Previous gynecologic or breast cancer, or ureterosigmoidoscopy	Institution of usual screening tests of annual rectal examination and FOBT and FS every 3–5 yr after diagnosis of underlying associated disease
Other gastrointestinal tract polyposis syndromes	Periodic examinations of upper and/or lower gastrointestinal tract, depending on cancer risk in specific syndrome

* FS indicates flexible sigmoidoscopy, either 60 cm or 35 cm, which is preferred to rigid sigmoidoscopy; and FOBT, fecal occult blood test.
† Colonoscopy refers to total colonoscopy to the cecum; in some cases double-contrast barium enema examination plus flexible sigmoidoscopy may be substituted.
(From Fleischer DE, et al: Detection and surveillance of colorectal cancer. JAMA 261:580–586, 1989, Table 1, with permission.)

20. What is the differential diagnosis of generalized lymphadenopathy?

*Causes of Generalized Lymphadenopathy**

INFECTIONS[†]		NEOPLASMS
Bacterial		Lymphoma
Scarlet fever	Tuberculosis	Acute lymphocytic leukemia
Syphilis	Atypical mycobacteria	Chronic lymphocytic leukemia
Brucellosis	(Melioidosis)	Other lymphoproliferative disorders
Leptospirosis	(Glanders)	Immunoblastic lymphadenopathy
Viral		Reticuloendothelioses
HIV (including AIDS)	Rubella	
Ebstein Barr virus	(Dengue fever)	MISCELLANEOUS
Cytomegalovirus	(West Nile fever)	Sarcoidosis
Hepatitis B	(Epidemic hemorrhagic fever)	Other chronic granulomatous disorders
Measles	(Lassa fever)	Systemic lupus erythematosus
Parasitic		Rheumatoid arthritis
Toxoplasmosis	(African tyrpanosomiasis)	Hyperthyroidism
(Kala azar)	(Filariasis)	Lipid storage diseases
(Chagas disease)		Generalized dermatitis
Rikettsial	**Fungal**	Serum sickness
(Scrub typhus)	Histoplasmosis	Phenytoin administration

* Parentheses indicate infections that are uncommon or not reported in the United States.
† Other infections that characteristically may produce regional lymphadenopathy (e.g., tularemia, Lyme disease, lymphogranuloma venereum) may rarely cause generalized lymphadenopathy.
(Modified from Libman H: Generalized lymphadenopathy. J Gen Intern Med 2:48–58, 1987, Table 1, with permission.)

21. Which disease is associated with pagophagia (ice-eating)?

Pagophagia is associated with iron deficiency anemia (IDA). Patients with IDA may also crave other food and nonfood substances (pica). Although this behavior is rarely volunteered by patients, it is found in approximately 50% of such patients. The pica of IDA responds to iron repletion therapy.

Rector WG: Pica: Its frequency and significance in patients with iron-deficiency anemia due to chronic gastrointestinal blood loss. J Gen Intern Med 4:512–513, 1989.

22. What is the risk of recurrence after a first unprovoked seizure?

In a study of 224 patients with a first unprovoked seizure the overall recurrence rate was 16% at 12 months, 21% at 24 months, and 27% at 36 months. Patients with a history of prior neurological insult had a higher rate of recurrence (34%), all of which occurred within 20 months. Among those without a history of neurological insult ("idiopathic"), patients free of recurrence at 36 months did not have a subsequent seizure. Among the idiopathic cases, recurrence risk was higher in those with generalized spike-wave EEGs (50% at 18 months) and in those who had a sibling with seizures.

Hauser WA, et al: Seizure recurrence after a first unprovoked seizure. N Engl J Med 307:522–527, 1982.

23. What are the four stages associated with alcohol withdrawal?

1. **Tremulousness** occurs 8 to 12 hours after cessation of drinking. The patient manifests a tremor that is aggravated by intention or agitation. This stage may be accompanied by nausea and vomiting, insomnia, headache, diaphoresis, tachycardia, and anxiety. The symptoms usually subside within 24 hours unless the patient progresses to the next stage.

2. **Alcoholic hallucinosis** usually occurs 12 to 24 hours after the cessation of drinking, but may take 6 to 8 days to develop. The patient will experience auditory or visual hallucinations alternating with periods of lucidity. The symptoms of the first stage will continue and become more severe.

3. **Grand mal seizures** or "rum fits" occur in 90% of cases between 6 and 48 hours of cessation of drinking. The seizures are generalized and usually multiple. This stage occurs in 3–4% of untreated patients.

4. **Delirium tremens** usually occurs 3 to 4 days following the cessation of drinking, but may not develop for up to 2 weeks. It manifests as confusion, hallucinations, tremors, and signs of autonomic hyperactivity (including fever, tachycardia, dilated pupils, and diaphoresis). It is a medical emergency and carries a mortality of 5–15% despite treatment. Death is usually due to cardiovascular collapse.

24. What is the LD_{50} for ethanol?

The LD_{50} for ethanol is 500 mg/dl. This is the serum level which will be lethal in 50% of patients who ingest a sufficient quantity of ethanol to achieve such a high serum level. The amount of orally ingested ethanol needed to produce this serum level varies with the size of the person, the rates of ingestion, absorption, hepatic metabolism, and other factors. The healthy 70 kg person can metabolize about 10 g of ethanol an hour.

25. What body organs are directly affected by chronic alcohol abuse?

Alcohol has been noted to have pathological effects in nearly every organ system.

Organ System	Effects of Alcohol Abuse	
CNS	Alcohol withdrawal "blackouts"	Hallucinations
	Dementia	Seizures
	Wernicke-Korsakoff syndrome	Peripheral neuropathy

Table continued on next page.

Organ System	Effects of Alcohol Abuse (Continued)	
Gastrointestinal	Esophageal varices	Neoplasm
	Esophagitis, gastritis	Cirrhosis
	Vitamin deficiencies (niacin, B_{12}, thiamine)	Chronic pancreatitis
Cardiovascular	Arrhythmias	Cardiomyopathy
	Congestive heart failure	Hypertension
Pulmonary	Pneumonia (aspiration)	Tuberculosis
Genitourinary	Impaired spermatogenesis	Testicular atrophy
	Impotence/infertility	Amenorrhea
Musculoskeletal	Myopathy	Rhabdomyolysis
	Higher incidence of gout	Osteonecrosis
Endocrine	Increased cortisol	Hyperglycemia
	Decreased T4 and T3	
Hematopoietic	Impaired granulocyte function	Anemia (iron deficiency,
	Thrombocytopenia	B_{12} and folate deficiency, sideroblastic)

26. How quickly can a healthy person clear ethanol from his or her body?

A normal person can metabolize 150 mg of ethanol per kilogram of body weight per hour. In a normal 70 kilogram person, this leads to a decrease in blood ethanol level of approximately 20 mg/dl/hr.

27. What laboratory data support a diagnosis of liver disease due to chronic alcohol abuse?

- Elevation in gamma-glutamyl transpeptidase (GGT)
- SGOT:SGPT ratio $\geq$ 2:1
- Hypoalbuminemia
- Prolonged prothrombin time (PT)
- Low blood urea nitrogen (BUN)
- Low glucose
- Thrombocytopenia
- Macrocytosis of red blood cells

28. What constellation of symptoms comprise the Wernicke-Korsakoff syndrome?

This syndrome most commonly occurs in the malnourished, alcoholic patient, and includes the following symptoms:

Symptoms of the Wernicke-Korsakoff Syndrome

Ocular	**Altered mental status**
Horizontal/vertical nystagmus	Alcohol withdrawal
Paralysis of conjugate gaze	Global confusion (apathetic, inattentive, lethargic,
External rectus muscle paralysis	slurred speech, irrational)
	Korsakoff's amnesic psychosis
Ataxia	• Anterograde amnesia (impairment of learning
Stance and gait are affected	new ideas)
Cannot walk without assistance	• Past memory disturbances (confabulation)

29. Which drugs can cause gingival hyperplasia?

Phenytoin, cyclosporine, and nifedipine should be suspected in any patient with gingival hyperplasia.

Butler RT, et al: Drug-induced gingival hyperplasia: Phenytoin, cyclosporine and nifedipine. J Am Dent Assoc 114:56–60, 1987.

30. Which laboratory tests should be done in the evaluation of a person with dementia or delirium?

Laboratory Tests Used to Evaluate Cognitive Impairment

Complete blood count (CBC)	Erythrocyte sedimentation rate (ESR)
Chemistry panel	Serologic test for syphylis (VDRL)
Serum thyroxine (T_4)	Vitamin B_{12}
Serum folate	Urinalysis
ECG	Chest x-ray
CT scan (in selected pts.)	MRI scan (in selected pts.)
EEG (in selected pts.)	Lumbar puncture (in selected pts.)

(From Ramsdell JW, et al: Evaluation of cognitive impairment in the elderly. J Gen Intern Med 5:55–64, 1990, Table 7, with permission.)

31. How do you convert deciliters to milliliters, grains to milligrams, teaspoons to milliliters, etc.?

Useful Calculations and Conversions

- Swallow (avg) adult ≈ 10 ml   Child ≈ 5 ml
  (not a mouthful)

- 1 teaspoon (tsp) = 5 ml   1 tablespoon (Tbsp) = 15 ml

- Grain   = 64.8 mg
  1/65 grain   = 0.015 grain   = 1 mg
  1/150 grain   = 0.0067 grain = 0.3 mg
  1/400 grain   = 0.0025 grain = 0.15 mg

- Percent solution   1% solution   = 1 gram/100 ml
                                       = 10 mg/1 ml
                                       = 10 grams/liter

- Milligram percent (mg%) 1 mg%   = mg/100 ml
                                     = 10 mcg/ml
                                     = 1 mg/dl
                                     = 10 mg/liter

- Deciliter (dl) = 100 milliliters
  1 mg/dl = 1 mg/100 ml = 1 mg% = 10 mcg/ml

- Part per million (ppm) = 1 part in a million
  1 ppm = 1 mg/liter = 0.1 mg% = 1 mcg/ml

- Milligram (mg)   = 0.001 grams
  1 mg   = 1000 mcg
                   = 0.015 grain

- Microgram (μg)(mcg)   = 0.001 mg
  1 mcg/ml   = 0.1 mg%
                        = 0.1 mg/dl
                        = 1 mg/liter

- Nanogram   = 0.001 micrograms
  1 ng/ml   = 0.001 mcg/ml
                  = 0.1 mcg%
                  = 0.1 mcg/dl
                  = 1 mcg/liter
                  = 0.001 mg%

- Milliequivalent (mEq)
  1 mEq   = $\dfrac{\text{molecular weight gm}}{\text{valence} \times 1000}$

  1 mEq/L   = $\dfrac{\text{mg/L} \times \text{valence}}{\text{molecular weight}}$

  mg/100 ml = $\dfrac{\text{mEq/L} \times \text{molecular weight}}{10 \times \text{valence}}$

(From Flomenbaum NE, Roberts JR: Emergency department reference guide, 2nd ed. New York, Cahners Publishing co., 1989, p 20, with permission.)

32. What is St. Anthony's fire, St. Guy's Dance, St. Hubert's disease?

The following is a list of diseases and syndromes named after the saints:

Saint Syndromes

PATRONYMIC NAME	DISEASE OR SYNDROME
1. St. Agatha's	Mastopathic inflammatory disease
2. St. Aignan's or Agnan's	Favus ringworm, tinea
3. St. Arman's	Pellagra
4. St. Anthony's	
a. St. Anthony's dance	Chorea (see also St. Vitus)
b. St. Anthony's fire	Ergotism (epidemic gangrene and psychotic alterations)
c. St. Anthony's fire	Erysipelas

Table continued on next page.

Saint Syndromes (Continued)

PATRONYMIC NAME	DISEASE OR SYNDROME
5. St. Apollonia's	Toothache
6. St. Avertin's	Epilepsy
7. St. Avidus'	Deafness
8. St. Blasius'	Quinsy (peritonsillar abscess)
9. St. Dymphna's	Mental derangements
10. St. Erasmus'	Colic pain
11. St. Fiacre's or Flacre's	Hemorrhoids
12. St. Francis'	Erysipelas
13. St. Gervasius'	Juvenile or adult rheumatic pains
14. St. Gete's	Carcinoma
15. St. Giles'	Leprosy
16. St. Gothard's	Ancylostomiasis (hookworm disease)
17. St. Guy's dance	Chorea
18. St. Hubert's	Rabies
19. St. Ignatius'	Pellagra
20. St. Kilda's	Colds, infections
21. St. Louis'	Encephalitis
22. St. Main's	Scabies
23. St. Martin's	Alcoholism
24. St. Mathurin's	Idiocy
25. St. Modestus'	Chorea
26. St. Roch's or Roche's	Plague
27. St. Sebastian's	Plague
28. St. Valentine's	Epilepsy
29. St. Vitus' dance	Chorea
30. St. Zachary's	Mutism

(From Magalini SI, Euclide S: Dictionary of Medical Syndromes, 2nd ed. Philadelphia, J.B. Lippincott, 1981, p 728, with permission.)

33. What is the classic tetrad in Henoch-Schonlein purpura (HSP)?

The classic tetrad of HSP consists of palpable purpura, arthralgia or arthritis, abdominal pain, and hematuria.

34. What is spontaneous bacterial peritonitis (SBP) and how do you make the diagnosis?

SBP is seen in patients with liver disease and ascites. It is peritonitis without an obvious cause for peritoneal contamination (such as trauma, perforation, etc.). It usually presents as fever and abdominal pain or tenderness, but it may be asymptomatic and should be looked for in any patient with ascites who presents with a sudden onset of hypotension or hepatic encephalopathy. It can be diagnosed by demonstrating an ascitic fluid white blood cell count $> 500/mm^3$, with $> 50\%$ polymorphonuclear leukocytes on differential count. The infecting organism can be identified on Gram stain and on culture of the ascitic fluid.

35. In what setting does SBP occur and what are the most common bacterial organisms involved?

SBP is an infection of pre-existing ascites in the absence of any obvious intra-abdominal source. It occurs most frequently in patients with Laennec's cirrhosis but has also been described in patients with other types of liver disease such as chronic active hepatitis, acute viral hepatitis, and metastatic disease. Children with ascites due to nephrosis are also at risk.

Bacteriology in 253 Cases of Spontaneous Bacterial Peritonitis

CAUSATIVE BACTERIA	CASES (%)
Gram-negative bacilli	175 (69)
E. coli	119 (47)
Klebsiella sp.	28 (11)
Other	28 (11)
Gram-positive cocci	76 (30)
Streptococci—all species	65 (26)
S. pneumoniae	21 (8)
Enterococci	13 (5)
Other	31 (12)
Staphylococci	11 (4)
Anaerobes/microaerophils	13 (5)
Miscellaneous	3 (1)
Polymicrobial	20 (8)

(From Wilcox CM, Dismukes WE: Spontaneous bacterial peritonitis. A review of pathogenesis, diagnosis, and treatment. Medicine 66:447–456, 1987, with permission.)

36. What are the common causes of dementia?

Common Causes of Dementia

1. Diffuse parenchymal diseases of the central nervous system
   Alzheimer's disease (presenile or senile form)
   Parkinson's disease
2. Vascular disease
   Stroke
   Multi-infarct dementia
3. Drugs and Toxins
   Antidepressants   Lithium
   Anticholinergics   Alcohol
   Benzodiazepines   Barbiturates
   Phenytoin   Beta-blockers
   Most antihypertensive agents
4. Metabolic disease
   Renal failure   Hyponatremia
   Volume depletion   Hypo- and Hyperglycemia
   Hepatic failure   Hypothyroidism
   Hypopituitarism   Addison's disease
   Hypo- and Hyperparathyroidism   Severe anemia
5. Systemic illnesses
   Prolonged, sustained hypertension   Endocarditis
   Meningitis   Syphilis
6. Intracranial conditions
   Normal pressure hydrocephalus   Brain abscess
   Subdural hematoma   Tumor
7. Deficiency states
   Vitamin B_{12} deficiency   Pellagra
   Folate deficiency

(From Ramsdell JW, et al: Evaluation of cognitive impairment in the elderly. J Gen Intern Med 5:55–64, 1990, Table 5, with permission.)

37. What is Bell's palsy?
Bell's palsy is a demyelinating viral inflammatory disease that is the most common ailment of the facial nerve (CN VII). It is characterized by the following:

Bell's Palsy

Onset:	Usually preceded by viral prodrome Onset is acute
Duration:	Approximately 5 days Peak symptoms at 48 hours
Findings:	Unilateral Loss of facial expression Widened palpebral fissure Diminished taste Difficulty in chewing (food collects between lips and teeth) Hypesthesia in one or more branches of the fifth cranial nerve Hyperacusis
Treatment:	Protect the affected eye Prednisone (if patient presents within the first 2 days) The symptoms are self-limited

Adaur KK: Current concepts in neurology: Diagnosis and management of facial paralysis. N Engl J Med 307:348–351, 1982.

38. What are the leading etiologies of cerebrovascular accidents (CVA)?

- Embolism
- Atherosclerotic disease
- Lacunar infarcts
- Hypertensive hemorrhage
- Ruptured aneurysms/arteriovenous malformation

CVAs are the third leading cause of adult deaths. The major risk factors include hypertension, cardiovascular disease, advanced age, diabetes mellitus, migraine headaches, and the use of oral contraceptive agents.

39. What are the treatable causes of dementia?

Treatable Causes of Dementia

Medications
Psychoactive agents:
   Tricyclic antidepressants
   Tranquilizers
   Lithium carbonate
   Sedatives
Methyldopa
Clonidine
Propranolol
Phenytoin
Barbiturates
Corticosteroids
Digitalis
Quinidine
NSAIDs
Cimetidine
Diuretics

Metabolic derangements
Hepatic encephalopathy
Hypercalcemia
Hyponatremia
Uremia

Chemical intoxication
Alcohol
Carbon monoxide
Lead
Arsenic
Mercury
Organophosphates
Trichloroethylene

Endocrinopathies
Hypo- or hyperthyroidism
Addison's disease
Cushing's disease
Hypoglycemia
Panhypopituitarism

Intracranial lesions
Subdural hematomas
Cerebrovascular accidents
Brain tumor
Brain abscess
Multiple sclerosis
Hydrocephalus

Infectious etiologies
Neurosyphilis
Meningitis
Abscess

Miscellaneous
Depression
Pellagra
Wernicke-Korsakoff syndrome
Schizophrenia
Changes in environment:
   Nursing home placement
   Hospitalization

40. What are the types and causes of peripheral neuropathies in the adult?

Motor	Sensory	Sensorimotor	
Guillain-Barré syndrome	Alcohol	Diabetes mellitus	Alcohol
Porphyria	Diabetes mellitus	Uremia	Inherited neuropathies
Lead poisoning	Vascular disease	Chronic inflammatory	Metronidazole
Sulfonamides	Neoplasm	polyradiculopathy	Colchicine
Amphotericin B	Uremia	Clofibrate	Chlorambucil
Dapsone	Arsenic	Chlorpropamide	Tolbutamide
Imipramine		Phenytoin	Ergotamine
Amitriptyline		Nitrofurantoin	Streptomycin
Gold		Ethambutol	Ethionamide
		Penicillamine	Gold
		Indomethacin	Phenylbutazone

Farrante JA: Focusing on peripheral neuropathies. Emerg Med 22:57–62, 1990.

41. Which common viral illnesses are frequently seen in adults?
- Influenza A > influenza B
- Respiratory viruses
    Rhinoviruses
    Coronaviruses
    Respiratory syncytial virus (RSV)
    Parainfluenza
    Adenoviruses
- Epstein-Barr virus (EBV)
- Herpes simplex virus I and II (HSV)
- Varicella-zoster virus
- Cytomegalovirus (CMV)

42. Which organism is responsible for the cellulitis of marine water workers?
Vibrio vulnificus is ubiquitous in coastal waters. It is found in zooplankton and shellfish, and causes infection by penetrating into minor abrasions or lacerations. *Vibrio vulnificus* is invasive and can result in necrotizing vasculitis and gangrene.

Johnston JM, et al: Vibrio vulnificus: Man and sea. JAMA 253:2850–2853, 1985.

43. What are common etiologies of pneumonia?

Common Etiologies of Pneumonia

Bacterial	Viral
S. pneumoniae	Influenza A or B
H. influenzae—type B	Parainfluenza
Gram negative bacilli	Adenovirus
(klebsiella, pseudomonas, *E. coli*, proteus)	Cytomegalovirus (CMV)
Mixed flora	
Anaerobic bacteria (aspiration)	**Fungal**
S. aureus	Cryptococcus
	Aspergillus
Atypical	Histoplasmosis
Mycoplasma	Candida
TWAR chlamydia	Coccidioides
Legionnaire's disease	

44. What are the predisposing factors to acquiring the toxic shock syndrome (TSS)?

TSS is secondary to an infection caused by *Staphylococcus aureus*. It should be considered in any patient presenting with fever, rash, and hypotension. Risk factors include:

High absorbency tampons

Diaphragm placement for contraception

Postoperative wounds:
- Breast augmentation
- Caesarean section
- Indwelling catheters

Cutaneous infections (especially in the axillary or perianal areas)
- Cellulitis
- Burns
- Insect bites
- Abscess

Chunha BA: Case studies in infectious diseases: Toxic shock syndrome. Emerg Med 21:119–126, 1989.

45. Which organisms are most commonly implicated in infective endocarditis?

Streptococcus species	40%
Staphylococcus aureus	20%
Enterococci	10%
Staphylococcus epidermidis	8%
Gram negative bacilli	7%
Fungi	4%
Culture negative	10%

46. What are the features of cat scratch fever?

Who: Children represent 75% of the cases

When: Following a cat scratch, bite, or just close contact with a cat (in 93% of cases). Usually occurs in the fall or winter months.

What: Pleomorphic, gram negative, bacillary organism

Symptoms: Primary lesion: raised, slightly tender papule or pustule that
- may be single or multiple.
- appears 3–10 days after contact with cat.

Regional lymphadenopathy including axillary (most common), cervical, preauricular, submandibular, inguinal, femoral, and epitrochlear nodes

Other symptoms and signs: Fever, headache, malaise, rash, anorexia, emesis, splenomegaly, sore throat

Diagnosis: Exclude other possibilities

History of contact with a cat

Primary lesion on skin

Regional lymphadenopathy

Positive intradermal skin test

Skin or lymph node biopsy with demonstration of the bacillus

Therapy: Penicillin, erythromycin, cephalosporins, or clindamycin

(Note: The disease is usually self-limited and will resolve spontaneously in 1–2 months.)

47. Which groups are most susceptible to infection by the herpes zoster virus?

Elderly (over age 60)

Patients with Hodgkin's and non-Hodgkin's lymphoma

Immunocompromised patients
- cancer
- organ transplant
- AIDS and HIV infection

Patients on high dose steroid therapy

Weller TH: Varicella and herpes zoster. N Engl J Med 39:1362–1368, 1434–1440, 1983.

48. Which areas of the GI tract can be involved in Crohn's disease?
Crohn's disease had been reported to affect all areas from the small bowel to the anus. The major site of involvement is the colon.

49. What is the most common cause of diarrhea?
Most commonly, diarrhea is a result of infectious etiologies. Enterotoxigenic *E. coli* is the most frequently documented pathogen, but there are a host of viral, bacterial, protozoal, and parasitic causes.

50. What is the significance of projectile emesis?
Projectile emesis is characterized by the forceful expulsion of material from the mouth. It is most commonly observed in gastric outlet obstruction but may also occur in cases of increased intracranial pressure.

51. What are the more common etiologies of GI hemorrhage?

Upper GI hemorrhage	Lower GI hemorrhage
Peptic ulcer disease	Angiodysplasia (A-V malformation)
Erosive gastritis	Carcinoma
Varices	Diverticulosis
Esophagitis	Inflammatory bowel disease
Mallory-Weiss tear	Hemorrhoids
Polyps	

Gregory PR, et al: Upper gastrointestinal bleeding: Accuracy of clinical diagnosis and prognosis. Dig Dis Sci 26(Suppl):65, 1981.

52. What are the symptoms suggestive of peptic ulcer disease (PUD)?
PUD is suggested by epigastric pain that is described as deep, aching, or "gnawing"; is relieved with food or antacids; and awakens the patient at night.

53. What precipitates hepatic encephalopathy?
Hepatic encephalopathy is a syndrome comprised of altered mentation (lethargy, obtundation), fetor hepaticus (the peculiar odor of the breath in patients with liver disease), and asterixis (the "wrist-flapping" tremor) occuring in the patient with underlying hepatic insufficiency. The causes are multifactorial and include:
Factors causing increased blood ammonia:
GI hemorrhage
Increased dietary protein
Constipation
Metabolic alkalosis
Onset of renal insufficiency (dehydration, diuretics, or acute tubular necrosis)
Insufficient treatment with laxatives and lactulose
Factors leading to worsened hepatic insufficiency:

Sedatives and tranquilizers	Hepatorenal syndrome
Analgesics	Progressive hepatocellular dysfunction
Viral hepatitis	Ethanol use

Systemic factors:

Infections	Hypercarbia
Electrolyte abnormalities	Hypokalemia
Hypoxemia	

Fraser CL: Hepatic encephalopathy. N Engl J Med 313:865–873, 1985.

54. What are common causes of jaundice in the adult population?

Biliary tract obstruction:
- Gallstone
- Tumor
- Pancreatic neoplasm

Congestive heart failure

Hepatocellular carcinoma

Hepatocellular dysfunction:
- Hepatitis

  Viral

  Alcohol induced

  Drug induced
- Cirrhosis

5. What are common etiologies of acute pancreatitis?

Etiologies of Acute Pancreatitis

Cholelithiasis	Alcohol abuse
Idopathic	Postoperative (abdominal surgery)
Drug-induced	Hyperlipidemia (Types I or V)
Hydrochlorothiazide	Infection
Sulfonamides	Viral infection (mumps)
Tetracyclines	*S. Typhi*
Estrogens	Streptococcus
Ethanol	Pancreatic neoplasm
6-mercaptopurine	

Singer M, et al: A review of the classification of pancreatitis. Gastroenterology 89:683–685, 1985.

56. Which drugs are frequently abused in the U.S.?

Alcohol

Marijuana

Cocaine/crack

PCP (phencyclidine)

Prescription medications
- Tricyclic antidepressants
- Sedative-hypnotics
- Narcotic analgesics
- Anxiolytic agents
- Diet aids (amphetamines)

Heroin

Poly-drug abuse is common among all individuals who abuse drugs, regardless of socioeconomic levels.

57. What are the pathogenetic mechanisms of death in overdoses of tricyclic antidepressant medications?

Tricyclic antidepressants are the third most frequent cause of drug-related deaths. More than two-thirds of the deaths are in women. The agents most commonly implicated are amitriptyline, desipramine, and nortriptyline. The pathogenesis of death includes:

Respiratory arrest

Cardiovascular arrhythmias
- Ventricular fibrillation
- Prolonged QRS
- Asystole

Intractable seizures

CNS depression/coma

Marshall J, et al: Cardiovascular effects of tricyclic anti-depressants. Therapeutic usage, overdose and management of complications. Am Heart J 103:3–20, 1982.

58. What are the antidotes available for overdoses of acetaminophen, narcotics, anticholinergic agents, methanol, phenothiazines, cyanide, and organophosphates?

Antidotes Available for Specific Drugs

DRUG	ANTIDOTE AND DOSAGE:
Acetaminophen	N-acetylcysteine: 140 mg/kg initially, followed by 70 mg/kg every 8 hours for 17 doses
Narcotics	Naloxone (Narcan): 0.4–2.0 mg IV. Can be repeated at 2–3 minute intervals
Anticholinergic agents	Physostigmine: 2 mg by slow IV. Repeat in 20 minutes if no improvement, followed by 1–2 mg IV for recurrent symptoms.
Methanol and ethylene glycol	Ethanol (absolute): 1 cc/kg in D5W IV over 15 minutes. Maintenance dose: 125 mg/kg/hr IV in D5W.
Phenothiazines, haloperidol, and loxitane	Diphenhydramine: 25–50 mg; or benztropine: 1–2 mg (may be given IV or IM).
Cyanide	Sodium nitrite: 300 mg IV; or sodium thiosulfate; 12.5 gm
Organophosphates (insecticides)	Atropine sulfate: 2–5 mg IV. Repeat every 10–30 minutes to maintain a decrease in bronchial secretions. After atropine, pralidoxime: 1 mg IV for 2 doses. Repeat every 8–12 hours for 3 doses if the muscle weakness is not relieved.

Guzzardi LJ: Role of the emergency physician in poisoning. Med Clin North Am 2(1):10–11, 1982.

59. Which organs are frequently damaged by intravenous drug abuse (IVDA)?
In descending order, the damage is most frequently seen in the lung, heart, and kidneys.

60. What should be the initial steps in the assessment and treatment of a patient with a suspected drug overdose?
- Control airway.
- Check vital signs (blood pressure, respiratory rate, pulse rate, and temperature).
- Stabilize any abnormalities in vital signs.
- Check mental status/level of consciousness.
- Obtain blood for laboratory studies (chemistries, arterial blood gases, toxic screen).
- IV fluid: D5W with thiamine ± naloxone.
- Quick physical examination (heart, lungs, abdomen, neurological).

Goldfrank LJR, et al: Management of overdose with psychoactive medications. Med Clin North Am 2(1):65, 1982.

61. What are the common infectious diseases observed among IV drug abusers?
Patients who are IV drug abusers run a high risk of acquiring serious infections from all classes of pathogens and any organ system may be affected. These include:

Common Infections in IV Drug Abusers

Central Nervous System	Lungs	Heart
Meningitis	Pneumonia	Endocarditis
Abscess	• *S. aureus*	• *S. aureus* (>50% of cases)
	• Aspiration (anaerobes)	• Gram negative bacilli
Eye	• Gram negative bacilli	• Enterococcus
Endophthalmitis	Abscess	• Candida species
	Septic pulmonary eboli	• Polymicrobial
	Empyema	
	Tuberculosis	

Table continued on next page.

Common Infections in IV Drug Abusers (Continued)

Abdomen	Muscle	HIV Infection
Hepatitis B (#1 infection in IV drug abusers)	Necrotizing fascitis Pyomyositis	AIDS, ARC, etc. AIDS-related:
Skin	**Joints**	• *Pneumocystis carinii* pneumonia (PCP)
Cellulitis	Osteomyelitis	• Cytomegalovirus (CMV)
• *S. aureus*	Septic arthritis	• Toxoplasmosis
• Streptococci	**Genitourinary**	• Cryptococcus meningitis
• Gram negative bacilli	Sexually transmitted diseases	• *Mycobacteria*
Suppurative phlebitis	Renal abscesses	*avium-intracellulare*

Dobkin JF: Infections in parenteral drug abusers. In Mandell GL, Douglas RG, Bennett JE: Principles and Practice of Infectious Disease, 3rd ed. New York, Churchill Livingstone, 1990, pp 2276–2280.

62. What are the etiologies of common cardiac arrhythmias observed in the adult population?

Arrhythmia	Rate	Etiologies
Sinus tachycardia	100–160	Fever, pain, drugs, hyperthyroidism, hypotension
Paroxysmal supraventricular tachycardia (PSVT)	130–220 (usually 160)	Pre-excitation syndrome (i.e., Wolff-Parkinson-White syndrome), AV nodal re-entry, congenital abnormalities, atrial septal defect, concealed accessory bypass tracts
Atrial flutter	250–350	Mitral valve disease, COPD, pulmonary embolus, alcohol abuse, organic heart disease, MI, cardiac surgery
Atrial fibrillation	Atrial = 350–500 Ventricular = 100–160	Myocardial ischemia/infarction, organic heart disease, rheumatic heart disease, alcohol abuse, CHF, elderly patients, febrile illness, hyperthyroidism, chest surgery
Ventricular tachycardia	120–280	Ischemic heart disease, myocardial infarction, mitral valve prolapse, cardiomyopathy, hypercalcemia, hypokalemia, hypomagnesemia, hypoxemia

63. Which heart valves are most frequently affected in rheumatic heart disease?
In descending order of frequency: Mitral > Aortic > Tricuspid > Pulmonary.

64. What is the mechanism of Cheyne-Stokes breathing in the patient with severe CHF?

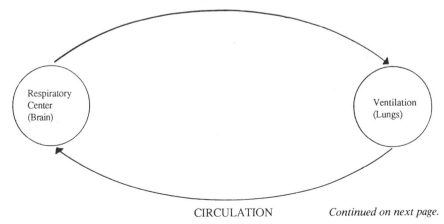

NERVES

Respiratory Center (Brain)

Ventilation (Lungs)

CIRCULATION

Continued on next page.

By using the diagram (see previous page), it is easier to understand the mechanism behind Cheyne-Stokes breathing. In the patient with left ventricular failure, the circulation time between the lungs and the respiratory center of the brain is lengthened. This delay causes the system to respond sluggishly, forming the basis of the oscillations in breathing patterns observed in Cheyne-Stokes respiration. Cheyne-Stokes breathing is characterized by periods of apnea alternating with hyperpnea. During apnea the PCO_2 rises and the PO_2 falls, causing stimulation of brain centers. The end result is hyperventilation. This results in a fall in the PCO_2, which results in suppression of the respiratory drive and another period of apnea ensues. The key to its development is the slow circulation time due to CHF, thereby altering the normally rapid feedback mechanism.

Lange RL, et al: The mechanism of Cheyne-Stoke respiration. J Clin Invest 41:42–52, 1962.

65. Which classes of medications should be given cautiously to persons whose ECGs reveal prolongation of the QT interval?

Anti-arrhythmics:

Class IA
- Quinidine
- Procainamide
- Disopyramide

Class IC
- Flecainide
- Encainide
- Lorcainide

Class III
- Amiodarone

Others:
- Phenothiazines
- Tricyclic anti-depressants
- Diuretics

66. What special management does a nontransmural or "non–Q-wave" MI require?
A nontransmural or non–Q-wave MI has a better short-term prognosis, but these patients are at risk for an extension of the infarction area, early onset of postinfarction pain, and an overall higher late mortality rate.

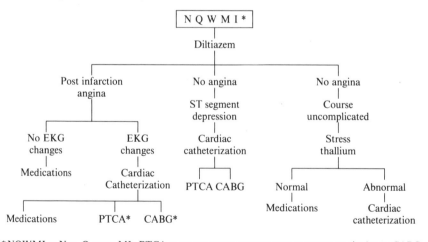

*NQWMI = Non–Q-wave MI; PTCA = percutaneous transvenous coronary angioplasty; CABG = coronary artery bypass grafting

Schechtman K: Predictors of mortality following non–Q-wave myocardial infarction. Cardio pp 98–106, 1990.

67. What symptoms indicate the need for corrective surgery in a patient with aortic stenosis?
In order of *decreasing* severity: (1) heart failure, (2) angina, (3) syncope.

68. When do ventricular premature depolarizations (VPDs) (or premature ventricular contractions [PVCs]) warrant medical therapy?

VPDs are usually not associated with an increased risk of sudden death. Although they occur in persons with otherwise normal hearts, they are more common in ischemic heart disease, cardiomyopathies, and the elderly. Treatment is advised in cases of:

- Frequent, repetitive ventricular ectopy
- Coronary artery disease (CAD)
    Angina
    Postmyocardial infarction
- Clinically significant valvular disease
- Mitral valve prolapse associated with syncope and/or ventricular tachycardia
- Cardiomyopathies
- Severe associated symptoms
- Syncope

69. What is torsades de pointes?

Torsades de pointes ("twisting of the points") is a polymorphic ventricular tachycardia characterized by QRS complexes that change in amplitude and electrical polarity, appearing to "twist" around the isoelectric line. A prolonged QT interval must be present. There may also be U waves.

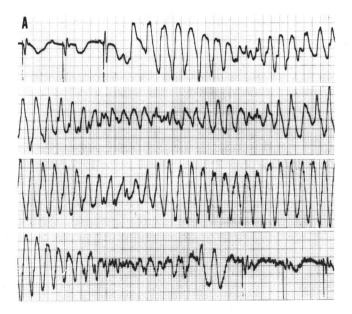

Torsades de pointes. *A,* Continuous recording monitor lead. A demand ventricular pacemaker (VVI) had been implanted because of type II second degree AV block. After treatment with amiodarone for recurrent ventricular tachycardia, the Q-T interval became prolonged (about 640 msec during paced beats), and the patient developed episodes of torsades de pointes. In this recording, the tachycardia spontaneously terminates and a paced ventricular rhythm is restored. Motion artifact is noted at the end of the recording as the patient lost consciousness. (From Zipes DP: Specific arrhythmias: Diagnosis and treatment. In Braunwald E (Ed): Heart Disease: A Textbook of Cardiovascular Medicine, 3rd ed. Philadelphia, W.B. Saunders Company, 1988, Fig. 22–36, p 699, with permission.)

Etiologies of this arrhythmia include:

Psychotropic drugs
- Phenothiazines
- Tricyclic antidepressants
- Lithium

Quinidine

Amiodarone

Disopyramide

Procainamide

Third degree heart block

Hypokalemia

Hypomagnesemia

Myocardial ischemia

Myocarditis

CNS lesions

Trauma

Tumors

Subarachnoid hemorrhage

Severe bradycardia

Saffer J, et al: Polymorphous ventricular tachycardia associated with normal and long Q-T intervals. Am J Cardiol 49:2021–2029, 1982.

70. What are the risk factors for the development of coronary artery disease (CAD)?

Hypertension

Hyperlipidemia

Tobacco use

Diabetes mellitus

Family history of CAD in those < age 55

Obesity

Sedentary lifestyle

Increasing age

Male sex

Grundy SM, et al: Coronary risk factors statement for the American public. Circulation 72(5):1135A–1139A, 1985.

71. What hormonal change occurs in women that increases their risk of CAD?

Menopause. Studies have shown that the risk of CAD, while lower in premenopausal females than in age-matched males, rapidly increases in postmenopausal females.

Gardan T, et al: Menopause and coronary heart disease: The Framingham study. Ann Intern Med 89:157–161, 1978.

72. A 35-year-old black male with past history of nephritic syndrome is admitted for elective knee surgery. He has been taking ibuprofen for 3 weeks. His admission serum creatinine is 3 mg/dl. What points help you to differentiate acute renal failure (ARF) from chronic renal failure (CRF)?

This patient with a previous history of nephritic illness has been taking a nonsteroidal anti-inflammatory drug (NSAID) and has a moderate degree of renal insufficiency. This could be ARF induced by the NSAID or could be an unrecognized progressive CRF. Urinary sediment can be useful in this situation. Acute interstitial nephritis is associated with red and white blood cell casts, whereas CRF is associated with broad casts (usually two to three times the diameter of a white blood cell). The presence of significant anemia, hyperphosphatemia, hypocalcemia, and changes of renal osteodystrophy are suggestive of advanced CRF. The most important confirmation of chronicity is demonstration of shrunken or small kidneys by ultrasound, IVP, or CT scanning.

73. What is the mechanism of acute renal failure secondary to NSAIDs?

The NSAIDs inhibit cyclo-oxygenase, an enzyme responsible for synthesizing prostaglandins from arachidonic acid. The intrarenal production of prostaglandins, especially PGE2, contribute significantly to the maintenance of renal blood flow (RBF) and glomerular filtration rate (GFR) in states of diminished effective arterial blood volume. In any of the prerenal states, angiotensin II and norepinephrine production is increased, which in turn increases renal vasodilator prostaglandin synthesis and thus leads to improvement of renal ischemia. The NSAIDs have the potential to significantly lower RBF and GFR in certain disease states (such as hypovolemia, CHF, nephrotic syndrome, and lupus nephritis) and produce acute renal failure.

An acute interstitial nephritis associated with nephrotic syndrome may also occur, particularly after the use of fenoprofen.

74. What patients are at highest risk of NSAID-induced renal failure?

The patients at highest risk for developing NSAID-induced renal failure include:

- Elderly patients
- Diabetic patients
- Patients receiving angiotensin converting enzyme (ACE) inhibitors and/or beta blockers
- Patients receiving more than one of the NSAIDs (i.e., aspirin and indomethacin)
- Patients on diuretics or patients who are dehydrated
- Patients with underlying CHF

75. Which conditions related to pregnancy predispose to acute renal failure (ARF)?

Although the incidence has markedly declined with control of septic abortions and antenatal care, ARF is not uncommon in pregnancy. Toxemia of pregnancy, antepartum hemorrhage, and postpartum hemorrhage are associated with an increased risk of ARF. The other predisposing factors are postpartum sepsis, abortion, postpartum hemolytic uremic syndrome, and amniotic fluid embolism. In addition, acute fatty liver and urinary tract obstruction are occasionally associated with ARF during pregnancy.

76. What are the physiological changes in the kidney during pregnancy?

Pregnancy is associated with an increase in GFR of about 50% and a mild decrease in plasma creatinine and BUN. There is a slight increase (about 1 cm) in kidney size, and dilation and tortuosity of the ureters. It was thought that these changes were secondary to pressure by the gravid uterus, but it is now known that these changes can be related to increased progesterone levels. Other physiological changes include increased uric acid clearance resulting in slight hypouricemia.

77. What are the effects of aging on the kidney?

- Diminished glomerular filtration rate (GFR)
- Decreased creatinine production (due to decreased muscle mass)
- Obstructive uropathy (due to benign prostatic hypertrophy)
- Urinary incontinence

78. What are the most common etiologies of acute renal failure in hospitalized patients?

- Hypoperfusion (approximately 50%)

  Dehydration   Sepsis

  CHF   Arrhythmia
- Postoperative renal failure
- IV contrast dye
- Drugs (especially aminoglycosides)
- Obstruction
- Hepatorenal syndrome

Hou SH, et al: Hospital acquired renal insufficiency: A prospective study. Am J Med 74:243–248, 1983.

79. Which antihypertensive agent is contraindicated in bilateral renal artery stenosis?

Angiotensin converting enzyme (ACE) inhibitors, especially captopril, may cause acute renal failure in these patients. Kidney function is usually quickly restored on discontinuation of the drug. In bilateral renal artery stenosis or stenosis to a solitary kidney, the renal perfusion pressure (and thus the GFR), depends upon the local renin-angiotensin system. When the system is blocked by captopril, a marked decrease in the efferent arterial pressure with subsequent decrease in renal perfusion pressure results, causing a diminished GFR.

Hricik DE, et al: Captopril-induced functional renal insufficiency in patients with bilateral renal artery stenosis or renal artery stenosis in a solitary kidney. N Engl J Med 308:373–376, 1983.

80. What does the presence of eosinophils in the urine denote?

Normal urine does not contain eosinophils, so their presence in a urine sample points to renal disease. The contribution of eosinophils to the immune response is not clearly known, but they are activated by antigens and antigen-induced hypersensitivity reactions. Eosinophils in the urine are characteristic of tubulointerstitial disease (i.e., interstitial nephritis), especially if they comprise >5% of the total number of white blood cells in the sample.

Eosinophils in the urine are seen in:
- Interstitial nephritis
- Urinary tract infections
- Kidney transplant rejection
- Acute tubular necrosis
- Hepatorenal syndrome

Carwin HL, et al: Clinical correlates of eosinophiluria. Arch Intern Med 145:1097–1099, 1985.

81. What comprises the hyporeninemic-hypoaldosteronism syndrome?

This syndrome features:
1. Low serum aldosterone levels (due to impaired secretion)
2. Low serum renin levels
3. Hyperkalemia (which is more severe than expected by the degree of renal insufficiency)

The average patient with the syndrome has the following characteristics:

Mean age	65 years
Asymptomatic hyperkalemia	75%
Chronic renal insufficiency	70%
Diabetes mellitus	50%
Cardiac arrhythmias	25%
Normal aldosterone response to ACTH	25%

82. In chronic renal failure patients, what is the importance of the $Ca^+ \times PO_4^-$ product (calcium-phosphate product)?

When the value of the product of the serum concentrations of calcium and phosphate exceeds 70, metastatic calcifications are more likely to occur. Calcium phosphate ($CaPO_4$) may precipitate out of the plasma and deposit in arteries, soft tissues, periarticular areas, and viscera.

Alfrey AC, et al: Extraosseous calcification. J Clin Invest 57:692–699, 1976.

83. Which organisms typically colonize the bronchioles of a patient who chronically abuses tobacco?

Hemophilus influenzae
Streptococcus pneumoniae
Branhamella catarrhalis
A variety of respiratory viruses

Tager A, et al: Role of infections in chronic bronchitis. N Engl J Med 292(11):563–571, 1975.

84. What is Hampton's hump?

Hampton's hump is a radiographic finding that is highly suggestive of a pulmonary infarction. It is a dense, homogeneous, wedge-shaped consolidation occurring in the middle and lower lobes. The base is contiguous with the pleura, but the apex points, in a convex fashion, towards the hilum. This gives the appearance of a "hump." Named after Aubrey Otis Hampton, U.S. radiologist, 1900–1955.

85. Which lung neoplasm is most prevalent among nonsmokers?

Ninety percent of all persons who develop lung cancer smoke. However, adenocarcinoma is the most common cancer seen in nonsmokers. It usually originates in the periphery of the lung and characteristically metastasizes to the lung, adrenal glands, liver, and brain.

86. What are the common etiologies of diffuse bilateral interstitial lung infiltrates?

- Pulmonary edema
- Miliary tuberculosis
- *Pneumocystis carinii* pneumonia
- Lymphangitic spread of carcinoma (breast, gastric)
- Sarcoidosis
- Lymphoma
- Drugs/toxins
  Nitrofurantoin
  Amiodarone
  Sulfonamides
  Zidovudine (AZT)
  Bleomycin
  Methotrexate
  Cyclophosphamide
  Chlorambucil
- Idiopathic

Crystal RG, et al: Interstitial lung disease of unknown cause. N Engl J Med 310:154–166, 235–244, 1984.

87. What is the erythrocyte sedimentation rate (ESR) and what causes it to be increased or decreased?

The ESR is a nonspecific index of inflammation. The normal values for patients under age 50 is 0–15 mm/hr in men and 0–20 mm/hr in women. The normal values increase with age and may reach values higher than the above-stated ranges in individuals over age 60, even in the absence of disease.

Whether the ESR is normal, increased, or decreased depends on the sum of forces acting on the RBCs. These include the downward force of gravity (dependent of the mass of the RBC), the upward buoyant forces (dependent on the density [mass/volume] of the RBC), and the bulk plasma flow (created by the downward moving RBCs). The ESR is affected by the following conditions:

Conditions that Increase and Decrease the Erythrocyte Sedimentation Rate

INCREASE	DECREASE
Inflammatory disorders	Increased serum viscosity
Hyperfibrinogenemia	Hypofibrinogenemia
Rouleaux formation	Sickle cell disease
Anemia (hypochromic, microcytic)	Leukemoid reaction
Pregnancy	Polycythemia
Hyperglobulinemia	Spherocytosis
Hypercholesterolemia	Anisocytosis
	High dose corticosteroids
	CHF
	Cachexia

The ESR is of little value in screening asymptomatic patients. It also is of little value in screening for malignancy, since it is often normal in patients with cancer. It is indicated in the diagnosis and monitoring of temporal arteritis and polymyalgia rheumatica. It may also be of value in monitoring the course and therapy of rheumatoid arthritis, Hodgkin's disease and other malignancies, and other inflammatory disorders.

88. What are the differences between presentation and prognosis of *Pneumocystis carinii* pneumonia (PCP) in the patient with AIDS and other types of immunocompromised patients (see also Ch. 13)?

	AIDS Patient	*Non-AIDS Patient*
Onset:	Insidious over weeks–months	Explosive, acute over 1–2 weeks
Symptoms:	Dyspnea, cough, fever, RR approx 24	Dyspnea, cough, fever, RR approx 38
Frequency:	Most common AIDS-related infection (>60%)	<30%
Recurrence:	30+%	<10%
Survival:	57%	50%
Diagnosis:	Bronchoscopy	Open lung biopsy
Treatment:	TMP/sulfa,* pentamidine (TMP/sulfa prophylaxis)	TMP/Sulfa

*TMP/sulfa = trimethoprim/sulfamethoxazole
Kouacs JA, et al: Pneumocystis carinii pneumonia: A comparison between patients with the acquired immune deficiency syndrome and patients with other immunodeficiencies. Ann Intern Med 100:663–675, 1984.

89. Which skin cancer is most common in adults?
Basal cell carcinoma (epithelioma) is the most common skin cancer. It occurs four to ten times as frequently as squamous cell carcinoma. The primary risk factor is excessive sun exposure, especially in fair-skinned individuals. Ninety percent of the tumors occur in sun-exposed areas of the skin. Metastasis is very rare and the prognosis is usually excellent, although deaths from local extension do occur. Removal of the tumor, by a variety of means, is usually curative.

90. Which skin cancer is associated with the highest mortality? What are its risk factors?
Melanoma causes the largest number of deaths related to skin cancer.

Risk Factors in Melanoma (in Descending Order)

Changing mole
Adulthood (age > 50 years)
Irregular pigmented lesions
    Dysplastic moles
    Lentigo maligna
Congenital nevus
White race
Previous cutaneous melanoma
Positive family history
Immunosuppression
Sun sensitivity
Excessive sun exposure

Rhodes AR, et al: Risk factors for cutaneous melanoma. JAMA 258:3146–3154, 1987.

91. What are actinic keratoses and in whom do they occur?

What:	Precancerous skin lesions: erythematous or tan plaques with an adherent scaly surface.
Whom:	Most common in elderly patients
Where:	Sun exposed areas: • face, dorsa of hands, forearms • balding scalp
Treatment:	Medical: 1–5% topical 5-fluorouracil Surgical: excision

92. Are tinea versicolor and vitiligo manifestations of the same disease?

No. The differences are shown in the following table:

	Vitiligo	Tinea
Etiology:	?Autoimmune	Fungal infection
Pathology:	Destruction of melanocytes	Decreased melanosomes in the stratum corneum
Incidence:	1%	Common
Age onset:	Young adults	Young adults
Description:	Macular depigmented areas. Absence of melanin	Small hypopigmented-to-tan macules with a bran-like scale
Associated conditions:	Grave's disease Pernicious anemia Diabetes mellitus Addison's disease	Seborrhea
Therapy:	Trioxsalen with sun exposure for a minimum of two times a week.	Selenium sulfide, sulfur ointments, ketoconazole, salicylic acid

Hertz KG, et al: Autoimmune vitiligo. N Engl J Med 297:634–637, 1977.

93. What are the differences between a chancre and chancroid?

	Chancre	Chancroid
Etiology:	Syphilis	A disease itself
Organism:	T. pallidum	H. ducreyi
Description:	Painless papule that rapidly erodes. Edge feels cartilaginous. Indurated	Painful, superficial ulcer with ragged edges. Base is covered by necrotic exudate
Location:	Penis, cervix/labia, anus/rectum in homosexuals	Preputial orifice, prepuce, frenulum in women
Treatment:	Penicillin G, tetracycline	Trimethoprim/sulfamethoxazole, erythromycin

94. What are petechiae?

Small, 1–3 mm round, reddish or brown lesions that do not blanch. They are caused by hemorrhage into the skin. They are commonly seen in platelet disorders and vasculitic processes.

95. When should a mole be removed?

Indications for Removal of a Mole

Change in size or diameter	Onset of bleeding, itching, or pain
Color becomes darker or lighter	Increase in height
Development of irregular borders	Congenital moles after one reaches
Elevation of the surface	adulthood (>50 years)

Rhodes AR, et al: Risk factors for cutaneous melanoma. JAMA 258:3146–3154, 1987.

96. What are cutaneous manifestations of hyperthyroidism?

Cutaneous Manifestation of Hyperthyroidism

Warm, moist, "velvety" texture of skin	Vitiligo
Increased palmar/dorsal sweating	Altered hair texture
Facial flushing	Alopecia
Palmar erythema	Pretibial myxedema

97. Which cardiac abnormality is a common cause of CHF in the elderly hypertensive patient?

Hypertensive hypertrophic cardiomyopathy commonly causes CHF in the elderly. The disease is characterized by:
- Severe concentric cardiac hypertrophy
- Small left ventricular cavity
- Elevated left ventricular ejection fraction (LVEF)

Tapale J, et al: Hypertensive hypertrophic cardiomyopathy of the elderly. N Engl J Med 312: 277–283, 1985.

98. Headaches in an elderly patient should always alert one to the possibility of which illness?

Temporal (giant cell) arteritis should be considered in any patient over the age of 50 with a headache. Untreated temporal arteritis can result in irreversible monocular blindness.

Symptoms of temporal arteritis include:
- Throbbing, unilateral headache
- Claudication of jaw when chewing and/or talking
- Decreased vision
- Fever
- Weight loss
- Pain and stiffness in the muscles and joints (15–20% patients have polymyalgia rheumatica)

Perovtka S, et al. Emergency care: Evaluation of headache and exclusion of serious etiologies. Modern Med 58:67–75, 1990.

99. What are the leading causes of blindness in the elderly?

Cataracts	Temporal arteritis
Glaucoma	*Chlamydia trachomatis*
Diabetes	Retinopathies

100. What are the different presentations of insulin-dependent diabetes mellitus (IDDM) versus non-insulin-dependent diabetes mellitus (NIDDM).

	IDDM	*NIDDM*
Age:	<40 years	>40 years, elderly
Onset:	Short period	Insidious, found incidentally on lab tests
Complications:	Diabetic ketoacidosis	Hyperosmolar coma
Body habitus:	Normal, thin	Obese
Pathology:	Islet cells destroyed	Insulin resistance, low insulin secretion, islet cells intact
Ketosis prone:	Yes	No
Therapy:	Insulin	Oral hypoglycemic agents, weight loss, balanced diet, perhaps insulin

101. Why are oral agents useful in the treatment of NIDDM?

Patients with NIDDM still have functioning beta cells in the islets of Langerhans of the pancreas. Therefore, there remains some endogenous insulin production. The oral hypoglycemic agents' primary mechanism of action is thought to include:
- Stimulation of insulin release from islet cells
- Increased insulin receptors in target tissues
- Improving the action of insulin

Ferner RE: Diabetes mellitus: Oral hypoglycemics. Med Clin North Am 72(6):1323–1335, 1988.

102. What are the end-organ effects of chronically elevated blood glucose?

End-organ Effects of Chronic Hyperglycemia

Skin:	**Kidneys:**
Dermopathy	Renal insufficiency
Diabetic foot ulcers	End stage renal disease (ESRD)
Lower susceptibility to skin	Nephrotic syndrome
infections	Repeated urinary tract infections
Eyes:	**CNS:**
Cataracts	Coma (as a result of diabetic ketoacidosis
Retinopathy	or hyperosmolar coma)
	Personality changes
Peripheral nerves:	Autonomic insufficiency
Peripheral neuropathy	
Mononeuropathy—median nerve	**Cardiovascular:**

Mononeuropathy—median nerve	Increased risk of CAD	Elevated total cholesterol
GU:	Silent myocardial ischemia	Lowered HDL cholesterol
Impotence	Cardiomyopathy	Hypertension
Retrograde ejaculation	Hypertriglyceridemia	Peripheral vascular disease

103. What tips on foot care should the diabetic receive?
- Check feet daily
- Wear cushioned shoes that fit properly (jogging shoes are great!)
- Never go barefoot
- Report redness, breakdown, or trauma to a physician immediately
- Soak in warm water 15–20 minutes daily, followed by lubrication with lotion
- Test bath water temperature with hands, not feet
- Calluses should be treated by a physician, nurse, or podiatrist (no bathroom surgery!)
- Trim nails squarely (do not round edges)

104. What is the strict definition of hypoglycemia?
Documented low blood sugar accompanied by symptoms that resolve with the ingestion of food. Symptoms include:

Anxiety	Trembling
Nervousness	Difficulty thinking
Headache	Sweating
Tachycardia	Confusion

Field JB: Hypoglycemia. Hosp Pract 187–194, Sept. 15, 1986.

105. What are consistent laboratory findings in adrenal insufficiency?
Hyponatremia (rarely <120 meq/l)
Hyperkalemia (rarely >7 meq/l)
Hypocarbia (HCO_3 approximately 15–20 meq/l)
Hypoglycemia
Elevated BUN
Elevated eosinophils
Elevated lymphocytes

106. Which metabolic derangement can cause obstructive sleep apnea?
Hypothyroidism that is severe enough to cause myxedema can lead to sleep apnea. The upper airway constriction is caused by myxedematous swelling of the face, tongue, and pharyngeal structures.

Orr WC, et al: Myxedema and obstructive sleep apnea. Am J Med 70:1061–1066, 1981.

107. What complaints in an elderly hypothyroid patient most commonly bring them to medical attention?
Constipation
Lethargy, easy fatigability
Difficulty in thinking
Cold intolerance
Bartuska DG: Thyroid disease in the news. Contemp Intern Med June 1989, pp 23–32.

108. What protection does the heterozygous sickle cell gene give?
The high frequency of the sickle cell gene in areas where malaria is endemic is an example of balanced polymorphism. The sickle cell gene protects the host from lethal *P. falciparum* malaria. The actual mechanism is still not fully understood, but it is postulated that the entry of the parasite into the host cell lowers red blood cell oxygen saturation. This desaturation leads to sickling and arrests the maturation of the parasite. The sickled cells are cleared by the phagocytic system.
Luzzatto L: Genetics of red cells susceptibility to malaria. Blood 54:961–976, 1979.

109. What are the different types of crises in sickle cell disease?
1. **Vaso-occlusive (painful):** The typical "sickle crisis" whose symptoms depend on location of occlusion.
2. **Aplastic:** Bone marrow suppression due to infection.
3. **Sequestration:** Seen in younger patients (age 1–5) while the spleen is still intact.
4. **Hemolytic:** Look for G6PD deficiency or malaria.
5. **Megaloblastic:** Seen in conditions of increased folate requirements (as in pregnancy).

110. How quickly does a megaloblastic bone marrow recover after adding the deficient vitamins to the patient's diet?
Within 6–8 hours after ingesting even small amounts of vitamin B_{12} or folate, the bone marrow begins to normalize.

111. Which drugs are most commonly implicated in drug-induced immune thrombocytopenia?

Antibacterials:
Sulfonamides
Rifampin
Trimethoprim
Ampicillin
Cephalosporins
p-Aminosalicylate
Nitrofurantoin
Isoniazid (INH)

NSAIDs:
Aspirin
Indomethacin
Phenylbutazone
Clinoril
Acetaminophen

Anticonvulsants:
Carbamazepine
Phenytoin
Sodium valproate
Diphenylhydantoin
Phthalazinol

Antihypertensives:
Methyldopa
Chlorothiazide
Hydrochlorothiazide
Diazoxide
Furosemide

Cinchona alkaloids:
Quinidine
Quinine

Miscellaneous
Heroin
Chlorpropamide
Bleomycin
Desipramine
Gold
Heparin
Cimetidine
Digitoxin

112. What are the differential diagnoses of macrocytic and microcytic anemias?

Macrocytic Anemia	Microcytic Anemia
Liver disease	Iron deficiency (most common
Vitamin B_{12} deficiency	type of anemia worldwide)
Folate deficiency	Hemoglobinopathies
Myelodysplastic syndrome	• Thalassemia
Drugs that impair DNA synthesis	• Sickle cell
• 6-Mercaptopurine	• SC disease
• Zidovudine (AZT)	Sideroblastic anemias
• 5-Fluorouracil	Anemia of chronic disease
• Hydroxyurea	

113. What are the characteristics of anemia of chronic disease?

Low serum iron	Hematocrit range 27–35%
Elevated or normal ferritin	Associated malignancy, or infectious
Low total iron binding capacity (TIBC)	or inflammatory disease

Lu GR: The anemia of chronic disease. Semin Hematol 20(2):61–80, 1983.

114. Which enzyme is usually elevated in lymphoma?

Lactate dehydrogenase (LDH) is elevated in many lymphomas and other lymphoproliferative disorders. The source is postulated to be tumor cells, and LDH is used as a measurement of disease activity.

Schneider RJ, et al: Prognostic significance of serum LDH in malignant lymphoma. Cancer 46:139–143, 1980.

115. Neutropenia is most commonly observed in which race of people?

Africans, West Indian blacks, and African Americans. This is not a genetic trait but rather an acquired one. The neutropenia probably results from an abnormal release of neutrophils by the bone marrow. The white blood cell count ranges 3000–4000 in African Americans. There is a normal response to infections, steroids, and pregnancy.

Exeilo GC: Non-genetic neutropenia in Africans. Lancet 2:1003–1004, 1972.

116. Which types of infections are asplenic patients most prone to develop?

Asplenic patients, either due to the anatomic absence of a spleen or functional asplenia, are prone to develop infections from encapsulated organisms. These include:
- *Streptococcus pneumoniae*
- *Hemophilus influenzae*
- *Neisseria meningitidis*

117. What criteria must be met to make the diagnosis of systemic lupus erythematosus (SLE)?

SLE is a chronic, inflammatory disease that results from an immunoregulatory disturbance. It is characterized by an exaggerated production of autoantibodies. There is a marked female predominance of the disease, with a female:male ratio of 9:1. To make a definitive diagnosis, four of the following 11 criteria must be met.

Diagnostic Criteria for SLE

1. Immunological disorder	(a) +LE cell preparation, *or* (b) anti-DNA antibody, *or* (c) anti-Sm antibody, *or* (d) falsely positive serological test for syphilis for at least 6 months.
2. Antinuclear antibody	Abnormal titer by immunofluorescence or equivalent test in the absence of "drug-induced lupus" syndrome.

Table continued on next page.

Diagnostic Criteria for SLE (Continued)

3. Malar rash	A fixed erythema over the malar eminence (flat or raised, sparing the nasolabial folds).
4. Discoid lupus	Erythematous. raised patches with adherent keratotic scaling and follicular plugging. Older lesions may scar.
5. Photosensitivity	Skin rash occurs in reaction to sun exposure.
6. Oral ulcers	Painless oral or nasopharyngeal ulcers.
7. Arthritis	Nonerosive arthritis involving two or more peripheral joints, characterized by edema, effusions, or tenderness.
8. Serositis	(a) Pleuritis by exam or history of pain, *or* (b) Pericarditis by ECG or rub or effusion.
9. Renal disorder	(a) Persistent proteinuria > 0.5 gm/day or greater than 3+ if not quantified, *or* (b) cellular casts: RBC, WBC, hemoglobin, granular, tubular, or mixed types.
10. Neurological disorder	(a) Seizures in the absence of other cause, *or* (b) psychosis in the absence of other cause.
11. Hematological disorder	(a) Hemolytic anemia with reticulocytosis, *or* (b) leukopenia, with count $< 4,000/mm^3$ on two or more occasions, *or* (c) lymphopenia, with count $< 1,500/mm^3$ on two or more occasions, *or* (d) thrombocytopenia, with count $< 100,000/mm^3$ in the absence of other cause (i.e., drugs).

(From Schumacher HR (ed): Systemic lupus erythematosus. In Primer on the Rheumatic Diseases, 9th ed. Atlanta, The Arthritis Foundation, 1988, pp 96–111, with permission.)

118. What are the three phases of discoloration in Raynaud's phenomenon?

Color	Phases
Pallor (white)	Vasospasm
Cyanosis (blue)	Digital ischemia
Rubor (red)	Reperfusion

119. What criteria are necessary to diagnose rheumatoid arthritis?
Rheumatoid arthritis boasts a worldwide distribution, affecting somewhere between 0.3%–1.5% of the U.S. population. Those affected most commonly are women between the 4th and 6th decades. To make a definitive diagnosis at least five of the following 11 criteria must be met.

Criteria for Diagnosing Rheumatoid Arthritis

1. Swelling in at least one joint for more than 6 weeks

2. Swelling in at least one other joint

3. Pain on motion or tenderness at one or more joints

4. Morning stiffness

5. Symmetric joint involvement (excludes the terminal interphalangeal joints)

6. Subcutaneous nodules (extensor surfaces)

7. X-ray changes:
   • erosions
   • bony decalcification
   • other typical changes of RA

8. Positive (+) rheumatoid factor (by any method)

9. Characteristic histologic changes in the synovial membrane:
   • villous hypertrophy
   • increased chronic inflammatory cells
   • cell necrosis

10. Characteristic histologic changes in the nodules:
   • chronic inflammatory cell infiltration
   • granulomas

11. Poor mucin precipitate from synovial fluid

Interpretation:
7 criteria = classic rheumatoid arthritis
5 criteria = definite rheumatoid arthritis
3 criteria = probable rheumatoid arthritis
2 criteria = possible rheumatoid arthritis

(From Schumacher HR (ed): Primer on the Rheumatic Diseases, 9th ed. Atlanta, The Arthritis Foundation, 1988, pp 207–208, with permission.)

120. A 19-year-old girl is admitted with salicylate poisoning. What are the acid-base disturbances that are seen in this condition if serial arterial blood gases are monitored?

Acute salicylate intoxication is characterized by profound effects on acid-base balance. Early in the course of intoxication, there is a primary respiratory alkalosis resulting from direct stimulation of the respiratory center in the medulla by salicylates. This causes an increase in pH and fall in P_aCO_2. A compensatory metabolic acidosis due to renal excretion of bicarbonate may be seen, which tends to bring the pH back toward normal. In young adults and children (especially with toxic doses), a primary metabolic acidosis ensues due to:

1. Impaired hepatic carbohydrate metabolism leading to accumulation of ketones and lactate in plasma.

2. Accumulated salicylic acid itself, which displaces several mEq of bicarbonate.

3. Dehydration and hypotension impair renal excretion of inorganic acids and cause further metabolic acidosis.

The resulting primary metabolic acidosis is normochloremic and associated with a high anion gap. The continuation of primary respiratory alkalosis and metabolic acidosis should give a clue to the diagnosis of acute salicylate intoxication. In more severe cases, primary respiratory acidosis occurs due to the depression of the respiratory center at very high salicylate levels.

121. Which hepatic disorders are associated with pregnancy? How are they diagnosed and treated?

Hepatic Disorders during Pregnancy

DIAGNOSIS	SYMPTOMS	LABORATORY FINDINGS	TREATMENT
Viral hepatitis	Most common etiology of jaundice during pregnancy Symptoms same as nonpregnant	Marked transaminase elevation Serologic markers Ultrasound: normal	Newborn immuno- prophylaxis at time of delivery
Intrahepatic cholestasis of pregnancy	Third-trimester pruritus without other symptoms	Bilirubin usually < 6 mg/dl Alkaline phosphatase 4 to 8 times normal Mild transaminase elevation Ultrasound: normal	Cholestyramine, 4–24 g/day Vitamin K
Preeclampsia	Second to third trimester	Hypertension, edema Bilirubin usually < 6 mg/dl Transaminase 5 × normal Microangiopathic hemolytic anemia, thrombocytopenia Ultrasound: normal; subcapsular hemorrhage	Delivery
Acute fatty liver	Third trimester	Abdominal pain, nausea, vomiting, hypertension Moderate transaminase increase Protime prolonged Hypoglycemia Leukocytosis, thrombocytopenia Ultrasound: increased echogenicity	Delivery

(From Carson JL, Elliot DL: Care of the pregnant patient with medical illness. J Gen Intern Med 3:577–588, 1988, Table 3, with permission.)

122. What is the carcinoid syndrome?

The carcinoid syndrome is a symptom complex caused by carcinoid tumors, which are the commonest endocrine tumors of the digestive tract. These tumors arise from enterochromaffin cells and have the ability to produce a wide variety of biologically active amines and peptides, including serotonin, bradykinin, histamine, ACTH, prostaglandins, and others. Because the liver, via the portal circulation, receives blood from the digestive tract and clears these products from the blood prior to their entry into the systemic circulation, most patients will not manifest symptoms until hepatic metastases occur.

The patients usually present with "cutaneous flushing" episodes, which typically are red in the beginning and then become purple, start on the face and then spread to the trunk, and last several minutes. These episodes are accompanied by increases in heart rate and decreases in blood pressure. They are initiated by alcohol, food stress, or palpation of the liver, or may be triggered by the administration of catecholamines, pentagastrin, or reserpine. The tumors can also cause diarrhea, crampy abdominal pain, obstruction, GI bleeding, and malabsorption.

123. What is the frequency of asymptomatic bacteriuria in patients over the age of 65, and is treatment necessary?
Asymptomatic bacteriuria is present in at least 20% of women and 10% of men over the age of 65. Treatment is not necessary unless it is associated with an obstructive uropathy.

Boscia JA, et al: Asymptomatic bacteriuria in the elderly. Infect Dis Clin North Am 1:893–905, 1987.

124. What are the two theories of site-specific tumor metastases?
Certain tumors exhibit site-specific metastases, which is the tendency of those tumors to preferentially spread to certain sites. The two theories proposed to explain this phenomenon, both of which are valid in selected cases, are:

1. **The "seed & soil" hypothesis** was proposed by Stephen Paget in 1889 and hypothesizes that certain tumors are predisposed to spread to specific tissues that have the ability to support the tumor's growth.

2. **The "mechanical" hypothesis** was proposed by James Ewing in 1928 and theorizes that certain tumors are predisposed to spread to specific tissues because they lie in the path of blood flow that carries tumor cells away from the primary site.

Zetter BR: The cellular basis of site-specific tumor metastases. N Engl J Med 322:605–612, 1990.

125. What are the common causes of delirium?

Common Causes of Delirium

1. **Drugs:**
   Sedative-hypnotics; phenothiazines; tricyclic antidepressants; lithium; narcotics; propoxyphene; pentazocine; antihypertensives; anticholinergics (other than psychotropic ones); diuretics; digitalis; anti-parkinsonian drugs; chlorpropamide; cimetidine; steroids; indomethacin; cancer chemotherapeutics; L-dopa; alcohol (intoxication and withdrawal).

2. **Metabolic disorders:**
   Electrolyte imbalances; acid-base disorders; hepatic encephalopathy; renal failure; respiratory failure; endocrinopathies; hypo- and hyperthermia; hypo- and hyperglycemia.

3. **Systemic illnesses:**
   Cardiac failure; arrhythmias; MI; pulmonary embolism; infection (especially pulmonary, renal, bacteremia, meningitis, and encephalitis); deficiency states.

4. **Cerebrovascular disorders:**
   Stroke; transient ischemic attack (TIA); subdural hematoma; cranial arteritis; cerebral vasculitis.

5. **Neoplasms:**
   Intracranial; extracranial.

6. **Stress:**
   Trauma; burns; surgery; sensory deprivation.

7. **Central nervous system diseases:**
   Neoplasm, trauma, epilepsy (ictal and post-ictal states).

(From Ramsdell JW, et al: Evaluation of cognitive impairment in the elderly. J Gen Intern Med 5:55–64, 1990, Table 6, with permission.

126. What is the classic pentad seen in Lyme disease?

Lyme disease, named after a town on the Connecticut shoreline where first identified in 1975, is a tick-borne infectious disease caused by the spirochete *Borrelia burgdorferi*. Occurrences are more common in the summer and fall seasons.

Clinical Pentad of Lyme Disease

Rash (erythema chronicum migrans)	Myalgias
	Fever
Headache	Chills

127. What are the clinical stages observed in Lyme disease?

Clinical Stages of Lyme Disease

STAGE	TIMING	SYMPTOMS
Stage 1	3–20 days after tick bite	Erythema chronicum migrans (ECM), headache, lethargy, malaise, fever, chills.
Stage 2	2–3 months after tick bite	**Cardiac symptoms:** prolonged PR interval, AV block, palpitations, and syncope. These symptoms can last 6 months or more.
		Neurological symptoms: usually these symptoms occur while ECM is still present. Include headache, stiff neck, photophobia, cranial nerve palsies (Bell's palsy), radiculoneuritis, encephalitis.
Stage 3	1–22 weeks after tick bite	Arthritis: asymmetric mono- or oligoarticular pattern. May have several recurrences of short (1–6 weeks) duration that primarily affect the large joints (i.e., the knees).

(Steere AC, et al: The early clinical manifestations of Lyme disease. Ann Intern Med 99:76–82, 1983.

128. How do you differentiate the common tachyarrhythmias?

Question	Sinus Tachycardia	Paroxysmal Atrial Tachycardia	Atrial Fibrillation	Atrial Flutter	Ventricular Tachycardia
Rate	100–200	169–190	160–190	140–160	100–230
Rhythm	Regular	Regular	Irregular	Regular	Slightly irregular
QRS shape	Normal[1]	Normal[1]	Normal[1]	Normal[1]	Abnormal
Atrial activity	Sinus P wave[2]	Absent or nonsinus P wave[2]	Absent	Flutter waves	Sinus P waves[2]
P-QRS relation	Yes	May be masked by rapid ventricular rate	No	May be masked by rapid ventricular rate	No
Carotid massage	Slows	No response, or converts to sinus rhythm	No response	Increased block	No response

[1] Unless intraventricular conduction disturbance.
[2] Sinus P waves are upright in lead II and occur at least 0.12 seconds before the QRS complex begins. (From Gottlieb AJ, et al: The Whole Internist Catalog. Philadelphia, W.B. Saunders, 1980, p 158, with permission.)

129. What are the manifestations of digitalis toxicity?

Manifestations of Digitalis Toxicity

1. **Arrhythmias:** the most dangerous and unfortunately often the first manifestation. Many different brady- and tachyarrhythmias have been described. The more common include supraventricular tachycardia (SVT) with atrioventricular (AV) block, ventricular ectopy, AV block, and sinoatrial (SA) or AV nodal exit block.
2. **Neurologic:** headache, fatigue, lethargy, confusion, delirium, seizures, and malaise.
3. **Gastrointestinal:** nausea, vomiting, diarrhea, anorexia.
4. **Visual:** disturbed color vision (greenish or yellow tinting, halos around objects)
5. **Endocrine:** gynecomastia in males.

130. What causes the hyperpigmentation of chronic venous stasis?

The breakdown of red blood cells as they pass through small blood vessels in the dermis, over a long period of time, leads to the hyperpigmentation changes.

BIBLIOGRAPHY

1. Andreoli TE, et al (eds): Cecil Essentials of Medicine, 2nd ed. Philadelphia, W.B. Saunders, 1990.
2. Hurst JW (ed): Medicine for the Practicing Physician, 2nd ed. Boston, Butterworths, 1988.
3. Kelley WN, et al (eds): Textbook of Internal Medicine. Philadelphia, J.B. Lippincott, 1989.
4. Noble J (ed): Textbook of General Medicine and Primary Care. Boston, Little, Brown, 1987.
5. Rubenstein E, Federman D (eds): Scientific American Medicine. New York, Scientific American Medicine, 1991.
6. Schroeder SA, et al (eds): Current Medical Diagnosis & Treatment. East Norwalk, CT, Appleton & Lange, 1990.
7. Stein JH (ed): Internal Medicine, 3rd ed. Boston, Little, Brown, 1990.
8. Wilson JD, et al (eds): Harrison's Principles of Internal Medicine, 12th ed. New York, McGraw-Hill, 1991.
9. Wyngaarden JB, Smith LH (eds): Cecil Textbook of Medicine, 18th ed. Philadelphia, W.B. Saunders, 1988.

2. ENDOCRINE SECRETS

Douglas W. Axelrod, M.D., Ph.D.

> *It would indeed be rash for a mere pathologist to venture forth on the uncharted sea of the endocrines, strewn as it is with the wrecks of shattered hypotheses, where even the most wary mariner may easily lose his way as he seeks to steer his bark amid the glandular temptations whose siren voices have proved the downfall of many who have gone before.*
>
> William Boyd (1885–1972)
> *Pathology for the Surgeon, 7th edition, Ch. 32*

GENERAL

1. Who was William of Ockham (or Occam)? What was his Razor? Of what did he die?
William of Ockham, known as Doctor Invincibilis, was a 14th century philosopher. His "Razor," a philosophical means of choosing doctrinal postulates, was *Essentia non sunt multiplicanda praetor necessitatum,* or "Entities (or postulates) are not to be multiplied without necessity." We use Occam's Razor to choose the fewest etiologies to explain multiple problems.
William of Ockham died of multiple causes (Axelrod's Corollary to Ockham's Razor).

2. What does Lao-tzu (founder of Taoism and author of *Tao Tê Ching*) say about the differences between endocrinology, neurology, and immunology?
"Once the whole is divided, the parts need names." Needless adherence to disciplinary or doctrinal lines subverts the inherent connections among these disciplines and leads to an incomplete understanding of the total organism, the whole.

3. What is the most important thing in approaching a patient (according to Zen Master Ikkyu)?
"Attention." Before one takes the history or does the physical, one should *attend* fully to the patient and thereby maximize the appreciation of the sensory data that are incoming. Failure to do so leads to the prejudicial selection of data and may bring about an erroneous or incomplete diagnosis.

DIABETES AND METABOLISM

4. How does one calculate caloric needs in prescribing a diet?
One may make an initial estimate of caloric needs by multiplying the patient's weight by the energy use per kilogram based on activity level. Bed rest is estimated to use 20–25 calories/kg/day; desk work uses 30; work including walking uses up to 35; very active physical labor uses 40–50. These estimates may be used as a first approximation but should be adjusted as the patient demonstrates his or her own caloric needs.

5. How many calories must one lack each day to lose 1 pound a week?
One pound of fat stores approximately 3500 calories. Thus, one must establish a deficit of 500 calories each day to lose 1 pound of fat each week. Of course, overall weight loss entails a day-to-day balance of salt, water, and muscle, as well as fat, so that this calculation may not match changes in the actual measured body weight.

6. What are the current recommendations for the distribution of dietary nutrients?

Distribution of Dietary Nutrients

Protein	20%
Fat	30%
Carbohydrate*	45–50%

*The carbohydrate portion is preferably made up of complex carbohydrates.

7. What is c-peptide?

C-peptide is the fragment that is clipped out of the center of the original insulin polypeptide after sulfhydryl bonding has connected what will become the alpha and beta chains. It is secreted from the pancreatic beta cells with insulin on an equimolar basis and may be used in assessing endogenous insulin secretion.

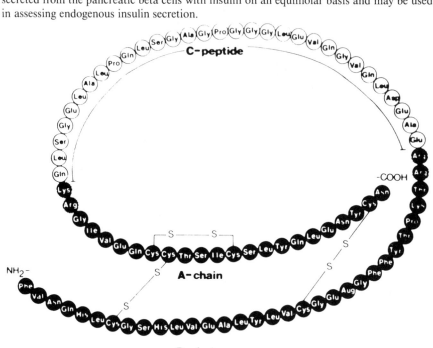

Amino acid sequence and covalent structure of human proinsulin. (From Skyler JS: Insulin dependent diabetes mellitus. In: Kohler PO (ed): Clinical Endocrinology. New York, John Wiley, 1986, p 505, with permission.)

8. What factors influence glucose control? Which factors may be modulated?

Glucose control is an overall result of the balance between glucose production and disposal. Glucose production is controlled by gluconeogenic substrate supply and the hormonal environment, including insulin, growth hormone, cortisol, glucagon, and catecholamines.

Glucose disposal may be divided into two processes. The first is cellular uptake, governed by actual caloric needs created by exercise and by circulating insulin. Second, disposal is also controlled, in part, by renal losses when the circulating glucose concentration exceeds the maximum renal threshold (T_{max}).

In the diabetic patient, production may be modulated by diet, exercise, insulin, or hypoglycemic agent selection, and the avoidance of stressors.

9. What is the average hepatic glucose production per day? What does this suggest about hyperglycemia attributed to routine intravenous fluids?

Within the first 24 hours of fasting, the liver generates roughly 180 grams of glucose for metabolic support. The usual regimen of 125 ml/hour of 5% dextrose would provide 150 grams of glucose per day. Obviously this amount should be easily tolerated. Hyperglycemia in this setting cannot be attributed to the intravenous fluids used.

10. Where does the major clearance of insulin occur?

Insulin has approximately 50% clearance on first pass through the liver. Once in the periphery, roughly 30% of the remainder is cleared by the kidney.

11. What is the difference between type I and type II diabetes?

Type I diabetes is defined as that form of glucose intolerance in which diabetic ketoacidosis (DKA) will ensue without exogenous insulin. Type II diabetes is that form of glucose intolerance in which DKA does not occur (barring extraordinary stress). These two forms have similarity to the former designations "juvenile onset" and "adult onset" diabetes, respectively. Note that the type of diabetes is not dependent on whether or not the patient uses insulin.

12. What are some causes of secondary diabetes?

Causes of Secondary Diabetes

Processes causing reduced insulin secretion:	Processes producing impairment of insulin action:
Pancreatitis or pancreatectomy	Insulin receptor defects
Cystic fibrosis	• With acanthosis nigricans
Hemochromatosis	• Insulin receptor antibodies
Pheochromocytoma	Anti-insulin antibodies
Somatostatinoma	Diseases producing excess anti-insulin hormones
Aldosteronoma	• Pheochromocytoma
Hypokalemia	• Cushing's syndrome
	• Acromegaly
	• Glucagonoma
	• Thyrotoxicosis

Diseases producing secondary diabetes by unknown mechanism:

Muscular dystrophy	Friedreich's ataxia	Chromosomal abnormalities
Myotonic dystrophy	Lawrence-Moon-Biedl	• Klinefelter's syndrome
Acute intermittent porphyria	syndrome	• Turner's syndrome
Glycogen storage disease, type I	Progeria	• Down's syndrome
Hyperlipidemia	Prader-Willi syndrome	Sexual ateliotic dwarfism

(From Garber AJ: Diabetes mellitus. In: Stein JH (ed): Internal Medicine, 3rd ed. Boston, Little, Brown, 1990, p 2244, with permission.)

13. How do you make the diagnosis of type II diabetes?

The diagnosis is made by demonstrating one of the following diagnostic criteria:

1. Classic symptoms of uncontrolled diabetes (polydypsia, polyuria, rapid weight loss) along with unequivocal elevation of random blood sugar (>200 mg/dl).

2. Fasting venous plasma glucose greater than 140 mg/dl on more than one occasion.

3. Fasting venous plasma glucose greater than 115 mg/dl.

and

Oral glucose tolerance test with 2-hour value and one other value both at least 200 mg/dl.

14. How does one sort out the terms "insulin dependent," "insulin requiring," and "insulin using"?

You must bear in mind the definitions of type I and II diabetes. The person using the terms "insulin-dependent" and "insulin-requiring" may mean the patient lapses into diabetic keto-acidosis (DKA) without insulin, indicating type I diabetes. Alternatively, however, the person may mean that the patient cannot be rendered euglycemic without the use of insulin. "Insulin-using" is a useful term when used to describe a type II diabetic, suggesting that the patient has failed control on diet and/or oral agents, and has therefore been placed on insulin therapy. These descriptions are prone to misinterpretation and should not be used as diagnostic terms.

15. In diabetic ketoacidosis (DKA), what are the usual deficits of sodium, potassium, and water?

	Total	*Per Kg-Body-Weight*
Water	5–11 liters	100 ml
Sodium	300–700 meq	7 meq
Chloride	350–500 meq	5 meq
Potassium	200–700 meq	5 meq
Phosphate	70–100 mMole	1 mMole

16. Continuous intravenous insulin is the usual means of insulin administration. What dose should be used?

After intravenous bolus of 0.1 U/kg, infusion should begin at 0.1 U/kg/hour. After this rate is initiated, blood glucose should be carefully followed and insulin administration tailored to the individual patient.

17. How does one convert to intermittent insulin after intravenous therapy?

One may begin a regimen of intermediate and short-acting insulins, beginning with 75% of the intravenous dose administered over the previous 24 hours. On discontinuing intravenous insulin, be sure to give the subcutaneous insulin for a long enough period prior to stopping the intravenous insulin, to allow the subcutaneous insulin to act.

18. When would one choose human insulin over another source?

Patients started on insulin should be started on human insulin. Patients experiencing lipo-dystrophy or in whom insulin resistance becomes problematic may benefit from switching to human insulin. Otherwise, there is no pressing reason to change insulin species in a well-controlled diabetic.

19. What accounts for the high frequency of recurrent diabetic ketoacidosis (DKA) in the alcoholic or malnourished patient? How might this complication be avoided?

Such patients are often depleted of potential glucogenic substrates, with low liver glycogen stores and even frank muscle wasting. If adequate glucose is not administered during the first 24–48 hours of therapy, there will be a tendency for recrudescence of the ketosis, burning adipose tissue because of the lack of gluconeogenic substrate. This may be prevented by glucose loading during this period, using insulin to ensure repletion of glycogen. Also, you should avoid cutting back on glucose therapy in an attempt to modulate circulating glucose levels. This should be accomplished by using insulin.

20. How is the management of hypertension different in the diabetic? Why?

Hypertension is implicated in accelerating the microangiopathy of diabetes, particularly the retinopathy and nephropathy. Therapy should therefore be more aggressive, initiated at a blood pressure 5–10 mmHg less than conventional therapeutic guidelines would indicate.

21. What are the antihypertensives of choice in diabetes? Which should be avoided and why?

In the diabetic the antihypertensives chosen should not worsen glucose or lipid control. They should not block normal "alerting" or counterregulatory mechanisms if hypoglycemia should occur. Finally, they should not antagonize common neurologic defects in diabetes, such as autonomic insufficiency and impotency.

Among the most-used agents in hypertensive diabetics, angiotensin-converting enzyme (ACE) inhibitors have been shown to slow the progression of diabetic nephropathy. Calcium channel blocking agents provide pressure reduction without adverse effects on lipids, glucose control, or autonomic interference. The newer alphha-blocking agents may also provide smoother control and an improved lipid profile.

Beta-blocking agents should be used with extreme care because of their blockade of hypoglycemic responses, degraded lipid profile, and incidence of impotence. Thiazide diuretics may also create worsened glucose and lipid profiles.

22. What are the kinetics of action of regular, NPH, and ultralente insulin?

Type	Onset (hr)	Peak (hr)	Duration (hr)
Regular	¼–1	2–5	4–8
NPH*	1–4	4–12	12–24
UltraLente	3–5	10–30	24–36

* Neutral protamine Hagedorn.

23. What steps can be taken to avoid or slow the progression of diabetic nephropathy?

Excellent glucose control, excellent blood pressure control, angiotensin-converting enzyme (ACE) inhibitors, and protein restriction all aid in preventing diabetic nephropathy.

24. How often should diabetics see an ophthalmologist? (Hint: segregate by type.)

Type I diabetics should see an ophthalmologist after 5 years of disease and at least yearly thereafter. Type II diabetics should start yearly check-ups at diagnosis.

25. To what ear infection is the diabetic predisposed? How is it treated?

Malignant otitis externa, an infection of the external auditory canal due to *Pseudomonas aeruginosa*, is mainly seen in elderly diabetic patients. It is an invasive and necrotizing infection with a high mortality, mainly due to meningitis. The typical clinical presentation consists of pain in the ear with or without a purulent drainage, swelling of the parotid gland, trismus, and paralysis of the 6th through the 12th cranial nerves. Treatment consists of anti-pseudomonal antibiotics with or without surgical debridement.

26. What should you think of when a diabetic's insulin requirement drops?

Success in weight control, improved exercise program, change in type or brand of insulin, or decrease in renal function (lessened insulin clearance) can lead to a drop in insulin requirements.

27. What is a reliable sign that the house officer has done a good job in seeing a diabetic patient in clinic?

The patient has his or her shoes off. A careful examination of the feet of a diabetic is a necessary part of comprehensive care. The patient must be taught to self-examine the feet and to administer proper foot care.

28. What is the indication for multiple injection regimens for diabetes?

Inability to maintain pre- and postprandial glucose levels to near-normal on single-dose regimens.

29. What are the indications for use of an insulin pump?

Patient and physician preference may lead a patient to use a pump instead of an intensive regimen (preprandial regular insulin plus intermediate or long-acting insulin). Failure of a well-monitored and executed intensive subcutaneous regimen is a reasonable indication for a pump. Pregnant patients often do well with insulin pumps.

30. What are the complications of multiple-injection regimens as compared to an insulin pump?

"Tight" glucose control may lead to loss of autonomic and cognitive appreciation of hypoglycemia ("hypoglycemic unawareness"). The lack of a depot of subcutaneous insulin leads to rapid loss of control in the event of pump failure. This carries the potential for rapid hyperglycemia.

31. What is the most important aspect of diabetic care?

Education. The diabetic patient will learn to know him/herself better than any member of the diabetes treatment team. The better the patient is educated, the better he or she will do.

32. What is the Somogyi phenomenon, and what are its signs and symptoms?

This process is hyperglycemia following hypoglycemia, known parochially as "The Bounce." The overuse of insulin with attendant hypoglycemia causes counterregulatory stress-hormone secretion, most notably glucagon, growth hormone, cortisol, and catecholamines. These agents lead to a rebound hyperglycemia, which may be confused with under-insulinization and result in mistaken therapy with larger doses of insulin.

This hypoglycemia and rebound hyperglycemia phenomenon often occur at night, with high glucose on awakening. The symptoms include poor sleep, nightmares, nighttime diaphoresis, and morning headache. The signs include hyperglycemia with positive urine ketones, the latter related to the hypoglycemia and fatty acid released. Early-morning home blood glucose surveillance may document the hypoglycemic pattern.

33. How may type II diabetics by treated?

Diet, exercise, hypoglycemia agents, and insulin can be used.

34. What hypoglycemic agents are currently most useful? What may lead you to choose one over another?

Characteristics of Oral Hypoglycemic Agents

GENERIC NAME	BRAND NAME	STRENGTH (mg)	ONSET (hr)	DURATION (hr)	DOSAGE RANGE	MAJOR TOXICITY
Tolbutamide	Orinase	500	0.5	6–12	500–3000	Photosensitivity
Chlorpropamide	Diabinese	100, 250	1.0	60–90	100–500	Hypersensitivity, jaundice, rash, pancytopenia, hyponatremia
Acetohexamide	Dymelor	250, 500	0.5	12–24	250–1500	GI disturbance, headache, rash
Tolazamide	Tolinase	100, 250, 500	4–6	10–18	100–1000	GI disturbance
Glyburide	Micronase	1.25, 2.5, 5	1.0	18–24	2.5–20	Hypoglycemia
Glipizide	Glucotrol	5, 10	0.5	12–24	5–40	Hypoglycemia

(From Garber AJ: Diabetes mellitus. In: Stein JH (ed): Internal Medicine, 3rd ed. Boston, Little, Brown, 1990, p 2249, with permission.)

Glipizide and glyburide are the most potent agents available with the fewest side-effects. The differences between these agents are actively debated. However, with a longer half-life, glyburide may not be indicated in the elderly, in whom a higher incidence of hypoglycemia has been reported using this agent.

35. What is the difference between fasting and reactive hypoglycemia? What are the types of reactive hypoglycemia?
Fasting hypoglycemia develops in the absence of substrate intake and is aggravated by prolonged fasting. Reactive hypoglycemia occurs within a characteristic time after eating.
   Three forms of reactive hypoglycemia have been discribed:
   1. The alimentary form, most often seen in dumping syndrome, shows rapid increase in blood glucose followed by a rapid decrease.
   2. Early type II diabetes often shows a slower-than-normal rise in blood glucose, which rises to supranormal levels, followed by an exaggerated drop in glucose at 3 to 5 hours.
   3. The idiopathic form does not show the exaggerated increase in blood glucose prior to a late fall to subnormal levels. This group may contain defects in gluconeogenic enzymes as well as in insulin and other gut hormone release.

36. How is c-peptide useful in assessing the etiology of fasting hypoglycemia?
C-peptide is absent in commercial insulin preparations. High endogenous insulin levels should be accompanied by high c-peptide levels. High insulin levels with low c-peptide levels are strongly suggestive of exogenous insulin use.

37. What is the biochemical mechanism for alcohol-induced hypoglycemia?
The oxidation of alcohol to acetaldehyde increases the NADH:NAD ratio, which in turn pushes the lactate:pyruvate redox pair toward lactate. Low pyruvate levels slow gluconeogenesis, and this can lead to hypoglycemia.

38. What is hemoglobin A1-C? What does it reflect?
Hemoglobin A1-C (glycohemoglobin) is hemoglobin glycosylated by nonenzymatic means. The percentage of glycohemoglobin in the circulation is indicative of the average ambient glucose concentration over the prior 4–8 weeks. The measurement of hemoglobin A1-C can be used as an indicator of the degree of glucose control over that time period.

PITUITARY

39. How is prolactin secretion regulated and how is it different from the other anterior pituitary hormones? And while you're at it, name them.
Prolactin is primarily controlled by negative feedback from the hypothalamus via the portal system. Prolactin inhibitory factor (PIF) has been identified as dopamine, so that dopamine and dopamine agonists suppress the secretion of prolactin. Thyrotropin releasing hormone (TRH) is a mild positive modulator of prolactin secretion; however, the major control is exerted by negative feedback.
   The other anterior pituitary hormones are positively stimulated by hypothalamic-releasing hormones: **luteinizing** and **follicle-stimulating hormones** (LH and FSH) by gonadotropin releasing hormone (GnRH), **thyrotropin** by thyrotropin-releasing hormone (TRH), **growth hormone** (GH) by growth-hormone-releasing hormone (GH-RH) (and negatively by somatostatin), and **ACTH** by corticotropin-releasing hormone (CRH).

40. What is the usual presentation for prolactinoma in women? In men?
Women usually present with interference of the menstrual cycle and by galactorrhea (the amenorrhea-galactorrhea syndrome). These changes are effected by relatively low prolactin levels, characteristically seen in very small prolactinomas.

Men usually present with impotence or with effects from the tumor mass. These changes are seen much later than those characterizing the presentation in women and are associated therefore with larger tumors.

41. What are the therapeutic options for prolactinomas?
Bromocriptine, a dopamine agonist, is very effective in shrinking prolactinomas, even those of very large size. Surgery is usually reserved for women wishing pregnancy and in whom the tumor is large enough to cause concern should it expand during pregnancy. Larger tumors have a high recurrence rate after surgery.

42. What medical therapies may be used in acromegaly?
A long-acting somatostatin analogue, Sandostatin (octreotide), is now undergoing evaluation and appears useful in decreasing tumor size and function. Some growth hormone secreting tumors may also respond to bromocriptine, but the response is unreliable.

43. What is the utility of IGF-1 (somatomedin C) in the management of acromegaly?
Monitoring IGF-1 (insulin-like growth factor-1) allows assessment of the efficacy of initial therapy and in follow-up in the post-therapeutic period.

44. Which circulating protein may be helpful in diagnosing a gonadotropin-secreting pituitary tumor?
The alpha subunit, which is common to the glycoprotein hormones LH, FSH, and TSH, is elevated in many of these cases.

45. Why would a woman with hypothyroidism have galactorrhea?
If her hypothyroidism is primary, that is, owing to thyroid gland dysfunction, the lack of feedback at the hypothalamus leads to an elevation of TRH, which is also a positive modulator of prolactin release.

46. What causes panhypopituitarism?

Etiologies of Hypopituitarism

Tumors	Infarction *(Cont.)*	Miscellaneous causes
Pituitary adenomas	Epidemic hemorrhagic fever	Pituitary abscess
Craniopharyngiomas	Malaria	Aneurysm
Metastatic carcinoma	Arteritis	Radiation therapy
Primary pituitary carcinoma	Sickle cell anemia (crisis)	Congenital absence
Meningioma	Shock syndrome	of the pituitary
Infarction	Infiltrative disease	Therapeutic ablation
Pituitary adenomas	Sarcoidosis	Hypothalamic disease
(pituitary apoplexy)	Eosinophilic granuloma	
Postpartum pituitary necrosis	Leukemia	
(Sheehan's syndrome)	Lymphoma	
Diabetes necrosis	Lymphocytic hypophysitis	
Trauma with stalk section	Hemochromatosis	

(From Boyd, et al: Disorders of the hypothalamus and anterior pituitary. In: Kohler PO (ed): Clinical Endocrinology. New York, John Wiley, 1986, p 44, with permission.)

47. What is the precision with which antidiuretic hormone (ADH) release is related to osmolarity? How much volume must one lose to trigger ADH release?
An osmolarity change of less than 1% will produce changes in ADH secretion. A loss of 10–15% of circulating volume will trigger ADH secretion.

48. Why is cortisol deficiency associated with hyponatremia?
It appears that cortisol negatively modulates the release of antidiuretic hormone (ADH) and that its deficiency is associated with a syndrome of inappropriate antidiuretic hormone-like (SIADH-like) physiology.

This is to be distinguished from the hyponatremia and hyperkalemia seen in primary adrenal deficiency with both cortisol and aldosterone deficiency. In that setting, aldosterone deficiency leads to potassium retention and sodium loss. The loss of sodium and volume contributes to an appropriate increase in ADH.

49. What is DDAVP and how is it used?
DDAVP, also known desmopressin, is 1-desamino-8-D-arginine vasopressin, a long-acting ADH analogue, which may be administered intranasally, intravenously, or subcutaneously. Its long action allows it to be used intranasally on a once- or twice-daily basis for diabetes insipidus.

ADRENAL

50. How much cortisol can the normal adrenal axis make during stress in one day? How, then, should "stress steroids" be administered for those patients adrenally insufficient for surgery, in sepsis, etc.?
Estimates of maximal adrenal output range from 125 to 300 mg of cortisol per 24 hours. The usual approach for treatment of a high-stress period in a patient deemed adrenally insufficient is to administer 100 mg of hydrocortisone by vein every 6 to 8 hours. The use of amounts greater than this is not directed to physiologic adrenal replacement but rather for pharmacologic effects.

51. What is Cushing's syndrome? What is Cushing's disease?
Cushing's syndrome is the symptom complex produced by an excess of adrenal corticosteroids. Cushing's disease is the most common cause of Cushing's syndrome, accounting for approximately two-thirds of all cases. It is caused by pituitary overproduction of adrenocorticotropic hormone (ACTH), leading to bilateral adrenal hyperplasia. Other causes of Cushing's syndrome include excess cortisol production originating in the adrenal gland (adrenal adenoma, or carcinoma), excess production of ACTH from a nonpituitary source (ectopic ACTH syndrome), and iatrogenic or factitious ingestion of excess exogenous corticosteroids.

52. Is there an indication for a random cortisol or ACTH measurement in the diagnosis of Cushing's disease?
No. These tests are not reliable in the screening for Cushing's disease.

53. What are the signs and symptoms of Cushing's disease?

Signs and Symptoms of Cushing's Disease

Skin	Endocrine	Adipose tissue	
Atrophic, thin skin	Amenorrhea	Weight gain	
Easy bruising	Diabetes	Truncal obesity	
Broad, purple stria	Hypertension	Fat deposition in supraclavicular	
on hips, abdomen,	**Immune system**	area and dorsum of back	
axillae	Susceptible to infections	(buffalo hump)	
Hair loss	Poor wound healing	Moon facies	
Tinea versicolor			
	Skeleton	**Psychiatric**	**Sexual characteristics**
Muscles	Osteoporosis	Psychosis	Women: Hirsutism
Muscle wasting	Chronic backache	Paranoia	Deepened voice
Decreased strength	Bone pain	Mood swings	Clitoral enlargement

54. What are the most reliable findings in Cushing's syndrome?

The most reliable physical findings are purple striae and thinning of the skin. Proximal muscle weakness may also be striking and unexpected until tested.

55. How should one screen for Cushing's syndrome?

Screening may be performed by the low-dose dexamethasone suppression test (1 mg dexamethasone at midnight should suppress 8 a.m. cortisol to less than 5 g/dl) or collection of a 24-hour urine for urinary free cortisol (should be less than 100 g/24 hr). The dexamethasone suppression test may yield false positive results in depression, obesity, or in patients taking phenobarbital.

56. What is Addison's disease and what are its causes?

Addison's disease is primary adrenal insufficiency. It is due to a failure of the adrenals to produce sufficient amounts of adrenal corticosteroids. Autoimmune destruction is responsible in approximately 80% of cases and adrenal destruction by tuberculosis in approximately 20% of cases. Other rare causes include adrenal destruction by bilateral hemorrhage or infarction, tumor, infections other than TB, surgery, radiation, drugs, amyloidosis, sarcoidosis, hyporesponsiveness to ACTH, and congenital abnormalities. Symptoms of adrenal insufficiency require loss of more than 90% of both adrenal cortices.

57. What are the major symptoms and signs of Addison's disease?

The major symptoms are hyperpigmentation, weakness, fatigue, anorexia, weight loss, salt craving, nausea, diarrhea, and postural dizziness. The major signs are hyperpigmentation (most prominent on skin folds, extensor surfaces, pressure points, the buccal mucosa and gums, nipples, areolae, perivaginal and perianal mucosa, and newly formed scars), hyperkalemia (usually mild), weight loss, orthostatic hypotension, adrenal calcifications, and vitilgo.

58. What are the differences (and their explanations) in the presentation of primary versus secondary adrenal insufficiency?

Primary adrenal insufficiency (Addison's disease) is caused by failure or destruction of the adrenal glands, leading to underproduction of glucocorticoids and mineralocorticoids. This results in an increase in ACTH production by the pituitary. Its signs and symptoms are described above. Secondary adrenal insufficiency is caused by deficient production of ACTH, leading to underproduction of glucocorticoids. The manifestations are the same as those of Addison's disease except for the following:

　　1. Hyperpigmentation is not seen. This is a product of the hypersecretion of ACTH and its related peptides (including melanocyte-stimulating hormone), which is not present in secondary adrenal insufficiency.

　　2. Signs and symptoms due to a deficiency of mineralocorticoids are also not seen. Since mineralocorticoid acitvity is largely regulated by the renin-angiotensin system and not ACTH, these manifestations of Addison's disease are lacking in secondary adrenal insufficiency.

　　3. Other manifestations of hypopituitarism may be seen with secondary adrenal insufficiency.

　　4. Hypoglycemia is more commonly seen with secondary adrenal insufficiency due to the presence of combined ACTH and growth hormone (GH) deficiency.

59. How is adrenal axis reserve tested?

An insulin tolerance test (ITT) provokes hyperfunction of the entire axis by inducing hypoglycemia. If adequate hypoglycemia is produced, the test has some predictive capacity for subsequent stress. Patients with seizure disorders or cardiac disease may not be candidates for ITT-induced hypoglycemia. In these cases, metyrapone may be used.

60. What does metyrapone do? How is it used?

Metyrapone inhibits the 11-hydroxylase step of cortisol synthesis, causing accumulation of 11-deoxy-cortisol, which does not provide feedback inhibition at the hypothalamus. The administration of metyrapone will therefore cause an intact axis to hyperfunction, with accumulation of 11-deoxy-cortisol, which may then be measured. It is also important to measure cortisol, which should be low. If cortisol is not low, there has been inadequate enzyme inhibition, and the test is not adequate.

61. What is a reasonable means of weaning a patient off corticosteroids?

First the patient should be placed on a short-acting corticosteroid, such as prednisone or hydrocortisone on a BID basis. Next, the evening dose should be weaned down, leaving a solitary morning dose. By this time, hydrocortisone should be substituted for prednisone. As the morning dose is weaned toward a physiologic level (20 mg), the next morning's cortisol may be measured. When a normal a.m. cortisol is attained, daily supplementation may be stopped. However, the patient should still use supplements for stress until an insulin tolerance test or metyrapone test can document adequate hypothalamic-pituitary-adrenal axis response to stress.

62. How should an incidentally found adrenal mass be evaluated? What parameters are of importance?

A good history and physical examination may suggest oversecretion of catecholamines, corticosteroids, adrenal androgens, or mineralocorticoids. Hyperaldosteronism or Cushing's syndrome may also be suggested by baseline electrolytes. Hormonal screening for hyperaldosteronism, Cushing's syndrome, pheochromocytoma, and adrenal androgens (DHEA-sulfate) is appropriate. The tumor size may be predictive of malignancy. Tumors larger than 6 cm have an increased prevalence of malignancy.

In the absence of suggestive findings, repeat scanning may be done at a 6–12 month period to evaluate any changes in size.

63. What are the differences among the ACTH stimulation test, insulin tolerance test (ITT), and metyrapone tests? What are the appropriate settings for their use?

ITT and metyrapone tests evaluate the response of the entire adrenal axis. The ACTH stimulation test stimulates only the adrenal glands. This test will suggest adrenal insufficiency when there had been prolonged defect anywhere in the adrenal axis or when there had been direct adrenal damage.

64. What is the rapid ACTH stimulation test?

This test is used to assess adrenal function; 250 g of synthetic ACTH (cosyntropin, Cortrosyn) is administered to the patient and cortisol levels are measured at 0 and 60 minutes. A normal cortisol response to the ACTH rules out primary adrenal insufficiency. Lack of a normal response indicates decreased adrenal reserve but does not differentiate between primary and secondary adrenal insufficiency.

65. How do you differentiate primary and secondary adrenal insufficiency?

Plasma ACTH levels can be used in this differentiation. In the face of adrenal insufficiency, ACTH levels > 250 pg/ml are associated with primary adrenal insufficiency (usually 400–2000 pg/ml) and ACTH levels of 0–50 pg/ml are associated with pituitary ACTH deficiency (secondary adrenal insufficiency) (usually < 20 pg/ml).

66. Which aspect of the hypothalamic-pituitary-adrenal axis is last to return after suppression by exogenous corticosteroids?

Corticotropin-releasing hormone (CRH) from the hypothalamus is the last to return.

67. What is the presentation of partial 17-hydroxylase deficiency? How may it be diagnosed?
This will present as hirsutism in the female. ACTH-stimulated 17-OH-progesterone levels will be elevated.

68. What are the multiple endocrine neoplasia (MEN) syndromes? To what chromosome have they been mapped?
These syndromes, consisting of tumors of multiple endocrine tissues, demonstrate the autosomal-dominant segregation of endocrine neoplasms. MEN-I has been mapped to chromosome 11; MEN-II to chromosome 10.

The Multiple Endocrine Neoplasia Syndromes

MEN I:
   Parathyroid hyperplasia
   Pancreatic islet cell tumors
   Pituitary tumors

MEN IIA:
   Parathyroid hyperplasia
   Medullary carcinoma of the thyroid
   Pheochromocytoma

MEN IIB:
   Ganglioneuromas
   Medullary carcinoma of the thyroid
   Pheochromocytoma

69. Why is beta blockade of a pheochromocytoma a bad idea as initial therapy?
Pheochromocytomas may secrete epinephrine, norepinephrine, or both. Because beta-adrenergic activity dilates peripheral blood vessels, beta-adrenergic blockade in the presence of unopposed alpha-agonists may lead to net peripheral vasoconstriction and an exacerbation of the patient's hypertension.

70. What are the organs of Zuckerkandl? Who cares?
These are rests of chromaffin tissue located in the paraaortic sympathetic chain in which extra-adrenal pheochromocytomas may arise. Mrs. Zuckerkandl cared deeply.

71. What are the renin/aldosterone findings in primary hyperaldosteronism? What is the Ganguli test and how may it be useful in this setting?
Aldosterone will be high, renin will be low. The Ganguli test utilizes prolonged standing posture followed by Lasix loading to assess the renin:aldosterone responses to low-volume status.

Ganguli A, et al: Control of plasma aldosterone in primary aldosteronism: Distinction between adenoma and hyperplasia. J Clin End Metab 37:765–775, 1973.

72. How do you decide whether to treat hyperaldosteronism medically or surgically? What is the drug of choice and why?
Patients with unilateral aldosteronomas are best treated surgically. Patients who are poor operative risks, or in whom there is bilateral hyperplasia, are best treated with a specific aldosterone receptor antagonist, spironolactone.

73. What are the most common settings for hyporeninemic hypoaldosteronism?
Type II diabetes, interstitial nephritis, and AIDS.

THYROID

74. What is the weight of a normal adult thyroid gland?
A normal adult thyroid gland weighs between 15 and 20 grams.

75. What are the goals and limitations of the various tests of the thyroid gland?

Comparison of Thyroid Tests

TEST	GOAL	COMMENTS
Total T_4	T_4 level	Detects 90% of hyperthyroid cases; affected by alterations in TBG and can be misleadingly high or low; free T_4 is only a fraction of the total T_4.
Free T_4	Assessment of free T_4	Directly measures free T_4; independent of TBG* levels.
Serum T_3	T_3 level	Used to detect hyperthyroidism; misleadingly low in patients with nonthyroidal illness (i.e., low value does not usually indicate hypothyroidism. Do not confuse with RT_3U.
$RT_3U^\dagger$	Assessment of free T_4	Clarifies whether alterations in T_4 are the result of thyroid disease or alteration in T_4 binding proteins. Does *not* measure T_3.
Radioactive iodine uptake (RAIU)	Extent of thyroid function	Normal range must be determined for each population district. Difficult to distinguish low from low normal values when dietary iodine is high. Hyperthyroidism doesn't always cause high iodine uptake.
TSH level	Index of thyroid status	Most sensitive test for primary hyperthyroidism (TSH high before other tests show low T_4).
Thyroid scan	Functional status of nodular goiter	Often not needed in other types of thyroid disease.
Ultrasound	Status of single nodule	Reliably discriminates between cystic and solid nodules in 90% of cases.

*TBG = Thyroxine-binding globulin.
$^\dagger RT_3U$ = resin T_3 uptake test.
(From Rubenstein E, Federman DD (eds): Scientific American Medicine. New York, Scientific American, Inc., 1989, Ch. 3, Pt. I, p 5, with permission.)

76. What are the causes of hyperthyroidism?
Hyperthyroidism is a syndrome resulting from the response to excess thyroid hormone levels. The excess thyroid hormone can come from hyperfunction of the thyroid gland, inflammation, or destruction of all or part of the gland with resultant release of stored hormone, or from a source outside the thyroid. Separation of the causes on the basis of a low or high radioactive iodine uptake (RAIU) can help narrow the differential diagnosis.

Causes of Hyperthyroidism

1. Normal or high RAIU	2. Low RAIU
a. Graves' disease	a. Subacute thyroiditis
b. Toxic multinodular goiter	b. Hyperthyroiditis
c. Solitary toxic nodule	c. Factitious thyrotoxicosis
d. Hypothalamic-pituitary disease	d. Jod-Basedow phenomenon (iodine-induced thyrotoxicosis)
e. Choriocarcinoma or hydatidiform mole	e. Metastatic thyroid carcinoma
f. Tumor metastases to the thyroid	f. Struma ovarii (teratoma)

(From Kohler PO (ed): Clinical Endocrinology. New York, John Wiley, 1986, p 90, with permission.)

77. What are the major signs and symptoms of hyperthyroidism?

Signs and Symptoms of Hyperthyroidism

SYSTEM	SYMPTOMS	SIGNS
Increased metabolic rate	Heat intolerance, increased appetite, weight loss	Sweating, reduced mass of muscles and fat; rarely fever
Cardiovascular	Palpitation; may have symptoms of heart failure	Tachycardia; hypertension (esp. systolic); arrhythmia (esp. atrial fibrillation); heart murmur or rub
Neuromuscular	Fatigue, muscular weakness	Tremor; $\uparrow$ deep tendon reflexes; proximal muscle weakness; rarely paralysis
Neuropsychiatric	Nervousness, irritability, depression, difficulty sleeping	Emotional lability, frank psychosis
Ophthalmologic	Eye irritation and stare,[1] photophobia,[1] diplopia[1]	Stare, lid retraction, lid lag, Graves' ophthalmopathy (proptosis, extraocular muscle dysfunction, optic neuropathy, chemosis)[1]
Skin, hair, and nails	Alopecia, rash of pretibial myxedema,[1] ankle swelling, brittle nails	Smooth, soft, warm skin; hair of fine texture and easily removable; edema; pretibial myxedema in Graves' disease[1]; onycholysis
Respiratory	Dyspnea	$\uparrow$ respiratory rate
Gastrointestinal	$\uparrow$ frequency and softening of bowel movements	Usually normal; may have splenomegaly[1]
Reproductive	Oligoamenorrhea, impotence	Gynecomastia
Other	Anorexia, constipation	Lymphadenopathy[1]

$\uparrow$ = increased.
[1] These findings are not manifestations of increased circulating thyroid hormone levels but are related to the disturbance in the immune system that occurs in Graves' disease.
(From Kohler PO (ed): Clinical Endocrinology. New York, John Wiley, 1986, p 93, with permission.)

78. What is a thyroid storm?

Thyroid storm is a dramatic, life-threatening exacerbation of thyrotoxicosis. It is characterized by severe signs and symptoms of exaggerated thyrotoxicosis with hypermetabolism, excessive adrenergic response, diaphoresis, and fever that, if untreated, can lead to death from cardiovascular collapse. There is usually marked tachycardia, widened pulse pressure, agitation, and delirium (or coma).

Thyroid storm is usually not associated with thyroxine (T_4) or triiodothyronine (T_3) levels markedly higher than the "pre-storm" values, and so its diagnosis must be made on clinical grounds. Thyroid storm can be initiated by another acute illness, such as infection, surgery, trauma to the thyroid, or withdrawal of partially effective antithyroid therapy.

79. What is the treatment for thyroid storm?

The treatment of thyroid storm involves the use of propranolol to control the cardiovascular manifestations, intravenous (IV) saturated solution of potassium iodide (SSKI) to block the release of thyroid hormone, and prophylthiouracil (PTU) to block thyroid hormone synthesis. The peripheral conversion of T_4 to T_3 is partially blocked by PTU, propranolol, and hydrocortisone. Supportive therapy, IV fluids, antipyretics, cooling blankets, and sedatives also play a role. In extreme cases, plasmapheresis or peritoneal dialysis have been used to remove thyroid hormone. In all cases, a search for and treatment of the initiating condition should be included in the treatment.

80. What are the four basic mechanisms that lead to hypothyroidism?

Hypothyroidism is a clinical syndrome caused by the cellular responses to a deficiency of thyroid hormone. It can be produced by the following four mechanisms:

1. **Primary:** due to a pathologic process intrinsic to the thyroid gland, leading to defective production of thyroid hormone or destruction of the gland.

2. **Secondary:** due to a deficiency of thyroid stimulating hormone (TSH) stimulation of a normal thyroid gland.

3. **Tertiary:** due to a deficiency of thyrotropin-releasing hormone (TRH) from the hypothalamus.

4. **Peripheral resistance to the action of thyroid hormone:** a rare cause of hypothyroidism (Refetoff syndrome).

81. What are the causes of hypothyroidism?

Causes of Hypothyroidism

CLASSIFICATION	SPECIAL FEATURES
Primary	
1. Autoimmune (chronic thyroiditis, idiopathic, "burnt out" Graves' disease)	Thyroid antibodies positive in most cases; pernicious anemia and other primary endocrine deficiencies may coexist.
2. Postablative	After radioactive iodine or surgery.
3. Subacute thyroiditis	Transient phase, usually preceded by sore neck and thyrotoxicosis with low I^{131} uptake.
4. Drugs (iodides, lithium, thionamides)	Coexistent thyroiditis (autoimmune) prior to ablative therapy; recent history of drug administration.
5. Thyroid agenesis	Most common cause in neonates.
6. Thyroid dysgenesis	May cause juvenile hypothyroidism.
7. Dyshormonogenesis	Goiter, family history.
8. Head and neck irradiation	History of treatment with radiation.
9. Neoplasia	Primary or metastatic tumor (rare).
Secondary	Associated with low TSH;* impaired TSH response to TRH,* when present, is helpful in diagnosis; requires thorough evaluation for underlying cause of pituitary failure.
Tertiary	Same as secondary, except TSH response to TRH is usually preserved.
Peripheral resistance	Raised levels of thyroid hormone and TSH.

*TSH = thyroid-stimulating hormone; TRH = thyrotropin-releasing hormone.
(From Kohler PO (ed): Clinical Endocrinology. New York, John Wiley, 1986, p 105, with permission.)

82. What are the major signs and symptoms of hypothyroidism?

Signs and Symptoms of Hypothyroidism

SYSTEM	SYMPTOMS	SIGNS
Reduced metabolic rate	Cold intolerance ↓ appetite Weight gain	Obesity Hypothermia
Neuromuscular	Muscle cramps Stiffness in joints Paresthesias Weakness	Delayed deep tendon reflexes ↑ muscle mass and rigidity Myotonia Joint effusions

Table continued on next page.

Signs and Symptoms of Hypothyroidism (Continued)

SYSTEM	SYMPTOMS	SIGNS
Neuromuscular *(Cont.)*	In infants: Mental retardation Short stature	Carpal tunnel syndrome
Neuropsychiatric	Lethargy Reduced energy ↑ sleeping	Delirium Dementia Frank psychosis
Skin, hair, and nails	Dry skin Hair loss Straightened hair Brittle nails Edema	Cool, thin, scaling skin Alopecia Coarse hair Myxedema (esp. face and periorbital tissues)
Cardiovascular	Angina	Bradycardia Hypertension Cardiomegaly with effusion ("myxedema heart")
Ear, nose and throat	Hoarseness Hearing loss Altered taste/smell Vertigo	Deep voice Slow speech Conductive hearing loss Enlarged tongue
Respiratory	Dyspnea	Reduced inspiratory effort Pleural effusion
Gastrointestinal	Epigastric pain Constipation	Abdominal distention Rarely toxic megacolon
Reproductive	Infertility Impotence Galactorrhea In children: Precocious puberty Delayed puberty	Galactorrhea

(From Kohler PO (ed): Clinical Endocrinology. New York, John Wiley, 1986, p 109, with permission.)

83. What is the pathogenesis of Graves' disease?

Graves' disease is an autoimmune disease in which T lymphocytes produce antibodies to certain thyroid antigens. Thyroid-stimulating immunoglobulin (TSI) is an antibody to the TSH receptor on the thyroid cells, which results in stimulation of growth and function. The cause of the autoimmune process is not known.

84. What is the NO-SPECS classification for Graves' ophthalmopathy?

NO-SPECS Classification for Graves' Ophthalmopathy

CLASS	CHANGE
0	No signs or symptoms
1	Only signs
2	Soft tissue involvement
3	Proptosis
4	Extraocular-muscle involvement
5	Corneal involvement
6	Sight loss (visual acuity)

It should be noted that Graves' ophthalmopathy does not necessarily progress in order of the NO-SPECS classes.

85. What are the available antithyroid drugs used for hyperthyroidism? Which are safe in pregnancy?
Methimazole (tapazole) and propylthiouracil (PTU). Methimazole has been associated with aplasia cutis in the newborn and is therefore not used in pregnancy in the U.S.

86. What characteristics are predictive of spontaneous remission in Graves' disease?
Small thyroid gland, young patient, female, acute onset of disease, low antithyroid antibody titers.

87. What therapies are available for Graves' ophthalmopathy? What are their indications?
Medical therapy may include the use of corticosteroids and/or cyclosporine. Steroids may be useful in moderate-to-severe disease; cyclosporine may be useful as an adjunct in therapeutic failure.

Nonmedical therapy includes radiotherapy to the orbit and surgical decompression. These methods are usually reserved for the more severe complications, such as corneal involvement or visual compromise.

88. What are the antibody profiles in Graves' disease, Hashimoto's thyroiditis, and subacute thyroiditis?
Hashimoto's thyroiditis has increased prevalence of high titers of antimicrosomal and antithyroid antibodies. Graves' patients often have high titers of antithyroid antibodies and thyroid-stimulating immunoglobulin (TSI). Subacute thyroiditis is rarely associated with short-lived elevations of antithyroid antibodies, usually in low titers.

89. What is hashitoxicosis?
This term is used when Hashimoto's thyroiditis is associated with hyperthyroidism secondary to uncontrolled release of thyroid hormone.

90. What is Jod-Basedow phenomenon and the mechanism of occurrence?
Jod-Basedow phenomenon is hyperthyroidism resulting from an iodine load. It is usually seen in the setting of endemic goiter, multinodular goiter, or in the patients with Graves' disease previously treated with antithyroid drugs. Any source of iodine, including contrast media, iodine-containing expectorants, or kelp may induce this process.

91. What is the natural history of subacute thyroiditis? How is it treated?
There is usually a prodromal viral-like syndrome, followed 2 to 3 weeks later by thyroid or ear pain, sometimes with dysphagia. The thyroid is slightly enlarged, firm, and tender. The patient may range from euthyroid to thyrotoxic. The active phase lasts from days to months and may recur before final resolution.

Nonsteroidal anti-inflammatory drugs are usually sufficient for the painful aspect. Hyperthyroidism is usually treated with beta blockers. Antithyroid medications are poorly effective. More severe pain or active thyroiditis may be treated with a tapering dose of corticosteroids.

92. What historical and physical findings are suggestive of malignancy in a thyroid nodule?
Risk factors include positive family history and head or neck irradiation. Multinodular goiter or longstanding thyroiditis may also increase risk. A single node, fixation of the node, local lymphadenopathy, and involvement of the recurrent laryngeal nerve suggest malignancy.

93. How is papillary carcinoma of the thyroid staged and treated?
Stage I: Single or multiple intrathyroidal nodules. Opinions differ as to treatment. One position suggests simple lobectomy followed by suppressive thyroxine therapy. Alternatively, lobectomy with near-total contralateral lobectomy followed by ablative radioiodine has been suggested, particularly in multicentric disease or patients older than 40.

Stage II: Cervical metastasis, nonfixed, and without invasion. Treatment consists of near-total or total thyroidectomy and is followed by radioiodine ablation and thyroid replacement with follow-up iodine scanning.

Stage III: Local cervical invasion or fixed cervical metastases. Treatment consists of near-total thyroidectomy with resection of available neoplastic tissue, followed by radioiodine ablation and thyroid replacement with follow-up iodine scanning.

Stage IV: Metastases outside the neck. Treatment is as per Stage III, with body scanning after ablation to assess metastases outside the neck and with follow-up higher dose radioiodine therapy as indicated.

94. What is follow-up for thyroid carcinoma?
Physical examination, thyroid function tests, thyroglobulin levels, and whole-body radioiodine scanning are indicated at 6–9 months, 1 year, 3 years, and then at 5-year intervals thereafter.

95. What is struma ovarii?
Ectopic thyroid tissue in an ovarian teratoma producing a hyperthyroid state. It is one of the rare causes of low-uptake (by neck scanning) hyperthyroidism. Other causes of low-uptake hyperthyroidism are thyroiditis, Jod-Basedow phenomenon, and exogenous thyroxine.

96. What is Reidel's thyroiditis?
A rare thyroiditis in which the gland is found to have extensive fibrosis with adherence to adjacent structures, producing a characteristic "woody" consistency.

97. How is the TRH stimulation test useful in hyperthyroidism and hypothyroidism?
The pituitary gland will be less responsive to TRH in the presence of high circulating levels of thyroxine. A "flat" TRH stimulation test suggests that the patient's axis is suppressed. On the other hand, the pituitary will be hyperresponsive to TRH with low circulating T_4, allowing the assessment of subtle hypothyroidism or in interpreting an axis with altered binding proteins or thyroxine metabolism, such as in dilantin or amiodorone use.

98. What does "euthyroid sick" mean and what are the usual findings?
Euthyroid sick designates the changes in thyroid hormone levels in patients with severe systemic illness. T_4 and T_3 will decrease, with increased reverse T_3. Despite maintenance of a functional euthyroid state, T_4 to T_3 conversion is decreased, with shunting to reverse T_3. TSH is normal or at the upper limit of normal. Recovery may be associated with a self-limited rise in TSH.

99. What is the earliest means of detecting medullary carcinoma of the thyroid (MCT)? What is the best therapy?
Pentagastrin-stimulation testing. This will provoke an exaggerated rise in calcitonin even in very early MCT. Surgery is the best therapy and should seek for cure.

GONADS

100. What is the differential diagnosis for impotence in the male?
Impotence may have circulatory, neurogenic, hormonal, pharmacologic, and psychiatric components. A drug history, particularly noting antihypertensives and alcohol, may be key in evaluating the source. Studies on REM-associated erections may help differentiate between psychogenic causes and other reasons. Barring patients with drug-induced impotence or those with normal nocturnal erections, further evaluation of penile circulation and neurologic integrity may be indicated.

101. What is NPT?
"Nocturnal penile tumescence" (NPT) describes erections associated with REM sleep. This phenomenon is detected using penile strain gauges and electroencephalography (EEG) in a sleep lab.

102. What does the Lyon hypothesis have to do with a buccal mucosal scraping in a man with long arms and infertility?
The Lyon hypothesis predicts random inactivation of an X chromosome in XX women, producing the distinctive Barr body in somatic cells. Men should not have Barr bodies, but men with Kleinfelter's syndrome, XXY, will have them on a smear of buccal cells.

103. What does obesity have to do with a hypogonadal male who can't smell well?
These findings suggest Kallmann's syndrome, a defect in midline hypothalamic development that produces obesity, hypogonadotropic hypogonadism, and disordered smell.

104. What is the difference between hirsutism and virilization?
Hirsutism is excess hair only. Virilization includes increased androgen response, including increased muscle mass, lowered voice, clitoral enlargement, and behavioral changes.

105. What is the differential diagnosis for hirsutism in a woman?
Racial or familial predilection, polycystic ovarian syndrome, ovarian or adrenal neoplasm, and partial adrenal hyperplasia syndrome.

BONE

106. What are the mediators of humoral hypercalcemia of malignancy?
Interleukin 1, tumor necrosis factor, lymphotoxin, parathyroid hormone related protein, and prostaglandins can all contribute to hypercalcemia in patients with malignancy.

107. What is a diphosphonate (bisphosphonate)?
A molecule modeled on pyrophosphate, in which the bridging oxygen is substituted by a carbon, disallowing phosphatase activity. These molecules inhibit osteoclast activity and bone resorption.

108. What are the indications for medical therapy of Paget's disease of bone? What medicines are available?
Pain, deformity, nerve entrapment, and cranial involvement indicate the need for medical therapy. Calcitonin and diphosphonates are indicated for suppression of disease activity.

109. How may bone density be measured?
Density in the appendages may be measured by single photon beam densitometry. Axial bone mass may be measured by CT scanning, dual photon densitometry, and dual x-ray absorptiometry.

110. What can a bone biopsy tell you?
Bone biopsy can evaluate the normal microstructure of bone. The presence of normal laminar deposition of bone, prevalence of osteoclastic and osteoblastic activity, prevalence of osteoid, and adequacy of mineralization can all be assessed. Pre-labeling with tetracycline allows a determination of bone turnover rate. Special straining also detects aluminum accumulation.

111. What are osteopenia, osteoporosis, and osteomalacia?
Osteopenia is any pathologic decrease in bone mass. Osteoporosis is osteopenia with normal histology. Osteomalacia is osteopenia with disordered calcification, leading to accumulation of osteoid.

112. What is the differential diagnosis of osteoporosis?

Classification of Osteoporosis

Primary osteoporosis	**Secondary osteoporosis** *(Continued)*
Juvenile	Bone marrow disorders
Idiopathic (young adults)	Multiple myeloma
Involutional	Mastocytosis
	Metastatic carcinoma
Secondary osteoporosis	Connective tissue diseases
Endocrine diseases	Osteogenesis imperfecta
Hypogonadism	Homocystinuria
Hyperadrenocorticism	Ehlers-Danlos syndrome
Hyperthyroidism	Marfan's syndrome
Hyperparathyroidism	Miscellaneous causes
Diabetes mellitus	Immobilization
Gastrointestinal diseases	Chronic obstructive pulmonary disease
Subtotal gastrectomy	Chronic alcoholism
Malabsorption syndromes	Chronic heparin administration
Chronic obstructive jaundice	Rheumatoid arthritis
Primary biliary cirrhosis	
Severe malnutrition	
Anorexia nervosa	

(From Riggs BL: Osteoporosis. In DeGroot LJ (ed): Endocrinology, 2nd ed. Philadelphia, W.B. Saunders, 1989, p 1196, with permission.)

113. What is the principle of the intact parathyroid hormone (PTH) assay? Why is it particularly useful in renal failure?
Antibodies to one end of the PTH molecule are attached to solid phase, such as beads or the inside of the test tube. The patient's serum is then added, incubated, and washed out, leaving PTH attached to the solid phase. A radio-labeled antibody to the other end of the PTH molecule is then added. This antibody will only bind to intact PTH, the other end of which is attached to the solid phase. Any fragments bound to the solid phase will not be recognized by the second antibody. In this manner, only "intact" PTH produces a signal. Renal failure causes poor clearance of PTH fragments, which produce large signals on one-site PTH assays, but which do not interfere with the two-site assay.

114. How does magnesium deficiency cause hypocalcemia?
Magnesium deficiency inhibits PTH release from the parathyroid glands, as well as interfering with its action at bone and kidney.

115. How should surgery for sporadic primary hyperparathyroidism differ from surgery for multiple endocrine neoplasia (MEA)?
Sporadic hyperparathyroidism is almost always secondary to an isolated parathyroid adenoma, which leads to cure on its resection. MEA is associated with diffuse parathyroid hyperplasia and hyperfunction. The therapy of choice is resection of $3\frac{1}{2}$ glands, usually with implantation of the remaining $\frac{1}{2}$ gland in the sternomastoid muscle or forearm.

116. What is familial hypocalciuric hypercalcemia (FHH) and how may it be differentiated from hyperparathyroidism?
FHH is a familial-dominant disorder in which the calcium level is set higher than normal in the setting of high-normal PTH levels. Urine calcium levels are remarkably low, in contradistinction to those seen in hyperparathyroidism. No long-term morbidity is associated with FHH. All patients with suspected hyperparathyroidism should be checked for FHH by urine calcium determination.

117. How does sarcoidosis cause hypercalcemia?
Sarcoid tissue is able to hydroxylate 25-hydroxy-vitamin D to the active 1,25-dihydroxy form and produce an endogenous hypervitaminosis D.

118. What are the mediators of renal bone disease? How may it be treated?
Hyperparathyroidism results from the hyperphosphatemia, hypocalcemia, and decreased 1,25-dihydroxy-vitamin D seen in chronic renal failure. Phosphate binders, such as calcium carbonate, and 1,25-dihydroxy-vitamin D, can prevent this process. Aluminum toxicity is also seen in patients treated with aluminum hydroxide for phosphate binding.

LIPIDS

119. What are the lipoproteins and their composition?
The lipoproteins are composed of the nonpolar (and therefore water-insoluble) cholesterol esters and triglycerides (TG), surrounded by a layer of polar (and therefore water-soluble) proteins and lipids (unesterified cholesterol and phospholipids). This structure allows the entire particle to remain miscible in serum. The major lipoproteins are:

Lipoproteins

| TYPE | DIAMETER | ELECTRO-PHORETIC MOBILITY | COMPOSITION (%) | | | | |
| | | | PROTEIN | TG | CHOLESTEROL | | PHOSPHO-LIPID |
					FREE	ESTER	
Chylomicrons	5000A	Origin	1–2	85–95	1–3	2–4	3–6
VLDL	2000A	Pre-beta	6–10	50–65	4–8	16–22	15–20
LDL	250A	Beta	18–22	4–8	6–8	45–50	18–24
HDL	80A	Alpha	45–55	2–7	3–5	15–20	26–32

120. What is the phenotypic classification of hyperlipidemic disorders?

Phenotypic Classification of Hyperlipidemic Disorders

TYPE	ASSOCIATED LIPO-PROTEINS*	ASSOCIATED LIPIDS*	ASSOCIATED CONDITIONS	CAD RISK
I	Chylo	TG	Uncontrolled diabetes, hypothyroidism, Dysglobulinemias	→
IIa	LDL	Chol	Porphyria, hypothyroidism, biliary obstruction, nephrosis, pregnancy, dysglobulinemias	↑↑
IIb	LDL and VLDL	Chol and TG	Same as IIa	↑↑
III	LDL	TG and Chol	Hypothyroidism, ethanol use, dysglobulinemias diabetes	↑↑
IV	VLDL	TG	Diabetes, lipodystrophy, ethanol use, glucocorticoid use, chronic renal disease, pregnancy, estrogens, glycogen storage diseases	?
V	VDL and Chylo	TG and Chol	Ethanol use, pancreatitis, dysglobulinemias, diabetes	→

*Chylo = chylomicrons; LDL = low density lipoproteins; VLDL = very low density lipoproteins; Chol = cholesterol, TG = triglycerides.
(From Schonfeld G: Disorder of lipoprotein transport. In Besser GM, et al (eds): Endocrinology, 2nd ed. Philadelphia, W.B. Saunders, 1989, p 2444, with permission.)

121. What apolipoprotein directs LDL binding to its receptor?

Apolipoprotein B-100 directs LDL bonding to its cellular receptor and its subsequent uptake into the cell.

122. How can the types of hyperlipidemias be differentiated based on measurement of total serum cholesterol, triglycerides (TG), and LDL cholesterol?

With the measurement of serum cholesterol, TG, LDL, and inspection of the plasma, one can differentiate the different types of hyperlipidemias. After the plasma has been kept at 4°C for 16 to 24 hours, it is inspected for clarity and the presence of a creamy surface layer. The presence of an elevation in cholesterol (LDL particles) will not change the plasma from its normal clarity. The presence of hypertriglyceridemia (>400 mg/dl) due to increased VLDL will cause the plasma to appear turbid. Chylomicrons will also cause the plasma to appear turbid as opposed to its normal clarity. The presence of elevated chylomicrons leads to the formation of a floating, creamy layer on top of the plasma. The following table shows a practical approach to phenotyping the hyperlipidemias:

Lipids*	Plasma	Type
Chol ↑, TG →	Clear	IIa
Chol ↑, TG 200–400 mg/dl	Clear to turbid	LDL < 190: IV LDL > 190: IIb
Chol ↑, TG 400–1000 mg/dl	Turbid Turbid, creamy layer	IV V (suspect III)
Chol ↑, TG > 1000 mg/dl	Turbid, creamy layer Clear, creamy layer	V I
Chol →, TG ↑	Turbid	IV

* Chol = cholesterol; TG = triglycerides; ↑ = increased; → = normal
(From Schonfeld G: Disorder of lipoprotein transport. In Besser GM, et al (eds): Endocrinology, 2nd ed. Philadelphia, W.B. Saunders, 1989, p 2444, with permission.)

123. What are the physical examination signs found in patients with the various hyper-lipidemias?

Characteristic Signs in the Hyperlipidemias

SYSTEM	SIGN	DISORDER
Skin	Eruptive xanthoma	Types I and V, primary and secondary
	Palmar xanthoma	Type III
	Xanthelasma	Types II and III
	Tendinous xanthoma	Type II
Eye	Arcus cornea	All
	Cataract	LCAT deficiency
	Corneal opacity	Fish-eye disease
Oropharynx	Large, orange tonsils	Tangier disease
	Yellow mucosal plaques	Type II
Heart	Coronary artery disease	Types II–IV
	Aortic valvular disease	Homozygous Type II
GI	Abdominal pain	Types I and V
	Hepatosplenomegaly	Types I and V, LCAT deficiency
	Malabsorption	Abetalipoproteinemia
Renal	Glomerular disease	LCAT* deficiency
	Renovascular disease	Types II and III

Table continued on next page.

Characteristic Signs in the Hyperlipidemias (Continued)

SYSTEM	SIGN	DISORDER
Neuromuscular	Gait disturbance	Abetalipoproteinemia
	Peripheral neuropathy	Tangier disease, Types IV and V
Hematologic	Anemia, normocytic	LCAT deficiency
	acanthocytosis	Abetalipoproteinemia

*LCAT = lethicin-cholesterol acyltransferase.
(From Schonfeld G: Disorders of lipoprotein transport. In Besser GM, et al (eds): Endocrinology, 2nd ed. Philadelphia, W.B. Saunders, 1989, p 2445, with permission.)

124. What is the defect in familial hypercholesterolemia?

Familial hypercholesterolemia is an autosomal dominant disorder caused by a defect in the cellular receptor for low density lipoproteins (LDL). The homozygotic state is associated with very early (age in the 20s) and very severe atherosclerotic cardiovascular disease (ASCVD). Heterozygotes have one normal and one abnormal allele. They have a 50% reduction in the LDL receptor activity and also exhibit premature ASCVD.

The disease is due to the presence of one (or two) of at least 12 abnormal alleles that lead to the production of an abnormal LDL receptor. This can occur by:

1. Production of a completely nonfunctional receptor.

2. Production of a receptor with only 1–10% of normal function (most common variety).

3. Production of a receptor that successfully binds to LDL but cannot successfully transport the LDL into the cell (internalization defect). This is thought to be rare.

125. How can you estimate a patient's low density lipoprotein (LDL) from measurements of total cholesterol, high density lipoprotein (HDL), and triglyceride (TG)?

After measurement of total cholesterol, HDL, and TG, the serum LDL can be estimated using the formula:

$$LDL = (Total\ cholesterol) - (HDL) - (TG/5)$$

126. Who should have their cholesterol measured?

The current recommendation is for all adults age 20 and older to be tested at least once every 5 years as part of a general medical examination.

The Expert Panel: Report of the National Cholesterol Education Program Expert Panel on Detection, Evaluation and Treatment of High Blood Cholesterol in Adults. Arch Intern Med 148:36–69, 1988.

127. How is a patient initially classified with respect to cholesterol level? What is the plan for follow-up?

After a total serum cholesterol is measured the patient is placed into one of three groups:

Cholesterol	Group
<200 mg/dl	Desirable blood cholesterol
200–239 mg/dl	Borderline-high blood cholesterol
>240 mg/dl	High blood cholesterol

Patients with desirable levels should be retested within 5 years. Patients with borderline-high levels who do *not* have definite coronary artery disease (CAD) or two risk factors (male sex, family history of premature CAD, cigarette smoking, hypertension, low HDL cholesterol, diabetes mellitus, definite cerebrovascular or peripheral vascular disease, and severe obesity) should receive dietary recommendations and be retested within 1 year.

Patients with borderline-high levels who *do* have definite CAD or two risk factors and patients with high levels should have a lipoprotein profile measured and be treated based on the result.

The Expert Panel: Report of the National Cholesterol Education Program Expert Panel on Detection, Evaluation and Treatment of High Blood Cholesterol in Adults. Arch Intern Med 148:36–69, 1988.

128. What are elevated levels of LDL-cholesterol?

Since the risk of coronary artery disease (CAD) is causally related to the level of LDL cholesterol, the focus of treatment is aimed at decreasing this level. Once the patient is found to have a screening total cholesterol greater than or equal to 240 mg/dl, or 200–239 mg/dl with two or more risk factors for CAD, the LDL should be measured or calculated from measurements of total cholesterol, triglycerides, and HDL.

An LDL level of less than 130 is desirable, 130–159 is borderline high, and greater than 159 is considered high risk.

The Expert Panel: Report of the National Cholesterol Education Program Expert Panel on Detection, Evaluation and Treatment of High Blood Cholesterol in Adults. Arch Intern Med 148:36–69, 1988.

129. At what LDL-cholesterol level should you begin dietary therapy and drug therapy? What are the goals of therapy?

Therapy for Elevated LDL-Cholesterol

	Start Therapy	Goal of Therapy
Dietary therapy		
Without CAD or two risk factors	≥160	<160
With CAD or two risk factors	≥130	<130

The Expert Panel: Report of the National Cholesterol Education Program Expert Panel on Detection, Evaluation and Treatment of High Blood Cholesterol in Adults. Arch Intern Med 148:36–69, 1988.

130. What are the currently available lipid-lowering agents, their mechanism of action, and their side-effects?

Summary of Lipid-lowering Agents

AGENT	MECHANISM OF ACTION	BIOCHEMICAL SIDE EFFECTS	SYSTEMIC SIDE EFFECTS	DOSAGE RANGE (DAILY)
Cholestyramine Colestipol	Increases excretion of bile acids in the stool; increases LDL receptor activity	May prevent absorption of fat-soluble vitamins	Constipation, bloating	12 to 24 gm 15 to 30 gm
Nicotinic acid	Decreases plasma levels of free fatty acids; possibly inhibits cholesterol synthesis; decreases hepatic VLDL synthesis	Altered liver function tests; increased uric acid; increased glucose tolerance	Cutaneous flushing, pruritus, gastro-intestinal upset	3 to 6 gm
Clofibrate	Decreases hepatic VLDL synthesis; increases lipoprotein lipase activity	Altered liver function tests; increased CPK, potentiation of warfarin	Decreased libido, in-creased incidence of cholelithiasis and perhaps of gastrointestinal malignancy, myositis	1 to 2 gm

Table continued on next page.

Summary of Lipid-lowering Agents (Continued)

AGENT	MECHANISM OF ACTION	BIOCHEMICAL SIDE EFFECTS	SYSTEMIC SIDE EFFECTS	DOSAGE RANGE (DAILY)
Probucol	Enhances scavenger pathway removal of LDL	Decreased HDL	Diarrhea, nausea, flatulence	1 gm
Gemfibrozil	Reduces incorporation of free fatty acids into triglycerides	Potentiation of warfarin	Myositis, diarrhea, nausea, skin rash (rare)	1200 mg
Lovastatin	Inhibits HMG CoA reductase	Elevated transaminase levels at 3–10 months	Sleep disturb-ances, myositis syndrome	Starting dose 20 mg; range 40–80 mg

(From Hurst JW (ed): Medicine for the Practicing Physician, 2nd ed. Boston, Butterworth, 1988, p 928, with permission.)

131. What effect does alcohol use have on lipids?

Alcohol has several effects on serum lipid levels. It causes an increase in triglyceride levels but does not affect LDL levels. It does cause an increase in HDL levels through an unknown mechanism. This may lead to a reduction of the risk of CAD, although use of alcohol is not specifically recommended.

The Expert Panel: Report of the National Cholesterol Education Program Expert Panel on Detection, Evaluation and Treatment of High Blood Cholesterol in Adults. Arch Intern Med 148:36–69, 1988.

132. Other than alcohol, what factors can increase HDL levels?

The following have been found to elevate HDL levels:
1. Weight loss.
2. Aerobic exercise (however, mild to moderate exercise may have little effect).
3. Discontinuation of cigarette smoking.
4. Drugs (nicotinic acid, gemfibrozil).

133. What are prostaglandins (PG)?

PGs are oxygenation products of 20-carbon (eicosanoic) fatty acids that produce a wide variety of biologic effects. They are part of a group of compounds derived from eicosanoic fatty acids (called eicosanoids) that also includes thromboxanes and leukotrienes. PGs are produced by many different tissues. They have regulatory actions throughout the body. They are produced and exert their effects locally rather than systemically.

134. What are the causes of gynecomastia?

Causes of Gynecomastia

1. **Idiopathic**

2. **Physiologic**
   Puberty
   Aging
   Newborn

3. **Drugs**
   Drugs with estrogen activity (conjugated or synthetic estrogens, oral contraceptives, digitalis [digitoxin only, not digoxin])
   Drugs that stimulate estrogen synthesis or effect (clomiphene citrate, HCG,* LHRH)

Table continued on next page.

Causes of Gynecomastia (Continued)

3. **Drugs** *(Continued)*

   Drugs that decrease testosterone synthesis or effect (cimetidine, spironolactone, ketoconazole, cancer chemotherapeutic agents)

   Unknown mechanisms (methyldopa, marijuana, testosterone, isoniazid, diazepam, ethionamide, tricyclic antidepressants, d-penicillamine, ?heroin, ?phenothiazines, ?amphetamines)

4. **Tumors with increased HCG or estrogen formation**

   Choriocarcinoma (testicular or teratoma)

   Other testicular tumors

   Bronchogenic carcinoma

   Adrenal carcinoma

5. **Increased estrogen synthesis**

   Liver disease (may be combined with decreased androgens)

   Thyrotoxicosis

   Obesity (presumed)

   True hermaphroditism

   Familial

6. **Decreased androgen synthesis or androgen resistance**

   Testicular failure (orchitis, trauma or castration, granulomatous disease, myotonic dystrophy, and neurological disorders)

   Klinefelter's syndrome

   Defects in testosterone synthesis

   Congenital anorchism

   Androgen resistance syndromes

   Renal failure

7. **Altered testosterone and estrogen binding**

   Thyrotoxicosis

8. **Unknown mechanism**

   Starvation-refeeding

* HCG = human chorionic gonadotropin; LHRH = luteinizing hormone-releasing hormone.
(From Kohler PO (ed): Clinical Endocrinology. New York, John Wiley, 1986, p 373, with permission.)

BIBLIOGRAPHY

1. Besser GM, et al (eds): Endocrinology, 2nd ed. Philadelphia, W.B. Saunders, 1989.
2. DeGroot LJ (ed): Endocrinology, 2nd ed. Philadelphia, W.B. Saunders, 1989.
3. Kohler PO (ed): Clinical Endocrinology. New York, John Wiley, 1986.
4. Stern JH: Internal Medicine, 3rd ed. Boston, Little, Brown, 1990.

3. CARDIOLOGY SECRETS

Gabriel B. Habib, M.D. and Anthony J. Zollo, Jr., M.D.

The heart is the root of life and causes the versatility of the spiritual faculties. The heart influences the face and fills the pulse with blood.

Huang Ti (The Yellow Emperor) (2697–2597 B.C.)
Nei Chung Su Wen, Bk. 3, Sect. 9 (tr. by Ilza Veith in: The Yellow Emperor's Classic of Internal Medicine)

Harvey's discovery of the circulation of the blood was a beautiful addition to our knowledge of the animal economy, but on a review of the practice of medicine before and since that epoch, I do not see any great amelioration which has been derived from that discovery.

Thomas Jefferson (1743–1826)
Letter to Edward Jenner, May 14, 1806 (quoted by John Baron in: Life of Edward Jenner, Vol. II, Ch. 3)

PHYSICAL EXAMINATION

1. What are the cardiac physical examination findings in cardiac tamponade?
The clinical triad of cardiac tamponade, first described by the thoracic surgeon Claude S. Beck in 1935, consists of:
1. Hypotension
2. Elevated systemic venous pressure
3. Small quiet heart

This classic triad is commonly present in patients with cardiac tamponade due to penetrating cardiac injuries, aortic dissection, or intrapericardial rupture of aortic or cardiac aneurysm. These are currently uncommon causes of cardiac tamponade. Today, the most common causes of cardiac tamponade are neoplastic disease and idiopathic pericarditis followed by acute MI and uremia.

Presently, the commonest physical findings of acute cardiac tamponade are:

1. **Jugular venous distension,** still the most common physical finding in medical patients with cardiac tamponade. It is almost universally present except in patients with severe hypovolemia.

2. **Pulsus paradoxus,** defined as a decrease in systolic blood pressure in excess of 10 mmHg during quiet inspiration. Pulsus paradoxus is difficult to elicit in volume-depleted patients.

3. **Tachycardia,** with a thready peripheral pulse. Severe cardiac tamponade may restrict LV and RV filling enough to cause hypotension. More commonly, blood pressure may be maintained within normal limits by compensatory increase of heart rate. Therefore, hypotension is uncommon in most patients with cardiac tamponade, but a thready and rapid pulse is almost invariably present.

Kussmaul's sign, an inspiratory increase in systemic venous pressure, is commonly present in chronic constrictive pericarditis but is rarely detected in acute cardiac tamponade.

Beck CS: Two cardiac compression triads. JAMA 104:714, 1935.

2. What is the third heart sound (S₃)? What is a physiologic S₃?

An S_3 (or ventricular gallop) is a low-frequency sound that is heard just after the second heart sound (S_2). It is found in normal young patients (called a physiologic S_3). It is also found in association with a variety of pathologic conditions (pathologic S_3), including congestive heart failure (CHF), mitral valve prolapse, thyrotoxicosis, coronary artery disease, cardiomyopathies, pericardial constriction, mitral or aortic insufficiency, and left-to-right shunts.

The mechanism behind an S_3 is controversial. It has been suggested that it is due to an increase in the velocity of blood entering the ventricles (rapid ventricular filling). It usually represents myocardial decompensation when associated with heart disease.

3. What is an S₄?

An S_4 (or atrial gallop) occurs just before the first heart sound (S_1) and reflects decreased ventricular compliance (a stiff ventricle). It is associated with coronary artery disease, pulmonic or aortic valvular stenosis, hypertension, and ventricular hypertrophy from any cause.

4. How do we grade heart murmurs?

Grading System for Heart Murmurs

GRADE	PHYSICAL EXAMINATION FINDINGS
1	Barely audible intensity (i.e., only a cardiologist can hear it!)
2	Low intensity murmur (the upper-level resident can hear it)
3	Loud murmur (everyone can hear it)
4	Loud murmur with palpable thrill
5	Loudest murmur audible (but still does require that the stethoscope is placed on the chest)
6	Murmur loud enough to be heard with the stethoscope off the chest

5. What is paradoxical splitting of the second heart sound and what are its causes?

The second heart sound (S_2) is normally split into an aortic component (A_2) and pulmonary component (P_2) caused by the closing of the two respective valves. The degree of splitting varies with the respiratory cycle (physiologic splitting). With inspiration, the negative intrathoracic pressure leads to increased venous return to the right side of the heart and a decrease to the left side of the heart. This causes P_2 to occur slightly later and A_2 to occur slightly earlier, which leads to a widening of the splitting of S_2. With expiration, the negative intrathoracic pressure is eliminated and A_2 and P_2 occur almost simultaneously. Paradoxical splitting of S_2 refers to the situation in which the split of A_2 and P_2 seems to widen with expiration and shorten with inspiration (the opposite of normal). This is caused by P_2 preceding A_2 during expiration and is usually caused by conditions that delay A_2 by delaying ejection of blood from the left ventricle and therefore closure of the aortic valve. Causes include aortic insufficiency, aortic stenosis, hypertrophic obstructive cardiomyopathy, myocardial ischemia, left bundle branch block, or a right ventricular pacemaker.

6. What is the mechanism behind fixed splitting of S₂ and what are its causes?

Fixed splitting of S_2 refers to the physical examination finding in which the interval between A_2 and P_2 does not change with the respiratory cycle. It is typically associated with atrial septal defects or right ventricular dysfunction.

7. How do you examine the jugular venous pulse? What are its three waves?

To examine a patient's jugular venous pulse, the patient's chest should be elevated to the point where the pulsations are maximally visualized (usually 30 to 45 degrees of elevation).

Its height above the sternal angle (angle of Louis) can then be measured. Since the sternal angle is about 5 cm from the right atrium (regardless of elevation angle), central venous pressure can be estimated by adding 5 cm to the measurement. Normal central venous pressure is 5–9 cm H_2O.

The jugular venous pulse consists of three waves:

1. **a-wave:** produced by right atrial contraction and occurs just before the first heart sound.

2. **c-wave:** caused by bulging upward of the closed tricuspid valve during right ventricular contraction. (It is often difficult to see.)

3. **v-wave:** caused by right atrial filling just prior to opening of the tricuspid valve.

8. What are "cannon a-waves"?

"Cannon a-waves" are very large and prominent a-waves that occur when the atria contract against a closed tricuspid valve. Irregular "cannon a-waves" are seen in AV dissociation or ectopic atrial beats. Regular "cannon a-waves" are seen in a junctional or ventricular rhythm in which the atria are depolarized by retrograde conduction.

9. What is the most common cause of a systolic ejection murmur, best heard at the second right intercostal space, in an 82-year-old asymptomatic man? What other physical findings would help confirm your clinical diagnosis in this patient?

By far the most common cause of a systolic ejection murmur at the right intercostal space in an elderly man is aortic sclerosis. This valvular abnormality is characterized by thickening and/or calcification of the aortic valve, and, unlike valvular aortic stenosis, it is typically *not* associated with any significant transvalvular systolic pressure gradient.

On physical examination, aortic sclerosis can be differentiated from aortic stenosis as follows:

	Aortic stenosis	Aortic sclerosis
Diminished carotid upstroke	+	–
Diminished peripheral pulses	+	–
Late peaking of systolic murmur	+	–
Loud S4	+	–
Syncope, angina or heart failure	+	–
Loud systolic murmur and thrill	+	–

10. Dynamic auscultation is very useful in the differential diagnosis of cardiac murmurs. What are the effects of standing, squatting, and leg-raising on the intensity and duration of the systolic murmur in patients with idiopathic hypertrophic subaortic stenosis (IHSS)?

In IHSS, a decrease in the size of the LV increases the dynamic LV outflow obstruction, leading to an increase in the intensity of the murmur. A decrease in LV volume occurs upon assuming the standing posture.

In contrast, leg-raising and squatting increase venous return and thereby increase LV volume, decreasing the dynamic LV obstruction and the intensity of the murmur.

11. What is the mechanism of pulsus paradoxus? What medical diseases can present with pulsus paradoxus?

Pulsus paradoxus was first described by Kussmaul in 1873 as the apparent paradox of the disappearance of the pulse during inspiration despite persistence of the heartbeat. In fact, pulsus paradoxus is an exaggeration of the normal inspiratory decline in systolic blood pressure and LV stroke volume. The fall in intrathoracic pressure is rapidly transmitted through the pericardial effusion and results in an exaggerated increase in venous return to the right side of the heart. This, in turn, causes bulging of the interventricular septum toward the LV, thereby resulting in a smaller LV volume and LV stroke volume during inspiration.

The figure illustrates the marked decrease in systolic blood pressure during inspiration in a patient with cardiac tamponade.

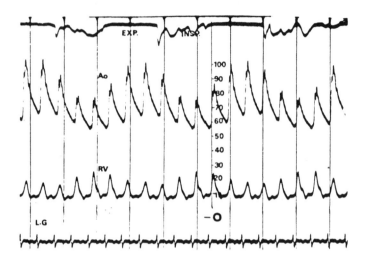

Recording of aortic (Ao) and right ventricular (RV) pressures in a patient with cardiac tamponade complicated by hypovolemia. *Pulsus paradoxus* is evident as a marked inspiratory decline in aortic systolic and pulse pressures during inspiration (INSP). RV pressure variation is out of phase with aortic pressure. Note that the RV waveform does *not* show a dip-and-plateau configuration. (From Shabetai R, et al: The hemodynamics of cardiac tamponade and constrictive pericarditis. Am J Cardiol 26:480, 1970, with permission.)

Pulsus paradoxus is *not* a sine qua non of cardiac tamponade. It may also be present in patients with severe chronic obstructive pulmonary disease complicated by the need for large negative intrathoracic pressures on inspiration. Interestingly, pulsus paradoxus is usually absent in chronic constrictive pericarditis.

ELECTROCARDIOGRAPHY

12. What is the classic ECG evolution of an acute transmural MI, with special reference to the sequence of ECG changes and their timing in relation to the onset of symptoms?
The ECG evolution of an acute MI consists of the following phases:

1. **Abnormal T-wave,** which is tall, prolonged, inverted, or upright. Hyperacute tall T-waves are typically seen in the first hour or two of MI evolution. The T-wave usually becomes inverted *after* ST-segment elevation has occurred and may remain inverted for days, weeks, or years.

2. **ST-segment elevations** in leads facing the infarcted myocardial wall, and "reciprocal ST depressions" in opposite leads. ST-segment changes are the most commonly recognized ECG signs of acute MI. ST-segment elevations rarely persist longer than 2 weeks except in patients with a ventricular aneurysm.

3. **Appearance of new Q-waves,** often several hours or days after onset of symptoms of MI. Alternatively the amplitude of the QRS complex is decreased. Evolution of Q-waves may occur earlier when thrombolytic therapy is administered.

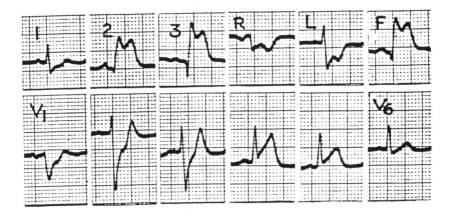

Acute **infero-apical** myocardial infarction. Note ST elevation in 2, 3, aVF, V₄, and V₅ with reciprocal depression in other leads. Q waves are developing in 2, 3, and aVF. (From Marriott HJL: Practical Electrocardiography, 8th ed. Baltimore, Williams & Wilkins, 1988, p 437, with permission.)

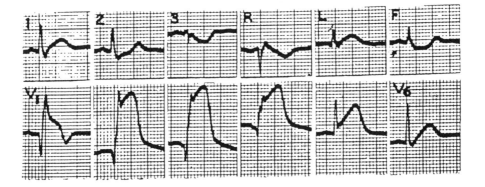

Acute **anterior myocardial infarction.** Note ST elevation in V₁₋₅, and loss of the normal upward concavity of the ST segment in 1, aVL and V₆, with reciprocal changes in 2, 3 and aVF. Q waves have developed in the right chest leads, and the pattern of RBBB has appeared, indicating septal involvement. (From Marriott HJL: Practical Electrocardiography, 8th ed. Baltimore, Williams & Wilkins, 1988, p 438, with permission.)

13. What are the ECG manifestations of atrial infarction?

Atrial Infarction: ECG Manifestations

1. Depressed or elevated PR segment
2. Atrial arrhythmias:
   a. Atrial flutter
   b. Atrial fibrillation
   c. AV nodal rhythms

14. Where does an S₃ occur in relation to the QRS complex? Where does the venous a-wave appear in the cardiac cycle?

The timing of the various arterial/venous pulsations, the heart sounds, pressure tracings, and ECG deflections are shown in the following figure:

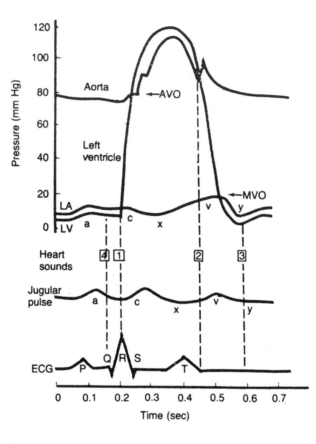

Simultaneous ECG, pressures obtained from the left atrium, left ventricle, and aorta, and the jugular pulse during one cardiac cycle. For simplification, right-sided heart pressures have been omitted. Normal right atrial pressure closely parallels that of the left atrium, and right ventricular and pulmonary artery pressures time closely with their corresponding left-sided heart counterparts, only being reduced in magnitude. The normal mitral and aortic valve closure precedes tricuspid and pulmonic closure, respectively, whereas valve opening reverses this order. The jugular venous pulse lags behind the right atrial pressure.

During the course of one cardiac cycle, note that the electrical events (ECG) initiate and therefore precede the mechanical (pressure) events and that the latter precede the auscultatory events (heart sounds) they themselves produce. Shortly after the P wave, the atria contract to produce the a wave; a fourth heart sound may succeed the latter. The QRS complex initiates ventricular systole, followed shortly by left ventricular contraction and the rapid build-up of left ventricular (LV) pressure. Almost immediately LV pressure exceeds left atrial (LA) pressure to close the mitral valve and produces the first heart sounds. When LV pressure exceeds aortic pressure, the aortic valve opens (AVO), and when aortic pressure is once again greater than LV pressure, the aortic valve closes to produce the second heart sound and terminate ventricular ejection. The decreasing LV pressure drops below LA pressure to open the mitral valve (MVO), and a period of rapid ventricular filling commences. During this time a third heart sound may be heard. (From Andreoli TE, et al (eds): Cecil Essentials of Medicine, 2nd ed. Philadelphia, W.B. Saunders, 1990, p 8, with permission.)

15. Which arrhythmias can be detected in young patients without apparent heart disease?
In a study of 24-hour continuous electrocardiographic (ECG) monitoring performed on 50 male medical students, severe sinus bradycardia (40 beats per minute or fewer), sinus pauses of up to 2 seconds, and nocturnal AV nodal block were frequently found. Frequent premature atrial or ventricular beats were not commonly found.

Brodsky M, et al: Arrhythmias documented by 24-hour continuous electrocardiographic monitoring in 50 male medical students without apparent heart disease. Am J Cardiol 39:390–395, 1977.

16. How do you differentiate between various types of supraventricular tachycardias (SVTs), namely, paroxysmal supraventricular tachycardia (PSVT), atrial flutter, and atrial fibrillation?
Atrial fibrillation (A fib) differs from all other SVTs by having totally disorganized atrial depolarizations without effective atrial contraction. Electrical activity may occasionally be detected on an ECG as small, irregular waves of variable amplitude and morphology. These rapid waves can occur at a rate of 350 to 600/min but are often difficult to recognize on a routine 12-lead ECG.

Atrial tachycardia (often called paroxysmal atrial tachycardia, or PAT) and **atrial flutter**, unlike A fib, demonstrate a regular ventricular rhythm and are characterized by regular and slower atrial rhythms. The flutter rate (i.e., the atrial rate) in atrial flutter ranges between 250 and 350 beats/min. The most common flutter rate is 300 beats/min and the most common ventricular rates are 150 and 75 beats/min, respectively. Atrial tachycardias have slower atrial rates ranging from 150 to 250 beats/min. The most common cause of PAT with block is digitalis toxicity.

Comparison of Atrial Fibrillation, Flutter and Tachycardia

	A FIB	A FLUTTER	A TACHYCARDIA
Atrial rate	>400	240–350	100–240
Atrial rhythm	Irregular	Regular	Regular
AV block	Variable	2:1, 4:1, 3:1, or variable	2:1, 4:1, 3:1, or variable
Ventricular rate	Variable	150, 75, 100, or variable	Variable

17. What is the importance of the findings of capture and fusion beats on ECG in the differentiation between ventricular tachycardia (V tach) and supraventricular tachycardia (SVT) with aberrancy?
A number of ECG findings have been reported to help in differentiating between V tach and SVT with aberrancy. These can be summarized as follows:

Distinguishing Features of Wide-complex Ventricular and Supraventricular Tachycardias

	Ventricular	Supraventricular
History of MI	+	–
Ventricular aneurysm	+	–
Fusion beats	+	–
Capture beats	+	–
Complete AV dissociation	+	–
Similar QRS when in sinus rhythm	–	+
RBBB* + QRS > 0.14 sec	+	–
LBBB* + QRS > 0.16 sec	+	–
Positive concordance in V1 to V6	+	–
LBBB + right QRS axis	+	–
Intermittent cannon waves	+	–

*LBBB/RBBB = left bundle branch block/right bundle branch block.

Three ECG findings are virtually pathognomonic of V tach: atrioventricular (AV) dissociation, capture beats, and fusion beats. A capture beat is a normally conducted sinus beat interrupting a wide-complex tachycardia. A fusion beat is a beat that has a QRS morphology intermediate between a normally conducted narrow beat and a wide-complex ventricular beat. The clinical hallmark of AV dissociation is the presence of intermittent cannon waves in the jugular neck veins.

18. Exercise stress ECG testing is a commonly performed noninvasive test aimed at assessing the risk of coronary artery disease (CAD). What are the medical contraindications to exercise ECG testing?

Exercise stress testing is widely used to detect and assess the functional significance of CAD. It has also been shown to predict survival in patients recovering from an acute myocardial infarction (MI). Risk stratification after acute MI is greatly affected by the results of exercise stress testing before hospital discharge. Since exercise stress testing is commonly requested by internists and family practitioners, it is imperative that contraindications be widely known and clearly understood so that use of this test is appropriate and safe. These include:

Contraindications to Exercise Testing

1. Myocardial infarction: acute or pending	6. Uncontrolled hypertension
2. Unstable angina	7. Uncontrolled cardiac arrhythmias
3. Acute myocarditis or pericarditis	8. Second- or third-degree AV block
4. Left main coronary artery disease	9. Acute noncardiac illness
5. Severe aortic stenosis	

19. What are the types of AV block?

1. **First-degree AV block:** Prolongation of the PR interval due to a conduction delay at the AV node.

2. **Second-degree AV block:** Manifested by dropped beats in which a P-wave is not followed by a QRS complex (no ventricular depolarization and therefore no ventricular contraction). It is divided into two types:
   a. **Type I** (Wenckebach phenomenon): The PR interval lengthens with each successive beat until a beat is dropped and the cycle repeats itself.
   b. **Type II:** The PR intervals are prolonged but do not gradually lengthen until a beat is suddenly dropped. The dropped beat may occur regularly, with a fixed number (X) of beats for each dropped beat (called an X:1 block). It is much less common than type I and is commonly associated with bundle branch blocks.

3. **Third-degree AV block** (complete heart block): The atria and ventricles are controlled by separate pacemakers. It is associated with widening of the QRS complex and a ventricular rate of 35–50 beats per minute.

20. What are the ECG changes in patients with hyperkalemia?

A tall, peaked, symmetrical T-wave with a narrow base (so-called tented T-wave) is the earliest ECG abnormality and is usually present in leads II, III, V2, V3, and V4. This is followed by shortening of the QT interval, widening of the QRS interval, ST-segment depression, flattening of the P-wave, and PR interval prolongation (see accompanying figure). Eventually, the P-waves disappear and the QRS complexes assume a configuration similar to a sine wave, eventually degenerating into V fib. Widening of the QRS complex can assume a configuration consistent with atypical right or left bundle branch block (BBB). This makes the recognition of hyperkalemia more difficult. Unlike typical RBBB configuration, hyperkalemia often causes prolongation of the entire QRS complex.

Sequence of ECG Changes in Experimental Hyperkalemia

Tall, symmetrical T-waves	K > 5.7 mEq/L
Reduced P-wave amplitude	K > 7.0 mEq/L
Prolongation of PR inverval	K > 7.0 mEq/L
Disappearance of P-waves	K > 8.4 mEq/L
Widening of QRS interval	K = 9–11 mEq/L
Ventricular fibrillation	K > 12 mEq/L

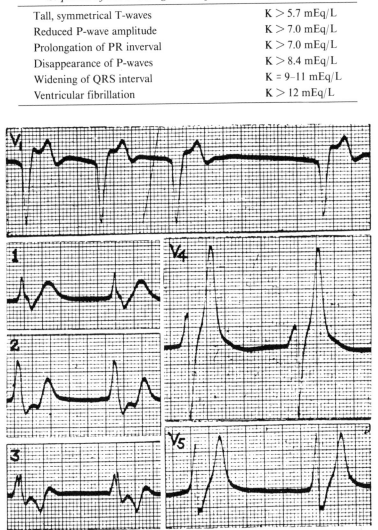

Hyperkalemia. This tracing shows evidence of advanced potassium intoxication: tall peaked T waves, absent P waves, widened QRS complexes and irregular rhythm. From a patient with serum potassium level of 8.1 mEq per liter. (From Marriott HJL: Practical Electrocardiography, 8th ed. Baltimore, Williams & Wilkins, 1988, p 526, with permission.)

21. What should make you suspect hypercalcemia by ECG? Are similar changes encountered in other conditions as well?

Hypercalcemia shortens the QT interval, particularly the interval between the beginning of the QRS complex and the peak of the T-wave. The abrupt slope to the peak of the T-wave is most characteristic of hypercalcemia. Other causes of shortened QT interval include digitalis. The figure below shows the ECG from a patient with hypercalcemia (calcium = 15 mg/dl) due to hyperparathyroidism.

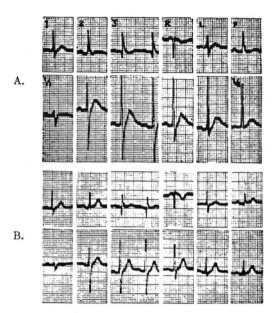

A.

B.

From a patient with **hyperparathy-roidism.** *A*, Before parathyroidectomy (serum calcium 15 mg). Note virtual absence of ST segment, early peak of T wave and relatively gradual down-slope of descending limb of T wave. *B*, After parathyroidectomy (serum calcium 10.7 mg). Note normal contour of ST-T pattern. (From Marriott HJL: Practical Electrocardiography, 8th ed. Baltimore, Williams & Wilkins, 1988, p 527, with permission.)

22. What is the normal range for P-R and Q-T intervals on a 12-lead ECG? Are these intervals related to heart rate, sex, or age?

The normal range for the P-R interval is 0.12 to 0.20 sec. It is not significantly related to age, sex, or heart rate. The normal range for the Q-T interval is also unrelated to age. The most important determinant of the Q-T interval is heart rate. As the heart rate increases, the Q-T interval shortens. To help evaluate a Q-T interval independently of heart rate, QTc (corrected Q-T interval) can be calculated. It is the ratio of measured Q-T interval over the square root of the R-R interval:

$$QTc \text{ (in seconds)} = \frac{Q\text{-}T \text{ (in seconds)}}{\sqrt{R\text{-}R \text{ interval (in seconds)}}}$$

The normal range for the QTc is 0.36 to 0.44 sec. A prolonged QTc is defined as QTc > 0.39 sec in men or > 0.44 sec in women.

Common causes of Q-T prolongation in adults include: hypokalemia, hypocalcemia, hypomagnesemia, or a type IA or IC antiarrhythmic drug such as procainamide, quinidine, disopyramide, flecainide, encainide, or lorcainide.

23. In the frontal plane, is a QRS axis of +120 degrees compatible with a diagnosis of left anterior hemiblock (or "left anterior fascicular block")?

The diagnosis of left anterior fascicular block (LAFB) requires the presence of a QRS of –60 to –90 degrees in the frontal plane. A frontal plane QRS axis of +120 degrees is consistent with right axis deviation and is therefore not compatible with a diagnosis of left anterior fascicular block.

Diagnostic Criteria for Left Anterior Fascicular Block

1. QRS Axis –60 to –90 degrees
2. Small q wave in lead I
3. Small r wave in lead III

24. Describe the ECG manifestations of RV hypertrophy.

Right Ventricular Hypertrophy

1. R-wave larger than S-wave in V1 or V2	4. Persistent rS pattern (V1–V6)
2. R-wave > 5 mm in V1 or V2	5. Normal QRS duration
3. Right axis deviation	

25. What are the causes of a prolonged Q-T interval?

Differential Diagnosis of Prolonged Q-T Interval

A. Congenital:
  1. With deafness: Jervell syndrome
  2. Without deafness: Romano-Ward syndrome

B. Acquired
  1. Drugs: Class IA/IC antiarrhythmics
  2. Electrolyte abnormalities: low K^+, Ca^{++}, Mg^{++}
  3. Hypothermia
  4. Central nervous system injury (least common cause)
  5. Liquid diets
  6. Coronary artery disease
  7. Cardiomyopathy
  8. Mitral valve prolapse

Prolongation of the Q-T interval is associated in certain patients with a definite increase in risk of V fib and death.

DIAGNOSIS

26. What are the differentiating features of cardiac and noncardiac causes of chest pain?

Cardiac Causes of Chest Pain

CONDITION	LOCATION	QUALITY	DURATION	AGGRAVATING/ RELIEVING FACTORS	ASSOCIATED SIGNS AND SYMPTOMS
Angina	Retrosternal, radiates to neck, left	Pressure, burning, squeezing	<10 min	Aggravated by exercise, cold, emotional stress, after meals. Relieved by rest, nitroglycerin	S_4, paradoxically split S_2, murmur of papillary muscle
Rest or crescendo angina	Same as angina	Same as angina	>10 min	Same as angina with gradually decreasing tolerance for exertion	Same as angina
Myocardial infarction	Substernal; may radiate like angina	Heaviness, pressure, burning, constriction	30 min or longer, variable	Unrelieved	Shortness of breath, diaphoresis, nausea, vomiting, weakness, anxiety
Pericarditis	Substernal or cardiac apex; may radiate to left arm	Sharp, stabbing, knifelike	Hours to days	Aggravated by deep breathing, rotating chest, or supine position. Relieved by sitting up and leaning forward.	Pericardial friction rub, cardiac tamponade, pulsus paradoxus
Dissecting aortic anuerysm	Anterior chest, back, abdominal	Excruciating, tearing, knifelike	Sudden onset, lasts for hours	Unrelated to anything	Lower blood pressure in one arm, absent pulses, murmur of aortic insufficiency, paralysis, pulsus paradoxus

Noncardiac Causes of Chest Pain

CONDITION	LOCATION	QUALITY	DURATION	AGGRAVATING/ RELIEVING FACTORS	ASSOCIATED SIGNS AND SYMPTOMS
Pulmonary embolism	Substernal or over area of pulmonary infarction	Pleuritic or like angina	Sudden onset, min. to >1 hour	May be aggravated by breathing	Dyspnea, tachypnea, tachycardia, hypotension, signs of right-sided CHF, rales, pleural rub, hemoptysis (with infarction)
Pulmonary hypertension	Substernal	Pressure		Aggravated by effort	Dyspnea, signs of pulmonary hypertension
Pneumonia with pleuritis	Over area of consolidation	Pleuritic, well localized		Aggravated by breathing	Dyspnea, cough, fever, dull to percussion, bronchial breath sounds, pleural rub
Spontaneous pneumothorax	Unilateral	Sharp, well localized	Sudden onset, hours	Painful breathing	Dyspnea, hyper-resonance, and decreased breath and voice sounds
Musculoskeletal	Variable	Aching	Short or long	Aggravated by movement, history of muscle exertion	Tender to pressure or movement
Herpes zoster	Dermatomal distribution		Prolonged	None	Rash appears in area of discomfort
GI disorders (esophageal reflux, ulcer)	Lower substernal, epigastric	Burning, colicky, aching		Precipitated by recumbency or meals, partial relief with antacids	Nausea, vomiting, food intolerance, melena, hematemesis, jaundice
Anxiety states	Often localized to a point, moves	Sharp, burning, variable	Variable	Situational anger, usually brief	Sighing respirations, often chest wall tenderness

(From Andreoli TE, et al (eds): Cecil Essentials of Medicine, 2nd ed. Philadelphia, W.B. Saunders, 1990, pp 12–13, Tables 2-2 and 2-3, with permission.)

27. A 31-year-old man complains of a sudden onset of sharp left chest pain, increased by deep inspiration and coughing. Physical examination, chest x-ray, and ECG are all normal. What is your differential diagnosis?

Differential Diagnosis of Pleuritic Chest Pain

1. Acute pleuritis (coxsackie virus A, B)	4. Pulmonary embolus or infarction
2. Acute pericarditis (coxsackie virus B)	5. Pneumothorax
3. Pneumonia (viral, bacterial)	

In this patient, the most likely clinical diagnosis causing pleuritic chest pain in the presence of a normal physical examination, chest x-ray and ECG is acute viral pleuritis or pericarditis.

28. A 56-year-old man presented to the Emergency Center with an acute onset of squeezing diffuse anterior chest pain associated with diaphoresis and dyspnea. What is your differential diagnosis and which tests would you request to help confirm your clinical suspicions?
The differential diagnosis of a squeezing, diffuse, anterior chest pain associated with diaphoresis and dyspnea consists of the following:

1. Acute myocardial infarction	4. Acute pericarditis
2. Angina pectoris	5. Acute pulmonary embolus
3. Acute aortic dissection	6. Acute pneumothorax

Among the above-listed diagnoses, the first three are most common and should be carefully considered in the diagnostic work-up of this patient. A 12-lead ECG is done to look for ST-segment elevations (evidence of acute myocardial injury due to infarction or pericarditis), ST-segment depressions (evidence of subendocardial ischemia), or T-wave changes. Determination of serial cardiac enzymes (creatine kinase [CK], and CK-MB isoenzyme) over the first 24–48 hours of hospitalization will help to confirm a diagnosis of acute MI. The absence of any ECG changes of acute MI or ischemia in a patient with severe anterior chest pain radiating to the back should suggest the clinical diagnosis of acute aortic dissection. Finally, a chest x-ray is helpful in the work-up of patients with acute chest pains to look for evidence of a pneumothorax, cardiac enlargement suggestive of cardiac failure, or a wedge-shaped pulmonary consolidation suggestive of acute pulmonary embolus.

29. What are the types of shock and their causes?

Classification of Shock States

TYPE	PRIMARY MECHANISM	CLINICAL CAUSES

Hypovolemic	Volume loss	Exogenous
		  Blood loss due to hemorrhage
		  Plasma loss due to burn, inflammation
		  Fluid and electrolyte loss due to vomiting,
		    diarrhea, dehydration, osmotic diuresis
		    (diabetes)
		Endogenous
		  Extravasation due to inflammation, trauma,
		    tourniquet, anaphylaxis, snake venom, and
		    adrenergic stimulation (pheochromocytoma)

Cardiogenic	Pump failure	Myocardial infarction, congestive heart failure,
		  cardiac arrhythmias, intracardiac obstruction
		  (including valvular stenosis)

Distributive (vaso- motor dysfunction)		

1. High or
     normal
     resistance
	Expanded venous
	  capacitance
		Hypodynamic septic shock due to gram-negative
		  enteric bacillemia; autonomic blockade; spinal
		  shock; tranquilizer, sedative or narcotic overdose

2. Low
     resistance
	Arteriovenous
	  shunting
		Pneumonia, peritonitis, abscess, reactive
		  hyperemia

Obstructive	Extracardiac
	  obstruction of
	  main blood
	  flow channels
		Vena caval obstruction (supine hypotensive
		  syndrome), pericarditis (tamponade), pulmonary
		  embolism, dissecting aortic aneurysm or aortic
		  compression.

(From: Weil MH, et al: Acute circulatory failure (shock). In Braunwald E (ed): Heart Disease: A Textbook of Cardiovascular Medicine, 3rd ed. Philadelphia, W.B. Saunders, 1988, p 569, with permission.)

30. Some patients exhibit ECG changes similar to those of MI but do not have any other definitive evidence of an MI. These patients are said to have ECG evidence of "pseudoinfarction." What is the differential diagnosis of pseudoinfarction?

Causes of Electrocardiographic Patterns of Pseudoinfarction

1. Left or right ventricular hypertrophy	5. Hyperkalemia
2. Left bundle branch block (LBBB)	6. Early repolarization
3. Wolff-Parkinson-White (WPW)	7. Cardiac sarcoid or amyloid
4. Hypertrophic cardiomyopathy	8. Intracranial hemorrhage

31. What is the diagnostic approach to a patient who presents to the CCU with clinical signs and symptoms suggestive of acute right ventricular (RV) MI? In particular, how would ECG help us in confirming this important clinical diagnosis?

About a third of patients with acute inferior wall MI develop an RV infarction. The clinical syndrome of RV MI should be suspected when the following clinical triad is present in a patient suffering from an inferior wall MI: (1) hypotension, (2) elevated jugular veins, and (3) clear lungs.

The clinical recognition of RV infarction is important. Confirmation of the clinical suspicion of acute RV MI can be obtained by performing a right-sided ECG. The presence of at least 1 mm of ST-segment elevation in lead V3R or V4R is characteristically present in RV MI. Further confirmation of the diagnosis of RV infarction can be derived from noninvasive assessment of RV systolic function using radionuclide techniques or two-dimensional echocardiography.

It is essential to avoid fluid restriction or diuresis in patients with RV infarction, as they depend on an adequate preload to maintain a normal left ventricular (LV) stroke volume. Depriving them of this optimal preload causes persistent hypotension and systemic hypoperfusion.

32. Your next-door neighbor, an 89-year-old woman, is brought to the Emergency Center (EC) after she was found unconscious in her backyard. She "woke up" a few minutes after her admission to the EC. Physical examination, neurologic examination, ECG, and chest x-ray are all normal. She feels fine and demands to be released. Would you admit her to the hospital? What is your differential diagnosis in this elderly woman?

Syncope, defined as a transient loss or impairment of consciousness, can be due to a wide variety of etiologies. The causes of syncope can be conveniently divided into two general categories: (1) cardiovascular and (2) noncardiovascular.

Patients most likely to have cardiovascular syncope are older patients, with or without a prior history of documented cardiac disease (manifested by angina pectoris, MI, or sudden cardiac death). Common cardiovascular causes of syncope include:

1. Tachyarrhythmias, such as V tach or SVT (A fib, atrial flutter, or PSVT).

2. Bradyarrhythmias, such as second- or third-degree (latter called complete) AV block, A fib with a slow ventricular response rate, or sinus bradycardia due to sick sinus syndrome.

3. LV outflow obstruction due to fixed lesions (valvular, subvalvular, or supravalvular aortic stenosis), or dynamic obstruction such as hypertrophic cardiomyopathy. Characteristically, these patients present with syncope during or immediately after exercise.

4. LV inflow obstruction due to severe mitral stenosis or a large left atrial myxoma.

5. Primary pulmonary hypertension.

It is desirable to hospitalize patients who are at high risk for cardiovascular syncope, since they have a much worse prognosis and may have potentially life-threatening complications of their underlying cardiovascular disease. Therefore, this elderly woman with syncope should be hospitalized, since she is at high risk for cardiovascular syncope.

33. Should a thorough work-up be done on all patients with syncope?

No. It has been well documented that routine use of expensive or invasive studies into the cause of syncope is not warranted. The etiology of syncope will be undetermined in 30–50% of cases even after a thorough (and often expensive) work-up. In up to 85% of the cases in which an etiology is identifiable, it will be identified, or at least suggested, by the initial history, physical examination, and ECG. Further studies should be ordered on the basis of the results of this initial evaluation.

34. What are the three types of cardiomyopathies and how are they distinguished?

Classification of Cardiomyopathy

TYPE	CHARACTERISTICS	SYMPTOMS AND SIGNS	LABORATORY DIAGNOSIS
Dilated (congestive)	Cardiac dilation, generalized hypocontractility	Left and right ventricular failure	X-ray: cardiomegaly with pulmonary congestion ECG: sinus tachycardia, nonspecific ST-T changes, arrhythmias, conduction disturbances, Q waves Echo: dilated LV, generalized decreased wall motion, mitral valve motion consistent with low flow Catheterization: dilated hypocontractile ventricle; mitral regurgitation
Hypertrophic	Ventricular hypertrophy, especially the septum, with or without outflow tract obstruction Typically good systolic but poor diastolic (compliance) ventricular function	Dyspnea, angina, presyncope, syncope, palpitations Large jugular a wave, bifid carotid pulse, palpable S_4 gallop, prominent apical impulse; "dynamic" systolic murmur and thrill, mitral regurgitation murmur	X-ray: LV predominance, dilated left atrium ECG: left ventricular hypertrophy, Q waves, nonspecific ST-T waves; ventricular arrhythmias Echo: hypertrophy, usually asymmetric (septum > free wall); systolic anterior motion of mitral valve; midsystolic closure of aortic valve Catheterization: provokable outflow tract gradient; hypertrophy with vigorous systolic function and cavity obliteration; mitral regurgitation
Restrictive	Reduced diastolic compliance impeding ventricular filling; normal systolic function	Dyspnea, exercise intolerance, weakness Elevated jugular venous pressure, edema, hepatomegaly, ascites, S_4 & S_3 gallops, Kussmaul's sign	X-ray: mild cardiomegaly; pulmonary congestion ECG: low voltage, conduction disturbances, Q waves Echo: characteristic myocardial texture in amyloidosis with thickening of all cardiac structures Catheterization: square root sign: M-shaped atrial waveform, elevated left and right-sided filling pressures

(From Andreoli TE, et al (eds): Cecil Essentials of Medicine. Philadelphia, W.B. Saunders, 1990, p 106, with permission.)

35. A 68-year-old man with hypertension presents to the Emergency Center with a 2-week history of progressive exertional dyspnea, orthopnea, and paroxysmal nocturnal dyspnea (PND). What is the differential diagnosis and how would physical examination assist in the assessment of this patient?

Differential Diagnosis of CHF in Hypertensive Patients

1. Coronary artery disease
2. Diastolic dysfunction associated with hypertension
3. Dilated cardiomyopathy (idiopathic or alcoholic)
4. Valvular heart disease (mitral regurgitation, aortic stenosis, aortic insufficiency)
5. Restrictive heart disease (amyloidosis)
6. Hypertrophic cardiomyopathy (idiopathic hypertrophic subaortic stenosis)

36. What are the mechanism and differential diagnosis of a hyperdynamic precordial impulse?

A hyperdynamic precordial impulse is described as a thrust of exaggerated height that falls away immediately from the palpating fingers. It is typically found in patients with a large stroke volume. The clinical conditions include thyrotoxicosis, anemia, beriberi, AV shunts or grafts, exercise, or mitral regurgitation. A hyperdynamic precordial impulse should be differentiated from the sustained apical impulse, a graphic equivalent of a heave, detected in the presence of LV hypertrophy due to hypertension or aortic stenosis.

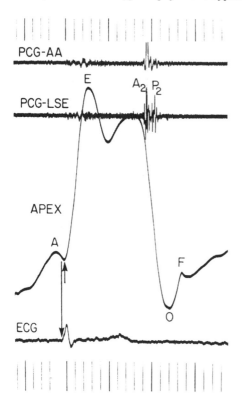

Left, Normal apexcardiogram. A low-amplitude *a* wave (A) in presystole follows the P wave of the ECG, which is not visible in this lead. The onset of the QRS (downward arrow) is followed after a brief electromechanical interval (0.02 sec) by the onset of the swift upward movement of the apex tracing (upward arrow), culminating in the E point at approximately the time of beginning ejection into the aorta. A generally declining curve during systole ends with an abrupt downward fall at the time of A_2. The nadir (0) is reached at approximately the time of mitral valve opening. The rapid filling wave (F) occurs during early diastolic filling of the left ventricle. (From Braunwald E (ed): Heart Disease: A Textbook of Cardiovascular Medicine, 3rd ed. Philadelphia, W.B. Saunders, 1988, p 58, with permission.)

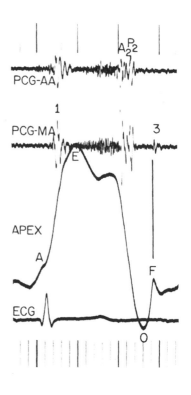

Right, Hyperdynamic apexcardiogram in mitral regurgitation. The configuration of the tracing in systole is qualitatively similar to a normal curve, although the amplitude was clearly exaggerated by palpation. The rapid filling wave (F) is higher than normal and terminates in a sharp point coincident with its audible counterpart, the third heart sound (3). (From Braunwald E (ed): Heart Disease: A Textbook of Cardiovascular Medicine, 3rd ed. Philadelphia, W.B. Saunders, 1988, p 58, with permission.)

37. What is the differential diagnosis of an abnormal early diastolic sound heard at the apex and lower left sternal border?

Differential Diagnosis of Early Diastolic Sound

1. Loud P_2
2. S_3 gallop
3. Opening snap
4. Pericardial knock
5. Tumor plop (atrial myxoma)

An early diastolic sound may be due to wide splitting of S_2, with or without a loud pulmonic closure sound. An ASD causes wide and fixed splitting of S_2. A loud P_2 usually indicates the presence of pulmonary hypertension, whether primary or secondary to chronic pulmonary disease.

Unlike other causes of an early diastolic sound, a third heart sound (S_3) can best be heard using the bell of the stethoscope. Unlike a physiologically split A_2–P_2, the A_2–S_3 interval does not change during respiration. Associated physical findings of CHF, such as pulmonary rales, distended neck veins, or edema are usually present along with an S_3.

An opening snap may be the only finding in a patient with mild noncalcified and pliable mitral valve. In such a patient, a loud S_1 is also commonly present. A diastolic rumble at the apex confirms the physical diagnosis of mitral stenosis.

In patients with chronic constrictive pericarditis, the sudden slowing of LV filling in early diastole associated with the restriction of a rigid pericardium, acting as "a rigid shell," causes the pericardial knock sound.

In some patients with large atrial myxomas protruding through the mitral valve during diastole, the sudden cessation of LV filling, caused by the tumor's obstruction to the flow of blood, creates an audible tumor plop. Cardiac auscultation in various positions helps to detect a tumor plop, since the extent of functional narrowing of the mitral valve by the tumor is often related to body position. Likewise, cardiac symptoms in these patients are often related to body position.

38. In patients with mitral stenosis, what are the pathophysiology and significance of an opening snap? Does the presence of an opening snap imply a more- or less-severe degree of stenosis?

An opening snap is typically present only when the mitral valve leaflets are pliable and is therefore usually accompanied by an accentuated S_1. Diffuse calcification of the mitral valve can be expected when an opening snap is absent. If calcification is confined to the tip of the mitral valve, an opening snap is still commonly present.

The interval between the aortic closure sound and opening snap (called A_2–OS) is inversely related to the mean left atrial pressure. A short A_2–OS interval is a reliable indicator of severe mitral stenosis; however, the converse is not necessarily true.

39. What is the "figure 3" sign? What congenital cardiac disease is it most likely to suggest?

A routine chest x-ray may reveal a characteristic "3" sign. This is the result of poststenotic dilatation of the descending aorta and the dilated left subclavian artery. A barium swallow may reveal a reverse "3" sign. Along with rib-notching, the presence of the "3" sign is almost pathognomonic for aortic coarctation. The characteristic "3" sign is shown in the figure.

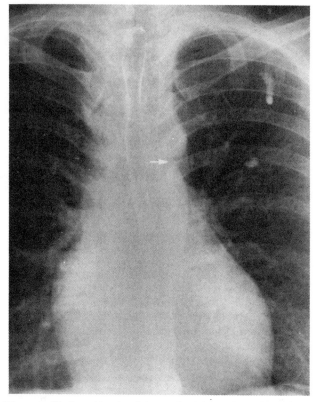

Coarctation of the aorta. The lateral border of the proximal descending aorta is composed of two arcs separated by a sharp indentation (arrow). The latter represents the site of coarctation. The upper bulge is formed by the dilated left subclavian artery, which obscures the aortic knob, and the lower bulge is caused by poststenotic dilatation of the aorta. The two bulges also indent the barium-coated esophagus. (From Baron MG: Obscuration of the aortic knob in coarctation of the aorta. Circulation 43:311, 1971, with permission.)

40. What are the *major* and *minor* Jones criteria for diagnosing acute rheumatic fever?

Rheumatic Fever: Major Jones Criteria

1. Carditis	4. Erythema marginatum
2. Polyarthritis	5. Subcutaneous nodules
3. Chorea	

Rheumatic Fever: Minor Jones Criteria

1. Fever	4. Elevated erythrocyte sedimentation rate
2. Arthralgia	or positive C-reactive protein
3. Prolonged PR interval	5. Previous rheumatic fever or rheumatic heart disease

The clinical diagnosis of acute rheumatic fever is made if two major criteria or one major and two minor criteria are present in a patient with a preceding streptococcal infection, as evidenced by (1) recent scarlet fever, (2) positive throat culture for group A streptococcus, and (3) increased ASO or other streptococcal antibody titer.

CORONARY ARTERY DISEASE

41. Is aspirin effective in the treatment of patients admitted to the Coronary Care Unit with unstable angina pectoris?

There is unequivocal evidence from two clinical trials, the VA and Canadian Cooperative trials, that aspirin reduces subsequent MI and mortality in unstable angina patients. Both mortality and MI are reduced by about 50% in aspirin-treated patients. Based on these results, aspirin is routinely administered in patients admitted to the Coronary Care Unit with unstable angina. On the other hand, there is no evidence to suggest a beneficial effect of aspirin in patients with chronic stable angina pectoris.

Lewis HD, et al: Protective effects of aspirin against acute myocardial infarction and death in men with unstable angina: Results of a Veterans Administration Cooperative Study. N Engl J Med 309: 396–403, 1983.

Cairns JA, et al: Aspirin, sulfinpyrazone, or both in unstable angina: results of a Canadian multicenter trial. N Engl J Med 313:1369–1375, 1985.

42. Which coronary artery is most commonly involved in patients with Prinzmetal's angina? Which ECG leads would most commonly show transient ST-segment elevations in these patients during episodes of chest pain?

The diagnosis of variant angina suspected clinically should be confirmed by obtaining a 12-lead ECG during episodes of angina. Characteristically, the ECG shows transient ST-segment elevations during episodes of chest discomfort or pain. These ECG changes are due to transient epicardial coronary spasm and are often complicated by arrhythmias or conduction disturbances. The ST-segment elevation is most commonly present in inferior leads, reflecting the frequency of involvement of the right coronary artery.

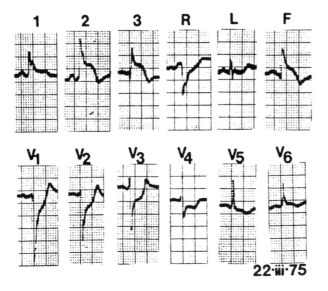

Electrocardiogram taken during angina demonstrates S-T segment elevation and reciprocal depression. (From Berman ND, et al: Prinzmetal's angina with coronary spasm. Angiographic, pharmacologic, metabolic and radionuclide perfusion studies. Am J Med 60:729, 1976, with permission.)

43. What are the most common precipitating factors for variant (Prinzmetal's) angina?

In patients with Prinzmetal's angina (named after Myron Prinzmetal), attacks do not typically occur following physical activity. More likely, anginal episodes occur at rest, at night, after emotional upsets, on exposure to cold weather or during or after meals. It is hypothesized that cold-induced angina may be due to coronary vasoconstriction,[1] and that a rapid rise in heart rate and blood pressure accompanying meals may increase myocardial oxygen consumption,[2] thus causing an imbalance between oxygen supply and demand in the myocardium.

1. Epstein SE, et al: Effect of a reduction in environmental temperature on the circulatory response to exercise in man. Implications concerning angina pectoris. N Engl J Med 280:7, 1969.

2. Goldstein RE, et al: Alterations in the circulatory response to exercise following a meal and their relationship in postprandial angina pectoris. Circulation 44:90, 1971.

44. Which test would you choose to perform in a patient presenting with recurrent oppressive chest pains at rest with associated ST-segment elevations?

Patients with a history of oppressive or squeezing chest pains occurring at rest and associated with transient ST-segment elevations should be suspected of having Prinzmetal's angina or variant angina. Of all available provocative tests for coronary vasospasm, the ergonovine test is the most sensitive and useful.[1] When administered IV in doses ranging from 0.05 to 0.40 mg, ergonovine is the most sensitive and specific test for provoking coronary artery spasm. A positive ergonovine test is defined by the induction of severe *focal* spasm in response to low doses of ergonovine administered by experienced personnel.

1. Winniford MD, et al: Ergonovine provocation to assess efficacy of long-term therapy with calcium antagonists in Prinzmetal's variant angina. Am J Cardiol 51:684, 1983.

45. What are the differences in efficacy and safety of the various classes of antianginal drugs used in the management of patients with vasospastic angina as compared to classic effort angina?

Three major classes of antianginal drugs are presently available: (1) nitrates (sublingual, oral, and IV), (2) beta-blockers, and (3) calcium blockers. Patients with Prinzmetal's angina differ from patients with effort angina (so-called classic or exertional angina) in their response to beta-blockers and calcium antagonists, but not in their response to nitrates.

Patients with both forms of angina respond promptly to nitrates. Although the response of patients with effort angina to beta-blockers is uniformly good, the response of patients with Prinzmetal's angina is variable. In some of these patients the duration of episodes of angina pectoris may be prolonged during therapy with propranolol, a noncardioselective beta-blocker.[1] In others, especially those with associated fixed atherosclerotic lesions, beta-blockers may reduce the frequency of anginal episodes.

Noncardioselective beta-blockers may, in some patients with variant angina, leave alpha-receptor-mediated coronary arterial vasoconstriction unopposed and thereby worsen anginal symptoms. In contrast to beta-blockers, calcium blockers are quite effective in reducing the frequency and duration of episodes of variant angina.[2] Along with nitrates, calcium blockers are presently the mainstay of treatment of Prinzmetal's angina because of their proven efficacy and safety.

1. Robertson RM, et al: Exacerbation of vasotonic angina pectoris by propranolol. Circulation 65:281, 1982.

2. Schroeder JS, et al: Prevention of cardiovascular events in variant angina by long-term diltiazem therapy. J Am Coll Cardiol 1:1507, 1983.

46. What is the value of treadmill exercise ECG testing in confirming the diagnosis of variant angina?

Exercise testing is the most common provocative test used by clinicians to confirm the clinical diagnosis of exertional angina pectoris. An exercise ECG test is considered positive for coronary artery disease if it shows at least a 1-mm ST-segment depression during exercise. Myocardial ischemia is induced in these patients by an increase in myocardial oxygen demand, primarily due to the increase in heart rate with exercise.

In patients with variant angina, myocardial ischemia is primarily due to a decrease in oxygen supply rather than to an increase in oxygen demand. Exercise testing is thus of limited diagnostic value in these patients. It may show ST-segment elevation, ST-segment depression, or no change in ST-segments during exercise.

47. A 78-year-old asthmatic man is brought to you for management of stable exertional angina of 3 years' duration. Past medical history reveals intermittent claudication after walking 50 yards. What is your approach to the management of this patient's anginal symptoms?
This is an elderly man with three medical problems:
1. Asthma
2. Intermittent claudication
3. Chronic stable angina.
The available antianginal drugs are:
    a. Nitrates
    b. Beta-blockers
    c. Calcium channel blockers.
The presence of asthma constitutes a contraindication for the use of beta-blockers. Cardioselective beta-blockers such as metoprolol (Lopressor) or atenolol (Tenormin) may be cautiously used in low doses. Noncardioselective beta-blockers are not safe in this patient.

The presence of peripheral vascular disease manifested by intermittent claudication is a contraindication for the use of any beta-blocker. Calcium antagonists and nitrates are thus antianginal drugs of choice in this patient.

48. Why is it desirable to admit to the Coronary Care Unit a patient with a prior history of chronic stable angina and recent increase in the frequency and duration of his or her anginal symptoms?
An increase in the frequency, duration, or intensity, or change in ease of relief with rest or nitroglycerin of previously stable exertional angina indicates the development of unstable angina pectoris. In view of the well-described propensity of unstable angina patients to develop life-threatening complications such as sudden cardiac death, acute MI, or refractory angina pectoris, they should be admitted to the hospital for ECG monitoring, observation, and initiation of effective antianginal and antiplatelet medications.

49. Which myocardial wall is frequently affected when, for example, a 48-year-old man presents with acute severe epigastric pain, anorexia, nausea, vomiting, and diaphoresis? Explain the rationale for such an unusual clinical presentation.
An exceptional clinical presentation of patients with acute inferior wall MI is that of epigastric pain associated with gastrointestinal symptoms, as in this patient. A less common clinical feature of acute inferior wall MI is hiccupping, which may, at times, be intractable.

These unique clinical manifestations of inferior wall MI are thought to be related to increased vagal tone and irritation of the diaphragm by the adjacent infarcted inferior wall.

50. Does early administration of thrombolytic therapy aimed at dissolving a coronary thrombus decrease mortality? If so, would you recommend thrombolytic therapy routinely (unless medically contraindicated) in MI victims admitted to the hospital within the first 6 hours?
The effect of intravenous (IV) thrombolytic therapy on myocardial infarct mortality is well-established. In the GISSI trial,[1] a large-scale, multi-center, randomized, clinical trial comparing IV streptokinase to placebo, 11,806 patients with acute MI presenting within 12 hours of symptom onset were enrolled. The hospital mortality was significantly reduced in patients treated within the first 6 hours. Most importantly, there was a remarkable 50% reduction in hospital mortality in patients treated within 1 hour of symptom onset. These

results illustrate the importance of early administration of IV thrombolytic therapy. This is best summarized by the commonly quoted phrase "Time Is Muscle."

Present standards of care for patients admitted with acute transmural MI include administration of IV thrombolytic therapy in all patients admitted within 6 hours of symptoms of an MI in the absence of contraindications to such therapy. The contraindications include bleeding disorders, severe uncontrolled hypertension, recent history of cerebrovascular accident, prolonged cardiopulmonary resuscitation (over 2–3 min), or active bleeding from a peptic ulcer or other source.

1. GISSI Trial: Effect of time to treatment on reduction in hospital mortality observed in streptokinase-treated patients. Lancet i:397–401, 1986.

51. When tissue plasminogen activator (t-PA) was compared to streptokinase (SK) in a major clinical trial, which drug was found to be more effective in achieving successful recanalization of a thrombosed coronary artery?

t-PA is a potent thrombolytic drug. In a multi-center clinical trial (TIMI, Phase I),[1,2] t-PA was shown to result in about twice as many successful reperfusions (due to clot lysis) compared to streptokinase.

1. Chesebro JH, et al: Thrombolysis in myocardial infarction (TIMI) trial, Phase 1: Comparison between intravenous tissue plasminogen activator and intravenous streptokinase. Circulation 76:142–154, 1987.

2. Dalen JE, et al: Six- and twelve-month follow-up of the Phase 1 thrombolysis in myocardial infarction (TIMI) trial. Am J Cardiol 62:179–185, 1988.

52. What is the most common cause of death in the first 48 hours after an acute MI? What therapy is proven to be effective in the prevention of this complication?

Ventricular fibrillation (V fib) is the most common cause of death in the first 48 hours after an MI. Other causes of death include cardiac rupture, pump failure due to massive infarction, acute mechanical complication such as ventricular septal rupture or acute mitral regurgitation, and cardiogenic shock.

ECG monitoring in coronary care units equipped to administer electrical cardioversion for ventricular tachycardia (V tach) or V fib has significantly reduced early mortality due to MI. Prophylactic administration of lidocaine has been documented to reduce the risk of primary V fib in the first 24 hours of infarction. However, mortality is essentially unchanged, since almost all episodes of primary V fib respond promptly to electrical defibrillation.

It is imperative to consider IV lidocaine prophylaxis in all patients admitted within 12 hours of the onset of symptoms. It is even more important to administer an adequate IV lidocaine loading dose of 2–3 mg/kg within the first 15–20 min to achieve a therapeutic lidocaine level as soon as possible. Patients admitted after 12 hours of infarct onset should not receive prophylactic lidocaine therapy.

Lidocaine Pharmacokinetics

Elimination half-life: 1–2 h	Reduced maintenance dose in:
Total IV loading dose: 2–3 mg/kg	1. Elderly patients
Maintenance infusion rate: 1–5 mg/min	2. Heart failure
Intramuscular (IM) dose: 4–5 mg/kg	3. Liver failure
	4. Cardiogenic shock

53. When is V fib complicating acute MI most likely to occur? Compare primary with secondary V fib.

Primary V fib occurs in the first few hours of the symptoms of an acute MI. The timing is as follows:

Timing of Primary Ventricular Fibrillation

50% of all episodes occur within 3 hours of MI onset
60% of all episodes occur within 4 hours of MI onset
70% of all episodes occur within 6 hours of MI onset
80% of all episodes occur within 12 hours of MI onset
All episodes of primary V fib occur within 48 hours

It is therefore mandatory to initiate IV lidocaine prophylaxis as soon as possible after the onset of symptoms. On the other hand, in patients admitted to the hospital after the first 12 hours of MI symptom onset, lidocaine prophylaxis is not necessary. Primary and secondary (so-called "complicating") V fib have different response rates to defibrillation and carry different prognostic implications.

Primary Versus Secondary Ventricular Fibrillation

	Primary V fib	Secondary V fib
Timing post-MI	<24 hours	>24 h
Successful response to defibrillation	90%	10–20%
Associated CHF or shock	–	+
Prognosis	Good	Poor

54. One of the most serious complications of non-Q-wave MI (previously called subendocardial MI) is recurrence of the MI. Which calcium antagonist, if any, has been shown to reduce the risk of reinfarction during hospitalization for a non-Q-wave MI?
Non-Q-wave MI is more likely than Q-wave MI to be complicated by early recurrent infarction. A recently completed randomized multicenter, prospective clinical trial—called the "Diltiazem Reinfarction Study (DRS)"—revealed a 50% reduction in recurrent infarction during hospitalization of patients with non-Q-wave MI treated with the calcium antagonist diltiazem compared to placebo. No published clinical trial has shown a reduction in reinfarction after non-Q-wave MI using any other calcium antagonist. Based on the results of the DRS study, administration of diltiazem in doses of 60–90 mg orally, every 6 hours, is recommended for patients admitted with a non-Q-wave MI.

Life-table cumulative reinfarction rates, according to treatment group. (From Gibson RS, et al: Diltiazem and reinfarction in patients with non-Q-wave myocardial infarction. Results of a double-blind, randomized trial. N Engl J Med 315:426, 1986, with permission.)

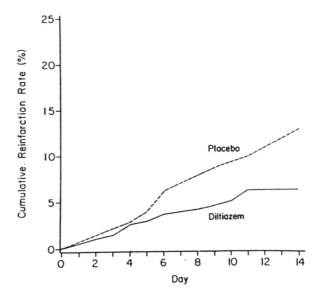

55. Cardiac rupture is almost always a fatal complication of acute MI. What are three risk factors for the development of this dreadful complication and what are its clinical features?

Myocardial Free-Wall Rupture: Risk Factors
1. Female sex
2. Hypertension
3. First MI

Features of Myocardial Free-Wall Rupture

1. LV to RV infarction ratio is 7:1
2. Seen in anterior or lateral wall MI
3. Usually with large MI (>20%)
4. Usually 3–6 days post-MI
5. Rare with left ventricular hypertrophy (LVH) or good collateral vessels

56. What is one unique complication of acute inferior wall MI that typically presents with hypotension, elevated neck veins, clear lungs, and a normal cardiac silhouette by chest x-ray? What is the appropriate management of this complication?

The clinical triad of hypotension, distended neck veins, and clear lungs in a patient with acute inferior wall MI is a classic triad of RV MI.

Confirmation of clinical suspicion of RV MI can be done by demonstrating at least 1 mm ST elevation in right-sided chest leads V3R or V4R. Clinical management of patients with RV infarction consists of volume expansion in combination with IV dopamine. It is most important in these patients to avoid giving any diuretics or preload-reducing drugs such as nitrates, as these would further worsen the low cardiac output state.

57. What is the single most important predictor of prognosis after acute MI?

The single most important predictor of 1- and 2-year survival post-MI is the left ventricular ejection fraction (LVEF), as shown in the accompanying figure. This is a more powerful predictor of survival after hospital discharge than frequency or complexity of ventricular premature beats (VPBs) detected by ambulatory monitoring.

The relative predictive power of LVEF and VPB frequency and complexity has been thoroughly evaluated. They were found to be *independent* predictors of survival post-MI. However, LVEF still remains the *single* most powerful predictor of survival post-MI.

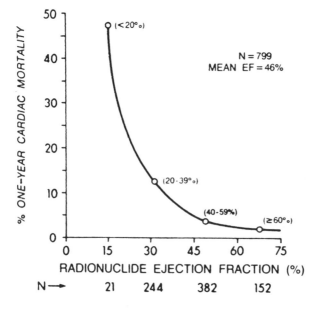

Cardiac mortality rates in four categories of radionuclide ejection fraction (EF) determined before discharge. N denotes the number of patients in the total population and in each category. Of 811 patients in whom the ejection fraction was recorded, 12 were lost to follow-up during the first year after hospitalization. (From The Multi-center Post-infarction Research Group: Risk stratification and survival after myocardial infarction. N Engl J Med 309:331, 1983, with permission.)

58. What is the differential diagnosis of a new systolic murmur and acute pulmonary edema appearing 3 days after admission to the Coronary Care Unit with acute anterior wall MI?
The differential diagnosis includes: (1) acute mitral regurgitation due to papillary muscle rupture[1] and (2) interventricular septal rupture.

Rupture of the posteromedial papillary muscle, associated with inferior wall MI, is more common than that of the anterolateral papillary muscle. Unlike rupture of the interventricular septum, which occurs with large infarcts, papillary muscle rupture occurs with a small infarction in about 50% of cases.

Differentiation between acute mitral regurgitation and ventricular septal rupture is difficult at the bedside. The location, severity, or radiation of the systolic murmur and presence or absence of a palpable systolic thrill do not reliably distinguish these two clinical diagnoses. Two-dimensional and Doppler echocardiography at the bedside can demonstrate the presence and severity of mitral regurgitation and localize the site of a ventricular septal defect (VSD). Further confirmation of the presence of a left-to-right shunt across a VSD can be obtained by a step-up in blood oxygen saturation from the right atrium to the pulmonary artery documented by blood sampling using a Swan-Ganz catheter. Both acute mitral regurgitation and septal rupture are potentially fatal complications of acute MI. They are most common 3 to 6 days post-infarction.

1. Nishimura, et al: Papillary muscle rupture complicating acute myocardial infarction: Analysis of 17 patients. Am J Cardiol 51:373, 1983.

59. What is the most likely cause of a persistent ST-segment elevation several weeks after recovery from a large transmural anterolateral wall MI?
Persistent ST-segment elevation is not an uncommon complication of large anterolateral transmural MI. It may be a manifestation of dyskinesis of the thinned-out infarcted myocardium. However, large infarcts may cause persistent ST-segment elevations in the absence of a ventricular aneurysm. The presence of persistent ST-segment elevations should suggest the presence of an LV aneurysm, and noninvasive confirmation of this diagnosis is best done by two-dimensional echocardiography or by radionuclide ventriculography.

60. Which MIs are most commonly complicated by LV aneurysms?
A ventricular aneurysm develops in 12–15% of survivors of an acute transmural MI. Aneurysms range from 1 to 8 cm in diameter. They are four times more common at the apex and anterior wall than in the inferoposterior wall, and are more common in patients with larger infarcts. The presence of an LV aneurysm is invariably associated with a markedly increased risk of death. Mortality is about six times higher than in patients with comparable global LV function. It is thought that death is often sudden, suggesting an increased risk of sustained V tach and V fib in these patients.

61. What is the mechanism of action of beta-blockers in reducing cardiovascular mortality in survivors of acute MI?
The mechanism of reduction in cardiovascular mortality with beta-blockers is a reduction in sudden cardiac deaths due to V fib. Thus, the protective effect of oral beta-blockers in post-MI patients is primarily due to their "anti-fibrillatory effects."

62. Beta-blockers are effective in the treatment of stable exertional angina pectoris. In the management of myocardial infarct (MI) survivors, would you recommend routine administration of oral beta-blockers even in those patients who are angina-free?
Several large-scale, multi-center, randomized, prospective, double-blind clinical trials conducted in the U.S. and abroad have shown a consistent reduction in total and cardiovascular mortality in survivors of acute transmural MI treated with oral beta-blockers for 1–3 years. The largest published U.S. beta-blocker post-MI trial is the Beta-Blocker Heart

Attack Trial (BHAT). This clinical trial randomized 3,837 MI survivors to either propranolol (180 or 240 mg/day) or placebo. At 3 years of follow-up, a 26% reduction in mortality was found in those patients treated with propranolol, compared to placebo-treated patients. The accompanying graph shows the life-table cumulative mortality curves for the propranolol- and placebo-treated groups.

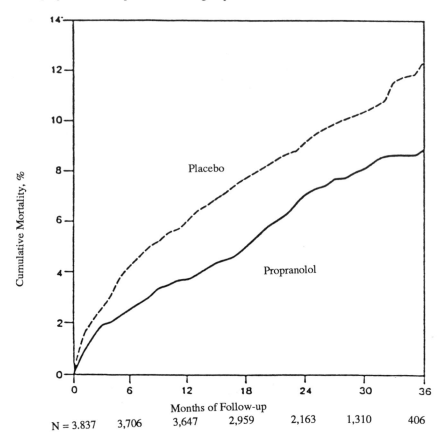

Life table cumulative mortality curves for groups receiving propranolol hydrochloride and placebo. N indicates total number of patients followed up through each time point. (From Beta-Blocker Heart Attack Trial Research Group: A randomized trial of propranolol in patients with acute myocardial infarction. I. Mortality results. JAMA 247:1707–1714, 1982, p 1709, with permission.)

Thus, regardless of the presence or absence of angina, we recommend routine administration of oral beta-blockers, propranolol (180–240 mg), timolol (10 mg bid), or metoprolol (100 mg bid), in survivors of a transmural MI, to be started 5–21 days post-MI and continued for up to 3 years.

63. A 67-year-old man has confined himself to bed for the last 3 to 4 days following what he thought were "flu-like" symptoms. A 12-lead ECG revealed new Q-waves in leads V1 to V6 and ST-segment elevation of 3 mm in leads V2 to V5, I, and aVL. His ECG from a routine clinic visit 2 weeks prior to the present incident was normal. What do you suspect in this patient? What tests would you order to confirm your suspicions? Is plasma creatinine kinase (CK) likely to be high in this patient?

This patient has ECG changes pathognomonic of the recent evolution of an extensive anterolateral MI, as evidenced by:

1. 3-mm ST-segment elevations in anterolateral leads V2 to V5, I, and aVL.
2. New Q-waves in all anterolateral chest leads.

The most likely clinical diagnosis in this patient is an acute, extensive anterolateral MI that occurred 3-4 days ago when he complained of "flu-like symptoms."

The laboratory confirmation of the clinical diagnosis of acute MI is routinely done by measuring serum CK levels at 6-hour intervals for 24-48 hours. Serum CK levels are elevated starting at 4-8 hours after symptom onset of acute MI, reach a peak at 18-24 hours, and normalize within 3-4 days. Since this patient sustained an acute MI 3-4 days ago, serum CK levels are likely to be normal.

In these late-comers, a measurement of LDH-1 isoenzyme or of the ratio of LDH-1 to LDH-2 is recommended. An LDH-1/LDH-2 ratio greater than 1.0 supports the clinical diagnosis of acute MI. Unlike serum CK, LDH is elevated at 1-2 days, reaches a peak at 3-6 days, and returns to normal 8-14 days after an acute MI. It is, therefore, the enzymatic method of choice to confirm a clinical diagnosis of acute MI that occurred 3-7 days before admission to a hospital.

64. What is Dressler's syndrome?

Dressler's syndrome, first described in 1854, is post-MI chest pain not due to coronary insufficiency. Its exact etiology is unclear, but it is characterized by inflammation of the pericardium and surrounding tissues. It occurs 2-10 weeks post-MI in 3-4% of cases and can be treated with corticosteroids and nonsteroidal anti-inflammatory agents (NSAIDs).

65. What is Bayes' theorem? How does it help us determine the value of exercise ECG testing in the detection of coronary artery disease (CAD)?

Bayes' theorem allows prediction of the presence or absence of CAD in a patient, given the prevalence of CAD in the population and the sensitivity and specificity of the diagnostic test used. In general, the ability of a noninvasive stress test (treadmill exercise ECG test, treadmill thallium myocardial scintigraphy, or bicycle exercise radionuclide ventriculography) to predict the presence or absence of CAD in patients with very low or very high pretest probability of CAD is poor. Thus, at both ends of the spectrum of pretest probability of CAD, noninvasive testing does not help the clinical decision to perform or not perform a definitive diagnostic test such as coronary arteriography for CAD. On the other hand, patients with a reasonable pretest probability of CAD are good candidates for noninvasive stress testing. An example of such a patient is a 67-year-old diabetic, hypertensive male smoker with atypical chest pain.

Probability of Coronary Artery Disease

PRETEST	AFTER TREADMILL ECG		AFTER TREADMILL THALLIUM
80%	Positive test: 95%	→	Positive test: 99%
		→	Negative test: 85%
	Negative test: 60%	→	Positive test: 90%
		→	Negative test: 30%

In the patient with typical exertional angina pectoris (associated with an 80% pretest probability of CAD), a negative treadmill ECG and thallium myocardial scintigraphy predict only a 30% probability of CAD. On the other hand, a positive treadmill thallium test in the same patient predicts a 90% probability of CAD. In such a patient, coronary angiography is recommended in the latter case (positive treadmill thallium test) but not in the former.

HYPERTENSION

66. A 45-year-old hypertensive woman has been treated with nifedipine 30 mg PO qid for chronic stable angina pectoris. She complains of ankle edema that worsened after the dose of nifedipine was recently increased. How would you manage this patient? Are diuretics indicated in this patient with ankle edema?
Edema is a common side-effect of chronic nifedipine treatment. Unlike other side-effects of nifedipine, edema is dose-dependent and commonly responds to decreasing nifedipine dose. It occurs in 10 to 30% of patients treated with nifedipine orally in daily doses of 30–120 mg. Characteristically, edema secondary to nifedipine is not associated with volume expansion and does not respond to diuretics.

67. What approach should be taken to the initial evaluation of possible secondary causes of hypertension? What is the value of such findings as postural hypotension, paroxysmal hypertension, or hypokalemia in the workup of these patients?
Initial evaluation of the hypertensive patient should be focused on historical or physical clues to one or more causes of secondary hypertension. Alcohol consumption, dietary salt intake, muscle weakness, paroxysmal episodes of palpitation, headache, sweating, nervousness, nausea or vomiting, prior known history of renal parenchymal disease, concomitant history of generalized atherosclerotic vascular disease, and documented postural hypotension should be carefully looked for, as they suggest various causes of secondary hypertension.

Paroxysmal hypertension and postural hypotension suggest pheochromocytoma. The presence of generalized atherosclerosis and abdominal or flank bruits suggest renal artery stenosis. Muscle weakness and unexplained hypokalemia should suggest aldosteronism. Prior history of renal parenchymal disease and the presence of an abnormal urine sediment suggest secondary hypertension due to parenchymal renal disease.

A careful history (including age at onset of hypertension and family history of hypertension), physical examination, and laboratory panel consisting of urinalysis, microscopy, CBC, blood electrolytes, serum creatinine, chest x-ray, and a 12-lead ECG should be obtained in all patients evaluated for hypertension.

68. Hypertensive patients are at higher risk for CAD. Does effective antihypertensive therapy decrease the risk of MI or angina pectoris?
Many large-scale prospective trials have been conducted to test the effect of antihypertensive therapy on total mortality, coronary heart disease morbidity, and mortality from renal failure and stroke. Although the incidences of heart failure, stroke, and total mortality were significantly reduced, the incidence of CAD manifestations such as angina or MI was not consistently reduced, despite effective blood pressure reduction.

Various hypotheses have been suggested to explain this apparent controversy. One of the more commonly accepted hypotheses, supported by the results of the Multiple Risk Factor Intervention Trial (MRFIT),[1] is that patients with ECG changes consistent with ischemia or LVH have an increase in CAD mortality, possibly due to the effects of diuretic-induced hypokalemia. Another hypothesis is the potentially detrimental effects of thiazide diuretics on blood lipid levels, increasing total cholesterol, and triglyceride and LDL cholesterol blood levels.

1. Multiple Risk Factor Intervention Trial Research Group: Multiple Risk Factor Intervention Trial: Risk factor changes and mortality results. JAMA 248:1465, 1982.

69. What should you recommend to a 42-year-old woman with an office blood pressure reading of 150/90? Would you initiate antihypertensive drug therapy in this patient?
Initiation of chronic antihypertensive drug therapy in a patient with a single office blood pressure measurement of 150/90 is not recommended. Unlike diastolic blood pressure, systolic blood pressure is subject to wider variations from one office visit to another and

from one examiner to another during a single office visit. Several factors may affect systolic blood pressure measurement and may thus result in the erroneous diagnosis of systemic hypertension. Among these factors are the patient's anxiety level, ambient temperature at the doctor's office, examiner (physician or nurse), time of day, physical activity preceding blood pressure measurements, size of cuff used, patient's posture (supine, sitting, or standing), and presence of coexistent medical problems such as fever, thyrotoxicosis, anemia, and AV fistula, to mention only a few.

Drug therapy for hypertension is recommended for sustained elevations of sitting blood pressure exceeding 140/90 on more than two clinic visits.

70. What class(es) of antihypertensive drugs would you prefer to use in a patient with a known history of CHF? Which drugs would you avoid?
The following classes of antihypertensive drugs are desirable in patients with CHF:

1. **Vasodilators** such as direct vascular smooth-muscle relaxing drugs (hydralazine and minoxidil), or angiotensin-converting enzyme inhibitors (captopril, enalapril, or lisinopril).

2. **Diuretics** such as thiazides.

Drugs that should be avoided in patients with hypertension and CHF are drugs with negative inotropic properties, such as:

1. **Calcium channel blockers** (verapamil or diltiazem).

2. **Beta-blockers** (propranolol, metoprolol, atenolol, etc.).

71. What is the interaction of alcohol consumption and hypertension?
Over 95% of all patients with hypertension (often called the "silent killer") in the U.S. have primary or essential hypertension. The most common causes of secondary hypertension include alcohol intake, oral contraceptive use, renal parenchymal disease, renovascular hypertension, and endocrine diseases.

The effect of alcohol consumption on blood pressure deserves special attention. Even small quantities of alcohol may raise blood pressure. A linear relationship between alcohol consumption and blood pressure has been described. A threshold effect has also been described, with a lower blood pressure observed in patients who consume 1 to 2 ounces of alcohol a day, compared to those who do not drink any alcohol. It is likely that alcohol causes hypertension by raising cardiac output and heart rate. The mechanism is probably a rapid rise in plasma epinephrine and cortisol levels.

Klatsky AL, et al: The relationship between alcoholic beverage use and other traits to blood pressure: A new Kaiser-Permanente study. Circulation 73:628, 1986.

CONGESTIVE HEART FAILURE

72. What are some of the common signs and symptoms of congestive heart failure (CHF)?
The signs and symptoms of CHF are listed in order of decreasing specificity:

Right Heart Failure	*Left Heart Failure*
Jugular vein distension	Chest x-ray with redistribution of perfusion
Hepatomegaly	or interstitial edema
Increased prothrombin time	Third heart sound (S_3)
Peripheral edema	Cardiomegaly
Increased SGOT, bilirubin	Pulmonary rales
Pleural effusion	Paroxysmal nocturnal dyspnea, orthopnea
Decreased albumin	Dyspnea on exertion
Abdominal discomfort	
Anorexia	
Proteinuria	

73. What is the differential diagnosis of CHF?

Isolated Right Heart Failure	Left or Biventricular Failure
Pulmonary embolus	Aortic stenosis
Tricuspid stenosis	Aortic insufficiency
Tricuspid regurgitation	Mitral stenosis
Right atrial tumor	Mitral regurgitation
Cardiac tamponade	Most cardiomyopathies
Constrictive pericarditis	Restrictive cardiomyopathy
Pulmonic insufficiency	Acute myocardial infarction (MI)
Right ventricular (RV) infarction	Myxoma
Intrinsic lung disease	Hypertensive heart disease
Ebstein's anomaly	Myocarditis
High cardiac output states (anemia,	Supraventricular arrhythmias
systemic fistulae, beriberi,	Left ventricular (LV) aneurysm
Paget's disease, carcinoid,	Cardiac shunts
thyrotoxicosis, etc.)	High cardiac output states

74. What factors can precipitate an exacerbation of formerly well-controlled chronic CHF?

Patients with well-controlled chronic CHF can experience sudden exacerbations. If this occurs, in addition to consideration of worsening of the underlying condition(s) that led to CHF in this patient, a precipitating factor must be searched for and corrected. These factors include:

Increased consumption of salt	Paget's disease
Fluid overload	Poor compliance with medications
Pulmonary emboli	Arrhythmias
Fever, infection	Elevated blood pressure
Anemia	High environmental temperature
Renal failure	Cardiac ischemia or MI
Pregnancy	Thyrotoxicosis

75. A 78-year-old man with a longstanding history of CHF presents with weakness, anorexia, nausea, and dizziness. The medical record reveals that he has been receiving digoxin 0.5 mg PO daily and furosemide 120 mg PO twice a day. What specific tests would you request in your evaluation?

Any patient receiving digitalis who presents with gastrointestinal complaints such as anorexia, nausea, or vomiting should be suspected of suffering from digitalis toxicity. Anorexia is often an early manifestation of digitalis intoxication. Interestingly, nausea and vomiting due to digitalis intoxication are thought to be mediated by stimulation of the area postrema in the medulla oblongata of the brainstem, rather than by any direct effects of digitalis on the gastrointestinal (GI) mucosa. These GI manifestations of digitalis intoxication are also observed in patients receiving excessive parenteral doses of digitalis. Not uncommonly, patients with chronic CHF complain of similar GI symptoms due to passive hepatic congestion or ascites. Differentiation of various causes of nausea and vomiting in such patients, on clinical grounds alone, can be very difficult.

Other manifestations of digitalis toxicity include:
1. **Neurologic symptoms:** headache, neuralgia, confusion, delirium and seizures.
2. **Visual symptoms:** scotomata, halos, altered color perception.
3. **Cardiac toxicity:**
   a. Ventricular or junctional tachyarrhythmias
   b. AV block
4. **Other manifestations:** gynecomastia, skin rash

By far the most life-threatening complications of digitalis intoxication are cardiac. Almost any arrhythmia can be a manifestation of digitalis intoxication. Cardiac arrhythmias commonly due to digitalis intoxication include paroxysmal atrial tachycardia (PAT) with AV block (Fig. A below), junctional tachycardia with or without AV block, and first-degree or Mobitz I second-degree AV block. The coexistence of increased automaticity of ectopic pacemakers with impaired AV conduction is very suggestive of digitalis intoxication (Fig. B on next page).

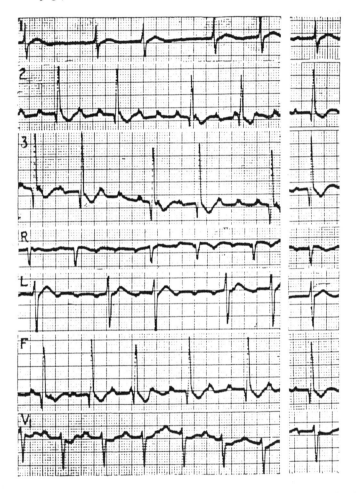

A. Paroxysmal atrial tachycardia with varying A-V block as a result of **digitalis intoxication.** Note that the P waves are almost normally directed (axis +90°), that the A-V conduction ratio varies and that the atrial rhythm is not precisely regular. The single column of complexes on the right is to show for comparison the form and direction of P waves (axis +60°) when sinus rhythm was restored. (From Marriott HJL: Practical Electrocardiography, 8th ed. Baltimore, Williams & Wilkins, 1988, p 488, with permission.)

The single most useful laboratory test to confirm the clinical suspicion of digitalis intoxication is a serum digoxin level. Even serum digoxin levels in the "therapeutic range" may be toxic in elderly patients or in patients with hypokalemia, hypercalcemia, acid-base disorders, or thyroid disorders.

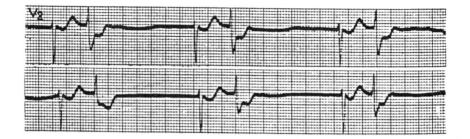

B. Digitalis intoxication. Note (1) atrial fibrillation with regular independent idionodal rhythm, (2) ventricular bigeminy with multiform ectopic QRS complexes and (3) S-T sagging in a lead with negative QRS complexes. (From Marriott HJL: Practical Electrocardiography, 8th ed. Baltimore, Williams & Wilkins, 1988, p 490, with permission.)

76. A large variety of cardiac drugs are presently available for use in the treatment of patients with CHF. Among these drugs are various classes of vasodilators (nitrates, hydralazine, prazosin or angiotensin-converting enzyme [ACE] inhibitors), digitalis, and diuretics. Which one or more of these drugs have been proven to decrease mortality?

Unlike digitalis or diuretics, some classes of vasodilators have been shown to reduce mortality in patients with CHF. Enalapril, an ACE inhibitor, was shown in a prospective randomized clinical study to reduce mortality in patients with severe CHF (NYHA Class IV). A combination of isosorbide dinitrate, a predominant venous vasodilator, and hydralazine, an arteriolar vasodilator, was shown in a VA randomized prospective clinical trial to reduce mortality of patients with moderately severe CHF (NYHA Class III and IV). Interestingly, not all vasodilators have been shown to decrease mortality in patients with CHF. In the VA trial, prazosin, a post-synaptic alpha-1 receptor blocker, did not alter mortality when compared to placebo. Therefore, although vasodilators, digitalis, and diuretics can improve symptoms and signs of CHF in most patients treated, only certain classes of vasodilators have been shown to reduce mortality in these patients.

The Consensus Trial Study Group: Effects of enalapril on mortality in severe congestive heart failure: Results of the Cooperative North Scandinavian Enalapril Survival Study (CONSENSUS). N Engl J Med 316:1429–1435, 1987.

Cohn JN, et al: Effect of vasodilator therapy on mortality in chronic congestive heart failure: Results of a Veterans Administration Cooperative Study. N Engl J Med 314:1547–1552, 1986.

INFECTION

77. What are generally accepted criteria for surgical intervention in infectious endocarditis?
1. Heart failure refractory to adequate medical therapy.
2. More than one major systemic embolic episode.
3. Persistent bacteremia despite appropriate antibiotics.
4. Severe valvular dysfunction by echocardiography.
5. Ineffective antimicrobial therapy (e.g., fungal endocarditis).
6. Resection of mycotic aneurysm.
7. Many cases of prosthetic valve endocarditis, especially with dehiscence or obstruction.
8. Development of persistent heart block or BBB, usually seen in the setting of aortic valve involvement and unrelated to drug therapy or ischemic heart disease.
9. Extravalvular myocardial invasion, such as myocardial abscess or pericarditis.

Dinubile MJ: Surgery in infective endocarditis. Ann Intern Med 96:650–659, 1982.

78. What are the infectious causes of culture-negative endocarditis?
There are many potential reasons why blood cultures may be negative in spite of the presence of infective endocarditis. They include prior administration of antibiotics, presence of uremia, and fastidious organisms. Nutritionally deficient streptococci, *Brucella* sp., intracellular organisms (rickettsia and chlamydia), fungi, anaerobes, and the HACEK group of organisms must also be considered when cultures are negative. The HACEK group includes *Hemophilus* sp., *Actinobacillus actinomycetemcomitans, Cardiobacterium hominis, Eikenella corrodens,* and *Kingella kingae.*

79. What does the new onset of conduction system abnormalities in the setting of endocarditis imply?
When conduction system abnormalities occur in the setting of infective endocarditis, one should suspect the presence of perivalvular and/or myocardial abscesses. Surgical drainage and valve replacement are usually necessary.

80. Some clinical manifestations of subacute bacterial endocarditis (SBE) are thought to be due to immune complex deposition within extracardiac organs rather than to direct bacterial invasion. What are these so-called immunologic manifestations of SBE?
Immunologic manifestations of infective endocarditis are thought to be mediated by the deposition of immune complexes within extracardiac structures, such as the retina, joints, fingertips, pericardium, skin, and kidney. Interestingly, these immunologic manifestations of endocarditis are reported almost exclusively in patients with a prolonged course of SBE. They include:

Immunologic Manifestations of Infective Endocarditis

1. **Roth spots:** cytoid bodies in the retina
2. **Osler nodes:** tender nodular lesions in the terminal phalanges
3. **Janeway lesions:** painless macular lesions on palms and soles
4. **Petechiae and purpuric lesions**
5. **Proliferative glomerulonephritis**

CONGENITAL HEART DISEASE

81. What are the most common congenital cardiac lesions to present in adulthood?
In adulthood, congenital cyanotic cardiac lesions are distinctly uncommon. By far the most common congenital cardiac lesions to present in adulthood are bicuspid aortic valve and atrial septal defect (ASD). ASDs alone account for about 30% of all congenital heart disease in adults. ASDs occur in the following types and frequencies:

Types and Frequencies of ASDs

1. Ostium secundum ASD	70%
2. Ostium primum ASD	15%
3. Sinus venosus ASD	15%

82. "Coeur-en-sabot" was coined by a French scientist in his first report of a congenital cardiac disease in 1888. Which congenital heart disease is it and what does the term coeur-en-sabot refer to in patients afflicted with this disease?
The term "coeur-en-sabot" (wooden shoe heart) was coined by E.L. Fallot, who first reported this cyanotic congenital heart disease. It describes the typical configuration of the cardiac silhouette on chest x-ray in patients suffering from tetralogy of Fallot. The four components of this malformation are:

1. Ventricular septal defect
2. Obstruction to RV outflow
3. Overriding of the aorta
4. RV hypertrophy.

The most distinctive radiographic finding in tetralogy of Fallot is RV hypertrophy. This results in a fairly classic boot (or "wooden shoe")- shaped configuration of the cardiac silhouette with prominence of the RV and a concavity in the region of the underdeveloped RV outflow tract and main pulmonary artery. This distinctive appearance of the cardiac silhouette is shown in the figure herewith.

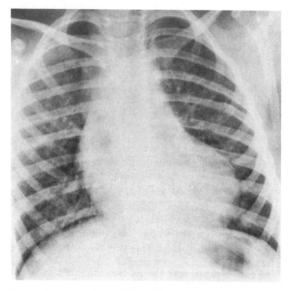

Bronchial collateral circulation in tetralogy of Fallot. The heart is slightly widened, the apex is rounded and elevated, the prominence of the normal main pulmonary artery is absent, and there is a right aortic arch. These findings are typical of tetralogy of Fallot. Although the pulmonary vasculature does not appear decreased, its pattern is definitely abnormal. The vessels do not radiate from the hilum, do not branch in an orderly fashion, and do not taper as they progress outward into the lungs. This pattern is characteristic of bronchial collateral vessels. (From Braunwald E (ed): Heart Disease: A Textbook of Cardiovascular Medicine, 3rd ed. Philadelphia, W.B. Saunders, 1988, p 162, with permission.)

83. What cardiac disease most commonly presents in adulthood with right bundle branch block (RBBB), first-degree AV block, and left axis deviation on ECG? Discuss the mechanism of these ECG findings.

The presence of complete or incomplete RBBB is an ECG hallmark of RV volume overload, often accompanied by rightward deviation of the QRS axis, except in patients with ostium primum atrial septal defect (ASD). Because of hypoplastic changes in the left anterior fascicle, patients with ostium primum ASD have left axis QRS deviation. Thus, the combination of RBBB and left axis QRS deviation is a fairly distinctive feature of ostium primum ASD, and is often accompanied by first-degree AV block.

CARDIAC SYNDROMES AND OTHER ENTITIES

84. What are the cardiac manifestations of ankylosing spondylitis? What is the most common associated valvular dysfunction encountered in this syndrome?

The incidence of cardiovascular involvement in ankylosing spondylitis ranges from 3 to 10%, depending on the duration of the disease. The characteristic cardiac involvement in ankylosing spondylitis consists of dilatation of the aortic valve ring and of the sinuses of Valsalva, as well as inflammatory changes in the aortic valve ring. The resultant clinical hallmark of cardiac involvement in patients with ankylosing spondylitis is aortic root dilatation and aortic regurgitation, often rapidly progressive and ultimately requiring aortic valve replacement. Echocardiography is the diagnostic technique of choice in the evaluation and follow-up of patients with ankylosing spondylitis and associated cardiac involvement.

Graham DC, et al: The carditis and aortitis of ankylosing spondylitis. Bull Rheum Dis 9:171, 1958.

85. What is the ECG triad of Wolff-Parkinson-White (WPW) syndrome?

Wolff-Parkinson-White Syndrome: ECG Triad

1. Short PR interval (<0.12 s)
2. Wide QRS complex (>0.12 s)
3. Delta wave or slurred upstroke of QRS complex

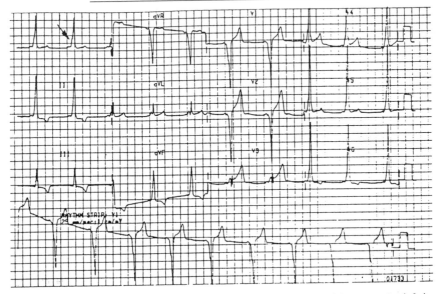

Right anteroseptal accessory pathway. The 12-lead ECG characteristically exhibits a normal to inferior axis. The delta wave is negative in V_1 and V_2, upright in lead I, II, AVL, and AVF, isoelectric in lead III, and negative in AVR. Location verified at surgery. Arrow indicates delta wave (lead I). (From Braunwald E (ed): Heart Disease: A Textbook of Cardiovascular Medicine, 3rd ed. Philadelphia, W.B. Saunders, 1988, p 686, with permission.)

86. What is the most common cause of death in Wolff-Parkinson-White (WPW) syndrome? Discuss the mechanism underlying sudden cardiac death in these patients.

Patients with a pre-excitation syndrome such as WPW are at risk for development of A fib with antegrade conduction along the accessory pathway. This tachycardia presents a potentially serious risk because it has a propensity to degenerate into V fib due to very rapid conduction over the accessory pathway.

Patients with accessory pathways and short refractory periods (less than 200 msec) are most prone to develop antegrade conduction of A fib along the accessory pathway and are therefore at risk for sudden cardiac death due to V fib.

Intermittent pre-excitation during sinus rhythm (best recognized by ambulatory ECG monitoring) and loss of conduction along the accessory pathway during exercise or during administration of ajmaline or procainamide suggest that the refractory period of the accessory pathway is long (over 250 msec). These patients are not at risk of developing very rapid ventricular rates when A fib or atrial flutter occur and are therefore not at risk of sudden cardiac death.

87. What are the cardiac manifestations of Marfan's syndrome? To what does the term "Marfan's syndrome–forme fruste" refer?

Marfan's syndrome is a generalized disorder of connective tissue that is inherited as an autosomal dominant trait. Cardiac abnormalities occur in over 60% of these patients and are almost always responsible for early death when it occurs. The most common cardiac lesion is dilatation of the aortic ring, sinuses of Valsalva, and ascending aorta. This leads to progressive aortic regurgitation and may be complicated by acute aortic dissection. The risk of dissection is markedly increased during pregnancy. Another common valvular dysfunction in Marfan's syndrome is mitral regurgitation due to a redundant myxomatous mitral valve (called "floppy" prolapsed mitral valve).

In contrast to adults, children with Marfan's syndrome are much more likely to have severe isolated mitral regurgitation than aortic root or aortic valve disease.

Mitral valve prolapse (MVP) in the absence of other systemic manifestations of Marfan's syndrome has been referred to as "Marfan's syndrome–forme fruste" in view of the similarity in the pathologic appearance of the myxomatous mitral valve in both disorders. Isolated MVP is more common than Marfan's syndrome.

88. Which age group, sex, and portion of the vascular system are most typically involved in patients with Takayasu's arteritis? How does it differ from that of atherosclerosis and giant cell arteritis?

Takayasu's arteritis is divided into three types involving different parts of the aorta, as shown in the figure. It typically affects young women. The female:male ratio is 8 to 1. In about three-fourths of all cases, onset is in the teenage years. This is in sharp contrast to atherosclerotic aortic disease, which usually affects older men, and giant cell arteritis, which usually affects women over the age of 50 years.

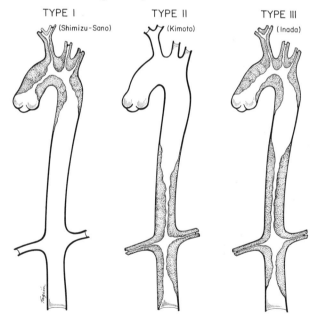

TYPE I	TYPE II	TYPE III
(Shimizu–Sano)	(Kimoto)	(Inada)

Types of Takayasu's arteritis. Type I involves primarily the aortic arch and brachiocephalic vessels. Type II affects the thoracoabdominal aorta and particularly the renal arteries. Type III combines features of both Types I and II. Types I and III may be complicated by aortic regurgitation. The eponyms for each type are noted. (From Braunwald E (ed): Heart Disease: A Textbook of Cardiovascular Medicine, 3rd ed. Philadelphia, W.B. Saunders, 1988, p 1563, with permission.)

	Takayasu's Arteritis	Atherosclerosis	Giant Cell Arteritis
Synonyms	Pulseless disease, reversed coarctation	—	Granulomatous arteritis
Age at onset	15–25 years	>50 years	>50 years
F:M ratio	8:1	1:4	2–3:1
Systemic prodrome	Fever, weight loss	None	Headache, fever
Site of involvement	Aortic arch, thoracoabdominal	Large arteries	Temporal arteries
Complications	Pulseless arms, aortic aneurysms, hypertension	Stroke, MI, claudication (legs)	Blindness, jaw or arm claudication, polymyalgia

89. What is the classic clinical prodrome that antedates the development of vascular disease in Takayasu's arteritis?

Prodromal Manifestations of Takayasu's Arteritis

1. Fever and night sweats	4. Arthralgias
2. Anorexia and weight loss	5. Pleuritic pain
3. Malaise and fatigue	

90. What is the holiday heart syndrome?

The holiday heart syndrome is characterized by the presence of supraventricular arrhythmias in alcoholic patients following an acute alcoholic binge. These arrhythmias are often transient and do not require long-term antiarrhythmic drug therapy. The most common arrhythmias in the holiday heart syndrome are A fib and A flutter. Digitalis and beta-blockers produce an effective and rapid therapeutic response. Supportive care is also essential to prevent alcohol withdrawal symptoms in these patients.

91. What is the most common location of an atrial myxoma? List the various cardiac chambers involved in a descending order of frequency.

Frequency of Location of Myxomas

1. Left atrium	86%
2. Right atrium	10%
3. Left ventricle	2%
4. Right ventricle	2%
5. Multiple locations	10%

The most common site of origin of atrial myxomas is the fossa ovalis. To prevent recurrence of myxoma, a wide resection of the fossa ovalis area of the interatrial septum is performed during surgical excision of atrial myxomas.

92. The incidence of acute rheumatic fever has dramatically decreased in the past two decades. What is presently the most common cause of chronic mitral regurgitation in the U.S.?

The most common cause of chronic mitral regurgitation in the U.S. today is mitral valve prolapse. This has replaced rheumatic heart disease, which was the most common cause of chronic mitral regurgitation in the 1950s and 1960s.

93. What are the physical examination findings in mitral regurgitation?
Mitral regurgitation is associated with an apical holosystolic murmur. The intensity and radiation of the murmur will vary with the cause and severity. Physical examination may also reveal a third heart sound (S_3), peripheral pulses with a quick upstroke and short duration, a widened pulse pressure, and a hyperdynamic precordium.

94. What is the treatment for mitral regurgitation?
Medical management of mitral regurgitation includes afterload reduction (to maximize "forward" cardiac output), salt restriction and diuretics (in the face of congestive heart failure), and digitalis (in the face of atrial fibrillation). Surgical management (mitral valve replacement) should be performed in patients refractory to medical management before they enter the severely symptomatic stage.

PACING

95. In an attempt to improve communication between different physicians, a three-letter code was created to describe the essential functions of a cardiac pacemaker. What is this code?

The Three-letter Pacemaker Code

---

1. **First position in the code:** refers to the chamber that is paced
2. **Second position in the code:** refers to the chamber that is sensed
3. **Third position in the code:** refers to the mode of response

The chamber that is paced or sensed may be:

    a. **The right ventricle** (referred to by the letter **V**)

    b. **The right atrium** (referred to by the letter **A**)

    c. **Both right ventricle and atrium** (referred to by the letter **D**)

Pacemakers that have sensing capabilities are usually demand pacemakers (they pace only when needed). In other words, they are not fixed-rate pacemakers.

The pacemaker mode of response is used only for demand pacemakers. It could be any of the following:

Pacemaker Mode of Response

    a. **Inhibited** (referred to by the letter **I**)
        Pacemakers with an inhibited mode of response (**I**) do not pace when a spontaneous depolarization (atrial or ventricular) is sensed by the pacemaker. Following a fixed interval, if no spontaneous depolarization is sensed, pacing occurs. The inhibited mode of response is most commonly used.

    b. **Triggered** (referred to by the letter **T**)
        Pacemakers with a triggered mode of response (**T**) pace shortly after a spontaneous depolarization is sensed. After a fixed interval, pacing will occur if no spontaneous depolarization is sensed.

    c. **Both** (referred to by the letter **D**)

The two most commonly used pacemakers today are:
    1. VVI, a pacemaker that can pace and sense the right ventricle (VV), and has an inhibited mode of response (I).
    2. DDD, so-called dual chamber AV sequential pacemaker, that can pace and sense either right ventricle or right atrium (DD) and that has both inhibited and triggered modes of response (D).

96. What are the reasons underlying the selection of "dual-chamber pacemakers" in certain cardiac patients?

Dual-chamber pacemakers (DDD) are more expensive, more difficult to implant, and require greater expertise from the clinician in charge of the patient's follow-up as compared to ventricular demand pacemakers (VVI). Insertion of a dual-chamber pacemaker is therefore reserved for patients who are not good candidates for ventricular demand pacemakers. These include older patients, patients with cardiac failure or left ventricular hypertrophy (LVH), and physically active young adults who would not tolerate fixed-rate ventricular pacing. On the other hand, patients who have a history of recurrent supraventricular tachycardia (SVT) are not good candidates for any pacing modality that involves atrial sensing, such as dual-chamber pacemakers. The latter would be better served by a simpler ventricular demand pacemaker (VVI).

97. One of the common complications of pacemakers that pace the ventricle only (so-called VVI or ventricular demand pacemakers) is pacemaker syndrome. What are the manifestations, pathophysiology, and management of this syndrome?

Artificial pacing of patients suffering from symptomatic bradyarrhythmias can be accomplished using ventricular demand pacemakers (VVI) or dual-chamber pacemakers (DDD). While most patients experience symptomatic improvement during ventricular demand pacing, some may report complaints of dizziness, palpitations, pounding sensation in the chest or neck, and/or dyspnea associated with ventricular pacing. This complication of ventricular pacing is called **pacemaker syndrome.** The underlying mechanism is thought to be related to loss of the normal AV synchrony during ventricular pacing. An improvement in cardiac output has been documented in various studies when the pacing modality was changed from ventricular to dual-chamber or AV sequential pacing.

It is likely that patients with left ventricular hypertrophy (LVH) or LV failure, or older patients who have a large atrial contribution to LV filling, would be most prone to develop pacemaker syndrome and may therefore be better candidates for AV sequential pacing using a DDD pacemaker.

Miller M, et al: Pacemaker syndrome: A non-invasive means to its diagnosis and treatment. PACE 4:503, 1981.

AORTA

98. What are the causes of acute, severe aortic regurgitation (AR)?

Causes of Acute Severe Aortic Regurgitation

Infective endocarditis
Dissecting aneurysm
Rupture or prolapse of aortic leaflet(s)
Traumatic rupture
Spontaneous rupture of myxomatous valve
Spontaneous rupture of leaflet fenestrations
Sudden sagging of a "normal" leaflet
Postoperative—faulty incision of a stenotic aortic valve

(From Morganroth J, et al: Acute severe aortic regurgitation. Ann Intern Med 87:225, 1977, with permission.)

99. Why is a wide pulse pressure, typically present in chronic severe aortic regurgitation (AR), unlikely to be observed in patients with acute aortic regurgitation?

The absence of a wide pulse pressure, as well as the concurrent absence of the characteristic arterial auscultatory signs of chronic AR, in patients presenting with acute AR is thought to be due to the much higher left ventricular end-diastolic pressure (LVEDP) in the acute form.

The acute development of a severe aortic valvular leak causes a much higher LVEDP in the normal-sized LV of patients with acute AR. Patients with chronic AR commonly have a dilated LV with increased compliance capable of accommodating large blood volumes without a significant rise of LVEDP.

Salient Hemodynamic Features of Severe Aortic Regurgitation

	Acute*	Chronic*
LV compliance	Not ↑	↑
Regurgitant volume	↑	↑
LV end-diastolic pressure	Markedly ↑	May be normal
LV ejection velocity	Not signif. ↑	Markedly ↑
Aortic systolic pressure	Not ↑	↑
Aortic diastolic pressure	→ to ↑	Markedly ↓
Systemic arterial pulse pressure	Slightly to moderately ↑	Markedly ↑
Ejection fraction	Not ↑	↑
Effective stroke volume	↓	→
Effective cardiac output	↓	→
Heart rate	↑	→
Peripheral vascular resistance	↑	Not ↑

* → = unchanged, ↑ = increased, ↓ = decreased.
(From Morganroth J, et al: Acute severe aortic regurgitation. Ann Intern Med 87:225, 1977, with permission.)

As a result of the rapid elevation of LVEDP in acute AR and its rapid equilibration with aortic pressure, the diastolic rumble of acute AR is much shorter and softer than that of chronic AR. Another auscultatory manifestation of the rapid rise of LVEDP is premature mitral valve closure. This is considered a reliable echocardiographic sign of acute AR.

100. What are the signs of chronic aortic regurgitation (AR) and what are their mechanisms?
Chronic AR is characterized by a dilated LV due to longstanding volume overload, with a large stroke volume and a wide pulse pressure. The peripheral arterial auscultatory signs of chronic regurgitation are primarily due to this wide pulse pressure of chronic AR.

Peripheral Arterial Signs of Chronic Aortic Regurgitation

1. **de Musset's sign:** bobbing of the head with each heartbeat
2. **Corrigan's pulse:** abrupt distension and quick collapse of femoral pulses (also called water-hammer pulse)
3. **Traube's sign:** booming systolic and diastolic sounds heard over the femoral pulse
4. **Muller's sign:** systolic pulsations of the uvula
5. **Duroziez's sign:** systolic murmur over femoral artery when compressed proximally and diastolic murmur when compressed distally
6. **Quincke's sign:** capillary pulsations of fingertips
7. **Hill's sign:** popliteal cuff systolic pressure exceeding brachial cuff pressure by more than 60 mmHg

101. What is the DeBakey classification of aortic dissections and what is its clinical and therapeutic significance?

The DeBakey classification of aortic dissections divides them into three groups based on location as shown in the figure. The most important clinical implication of this classification is the difference in therapeutic approach between different types. In general, DeBakey aortic dissections types I and II are best managed surgically, whereas DeBakey aortic dissections type III are best managed medically. These differences are based largely on the disparate natural history of proximal (DeBakey types I & II) and distal dissections (DeBakey type III). Even minimal progression of a proximal dissection can cause potentially fatal complications, such as cardiac tamponade, acute aortic regurgitation, or neurologic compromise. On the other hand, patients with distal aortic dissections often have advanced cardiovascular and cardiopulmonary disease and are therefore poor surgical candidates.

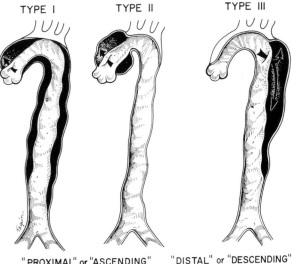

The DeBakey classification of aortic dissections. (From Braunwald E (ed): Heart Disease: A Textbook of Cardiovascular Medicine, 3rd ed. Philadelphia, W.B. Saunders, 1988, p 1554, with permission.)

102. What is the most common site of aortic coarctation? List various sites of aortic involvement and associated malformations in descending order of prevalence.

The most common sites of aortic coarctation are listed below in a descending order of frequency:

Sites of Aortic Coarctation

1. Postductal (adult-type coarctation)
2. Localized juxtaductal coarctation
3. Preductal (infantile-type coarctation)
4. Ascending thoracic aorta
5. Distal descending thoracic aorta
6. Abdominal aorta

The most frequent site of aortic coarctation in the adult, namely postductal coarctation, is illustrated in the accompanying figure.

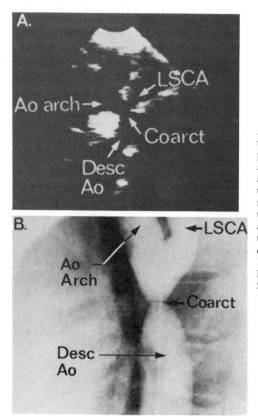

A, Two-dimensional echocardiogram obtained using the infraclavicular transducer position in a patient with coarctation of the aorta. A discrete area of narrowing in the aorta can be seen just distal to the takeoff of the left subclavian artery (LSCA). *B*, Aortography confirmed a discrete coarctation of the aorta. Areas of pre- and poststenotic dilatation are present. Coarct = coarctation of the aorta; Ao arch = aortic arch; Desc Ao = descending aorta. (From Braunwald E (ed): Heart Disease: A Textbook of Cardiovascular Medicine, 3rd ed. Philadelphia, W.B. Saunders, 1988, p 996, with permission.)

103. Which congenital cardiac lesions are associated with coarctation of the aorta?
Aortic coarctation is frequently not an isolated cardiac lesion. It is often associated with other congenital cardiac lesions.

Aortic Coarctation: Associated Malformations

1. Bicuspid aortic valve
2. Patent ductus arteriosus
3. Ventricular septal defect
4. Berry aneurysms of circle of Willis

DRUG THERAPY

104. Which antiarrhythmic agent is likely to initially worsen the arrhythmia it is used to treat? Why?
Bretylium, used parenterally for the treatment of serious ventricular tachyarrhythmias, causes an initial release of norepinephrine from adrenergic nerves followed by inhibition of norepinephrine release. It is this initial effect that can cause a transient increase in ventricular irritability and hypertension. This is commonly observed in digitalized patients.

105. What are the mechanisms of action and usual doses of vasodilating drugs?

Mechanisms of Action and Dosages of Vasodilators

AGENT	MECHANISM OF ACTION	VENOUS DILATING EFFECT	ANTERIOLAR DILATING EFFECT	USUAL DOSAGE
Nitroglycerin	Direct*	+++	+	25–500 μg/min IV
Isosorbide dinitrate	Direct*	+++	+	5–20 mg q 2 hr SL 10–60 mg q 4 hr PO
Hydralazine	Direct	–	+++	10–100 mg q 6 hr PO
Minoxidil	Direct	–	+++	10–40 mg/day PO
Sodium nitroprusside	Direct	+++	+++	5–150 μg/min IV
Epoprostenol (prostacyclin)	Direct	+++	+++	5–15 ng/kg/min IV
Phenoxybenzamine	Alpha-adrenergic blockade	++	++	10–20 mg q 8 hr PO
Phentolamine	Alpha-adrenergic blockade	++	++	50 mg q 4–6 hr PO
Prazosin	Alpha-adrenergic blockade	+++	++	1–10 mg q 8 hr PO
Trimazosin†	Alpha-adrenergic blockade and some other undetermined mechanism	+++	++	50–450 mg bid, PO
Captopril	Inhibition of angiotensin converting enzyme	+++	++	6.25–50.0 mg q 6–8 hr PO
Enalapril	Inhibition of angiotensin converting enzyme	+++	+++	5–20 mg bid, PO
Lisinopril	Inhibition of angiotensin converting enzyme	+++	++	10–40 mg/day PO
Nifedipine	Calcium channel blockade	+	++	10–40 mg q 6 hr PO 10–40 mg q 6 hr SL

* Nitrates may act by releasing the vasodilator prostacyclin.
† For investigational use only.
(From Rubenstein E, Federman D (eds): Scientific American Medicine. New York, Scientific American, Inc., 1988, Ch. 1 (Cardiovascular Medicine), Part II, Table 4, with permission.)

106. What is the mechanism of action of digitalis?

Digitalis and all the cardiac glycosides act by inhibiting Na^+-K^+ ATPase activity (the "sodium pump"). This blocks the transport of sodium and potassium across cell membranes, leading to an intracellular increase in sodium and decrease in potassium. The increase in intracellular sodium leads to an exchange for calcium. The increased intracellular calcium, the contractile element of muscle, leads to increased contractility (positive inotropic effect).

The antiarrhythmic effects of the cardiac glycosides are probably not due to any direct effect of the drug. Rather, they are mediated by an increase in vagal tone in the atria and AV junction.

107. What factors contribute to digitalis toxicity?

Contributing Factors in Digitalis Toxicity

Hypokalemia	Renal insufficiency (digoxin)	Drugs:
Hypercalcemia	Hepatic insufficiency	Quinidine Amiodarone
Hypomagnesemia	(digitoxin)	Verapamil (Others)

108. What are the elimination half-lives of digoxin and lidocaine? How do you use this information to guide you in the initiation of digoxin or lidocaine therapy?
Lidocaine is metabolized in the liver. Its elimination is prolonged in old age and during liver failure, heart failure, and cardiogenic shock. Because the elimination half-life of lidocaine is 1–2 hours in healthy individuals, initiation of IV infusion of lidocaine without a preceding bolus will not result in a steady-state serum lidocaine level until about 6 hours later. Thus, it is imperative to give an IV loading dose of 3 mg/kg over the first 15–20 min to bring the lidocaine blood level to a therapeutic range as soon as possible.

Digoxin elimination half-life is about 36 hours. In the absence of loading, a steady-state level would be reached in 5–6 days. It is therefore mandatory to give a loading dose of 0.75 mg within 6–24 hours to provide a steady-state serum digoxin level more rapidly. The duration of initial digitalization depends on the urgency of digitalis therapy. In patients with acute pulmonary edema, digitalization with a full IV loading dose of 0.75 mg should be completed within the first 4–6 hours, whereas in patients with chronic CHF, full oral digitalization can be performed over a period of 24–48 hours. Digoxin is primarily eliminated by the kidneys. The oral maintenance dose should be reduced in the presence of renal failure to avoid digitalis toxicity.

109. Patients maintained on digitalis commonly exhibit some changes on ECG referred to as "digitalis effect." What are these changes and how do they compare with those in patients with myocardial ischemia?
Digitalis is to the ECG what syphilis once was to medicine, a "great imitator." Digitalis can cause a variety of ECG abnormalities depending on the serum digoxin level. Administered in therapeutic doses, it causes a characteristic sagging of the ST segment and flattening and inversion of the T-waves. These changes typically occur in the inferolateral ECG leads and are commonly referred to as **digitalis effect.** These effects of digitalis on the ST and T-waves are difficult to distinguish from those of subendocardial myocardial ischemia. However, some subtle differences exist. Typically, horizontal or down-sloping ST-segment depression, sharp-angled ST-T junctions, and U-wave inversion are present in patients with subendocardial ischemia (coronary insufficiency, as in figures **A** and **B**). Less commonly, tall T-waves may be another subtle ECG sign of myocardial ischemia, as in figure **C**. The three figures show the ECG changes of coronary insufficiency. These should be compared with those of digitalis effect, shown in figure **D**.

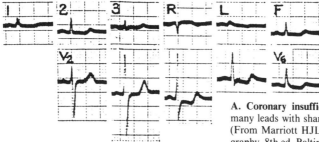

A. Coronary insufficiency. ST depression in many leads with sharp-angled ST-T junctions. (From Marriott HJL: Practical Electrocardiography, 8th ed. Baltimore, Williams & Wilkins, 1988, pp 451–452, with permission.)

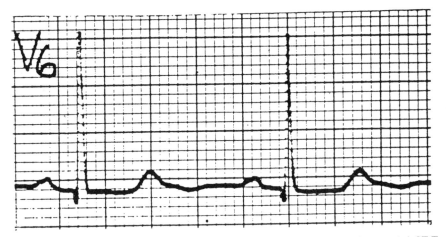

B. Coronary insufficiency—three subtle signs: horizontality of ST segments, sharp-angled ST-T junctions, U-wave inversion. (From Marriott HJL: Practical Electrocardiography, 8th ed. Baltimore, Williams & Wilkins, 1988, pp 451–452, with permission.)

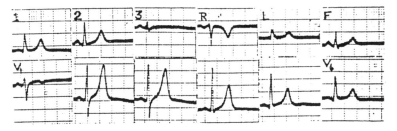

C. Coronary insufficiency. Abnormally tall precordial T waves are the only electrocardiographic sign of myocardial ischemia in this patient with typical angina (From Marriott HJL: Practical Electrocardiography, 8th ed. Baltimore, Williams & Wilkins, 1988, pp 451–452, with permission.)

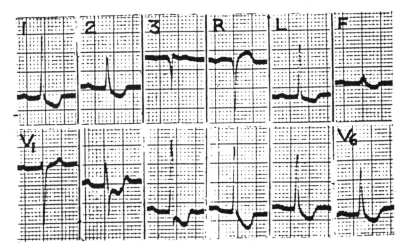

D. Digitalis effect. Note sagging ST segments in most leads with short Q-T interval. (From Marriott HJL: Practical Electrocardiography. Baltimore, Williams & Wilkins, 1988, p 478, with permission.)

110. In primary prevention trials aimed at reducing cardiovascular mortality with cholesterol-lowering drugs, which drugs have been shown to lower the risk of death from cardiac causes?

Two coronary primary prevention trials, the Lipid Research Clinic-Coronary Primary Prevention Trial (LRC-CPPT)[1] and the Helsinki Heart Study (HHS),[2] were designed to test the hypothesis that reduction of serum cholesterol decreases cardiovascular mortality. Both clinical trials showed that cholesterol-lowering drugs such as cholestyramine and gemfibrozil effectively reduce serum cholesterol and decrease cardiovascular mortality.

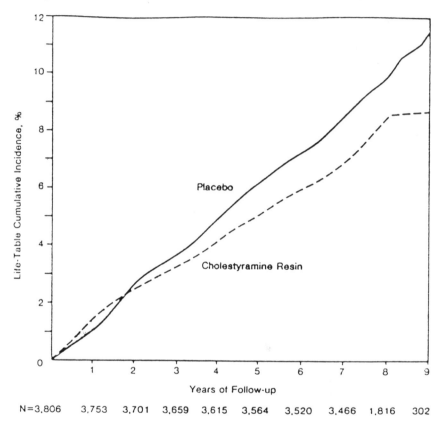

N=3,806　　3,753　　3,701　　3,659　　3,615　　3,564　　3,520　　3,466　　1,816　　302

Life-table cumulative incidence of primary end point (definite coronary heart disease death and/or definite nonfatal myocardial infarction) in treatment groups, computed by Kaplan-Meier method. N equals total number of Lipid Research Clinics Coronary Primary Prevention Trial participants at risk for their first primary end point, followed at each time point. (From Lipid Research Clinics Program: The Lipid Research Clinics Coronary Primary Prevention Trial Results. 1. Reduction in Incidence of Coronary Heart Disease. JAMA 251:351, 1984, with permission.)

A 1% reduction in serum cholesterol in the LRC-CPPT was associated with a 2% reduction in cardiovascular mortality. Overall, about a 10% reduction in serum cholesterol was accompanied by a 20% decrease in cardiovascular mortality. One of the most interesting findings in this clinical trial is that the reduction in cardiovascular mortality was highest in those patients who had the lowest reduction in serum cholesterol levels, supporting the causal relationship between cholesterol and cardiovascular disease.

Coronary Primary Prevention Trials: LRC-CPPT vs. HHS

	LRC-CPPT[1]	HHS[2]
Publication	JAMA 1984	NEJM 1987
Cholesterol-lowering drug	Cholestyramine	Gemfibrozil
Average daily dose	24 g	600 mg bid
Duration of follow-up	7.4 years	5 years
Reduction in cholesterol	8.5%	10%
Reduction in LDL cholesterol	13%	10%
Increase in HDL cholesterol	2%	10%
Reduction in CV mortality	19%	34%

1. Lipid Research Clinics Program: The Lipid Research Clinics Coronary Primary Prevention Trial Results. 1. Reduction in Incidence of Coronary Heart Disease. JAMA 251:351, 1984.
2. Frick MH, et al: Helsinki Heart Study: Primary-prevention trial with gemfibrozil in middle aged men with dyslipidemia. N Engl J Med 317:1237–1245, 1987.

Kaplan-Meier cumulative incidence (per 1000) and annual number of cardiac end points, according to treatment group and time. Data for the sixth year (stars) were derived from 305 person-years of observation for gemfibrozil and from 316 person-years of observation for placebo. (From Frick MH, et al: Helsinki Heart Study: Primary-prevention trial with gemfibrozil in middle aged men with dyslipidemia. N Engl J Med 317: 1237–1245, 1987, with permission.)

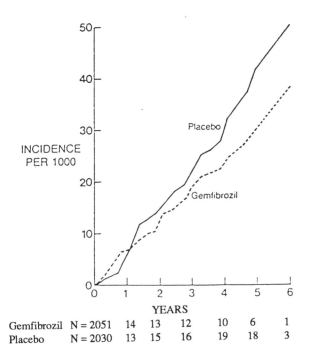

Gemfibrozil N = 2051	14	13	12	10	6	1
Placebo N = 2030	13	15	16	19	18	3

111. Most lipid-lowering drugs are aimed at lowering serum cholesterol levels by reducing the LDL fraction of cholesterol. Some lipid-lowering drugs are capable of raising the serum level of HDL cholesterol as well. Which lipid-lowering drug is most effective in raising HDL cholesterol levels? Is such an effect likely to affect coronary heart disease mortality?
Among all available lipid-lowering drugs, gemfibrozil results in the most marked increase in high-density lipoprotein (HDL) levels. A 600 mg dose, taken twice a day, resulted in a 10% increase in HDL in the Helsinki Heart Study (HHS). The HHS is a clinical trial in which 4,081 asymptomatic men with hyperlipidemia were randomly assigned to receive gemfibrozil or placebo over 5 years. Unlike patients in the Lipid Research Clinic-Coronary Primary Prevention Trial (LRC-CPPT), who received cholestyramine and experienced almost no change in the serum HDL level, gemfibrozil-treated patients experienced a 10%

increase in HDL and a remarkable 34% reduction in CHD mortality. The corresponding reduction in CHD mortality achieved in cholestyramine-treated patients was only 19%.

It is likely that the 10% increase in HDL cholesterol levels induced by gemfibrozil accounted for the additional 15% reduction in CHD mortality. This led to the so-called "HDL hypothesis," namely, that an increase in HDL alone can decrease the risk of death from coronary heart disease.

112. Cardioselectivity of a beta-blocking drug refers to its negligible blockade of bronchial beta-2 receptors at low doses. Which beta-blockers are cardioselective and what are the clinical implications of this pharmacologic property?

Cardioselective Beta-blockers	*Noncardioselective Beta-blockers*
1. Atenolol (Tenormin)	1. Propranolol (Inderal)
2. Metoprolol (Lopressor)	2. Timolol (Blocadren)
3. Acebutolol (Sectral)	3. Pindolol (Visken)
	4. Nadolol (Corgard)

Cardioselectivity refers to the predominant blockade of the beta-1 adrenergic receptors, which are mostly present in the heart. Cardioselective beta-blockers, in low doses, have minimal blocking effects on beta-2 receptors, the predominant beta receptors in the lungs. However, cardioselectivity is only relative. When administered in large doses, cardioselectivity is markedly diminished. Despite these limitations, cardioselective beta-blockers are much safer than noncardioselective beta-blockers in patients with obstructive lung disease.

113. What is the importance of intrinsic sympathomimetic activity (ISA) as it applies to beta-blockers? Which beta-blockers possess ISA?
ISA refers to the partial beta-adrenergic agonist properties of some beta-blockers. When sympathetic activity is low (at rest), these beta-blockers produce low-grade beta-stimulation. However, under conditions of stress (exercise), beta-blockers with ISA behave essentially as conventional beta-blockers without ISA. The clinical significance of ISA is not clearly established.

Pindolol and acebutolol demonstrated ISA. All other beta-blockers presently available do not have any significant intrinsic sympathomimetic activity.

114. Prior to elective cardioversion of a patient with A fib, a 2-week course of anticoagulation decreases the risk of thromboembolic events during and shortly after cardioversion. Is anticoagulation similarly required in a patient with A fib with a fast ventricular rate of 230/min and systolic blood pressure of 70 mmHg?
It is of paramount importance to weigh carefully the risks and benefits of cardioversion and anticoagulation prior to elective cardioversion. A 10–14 day period of adequate anticoagulation is desirable before elective cardioversion of a patient with A fib. However, the most important question to address before any therapeutic decision is made in a patient with A fib with a fast ventricular response rate is how urgent is cardioversion? Whenever there is clinical evidence of hemodynamic compromise, such as CHF, hypotension or systemic hypoperfusion, acute anginal symptoms, or acute MI, urgent cardioversion should be administered *immediately,* regardless of left atrial or LV size, systolic LV function, or prior anticoagulation.

The patient in question is a classic example of A fib with a fast ventricular response rate of 230/min and severe hypotension, in whom cardioversion should *absolutely not* be delayed. Electrical cardioversion should be immediately administered in this patient regardless of prior anticoagulation.

115. What is the initial management of acute pulmonary edema, with special reference to the use of digitalis, diuretics, and vasodilators?

It is essential to individualize your therapeutic approach to a patient with acute pulmonary edema. However, some general guidelines for therapy are helpful:

   1. IV diuresis with a loop diuretic such as furosemide (20 to 60 mg IV push, to be repeated as necessary). IV furosemide lowers venous tone and thus lowers pulmonary wedge pressure even *before* inducing effective diuresis.

   2. IV, cutaneous, or oral preload-reducing drug therapy. Nitrates are effective venodilators. In single oral doses of 40–60 mg (to be repeated three or four times daily), they are effective in lowering pulmonary capillary wedge pressure and thus improving congestive symptoms of dyspnea, orthopnea, paroxysmal nocturnal dyspnea, and nocturnal cough.

   3. IV digitalization is recommended in patients with acute pulmonary edema with or without associated A fib.

   4. Oxygen therapy, depending on results of arterial blood gas measurements.

   5. Bed rest and salt restriction.

   6. Afterload-reducing drugs are effective in ameliorating signs and symptoms of CHF. Angiotensin-converting enzyme (ACE) inhibitors such as captopril, enalapril, or lisinopril are effective afterload and preload-reducing drugs and can be administered orally in patients with overt CHF.

BIBLIOGRAPHY

1. Braunwald E (ed): Heart Disease: A Textbook of Cardiovascular Medicine, 3rd ed. Philadelphia, W.B. Saunders, 1988.
2. Hurst JW (ed): The Heart, 7th ed. New York, McGraw-Hill, 1990.
3. Marriott HJL: Practical Electrocardiography, 8th ed. Baltimore, Williams & Wilkins, 1988.
4. Johnson RA, et al: The Practice of Cardiology. Boston, Little, Brown, 1980.
5. Wilson JD, et al (eds): Harrison's Principles of Internal Medicine, 12th ed. New York, McGraw-Hill, 1991.

4. INFECTIOUS DISEASE SECRETS

Robert L. Atmar, M.D., Richard J. Hamill, M.D., and J. Todd Bagwell, M.D.

> *It is certainly a one-sided opinion—even though generally adopted at the moment—that all infectious agents which are still unknown must be bacteria. Why should not other microorganisms just as well be able to exist as parasites in the body of animals?*
>
> Robert Koch (1843–1910)
> *Zur Untersuchung von pathogenen Organismen, 1881, tr. by Max Samter*

1. What is Luria's law?
Three antibiotics equals one fungal infection.

Matz R: Principles of medicine. NY State J Med 77:99–101, 1977.

2. What useful role is played by the blood cells (amebocytes) of the horseshoe crab, *Limulus polyphemus?*
In 1956, Bang reported that gram-negative bacterial endotoxin caused gelation of a lysate prepared from the blood cells (amebocytes) of the *Limulus* crab. This limulus amebocyte lysate reaction is the basis of an assay now used to detect the presence of endotoxin in various body fluids, pharmacologic products, and medical devices.

Bang FB: A bacterial disease of *Limulus polyphemus*. Bull Johns Hopkins Hosp 98:325–350, 1956.

3. What is Vincent's angina?
Vincent's angina is a necrotizing pharyngitis caused by a mixture of anaerobes and spirochetes. *Streptococcus pyogenes* and *Staphylococcus aureus* may also play a role. Symptoms include an extremely sore throat, fever, and foul breath. Physical examination reveals pharyngeal ulcerations that are covered with a purulent exudate. Treatment with penicillin is curative.

4. Where and when was the last naturally occurring case of smallpox identified?
In Merka Town, Somalia in October 1977.

5. What are the tick-borne infectious diseases seen in the United States?

Tick-borne Infectious Diseases in the USA

DISEASE	ORGANISM
Lyme disease	*Borrelia burgdorferi*
Q fever	*Coxiella burnetii*
Colorado tick fever	An orbivirus
Rocky Mountain spotted fever	*Rickettsia ricketsii*
Tularemia	*Francisella tularensis*
Babesiosis	*Babesia microti*
Relapsing fever	*Borrelia duttoni* and other species

6. What is tick paralysis?
Tick paralysis is a complication of prolonged attachment of certain species of ticks (*Dermacentor andersoni* and *Dermacentor variabilis* in the U.S.). It is an ascending paralysis that begins in the lower extremities and rapidly progresses to involve the upper

extremities and head. It is thought to be caused by a neurotoxin in the tick's saliva, and it usually resolves quickly after the tick is removed.

7. Postsplenectomy sepsis is caused by which organisms?
Splenectomy predisposes patients to sepsis by encapsulated organisms, including:

Streptococcus pneumoniae	*Neisseria meningitidis*
Haemophilus influenzae	*Escherichia coli*

Occasional cases due to *Staphylococcus aureus* and *Capnocytophaga canimorsus* (DF-2) have been described.

Zarrabi HM: Serious infections in adults following splenectomy for trauma. Arch Intern Med 144:1421–1424, 1984.

8. Infective endocarditis due to *Pseudomonas aeruginosa* occurs almost uniformly in which risk group?
Pseudomonas aeruginosa causes infective endocarditis on native heart valves in intravenous (IV) drug abusers. It is also a rare cause of prosthetic valve endocarditis. The occurrence of *P. aeruginosa* endocarditis is subject to considerable regional variation. It is thought that the source of the organism is water that contaminates drug paraphernalia.

Cohen PS, et al: Infective endocarditis caused by gram-negative bacteria: A review of the literature, 1945–1977. Prog Cardiovasc Dis 22:205–242, 1980.

9. What are the causative organisms of prosthetic valve endocarditis (PVE) and their time of appearance relative to the valve replacement surgery?
Traditionally, prosthetic valve endocarditis has been classified according to the time of onset with respect to the replacement surgery. Two months after surgery is used as the division between early and late onset endocarditis:

Prosthetic Valve Endocarditis (PVE)

ORGANISM	EARLY PVE (%)	LATE PVE (%)	OVERALL (%)
Staphylococci			
S. epidermidis	35	26	29
S. aureus	17	12	14
Streptococci			
Group D streptococci (including enterococci)	3	9	7
S. pneumoniae	1	<1	1
Other (including viridans streptococci)	4	25	17
Gram-negative bacilli	16	12	13
Diphtheroids	10	4	7
Other bacteria	1	2	2
Candida	8	4	5
Aspergillus	2	1	1
Other fungi	1	<1	1
Culture negative	1	4	3
Total number			
Microorganisms	292	445	737
Patients	272	429	701

(From Mayer KH, et al: Evaluation and management of prosthetic valve endocarditis. Prog Cardiovasc Dis 25:43–62, 1982, with permission.)

10. What are the causes of biologic false-positive RPR (serologic test for syphilis)?
The causes of biologic false-positive RPRs (rapid plasma reagins) can be divided into those that are acute and those of chronic duration:

Acute (positive <6 months)	*Chronic* (>6 months duration)
Acute febrile illnesses	Chronic infections (lepromatous leprosy)
Recent immunizations	Autoimmune disease (e.g., SLE)
Pregnancy	Narcotics addicts who use drugs intravenously

When false-positive tests occur, the titer is usually low (i.e., < 1:8).

11. Do the specific treponemal serologic tests for syphilis (i.e., MHA-TP, FTA-ABS) return to undetectable levels after appropriate antimicrobial therapy for syphilis?

No. The treponemal tests remain positive for life after initial infection. The tests should not be used to assess the response to therapy.

12. What is the expected rate of fall of nontreponemal serologic tests after appropriate treatment of 1°, 2°, and early latent syphilis?

One should expect a fourfold decline in the VDRL or RPR at 3 months and an eightfold decline at 6 months.

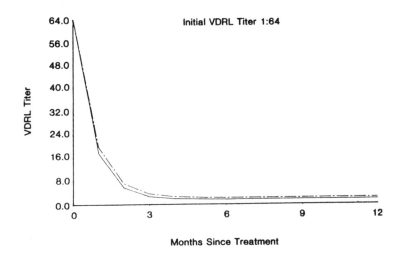

VDRL titer decline after treatment of primary or secondary syphilis with penicillin or tetracycline. (From Brown ST, et al: Serologic response to syphilis treatment. JAMA 253:1296–1299, 1985, with permission.)

13. What are the clinical settings and risk factors associated with *Candida* sp. infections?

Clinical Settings and Risk Factors for Candida *Infections*

CLINICAL SETTING	RISK FACTORS
1. Chronic mucocutaneous infections	a. Defects in T lymphocyte immunity, congenital (e.g., chronic mucocutaneous candidiasis) or acquired (e.g., AIDS) b. Qualitative defects in neutrophil function (e.g., myeloperoxidase deficiency)
2. Deeply invasive, disseminated infections	a. Peripheral neutrophil count < 500/mm³ b. Mucosal barrier breakdown (burn, cytotoxic agents, gastrointestinal surgery, IV catheter sites) c. Candidal overgrowth (broad spectrum antibiotics)
3. Colonization of a catheter with fever	a. Indwelling catheter

The difference between categories 2 and 3 may be clinically difficult to distinguish, and if there is doubt the patient should be treated for disseminated disease.

14. Endophthalmitis is present in what percentage of patients with candidemia?

Endophthalmitis has been reported to be present in 10–37% of candidemic patients and is an important clue that the infection is disseminated.

Brooks RG: Prospective study of *Candida* endophthalmitis in hospitalized patients with candidemia. Arch Intern Med 149:2226–2228, 1989.

15. Which species of *Candida* most commonly colonizes the skin?

C. parapsilosis commonly colonizes the skin, and its identification in blood cultures may suggest a contaminated intravascular line.

16. Which occupations are associated with *Erysipelothrix rhusiopathiae* infection?

Infection with *Erysipelothrix* is an occupational disease of fisherman, fish handlers, butchers, meat processing workers, poultry workers, farmers, veterinarians, and abattoir workers. There are two major clinical syndromes: (1) localized cutaneous and (2) disseminated/endocarditis.

Ninety percent of infections follow cutaneous inoculation with infectious material. The skin is indurated with distinct borders and a violaceous color. This gram-positive rod is very sensitive to penicillin. Cephalosporins are an alternative agent in penicillin-allergic patients.

Gorby GL, et al: Erysipelothrix endocarditis: Microbiologic, epidemiologic and clinical features of an occupational disease. Rev Infect Dis 10:317–325, 1988.

17. What are the infusion-related syndromes associated with IV vancomycin administration?

There are three infusion-related syndromes associated with vancomycin: (1) the "red-man syndrome," (2) the "pain and spasm syndrome," and (3) the occurrence of hypotension. The **red-man syndrome** is a histamine-mediated phenomenon that occurs with too rapid an infusion of vancomycin and is characterized by the development of erythema, hives, and pruritus across the upper trunk and face. The **pain and spasm syndrome** is characterized by throbbing chest pain that resolves when the antibiotic infusion is stopped. The pain is not secondary to myocardial ischemia. **Hypotension**, a very rare infusion-related syndrome, can usually be treated with antihistamines, although pressor agents are occasionally needed.

18. How is the "bedside" cold agglutinin test performed and what is the interpretation of a positive result?

Four to five drops of blood are added to a blood collection tube containing sodium citrate. The tube is immersed in an ice bath for 1–2 minutes. Floccular hemagglutination observed on the side of the tube is indicative of a positive reaction. Confirmation is provided if the agglutination disappears when the tube is warmed to 37°C. A positive test by this method correlates with a cold agglutinin titer of > 1:64, seen with *Mycoplasma pneumoniae* infections.

Griffin JP: Rapid screening for cold agglutinins in pneumonia. Ann Intern Med 70:701–705, 1969.

19. In what percentage of patients with acute infectious mononucleosis is the commercial Monospot test for detection of heterophil antibodies reactive?

Heterophil antibodies, as detected by the Monospot test, are present in approximately 90% of cases at some point in the illness.

20. What are the causes of a false-positive Monospot test?
Serum sickness, lymphoma, and acute hepatitis can give a false-positive result. One can distinguish false-positives from true-positives with differential adsorptions using guinea pig kidney and beef red cells as follows:

	Unadsorbed	Adsorption with Guinea Pig Kidney	Adsorption with Beef RBCs
Inf. mononucleosis	4+	3+	0
Lymphoma	3+	0	0
Serum sickness	3+	0	0
Hepatitis	3+	0	0
Normal	1+	0	1+

(From Schooley RT, Dolin R: Ebstein-Barr virus. In Mandell G, et al (eds): Principles and Practice of Infectious Diseases, 3rd ed. New York, Churchill Livingstone, 1990, p 1178, with permission.)

21. What is the differential diagnosis of exudative pharyngitis?
Exudative pharyngitis is caused by the following agents:

- Groups A, C, and G streptococci
- *Corynebacterium hemolyticum* and *Corynebacterium diphtheriae*
- Anaerobic bacteria
- *Yersinia enterocolitica*
- *Mycoplasma pneumoniae*
- Adenovirus, herpes simplex virus, and Epstein-Barr virus.

22. Patients with multiple myeloma are prone to develop infections owing to what types of organisms?
Infections in patients with myeloma demonstrate a biphasic pattern. Infections with *Streptococcus pneumoniae* and *Haemophilus influenzae* occur at the time of initial presentation of myeloma, early in the disease, and in patients who are responding to chemotherapy. Infections with *Staphylococcus aureus* and gram-negative bacilli (including *Escherichia coli, Pseudomonas aeruginosa, Klebsiella pneumoniae, Enterobacter* species, and *Serratia marcescens*) cause approximately 80% of infections seen after diagnosis of myeloma and 92% of deaths due to infections. These latter infections occur in patients with active and advancing disease and in those responding to chemotherapy in the period in which they are neutropenic.

Savage DG, et al: Biphasic pattern of bacterial infection in multiple myeloma. Ann Intern Med 96:47–50, 1982.

23. When examining a sputum specimen, what criteria should be used to indicate that a specimen originates from the lower respiratory tract and is adequate for culture?
Generally a sputum is considered adequate when there are fewer than 10 epithelial cells and more than 25 polymorphonuclear leukocytes per *low* power (100×) field. The presence of free alveolar macrophages (FAMs) also confirm the lower respiratory tract origin.

24. What is the differential diagnosis of trismus ("lockjaw")?
While tetanus is the best-known cause of trismus, the following disorders must be considered in a patient with tonic spasm of the masticatory muscles:

- Inflammatory lesions of the floor of the mouth, cheeks, pharynx or external auditory canal (peritonsillar or dental abscess, Ludwig's angina, trichinosis)
- Malignancies (sarcoma of the jaw, squamous cell carcinoma of the oral cavity)
- Psychiatric disorders (hysteric tetanus)
- Mechanical problems (temporomaxillary ankylosis, dislocation of the jaw)
- Strychnine poisoning (a late manifestation)
- Phenothiazines (part of a dystonic reaction)
- Encephalitis

25. What are the different clinical presentations of tetanus in the adult?

Tetanus may present in one of three clinical forms:

- *Generalized tetanus* is the most common form of the disease. This form is characterized by trismus, nuchal rigidity, dysphagia, irritability, and rigidity of the abdominal muscles.
- *Localized tetanus* is manifested by persistent rigidity of a group of muscles close to the site of injury. It occasionally progresses to generalized tetanus.
- *Cephalic tetanus* is a severe form of localized tetanus that occurs when the injury is on the head or neck. It usually presents with cranial motor nerve dysfunction (most commonly involving cranial nerve VII), and it has a poor prognosis.

26. If a patient with no prior history of tetanus vaccination recovers from an episode of tetanus, is he or she at risk for a second episode?

Yes. The occurrence of tetanus does not prevent second episodes of clinical disease from occurring, because the amount of toxin needed to produce the clinical syndrome is so small that it is usually not immunogenic. Hence, persons recovering from tetanus should be vaccinated with tetanus toxoid against future episodes of the disease.

27. What are the three types of antimicrobial resistance mechanisms displayed by *Staphylococcus aureus* for beta lactam antibiotics and their proposed mechanisms?

1. Plasmid-mediated production of extracellular enzymes (beta lactamases) that act on the beta lactam ring.

2. Chromosomally mediated resistance (methicillin-resistance or intrinsic resistance) that results from production of penicillin-binding proteins with altered affinity for beta lactam antibiotics.

3. Tolerance, defined by a minimal bactericidal concentration to minimal inhibitory concentration (MBC/MIC) ratio > 32, which results from an inability of beta lactam antibiotics to activate autolytic enzymes.

Sabath LD: Mechanisms of resistance to beta-lactam antibiotics in strains of *Staphylococcus aureus*. Ann Intern Med 97:339–344, 1982.

28. *Staphylococcus saprophyticus* is most commonly associated with which infectious problem?

Staphylococcus saprophyticus almost exclusively causes urinary tract infections, usually in young women. There is a high correlation between genitourinary mucosal colonization with this organism and the subsequent development of a urinary tract infection. Symptoms and findings on urinalysis are indistinguishable from patients who have infections due to enteric organisms. This bacterium accounts for 20% of urinary tract infections in women 16 to 35 years old.

Jordan PA, et al: Urinary tract infection caused by *Staphylococcus saprophyticus*. J Infect Dis 142:510, 1980.

29. What are the etiologic and epidemiologic associations in the toxic shock syndrome?

1. Approximately 70% of cases occur in women < 30 years old in association with their menstrual period.

2. Approximately 30% of cases are not associated with menses but occur in association with:

a. IV drug abusers	d. Surgical wound infections	f. Parturition
b. Homosexuals	e. Nonsurgical traumatic	g. Staphylococcal
c. Staphylococcal sepsis	wounds	pneumonia

The toxins elaborated by *S. aureus* are responsible for the clinical manifestations. There is a strong association between the toxic shock syndrome and recovery of *S. aureus* from vaginal cultures.

Broome CV: Epidemiology of toxic shock syndrome in the United States: Overview. Rev Infect Dis 11:S14–S21, 1989.

30. How is the diagnosis of toxic shock syndrome made?

The diagnosis of toxic shock syndrome is a clinical diagnosis based on the presence of certain signs and symptoms. The diagnostic categories are as follows:

Definite Toxic Shock Syndrome (All Criteria Must Be Present)

1. Temperature $\geq$ 38.9° C (102° F)
2. Rash (diffuse or palmar erythroderma) with desquamation of palms or soles 1–2 weeks after the onset of illness.
3. Hypotension—manifested by one of the following:
   a. Systolic blood pressure <90 mmHg
   b. Orthostatic decrease in systolic blood pressure $\geq$ 15 mmHg
   c. Orthostatic dizziness or syncope
4. Clinical or laboratory abnormalities in three or more organ systems
   a. Mucous membrane   e. Renal
   b. Gastrointestinal   f. Muscular
   c. Hepatic   g. Cardiovascular
   d. Central nervous system

Tofte RW, et al: Toxic shock syndrome in the United States: Evidence of a broad clinical spectrum. JAMA 246:2163–2167, 1981.

Probable Toxic Shock Syndrome (at Least Three [3] Criteria with Desquamation or at Least Five [5] Criteria without Desquamation)

---

1. Temperature $\geq$ 38.9° C (102° F)
2. Diffuse or palmar erythroderma (rash)
3. Hypotension, orthostatic dizziness, or syncope
4. Myalgia
5. Vomiting, diarrhea, or both
6. Mucous membrane inflammation (conjunctivitis, pharyngitis, or vaginitis)
7. Clinical or laboratory abnormalities in two or more organ systems
8. Reasonable evidence for the absence of other causes of the illness

---

Tofte RW, et al: Toxic shock syndrome: Evidence of a broad clinical spectrum. JAMA 246:2163–2167, 1981.

31. What is the significance of bacteremia or endocarditis due to *Streptococcus bovis*?

A strong association exists between lesions of the gastrointestinal tract, particularly bowel carcinoma, and *S. bovis* bacteremia or endocarditis. Patients in whom this organism is identified should have a thorough evaluation of the gastrointestinal tract performed.

Klein RS, et al: Association of *Streptococcus bovis* with carcinoma of the colon. N Engl J Med 297:800–802, 1977.

32. Infection with *Streptococcus agalactiae* is most commonly seen in which epidemiologic setting?

Infection with group B streptococci is seen in postpartum women and neonates.

33. How often is there a current or past history of diarrhea in patients with amebic liver abscess?

A history of past or present intestinal symptoms is obtained in less than 20% of patients with amebic liver abscess. The major presenting manifestations are those referable to the abscess itself or its extension and rupture into adjacent structures. *Entamoeba histolytica* is found in the stool in less than one-third of patients with an abscess.

34. Which part of the liver is most commonly involved in patients with amebic liver abscess?

Amebic liver abscesses are most commonly single lesions involving the right superior or superior-posterior aspect of the liver. The etiology of a suspected amebic liver abscess can be determined by the indirect hemagglutination or gel precipitin tests, which are positive in over 90% of patients with an amebic liver abscess.

35. Primary amebic meningoencephalitis due to *Naegleria fowleri* occurs in which epidemiologic setting?

Cases of primary amebic meningoencephalitis due to *Naegleria fowleri* occur predominantly in children or young adults in robust health who have been swimming, diving, or water skiing in small lakes, usually in the southern U.S. The organism is associated with fresh water that has heavy growths of algae and bacteria, which usually result from high concentrations of sewage components in the water.

John DT: Primary amebic meningoencephalitis and the biology of *Naegleria fowleri*. Ann Rev Microbiol 36:101–123, 1982.

36. Why should aminoglycoside antibiotics be given with careful monitoring to patients with neuromuscular diseases, such as myasthenia gravis?

Aminoglycoside antibiotics demonstrate neuromuscular blockade properties by inhibiting presynaptic release of acetylcholine and depressing postsynaptic sensitivity to acetylcholine. Patients with myasthenia gravis have shown increased sensitivity to the paralytic effects of these agents. The paralytic effects can be overcome with anticholinesterases and calcium.

37. How can you differentiate acute paralytic polio from the Guillain-Barré syndrome?

Acute paralytic polio and the Guillain-Barré syndrome may be clinically differentiated by the following criteria:

Presence of	Polio	Guillain-Barré
Fever	+	–
Acutely ill	+	–
Signs of meningeal infection	+	–
Symmetrical paralysis	–	+
Motor loss	+	+
Sensory loss	Rare	80%
Pattern of progression of paralysis	No pattern	Ascending
Duration of progression of paralysis	3–4 days	Up to 2 weeks in stages

38. What are the five different disease manifestations in humans caused by the dimorphic fungus *Histoplasma capsulatum*?

1. Acute pulmonary histoplasmosis
2. Disseminated histoplasmosis
3. Fibrosing mediastinitis
4. Chronic cavitary fibronodular pulmonary histoplasmosis
5. Histoplasmoma

Goodwin RA, et al: Histoplasmosis. Am Rev Respir Dis 117:929–955, 1981.

39. What is the reason postulated for recrudescence of herpes simplex viral infections in a small area and of varicella in a dermatomal region?

Both herpes simplex and varicella-zoster viruses cause latent infections in human sensory nerve ganglia. However, the cells that are latently infected are different. Herpes simplex virus causes a latent infection of individual neuronal cells. With reactivation, infection does not spread well from cell to cell but does spread easily to the skin. Hence, only a small area of skin is involved during reactivation.

Varicella-zoster virus, on the other hand, causes a latent infection in the satellite cells, and during reactivation the infection readily spreads throughout the sensory ganglia. The virus is then able to spread to all areas of the sensory dermatome.

Croen KD, et al: Patterns of gene expression and sites of latency in human nerve ganglia are different for varicella-zoster and herpes simplex viruses. Proc Nat Acad Sci USA 85:9773–9777, 1988.

40. What are the sexually transmitted diseases that cause genital ulceration with regional adenopathy?

Syphilis, genital herpes, chancroid, lymphogranuloma venereum, and granuloma inguinale are all sexually transmitted causes of genital ulceration with regional adenopathy.

Krockta WP, Barnes RC: Genital ulceration with regional adenopathy. Infect Dis Clin North Am 1:217–233, 1987.

41. What is hydrophobia and why is it significant in infectious diseases?

Patients with rabies encephalitis often have unusual painful pharyngeal spasms when exposed to water and as a consequence will avoid water. Hydrophobia is important as a helpful diagnostic clue in a patient with an early encephalitis, pointing towards the diagnosis of rabies.

42. What animal vectors are involved in human rabies?

Dogs account for more than 90% of reported human cases of rabies in areas of the world where domestic rabies is not well controlled. Other domestic animals contribute 5–10% worldwide and include cats, cattle, horses, sheep and pigs. In the U.S., the principal vectors or rabies are wild mammals, including the striped skunk, raccoon, and insectivorous bats. Small rodents (such as rats or mice), birds, and reptiles are not known to be reservoirs of rabies.

43. What is the "groove sign" and what is its significance in diagnosing genital ulcerative disease?

The "groove sign" is the occurrence of adenopathy above and below the inguinal ligament. Though it has been said to be pathognomonic of lymphogranuloma venereum, it is seen in only 15% or less of patients and also occurs in other infectious and neoplastic conditions.

Krockta WP, Barnes RC: Genital ulceration with regional adenopathy. Infect Dis Clin North Am 1:217–233, 1987.

44. What is the significance of perinatal transmission of hepatitis B and how often does it occur in offspring of women who are chronically hepatitis B surface antigen (HB$_s$Ag) positive?

Neonates who acquire hepatitis B infection in the perinatal period tend to become chronic carriers and are at significantly increased risk for the complications of cirrhosis and hepatocellular carcinoma. These complications are potentially preventible with passive and active immunization of the infant. Women who are HB$_s$Ag positive and hepatitis B "e" antigen (HB$_e$Ag) positive transmit the virus to their offspring 50–70% of the time, whereas those who are HB$_s$Ag positive, but HB$_e$Ag negative, transmit it approximately 10% of the time.

45. What criteria are suggestive of urinary tract infection on the microscopic examination of a clean-catch urine specimen?

Type of Urine	Method of Observation	Finding	Indication
Uncentrifuged	Hemocytometer	$\leq 10^3$ WBC/ml	Normal
		$> 10^4$ WBC/ml	Infection
	Low-power magnification (10 X objective)	> 2–3 WBC/field	Correlates with $> 10^4$ WBC/ml
	High-power magnification (45 X objective)	1–2 WBC field, bacteria	$\geq 10^5$ WBC/ml, $\geq 10^5$ bacteria/ml
	High-power magnification (45 X objective)	WBC cast	Suggests renal involvement (pyelonephritis)
Uncentrifuged or centrifuged	High-power magnification	a. WBC cast	Same as above
		b. RBC cast	Indicates glomerulonephritis

(From Musher DM: Urinary tract infection. In Dupont H, Pickering L (eds): Infectious Diseases Handbook. Menlo Park, CA, Addison-Wesley, 1986, p 450, with permission.)

46. Which organisms are likely to cause a chronic urinary tract infection with urinary pH ≥ 7.5?

Urinary pH is elevated in chronic urinary tract infections caused by organisms that are urease producers. *Proteus* sp. are the most common organisms that cause this clinical presentation, but *Klebsiella* and other urease producers may also present in this manner.

47. Linear calcifications seen in the wall of the urinary bladder on a KUB (kidneys and upper bladder) roentgenogram are indicative of which chronic infection?

Schistosoma haematobium infection may result in bladder wall calcifications as a result of the deposition of eggs in the submucosa and mucosa of the bladder. The consequent inflammatory response leads to scarring and calcium deposition.

48. Which antibiotics can be found in cyst fluid in patients with polycystic kidney disease?

Trimethoprim-sulfamethoxazole and chloramphenicol are found in significant concentrations in cyst fluid. Patients with polycystic disease and urinary tract infection may fail to improve with other antibiotics. Surgical aspiration or drainage of infected cysts may be necessary.

49. What factors are necessary for methenamine to function effectively as a urinary tract antiseptic?

Methenamine itself is not bactericidal but depends on hydrolysis, at an acid pH, to liberate ammonia and formaldehyde by the following reaction:

$$N_4(CH_2)_6 + \longleftrightarrow 4NH_{4+} + 6HCHO$$

Formaldehyde is the bactericidal agent. In order for this reaction to work optimally, urine pH needs to be less than 7.0. Urinary acidification (with cranberry or other juice) is usually administered in conjunction with methenamine.

In addition, there needs to be sufficient time for this hydrolysis to occur (usually on the order of hours). Consequently, the drug is ineffective in patients with indwelling bladder catheters.

50. Which organisms are weakly acid-fast positive?

Nocardia sp. and *Actinomyces* sp. are weakly acid-fast positive.

51. What are the most common etiologic agents in the acute sinusitis syndrome?

Microbial Etiology of Acute Community-acquired Antral Sinusitis

MICROBIAL AGENT	PERCENT OF CASES (RANGE)	
	ADULTS	CHILDREN
Bacteria		
S. pneumoniae	31 (20–35)	36
H. influenzae (unencapsulated)	21 (6–26)	23
S. pneumoniae and H. influenzae	5 (1–9)	—
Anaerobic bacteria (*Bacteroides* sp., *Pepto-streptococcus* sp., *Fusobacterium* sp., etc.)	6 (0–10)	—
S. aureus	4 (0–8)	—
S. pyogenes	2 (1–3)	2
M. catarrhalis	2	19
Gram-negative bacteria	9 (0–24)	2
Viruses		
Rhinovirus	15	—
Influenza virus	5	—
Parainfluenza virus	3	2
Adenovirus	—	2

(From Gwaltney JM: Sinusitis. In Mandell G, et al (eds): Principles and Practice of Infectious Diseases, 3rd ed. New York, Churchill Livingstone, 1990, p 510, with permission.)

52. What percentage of patients with pneumococcal pneumonia also have bacteremia?
Bacteremia occurs in 25–30% of individuals with pneumococcal pneumonia.

53. What are the radiographic changes associated with osteomyelitis?
1. Deep soft tissue swelling and obliteration of muscle planes are usually the earliest radiographic changes to be seen.
2. Periosteal reaction.
3. Cortical irregularity.
4. Rarification of bone.
5. Sequestrum (a devitalized area of bone that results from loss of vascular supply).
6. Involucrum (periosteal new bone formation that occurs in response to infection).

54. What is the most common bacterial species causing osteomyelitis in patients with sickle cell disease?
Approximately 80% of cases of osteomyelitis in patients with sickle cell disease are due to *Salmonella* species.
   Engh C, et al: Osteomyelitis in the patient with sickle cell disease. J Bone Joint Surg 53A:1, 1971.

55. How reliable are sinus tract cultures for determination of the etiologic agent causing chronic osteomyelitis?
The likelihood that a sinus-tract isolate will correspond with an operative isolate is high if *Staphylococcus aureus* is the organism isolated from a sinus tract culture (78%). However, only 44% of sinus tract cultures from patients with biopsy-proven *S. aureus* osteomyelitis will yield this organism. The predictive value of cultures growing the Enterobacteriaceae, *Pseudomonas aeruginosa,* and mixed cultures of *Streptococcus* species is less than 50%, and only a small number of cultures from sinus tracts of patients with chronic osteomyelitis caused by these organisms will yield the operative pathogen.
   Mackowiak PA, et al: Diagnostic value of sinus-tract cultures in chronic osteomyelitis. JAMA 239:2772–2775, 1978.

56. In a young, healthy patient who presents with *Pseudomonas aeruginosa* osteomyelitis of the calcaneus bone, what is the most likely cause of this disorder?
Pseudomonas osteomyelitis of the foot in an otherwise healthy patient is almost always a result of a puncture wound to the foot. Ninety percent of cases of osteomyelitis that result from puncture wounds to the feet are due to *P. aeruginosa.* The remaining 10% are due to various other gram-negative organisms, staphylococci, streptococci and atypical mycobacteria.
   Riley HD: Puncture wounds of the foot: Their importance and potential for complications. J Oklahoma State Med Assoc 77:3–6, 1984.

57. Bacterial endophthalmitis secondary to penetrating trauma to the eye is associated with which pathogens?

Organisms	Frequency
S. epidermidis, S. aureus, streptococci	60%
Bacillus sp.	25%
Gram-negative rods	10%
Fungi	5%

Bacillus cereus causes a particularly fulminant form of the disease, not uncommonly requiring enucleation. Fortunately, given all the episodes of trauma that occur to the eye, secondary infection is relatively uncommon.
   Davey RT Jr, et al: Post-traumatic endophthalmitis: The emerging role of *Bacillus cereus* infection. Rev Infect Dis 9:110–123, 1987.

58. Acute gastric anisakiasis results from what dietary habit?

Acute gastric anisakiasis is associated with the eating of sushi. It results from gastric mucosal penetration of the *Anisakis* larvae in individuals who have ingested raw fish. The most common fish involved is mackerel. Symptoms consist of the acute onset of severe epigastric pain, nausea, and vomiting that begin within 12 hours after ingestion. Treatment consists of endoscopic removal of the larvae.

Sugimachi K, et al: Acute gastric anisakiasis. Analysis of 178 cases. Arch Intern Med 253:1012–1013, 1985.

59. What is the most common cause of nonepidemic viral encephalitis in the U.S.?

Herpes simplex type 1 causes a focal encephalitis and is the most common cause of nonepidemic viral encephalitis in the U.S.

60. Who should receive prophylaxis after exposure to patients with *Neisseria meningitidis* meningitis?

Household contacts are at greatly increased risk of acquiring the disease and should receive prophylaxis. Individuals in closed populations such as military barracks, nursery schools, college dormitories, and chronic care hospitals are also at increased risk. Hospital personnel who have intimate exposure to infected patients should receive prophylaxis, but other personnel without such exposure need not be treated.

Centers for Disease Control: Meningococcal disease—United States. MMWR 30:113–115, 1981.

61. What is the classic definition that has been used for fever of undetermined origin (FUO)?

The classic definition of FUO as defined in criteria established in the classic article by Petersdorf and Beeson is:

1. Illness of more than 3 weeks duration. This eliminates any acute, self-limited illnesses.
2. Documented fever higher than 101°F (38.3°C) on several occasions.
3. Uncertain diagnosis after 1 week in the hospital to allow completion of routine laboratory examinations.

Petersdorf RG, Beeson PB: Fever of unexplained origin: Report of 100 cases. Medicine 40:1–29, 1961.

62. What are the major causes of fever of undetermined origin?

Causes of Fever of Undetermined Origin

I. Infection	**II. Cancer**
A. Generalized	A. Hematological
1. Tuberculosis	1. Lymphoma
2. Histoplasmosis	2. Hodgkin's disease
3. Typhoid fever	3. Acute leukemia
4. Cytomegalovirus	B. Tumors with propensity to cause fever
5. Epstein-Barr virus	1. Hepatoma
6. Miscellaneous:	2. Renal cell carcinoma
a. Syphilis	3. Atrial myxoma
b. Brucellosis	
c. Malaria	**III. Rheumatologic disorders**
B. Localized	1. Rheumatoid arthritis
1. Infective endocarditis	2. Systemic lupus erythematosus
2. Empyema	3. Vasculitis

Table continued on next page.

Causes of Fever of Undetermined Origin (Continued)

3. Intra-abdominal infection	IV. **Miscellaneous**
a. Peritonitis	1. Drug-induced
b. Cholangitis	2. Immune complex:SLE, RA
c. Abscess	3. Vasculitis
4. Urinary tract	4. Alcoholic liver disease
a. Pyelonephritis	5. Granulomatous hepatitis
b. Perinephric abscesses	6. Inflammatory bowel disease,
c. Prostatitis	Whipple's disease
5. Decubitus ulcer	7. Recurrent pulmonary emboli
6. Osteomyelitis	8. Factitious fever
7. Thrombophlebitis	9. Undiagnosed

(From Larson EB, et al: Fever of undetermined origin: Diagnosis and follow-up of 105 cases, 1970–1980. Medicine 61:269–292, with permission.)

63. What types of reactions to penicillin may be predicted by skin testing prior to antibiotic use?

Skin testing is predictive of IgE-mediated reactions. Such reactions, including accelerated urticaria or anaphylaxis, occur with varying frequency depending on the skin test result. Among patients with a positive skin test, the frequency of these reactions varies from 10% in those without a previous history of penicillin allergy to 50–70% in those with a past history of penicillin allergy. In patients with a negative skin test, accelerated urticaria occurs in only 1% and anaphylaxis does not occur.

Skin test reactivity is not predictive of other types of reactions, such as serum sickness, maculopapular rash, exfoliative dermatitis, hemolytic anemia, or interstitial nephritis.

64. What chest x-ray findings are very suggestive of thoracic actinomycosis?

1. Lesions extending through the chest wall.
2. Involvement of adjacent lobes by transgression through an interlobar fissure.
3. Periostitis or destruction of bones such as ribs or sternum adjacent to a pulmonary process.
4. Vertebral destruction, with disc space sparing, due to extension from mediastinal or thoracic involvement.

Flynn WM, et al: The roentgen manifestations of thoracic actinomycosis. Am J Roentgenol Radium Ther Nucl Med 110:707, 1970.

65. Which parasitic disease mimics pulmonary tuberculosis? How is it diagnosed?

The trematode lung fluke *Paragonimus westermani* can cause a pulmonary syndrome consistent with pulmonary tuberculosis. Chronic bronchitis, bronchiectasis, lung abscess, and pleural effusion are other clinical syndromes related to paragonimiasis. Examination of the sputum provides the opportunity for finding the characteristic operculated eggs (possessing a lid).

66. What is a Simon focus?

During primary infection with *Mycobacterium tuberculosis,* apical and subapical pulmonary foci may undergo necrosis at the time that delayed hypersensitivity develops. These foci may then develop tiny calcific deposits, within which latent but viable mycobacteria persist. These foci can later reactivate.

67. What is Pott's disease?

Percival Pott, an English surgeon, first wrote the classic description of the disease that bears his name in 1779. It refers to spinal tuberculosis.

68. What are the clinical features of genitourinary tuberculosis?

Clinical Features of Genitourinary Tuberculosis

Sterile pyuria	50%
Painless hematuria	40%
Fever	10%
Perinephric abscess	10%
Positive sputum culture	20–40%
Positive urine culture	80%

Smith AM, Lattimer JK: Genitourinary tract involvement in children with tuberculosis. NY State J Med 73:2325, 1973.

69. What is Poncet's disease?

Poncet's disease is a polyarticular arthritis that occurs during active *Mycobacterium tuberculosis* infection, in which no infections or other cause of the arthritis can be demonstrated. *M. tuberculosis* cannot be isolated from the affected joint spaces. The disorder is thought to have an immunological basis.

Dall L, et al: Poncet's disease: Tuberculous rheumatism. Rev Infect Dis 11:105–107, 1989.

70. What is the most important prognostic factor in tuberculous meningitis?

The patient's neurologic exam at clinical presentation appears to indicate what the outcome will be. Patients who are stuporous or hemiplegic have a mortality rate of approximately 80%. Patients with only meningismus and fever have a mortality rate of approximately 5–9%. Patients with a severe neurologic deficit should probably receive steroids.

Ogawa SK, et al: Tuberculous meningitis in an urban medical center. Medicine 66:317–326, 1982.

71. What is the differential diagnosis of eosinophilic meningitis?

- Central nervous system infection caused by parasites *(Toxoplasma gondii, Trypanosoma* sp., *Trichinella spiralis, Toxocara canis, Toxocara cati, Taenia solium, Fasciola hepatica, Paragonimus westermani, Angiostrongylus cantonensis,* and *Gnathostoma spinigerum)*
- *Mycobacterium tuberculosis*
- Fungi *(Coccidioides immitis* and *Histoplasma capsulatum)*
- Viruses (lymphocytic choriomeningitis [LCM] virus)
- Rickettsiae
- Neoplasia (leukemia, lymphoma, and meningeal tumors)
- Multiple sclerosis
- Hypereosinophilic syndrome
- Collagen vascular disease
- Allergic reaction to foreign body or direct instillation of drugs or contrast agents into the CSF
- Drug allergy (e.g., ibuprofen, ciprofloxacin).

Asperilla MO, et al: Eosinophilic meningitis associated with ciprofloxacin. Am J Med 87:589–590, 1989.

72. What percentage of patients with tuberculous meningitis will have a positive purified protein derivative (PPD) skin test?

The PPD skin test is positive in 50–95% of patients with tuberculous meningitis. Stated another way, the PPD is negative in up to 50% of patients with tuberculous meningitis.

Molavi A, LeFrock JL: Tuberculous meningitis. Med Clin North Am 69:315–331, 1985.

73. What are the three major clinical syndromes associated with *Aspergillus* sp. and how are they treated?

Aspergillus sp. may cause three clinical syndromes:

1. Allergic bronchopulmonary aspergillosis (ABPA), which is treated with cortico-steroids.

2. Aspergilloma (fungus ball), which is not treated unless complications such as significant hemoptysis warrant surgical resection.

3. Invasive aspergillosis, which is treated with antifungal therapy (amphotericin B) with or without surgical debridement.

74. The majority of cases of Rocky Mountain spotted fever (RMSF) occur in what region of the U.S.?

The majority of cases in the U.S. occur in the South Atlantic states. Despite its name, very few cases of RMSF occur in the Rocky Mountain states.

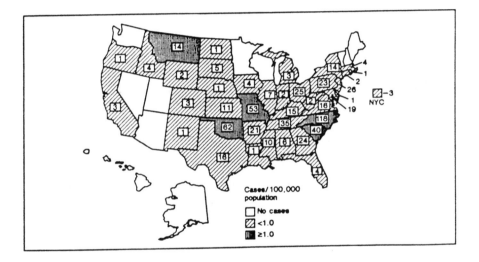

Reported cases and rates of Rocky Mountain spotted fever, by state—United States, 1989. (From Centers for Disease Control: Rocky Mountain spotted fever and human ehrliciosis, United States, 1989. MMWR 39(17):281–284, 1990.)

75. What is the Fitz-Hugh–Curtis syndrome and what organisms cause it?

The Fitz-Hugh-Curtis syndrome is a perihepatitis usually caused by either *Neisseria gonorrhoeae* or *Chlamydia trachomatis* and is thought to occur by spread of organisms from the fallopian tubes to the surface of the liver. This should be considered one of the causes of right-upper-quadrant pain in young, sexually active persons. It occasionally has been reported in males, probably as a result of bacteremic spread.

76. Are fever patterns helpful in establishing the cause of the fever?

There have been multiple classifications of fever patterns. For the most part, the pattern of fever is not helpful in establishing its cause. Two exceptions are fever secondary to cyclic neutropenia and fever secondary to malaria. Patients with cyclic neutropenia have fevers every 3 weeks, coincident with their neutropenia. Patients with malaria may have paroxysms of fever every 2 or 3 days, depending on the infecting parasite.

77. Which organisms most commonly cause infectious complications after a human bite?
Streptococci (alpha and Group A beta hemolytic), *Staphylococcus aureus, Eikenella corrodens, Peptostreptococcus* sp., *Bacteroides* sp., and *Fusobacterium* sp. are the most common organisms cultured from human bite wounds.

78. Which other organisms should be considered after dog or cat bites?
Pasteurella multocida and *Capnocytophagia canimorsus* (DF-2) may cause infection after dog or cat bites. Several other pathogens have been transmitted after bites by these animals, including rabies, tularemia (cats), brucellosis (dogs), EF-4 (dogs), and blastomycosis (dogs).

79. What is the Jarisch-Herxheimer reaction?
It is a self-limited systemic reaction that occurs within 1–2 hours after the initial treatment of syphilis with antimicrobial agents. It is particularly common in patients treated for secondary syphilis but can occur with treatment of any stage. The reaction consists of a rather abrupt and dramatic onset of chills, fever, myalgias, tachycardia, hyperventilation, vasodilation with associated flushing, and mild hypotension. It is probably due to the release of endotoxin or other pyrogens from the spirochetes.

80. Which agents should be considered in the differential diagnosis of necrotizing pneumonia?
Staphylococcus aureus, aerobic gram-negative bacilli (excluding *H. influenzae*), and anaerobes are the most likely agents to cause necrotizing pneumonia. *Aspergillus* sp. and *Mycobacterium tuberculosis* may also cause this clinical picture.

81. What is typhlitis?
Typhlitis is a necrotizing enterocolitis that may be seen in patients who are severely neutropenic from any cause. Signs and symptoms may mimic acute appendicitis with fever, and abdominal pain with rebound tenderness. The involved bowel, usually the cecum and terminal ileum, is edematous and has discrete areas of ulceration. It is thought that the bacteria that make up the normal gut flora are able to invade, proliferate, and produce local destruction due to the absence of neutrophils.
   Steinberg D, et al: Necrotizing enterocolitis in leukemia. Arch Intern Med 131:538–544, 1973.

82. What is blackwater fever?
Blackwater fever refers to the dark-colored urine ("black water") associated with the clinical syndrome of acute and massive hemolysis seen during *Plasmodium falciparum* malaria. It may be etiologically related to the therapeutic use of quinine.

83. Which species of malaria is associated with the occurrence of febrile paroxysms every 72 hours?
Febrile paroxysms occur every 72 hours during infection with *Plasmodium malariae.* The other species of malaria that infect man, *P. vivax, P. ovale,* and *P. falciparum,* have 48-hour erythrocyte cycles and therefore a 48-hour fever pattern.

84. Which species of malaria have exoerythrocytic stages from which late relapses may occur if not adequately treated?
P. vivax and *P. ovale* have exoerythrocytic stages in the liver from which relapse may occur months to years later.

85. What causes "swimmer's itch"?
Swimmer's itch is caused by the schistosome cercariae of several avian and mammalian hosts. Migratory birds, particularly ducks, harbor the adult worms and deposit the

organism in fresh water where snails become infected. Cercariae break out of the snails and penetrate the skin of warm-blooded animals. The cercariae are walled off and destroyed in the skin and evoke an acute inflammatory response that results in the associated pruritus.

86. What are Osler's nodes and in what situations may they be seen?
Osler's nodes are small, painful, nodular lesions (2–15 mm in size) that usually appear in the pads of the fingers or toes. They may be seen in association with infective endocarditis (subacute), gonococcal infections, marantic endocarditis, hemolytic anemia, systemic lupus erythematosus (SLE), and intra-arterial lines (distal to the cannulation site).

87. Which organism is associated with the consumption of water chestnuts?
The intestinal fluke *Fasciolopsis buski,* which is endemic in the Far East and Southeast Asia, causes infection in individuals who have ingested water chestnuts on which the metacercaria have encysted. The principal host of *F. buski* is the pig.

88. Extrusion of "sulfur granules" from a draining wound are characteristic of what infection?
Infection with *Actinomyces* sp. characteristically form external sinuses that discharge "sulfur granules." These consist of conglomerate masses of branching filaments of the organism cemented together and mineralized by host calcium phosphate stimulated by tissue inflammation.

89. What are the most common causes of bacterial meningitis in the adult?
S. pneumoniae is the most common cause of bacterial meningitis in the adult, followed by *N. meningitidis* and *H. influenzae.* The proportion of disease caused by other gram-negative bacilli has been increasing in recent years, whereas those cases due to staphylococci and other streptococci have been decreasing. In adults over the age of 60, *Listeria monocytogenes* becomes the second or third most common cause of meningitis.

90. How often is the Gram stain likely to be positive in patients with bacterial meningitis?
The Gram stain of the CSF in patients with bacterial meningitis demonstrates the etiologic agent in the majority of cases. The following table demonstrates the sensitivity of the Gram stain for each pathogen:

Organism	Positive (%)
N. meningitidis	66
S. pneumoniae	83
H. influenzae	76
L. monocytogenes	42

91. Rhinocerebral mucormycosis occurs most commonly in what setting?
Rhinocerebral mucormycosis is a rare fungal infection that occurs almost exclusively in patients with diabetes mellitus, particularly when poorly controlled or with ketoacidosis. Occasional cases have been described in patients with hematologic neoplasms, renal insufficiency, and in infants with severe diarrhea. The disease is characterized by black, necrotic lesions of the palate or nasal mucous membranes that rapidly involve the paranasal sinuses with extension into the brain. The organism has a particular predisposition to invade vascular structures.

Lehrer RI, et al: Mucormycosis. Ann Intern Med 93:93–108, 1980.

92. The intermediate stage of which tapeworm causes the clinical syndrome of cysticercosis?
Cysticercus cellulosae is the intermediate stage of *Taenia solium,* the pork tapeworm, and causes the clinical syndrome of cysticercosis.

93. Why are antistreptolysin O (ASO) antibodies of little help in the diagnosis of cutaneous infections by *Streptococcus pyogenes*?

The ASO response after skin infections is weak. This is probably a result of inactivation of streptolysin O by skin lipids. Antibody responses to DNAse B are brisk, as is the response to hyaluronidase. Antibodies to the latter two substances can be helpful in the serodiagnosis of streptococcal skin infections.

94. What is the most common cause of secondary pneumonia following illness due to influenza?

Streptococcus pneumoniae is the most common pathogen that causes pneumonia after influenza virus infection. However, the incidence of pneumonia caused by *S. aureus* is also increased. Therefore, this agent must also be considered when treating a patient with this clinical syndrome.

95. What are the symptoms of scombroid fish poisoning and what causes it?

Scombroid, or histamine fish poisoning, is characterized by symptoms of a histamine reaction: flushing, headache, nausea, vomiting, abdominal cramps, diarrhea, and dizziness. It is thought to be due to histamine formed in the fish meat, in addition to the presence of substances that inhibit the degradation of histamine.

Marrow JD, et al: Evidence that histamine is the causative toxin of scombroid fish poisoning. N Engl J Med 324:716–720, 1991.

96. What are the symptoms of ciguatera fish poisoning and what causes it?

Ciguatera fish poisoning is characterized by the onset of nausea, vomiting, diarrhea, abdominal cramps, and numbness or paresthesias of the structures of the oropharynx 1–6 hours following the ingestion of "poisoned" fish. Other symptoms may also be present, including shooting pains in the legs and pain in the teeth. It is caused by accumulation of ciguatoxin in the fish from the food chain. The source of the toxin in the food chain is a dinoflagellate *(Gambierdiscus toxicus).* The illness may last for days to months.

97. Which infectious diseases are associated with raw shellfish ingestion?

Raw shellfish may be the source of a number of pathogens. Viral diseases that may be acquired after raw shellfish ingestion include hepatitis A and Norwalk virus gastroenteritis. Bacterial pathogens include *Vibrio* sp. (cholera and noncholera), and, less commonly, *Campylobacter* sp., *Salmonella* sp., *Shigella* sp., and *E. coli.*

Eastaugh J, et al: Infectious and toxic syndromes from fish and shellfish consumption. Arch Intern Med 149:1735–1740, 1989.

98. What group of patients develops keratitis due to *Acanthamoeba*?

Acanthamoeba species cause a severe and difficult-to-treat keratitis in individuals who wear soft contact lenses. The incidence is much higher in those individuals who prepare their own saline solution and also in persons who wear their lenses in lakes and swimming pools.

Stehr-Green JK, et al: *Acanthamoeba* keratitis in soft-contact wearers: A case control study. JAMA 258:57–60, 1987.

99. What causes acute hemorrhagic conjunctivitis?

Acute hemorrhagic conjunctivitis is caused by enterovirus 70 and coxsackie A24 viruses. It is characterized by ocular pain, swelling of the eyelids, and subconjunctival hemorrhage. The incubation period is 1 day and the duration of illness is approximately 1 week. These facts distinguish it from adenovirus infection (epidemic keratoconjunctivitis), which has an incubation period of 5–7 days and may have symptoms present for 2–3 weeks.

100. What is the "hyperinfection" syndrome associated with *Strongyloides stercoralis*?

Hyperinfection syndrome due to *Strongyloides stercoralis* is the result of systemic dissemination by the filariform larval stage of the organism. This usually occurs in individuals who are immunocompromised, primarily due to defects in cell-mediated immunity. Such patients present with abdominal pain, diarrhea, vomiting, shock, fever, cough, and decreased mental status. Bacteremia is a frequent accompanying event, usually with enteric organisms, which are thought to accompany the larva as they migrate through the bowel wall.

Igra-Siegman Y, et al: Syndrome of hyperinfection with *Strongyloides stercoralis*. Rev Infect Dis 3:397–407, 1981.

101. How may the chills associated with the infusion of amphotericin B be treated?

IV meperidine (Demerol) is an effective treatment for the rigors associated with the administration of amphotericin B. Dantrolene, given orally or IV, is also said to be effective in anecdotal reports, but controlled studies of this therapy have not been reported.

102. What are hepatitis C and hepatitis E?

Hepatitis C and hepatitis E are two of the non-A, non-B hepatitis viruses. Hepatitis C is an RNA virus that is spread in a manner similar to the hepatitis B virus (by the parenteral route). It is probably the major cause of hepatitis associated with the administration of blood products. Hepatitis E is also an RNA virus, but it is spread in a manner more like the hepatitis A virus (by the fecal-oral route). It is a significant cause of epidemic hepatitis in Asia and Africa, and is increased in severity in pregnant women.

103. What is the window period during hepatitis B infection?

The window period occurs during acute infection when the patient no longer has detectable hepatitis B surface antigen (HB$_s$Ag) and does not yet have detectable antibody to the surface antigen (anti-HB$_s$Ag). However, the patient will have antibody to the core antigen (anti-HB$_c$) and should develop anti-HB$_s$Ag in the following month.

104. What is the delta agent and what condition is necessary for it to cause infection in man?

The delta agent is a defective RNA virus and is the causative agent of hepatitis D. It requires the presence of hepatitis B surface antigen for infection to occur, so that it is seen as a co-infection with acute hepatitis B infection or as a superinfection in a chronic carrier of hepatitis B. It is generally spread by the parenteral route in the U.S., but other modes of spread seem to occur in other parts of the world.

105. What are the infectious causes of parotitis?

Acute Viral Parotitis	Acute Suppurative Parotitis
Mumps virus	*Staphylococcus aureus*
Influenza	*Streptococcus pneumoniae*
Parainfluenza types 1 and 3	Enteric gram-negative bacilli
Coxsackie A and B	*Haemophilus influenzae*
ECHO	*Actinomyces* sp.
Lymphocytic choriomeningitis	*Mycobacterium tuberculosis*
	Anaerobic organisms
	Salmonella typhosa

McAnally T: Parotitis. Clinical presentations and management. Postgrad Med 71:87–99, 1982.

106. Which infectious agent occurs in nursery workers who handle sphagnum moss?

Outbreaks of sporotrichosis (lymphocutaneous infection due to *Sporothrix schenkii*) have occurred in nursery and forestry workers handling seedlings packed in sphagnum moss.

Disease has also been associated with contaminated hay, timbers, and thorny bushes, such as roses. It is a subacute or chronic mycosis of the skin and regional lymphatics. It occurs after the percutaneous introduction of *Sporothrix schenkii*. The source of the trauma that allowed entry of the organism may not be reported by the patient or be evident on physical examination.

Powell KE, et al: Cutaneous sporotrichosis in forestry workers. Epidemic due to contaminated sphagnum moss. JAMA 240:232, 1978.

107. What are the most common causes of infection in the first month following solid organ transplantation?

Infections in the first month following solid organ transplantation generally are not secondary to immunosuppression; they are the infections seen in most postoperative patients. Hence, urinary tract infections; pneumonia due to gram-negative bacilli, *Staphylococcus aureus*, or aspiration; bacteremia (catheter-related); and wound infections are most commonly seen. Herpes simplex infections, usually due to reactivation, may also be seen during this time, and pre-existing infections may be first recognized during this time (e.g., strongyloidiasis, tuberculosis, or systemic mycoses).

108. What are the most common pathogens in the second to sixth month following solid organ transplantation?

The pathogens seen during the second to sixth month following solid organ transplantation are more typical of the pathogens seen in immunocompromised hosts. Viral pathogens include cytomegalovirus, Epstein-Barr virus, varicella-zoster virus, papovavirus (BK and JC), and adenovirus. Herpes simplex virus infections continue to be a problem, and non-A, non-B hepatitis is seen during this period. Other pathogens include the following: aspergillus, nocardia, toxoplasma, cryptococcus, *Pneumocystis carinii*, legionella, and *Listeria monocytogenes*.

109. Which infectious diseases have been reported to be transmitted by blood transfusion?

Several infectious agents may be transmitted by blood transfusion. The most common transmissible pathogens are viruses, but other agents have also been implicated. Infectious agents that have been identified as being transmitted by blood transfusions include the following:

- Hepatitis A, hepatitis B, hepatitis D
- Non-A, non-B hepatitis (including hepatitis C)
- HTLV-1, HIV-1, HIV-2
- Cytomegalovirus (CMV), Epstein-Barr virus (EBV)
- Syphilis
- Babesiosis
- Toxoplasmosis
- Malaria
- American trypanosomiasis (Chagas disease).

Berkman SA: Infectious complications of blood transfusion. Blood Reviews 2:206–210, 1988.

110. What is a chagoma?

A chagoma (from Chagas) is the lesion caused by replication of *Trypanosoma cruzi* at the site of inoculation, i.e., at the site of the reduviid bug bite.

111. *Vibrio vulnificus* has been described primarily with which two clinical syndromes?

1. A cutaneous localized cellulitis after a localized inoculation.
2. A high-mortality sepsis syndrome with bacteremia usually after raw-oyster ingestion, seen in immunocompromised patients, especially cirrhotics.

Bouner JB, et al: Spectrum of Vibrio infections. Ann Intern Med 99:464, 1983.

112. What is erythema chronicum migrans (ECM), and why is it significant?

ECM is the skin rash that results from infection due to *Borrelia burgdorferi*, the causative agent of Lyme disease. The rash begins as a macule or papule at the site of an *Ixodes* tick bite, 4 to 20 days after the bite. Usually, it is located on the trunk or proximal extremity and is characterized by an erythematous border with central clearing. Skin lesions are often associated with systemic symptoms such as malaise, fatigue, headache, stiff neck, and fever.

Meyerhoff J: Lyme disease. Am J Med 75:663–670, 1983.

113. Which infections are seen in individuals associated with cats?

Toxoplasmosis	Cat scratch disease
Hookworm	Pasteurellosis (bite wound, usually)
Rabies	Toxocariasis (visceral larval migrans)
Strongyloidiasis	Tularemia
Dermatomycoses	

Elliot DL, et al: Pet-associated illness. N Engl J Med 313:985–995, 1985.

114. What is the bacteriology of clenched-fist injuries?

Bacteria isolated from clenched-fist injuries usually reflect those of the mouth or skin inoculated into the wound and consist of the following:

Aerobic bacteria:	Anaerobic bacteria:
Streptococcus (alpha-hemolytic; beta-hemolytic, group A and non-group A; gamma-hemolytic	*Acidaminococcus* sp.
	B. melaninogenicus
	B. oralis
S. aureus	*B. intermedius*
S. epidermidis	*B. ureolyticus*
E. corrodens	*B. ruminicola*
Neisseria sp.	*Bacteroides* sp. (non-*fragilis*)
Moraxella sp.	*Clostridium* sp.
H. influenzae	*Eubacterium* sp.
H. parainfluenzae	*F. nucleatum*
H. aphrophilus	*Peptococcus prevotii*
E. cloacae	*Peptococcus magnus*
Enterobacter sp.	*Peptostreptococcus anaerobius*
K. pneumoniae	*Peptostreptococcus micros*
Corynebacterium sp.	*Veillonella* sp.

(From Goldstein EJC: Clenched-fist injury infections. Infect Surg July, 1986, pp 384–390, with permission.)

115. What causes hand-foot-mouth disease and what are the clinical findings of this disease?

Hand-foot-mouth disease may be caused by a number of viruses in the picornavirus family. It has been most associated with coxsackie A16, but outbreaks have also been attributed to coxsackie A4, A5, A9, A10, B2, B5, and enterovirus 71. It is characterized by an ulcerative exanthem, usually occurring on the buccal mucosa, which is followed by a vesicular exanthem involving the hands and feet.

116. Which arm of the immune system is inhibited by corticosteroids, and what are the infectious consequences?

Corticosteroids predominantly influence cell-mediated immunity by interfering with mononuclear cell migration and bactericidal capacities. The consequences are increased numbers of infections with organisms that are normally controlled through cell-mediated immune mechanisms:

Viruses	Bacteria
Herpes simplex	Legionella species
Varicella-zoster virus	Salmonella species
Cytomegalovirus	Mycobacteria species
JC virus	*Listeria monocytogenes*
Fungi	**Parasites**
Cryptococcus neoformans	*Pneumocystis carinii*
Histoplasma capsulatum	*Strongyloides stercoralis*
Coccidioides immitis	*Toxoplasma gondii*

Fauci AS, et al: Glucocorticosteroid therapy: Mechanisms of action and clinical considerations. Ann Intern Med 84:304–315, 1976.

117. Which infectious diseases are associated with fecal leukocytes?
Fecal polymorphonuclear leukocytes (PMNs) are seen with:

Shigella
Enteroinvasive *Escherichia coli*
Salmonella enteritidis
Vibrio parahemolyticus
Clostridium difficile
Campylobacter jejuni
Entamoeba histolytica

Fecal mononuclear leukocytes are seen with:

Salmonella typhi
Yersinia enterocolitica
Campylobacter fetus

Guerrant RL: Principles and syndromes of enteric infection. In Mandell GL, et al (ed): Principles and Practice of Infectious Diseases, 3rd ed. New York, Churchill Livingstone, 1990, pp 837–851.

118. What is the differential diagnosis for fever and pulmonary infiltrates in a patient with Hodgkin's disease?
Patients with Hodgkin's disease can be infected with the normal respiratory pathogens such as *Streptococcus pneumoniae,* particularly following courses of chemotherapy. Classically, these patients are infected with organisms that are normally controlled by cell-mediated immunity:

Viruses	Bacteria
CMV	*Legionella* sp.
Adenovirus	*Nocardia* sp.
Herpes simplex virus	*Mycobacterium tuberculosis*
Fungi	**Parasites**
Cryptococcus neoformans	*Pneumocystis carinii*
Histoplasma capsulatum	*Strongyloides stercoralis*

In addition, noninfectious entities such as tumor invasion, hemorrhage, radiation pneumonitis, and drug reactions have to be considered.

Rosenow EC III, et al: Pulmonary disease in the immunocompromised host. Mayo Clin Proc 60:473–487, 610–631, 1985.

119. Which infectious agents have been implicated in cervical carcinoma?
Cancer of the cervix behaves epidemiologically as if it were a sexually transmitted disease. Strong epidemiologic associations exist between cervical infections with herpes simplex virus and *Chlamydia trachomatis*. However, the strongest association exists with infection due to human papillomavirus (HPV). HPV types 16 and 18 have the strongest link with subsequent malignancy.

120. What are the predisposing factors for the development of pyogenic liver abscess?
Fortunately, pyogenic liver abscesses are uncommon despite the frequency of intra-abdominal infections. The causes can be categorized by the following schema:

    a. Biliary: calculus, stricture, or tumor
    b. Portal: appendicitis, diverticulitis, or inflammatory bowel disease in the bed of the portal circulation (which may be associated with pylephlebitis, or inflammation of the portal vein)
    c. Contiguous structure infection: gallbladder
    d. Hematogenous spread via the hepatic artery
    e. Penetrating and nonpenetrating wounds of the liver
    f. Cryptogenic

Biliary disease is now the most common underlying condition. About one-fourth of cases are cryptogenic.

    Rubin RH, et al: Hepatic abscess: Changes in clinical, bacteriologic and therapeutic aspects. Am J Med 57:601–610, 1974.

121. What are the infectious causes of an eosinophilic pleural effusion?
    1. Bacterial pneumonia (usually *S. pneumoniae*)
    2. Fungi: *Cryptococcus neoformans, Histoplasma capsulatum,* and *Coccidioides immitis*
    3. *Mycobacterium tuberculosis*

Some authors feel that pleural fluid eosinophilia offers no help in differential diagnosis. Other common associations with eosinophils in the pleural fluid are with spontaneous pneumothorax or after repeated thoracenteses.

    Light RW, et al: Cells in pleural fluid. Arch Intern Med 132:854–860, 1973.

122. What are the two types of bone marrow toxicity associated with the use of chloramphenicol?
One form of toxicity is a reversible bone marrow suppression due to the inhibition of mitochondrial protein synthesis. It can be manifested by reticulocytopenia, anemia, leukopenia, or thrombocytopenia. Vacuolization of erythroid and myeloid precursors will be seen in the bone marrow. This form of toxicity is dose-related and seen most frequently in patients receiving more than 4 grams per day.

    The second type of toxicity is an idiosyncratic response, frequently manifested as an aplastic anemia. It is estimated to occur once in 25,000–40,000 patients who receive chloramphenicol. It may occur weeks to months after cessation of the drug.

123. Which viral illnesses are more severe in pregnancy?
Pregnant patients have been noted to have increased morbidity and/or mortality from infections due to varicella, influenza, hepatitis C, poliovirus, and measles. Rubella, while associated with increased fetal defects, has not been noted to be more severe in pregnancy.

124. What is the significance of the presence of a methylthiotetrazole (MTT) side chain in certain cephalosporins and which cephalosporins have one?
Methylthiotetrazole side chains are associated with an increased risk of bleeding after antibiotic administration and with the occurrence of disulfiram-like reactions after ethanol ingestion. Cefamandole, cefoperazone, cefotetan, and moxalactam all have MTT side chains.

125. Other than a history of allergy to the antibiotic, what is the most important contraindication to the use of imipenem?
Seizures occur in up to 1% of patients on imipenem. Patients with a history of pre-existing seizure disorder, recent head trauma, or chronic alcoholism are at increased risk for this

complication. Seizures are also seen in patients with renal failure when the dose is not adjusted. Treatment consists of withdrawal of the drug and anticonvulsants.

126. What are the two most important drug-drug interactions associated with ciprofloxacin?
Coadministration of ciprofloxacin with theophylline may result in an increase in theophylline levels and theophylline toxicity. Magnesium- and aluminum-containing antacids will decrease the bioavailability of ciprofloxacin when they are administered simultaneously. This may cause the peak serum levels to be in the subtherapeutic range for an otherwise susceptible organism.

127. What are important drug-drug interactions associated with erythromycin?
Erythromycin alters the metabolism of a number of drugs, resulting in increased drug effect and possible toxicity. These drugs include the oral anticoagulants, carbamazepine, phenytoin, corticosteroids, cyclosporine, theophylline, digoxin, and ergot alkaloids.

128. What are the mechanisms of resistance to acyclovir?
Acyclovir triphosphate is a potent inhibitor of viral DNA polymerase. It enters the infected cell as acyclovir and is phosphorylated to a monophosphate by viral thymidine kinase (TK). Further phosphorylation is accomplished by cellular enzymes. The major mechanism of resistance is alteration in viral TK. Alterations in the DNA polymerase as a cause of resistance are much less common.

129. In what percentage of patients with symptomatic giardiasis can the diagnosis be made by stool examination for the parasite?
The diagnosis of giardiasis can usually be made by careful examination of the stool for trophozoites or cysts. The diagnosis is confirmed 50–70% of the time after only one stool examination and over 90% of the time after examination of three stool specimens.

130. An immigrant from Mexico who presents with a seizure disorder and is found to have multiple, small, ring-like lesions on a CT of the head is likely to have what disorder?
Neurocysticercosis. This is the invasion of the human CNS by the larval form of the pork tapeworm, *Taenia solium*. CT scans typically demonstrate cystic lesions that do not usually enhance with contrast, and in many cases hydrocephalus is also seen. It is the most common cerebral parasitic infection in man.

   Loo L, et al: Cerebral cysticercosis in San Diego. Medicine 61:344–359, 1982.

131. What are the etiologic agents of the sexually transmitted diseases chancroid, lymphogranuloma venereum, and granuloma inguinale?
Chancroid:	*Haemophilus ducreyi*
Lymphogranuloma venereum:	*Chlamydia trachomatis*, serovars L1–3
Granuloma inguinale:	*Calymmatobacterium granulomatis*

132. What percent of older patients with salmonella bacteremia will have an endovascular source of infection?
Approximately 25% of patients over the age of 50 years will have an endovascular source of infection. Salmonella organisms tend to "seed" abnormal tissues (hematomas, tumors, cysts, stones, and altered endothelia such as aortic aneurysms) during bacteremia.

   Cohen OS, et al: The risk of endothelial infection in adults with *Salmonella* bacteremia. Ann Intern Med 89:931, 1978.

133. What is the serologic response to Epstein-Barr virus infection?

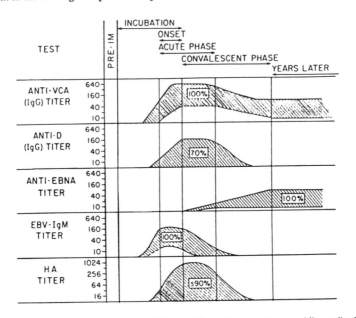

Antibody response to Epstein-Barr virus (EBV) specific antigens and heterophile antibodies as a function of time following primary infection. EBNA, Epstein-Barr nuclear antigens; HA, heterophile antibody; VCA, viral capsid antigens; ANTI-D, anti-early antigen, diffuse component; ANTI-EBNA, anti-Epstein-Barr nuclear antigen; EBV IgM, antiviral capsid antigen IgM antibody. (From Schooley RT: Chronic fatigue syndrome: A manifestation of Epstein-Barr virus infection? In Remington JS, Swartz MN (eds): Current Clinical Topics in Infectious Disease, Vol. 9. New York, McGraw-Hill, 1988, pp 126–146, with permission.)

This curve represents the typical sequence of serologic events following exposure to the Epstein-Barr virus. The incubation period ranges from 30–50 days. Antibody to viral capsid antigen (difficult to detect in some labs) can be demonstrated at the time of clinical presentation and is diagnostic of acute infection. The anti-Epstein-Barr virus nuclear antigen (anti-EBNA) characteristically occurs 3–4 weeks after the onset of clinical illness. Both the anti-VCA and anti-EBNA antibodies are present lifelong following infection.

(From Schooley RT: Chronic fatigue syndrome: A manifestation of Epstein-Barr virus infection? In Remington JS, Swartz MN (eds): Current Clinical Topics in Infectious Disease, Vol. 9. New York, McGraw-Hill, 1988, pp 126–146, with permission.)

134. Are *Listeria monocytogenes* infections usually associated with a peripheral blood monocytosis?

No, only rarely. The initial isolate was from a patient with a mononucleosis-like syndrome. In experimental animals (rabbits), monocytosis is frequently the rule.

135. Which four organisms may be confused with *Listeria monocytogenes,* either on Gram stain or on blood agar plates?

1. *Corynebacterium* species
2. β-hemolytic streptococci
3. Enterococcus
4. *Streptococcus pneumoniae*

One should always make certain this organism is not overlooked in clinical specimens submitted to the laboratory, especially spinal fluid.

136. How is disease due to *Corynebacterium diphtheriae* produced?

Certain strains of *C. diphtheriae*, when infected by a lysogenic bacteriophage, produce a toxin that enters cells and interrupts protein synthesis, resulting in neuritis and myocarditis.

137. What are the manifestations of human infection by *Dirofilaria immitis*, the dog tapeworm?

Most commonly, infection with *D. immitis* manifests as a solitary, noncalcified lung nodule less than 2 cm in diameter. Man is an unsuitable host for the development of the larvae to adulthood. Consequently, they die and embolize to the lung, where release of antigens leads to an endarteritis with subsequent distal pulmonary infarction.

Risher WH, et al: Pulmonary dirofilariasis. The largest single institution experience. J Thorac Cardiovasc Surg 97:303–308, 1989.

138. Infection with *Chlamydia psittaci* should be considered an occupational hazard of what groups of individuals?

The disease occurs in pet-shop employees, pigeon fanciers, zoo workers, veterinarians, and employees of poultry-processing plants. It is one of the causes of the atypical pneumonias.

139. What is the differential diagnosis of atypical lymphocytosis?

Differential Diagnosis of Atypical Lymphocytosis

Rubella	Epstein-Barr virus-induced mononucleosis
Roseola	Cytomegalovirus infections
Toxoplasmosis	Acute viral hepatitis
Mumps	Drug interactions

140. What is erythema nodosum leprosum?

Erythema nodosum leprosum is a complication of therapy seen in patients with the full lepromatous (LL) form of leprosy. It occurs most commonly within the first year of treatment. The problem is manifested as nodular skin lesions that histopathologically resemble Arthus-type reactions with localized vasculitis in the veins and arteries. The vasculitis is characterized by polymorphonuclear leukocytic and eosinophilic infiltrates. Erythema nodosum leprosum may also be associated with neuritis, polyarthritis, and immune-complex glomerulonephritis.

Jacobson RR, et al: The diagnosis and treatment of leprosy. South Med J 69:979–985, 1976.

141. What is the minimum inhibitory concentration (MIC)? What is the minimum bactericidal concentration (MBC)?

The MIC represents the minimum concentration of a given antibiotic that will inhibit the growth of a given pathogen but will not kill it. It is usually expressed in micrograms per milliliter. The MBC represents the minimum concentration of a given antibiotic that will kill a given pathogen.

142. What are the sites and mechanisms of action of the various classes of antibiotics? Which are bactericidal and which are bacteriostatic?

Mechanism of Action of Antimicrobial Agents

CLASS	SITE OF ACTION	EFFECT	CIDAL	STATIC
Penicillins, cephalosporins	Cell wall	Inhibit cross-linking of peptidoglycan, resulting in spheroplast formation	+	occ.*
Vancomycin	Cell wall	Block transfer of pentapeptide from cytoplasm to cell membrane	+	occ.
Polymyxin B, colistin	Cytoplasmic membrane	Bind phospholipid and disrupt cell membrane	+	
Aminoglycosides	Ribosome	Bind to 30^S subunit. thereby inhibiting attachment of messenger RNA; also affects transfer RNA	+	
Tetracyclines	Ribosome	Bind to 30^S subunit and inhibit binding of transfer RNA		+
Chloramphenicol	Ribosome	Bind to 50^S subunit and inhibit messenger RNA translation	occ.	+
Erythromycin, clindamycin	Ribosome	Inhibit messenger RNA translation	occ.	+
Rifampin	Nucleic acid synthesis	Impaired RNA formation by inhibiting DNA-dependent RNA-polymerase	+	occ.
Metronidazole	Nucleic acid synthesis	Damages nucleic acid structure	+	
Quinolones	Nucleic acid synthesis	Inhibit DNA gyrase	+	
Sulfonamides	Nucleic acid synthesis	Competitive inhibition of para-amino benzoic acid, thereby blocking formation of thymidine and purines		+

* occ. = occasionally.
(From Wyngaarden JB, Smith LH (eds): Cecil Textbook of Medicine, 18th ed. Philadelphia, W.B. Saunders, 1988, p 113, with permission.)

BIBLIOGRAPHY

1. Brown HW, Neva FA (eds): Basic Clinical Parasitology, 5th ed. East Norwalk, CT, Appleton & Lange, 1983.
2. Fields BN, Knipe DM (eds): Field's Virology, 2nd ed. New York, Raven Press, 1990.
3. Hoeprich PD, Jordan MC (eds): Infectious Diseases: A Modern Treatise of Infectious Processes, 4th ed. Philadelphia, J.B. Lippincott, 1989.
4. Howard RJ, Simmons RL (eds): Surgical Infectious Diseases, 2nd ed. East Norwalk, CT, Appleton & Lange, 1987.
5. Mandell GL, Douglas RG, Bennett JE (eds): Principles and Practice of Infectious Diseases, 3rd ed. New York, Churchill Livingstone, 1990.
6. Rubin RH, Young LS (eds): Clinical Approach to Infection in the Compromised Host, 2nd ed. New York, Plenum Publishers, 1988.

5. GASTROENTEROLOGY SECRETS

Karen L. Woods, M.D. and Patrice A. Michaletz, M.D.

The longer I live, the more I am convinced that the apothecary is of more importance than Seneca; and that half the unhappiness in the world proceeds from little stoppages, from a duct choked up, from food pressing in the wrong place, from a vexed duodenum or an agitated pylorus.

Sydney Smith (1771–1845)
Quoted by Lady Holland in A Memoir of the Rev. Sydney Smith, Ch. 6.

GASTROINTESTINAL BLEEDING

1. Describe the initial approach to the patient who presents with acute gastrointestinal (GI) bleeding.

The initial approach should include a rapid assessment to gauge the urgency of the situation. It is relatively simple to determine whether or not the patient is hemodynamically stable or unstable (vital signs normal, without a drop upon changing from recumbency to the sitting or standing position, versus orthostatic hypotension and tachycardia). The presence of GI bleeding should be confirmed by inspecting the stool for melena or hematochezia and the nasogastric (NG) aspirate for blood from the upper GI tract.

The site of bleeding can frequently be determined from the patient's complaints. Upper GI bleeding often presents with hematemesis combined with melena. The presence of hematochezia with a negative NG aspirate suggests a lower GI source of bleeding.

During this initial phase, blood should be obtained for a complete blood count (CBC), clotting studies, routine chemistry, and type and cross match, so if transfusions are necessary they can be given without delay. Clearly, the urgency of further management depends upon the results of this initial assessment. If the patient appears hemodynamically stable with minor bleeding, further management can be undertaken electively. However, if there are signs that the patient is having an acute, life-threatening bleed and is in an unstable condition, resuscitation and evaluation for the source must be undertaken immediately. This would include obtaining venous access with a large-bore intravenous (IV) cannula and immediately beginning fluids, such as normal saline or lactated Ringer's, to quickly improve the circulation and restore intravascular volume. Placement of an NG tube to assess rapidity of bleeding and to clear the stomach of blood for endoscopic evaluation should also be done at this time. Close monitoring of vital signs and urinary output in an Intensive Care Unit setting is important. Blood transfusions should be given as indicated for massive bleeding in the patient who is hemodynamically compromised. Once the patient has been stabilized, a search can then be carried out to localize the source of bleeding.

2. What are the common causes of upper GI bleeding?

Common sources of upper GI tract hemorrhage include duodenal ulcer, gastric ulcer, marginal ulcer following gastric ulcer surgery, Cushing's ulcers in the patient who has suffered a major burn or has been in the intensive care unit, esophageal or gastric varices in the cirrhotic patient or those with splenic vein thrombosis, and Mallory-Weiss tears (most commonly seen in the alcoholic population).

3. What questions addressed in history taking and the physical examination can help identify the source of an upper GI bleed?

Important questions that may point to a likely source include:

- Is there a history of prior bleeding episodes?
- Is there a family history of diseases that cause bleeding?
- Are there other superimposed illnesses that may lead to bleeding, such as cirrhosis, carcinoma, coagulopathy, a known connective tissue disorder, or amyloidosis?
- Has the patient had prior surgery of the intestinal tract, such as gastric surgery for peptic ulcer or the placement of an arterial bypass graft?
- Is the patient an alcoholic or does he take ulcerogenic drugs, such as aspirin or other nonsteroidal anti-inflammatory agents?
- Has the patient recently had a caustic ingestion?
- Was the bleeding episode preceded by abdominal pain, dyspepsia, or retching?
- Have there been recent nose bleeds?

4. Is examination of the skin helpful in identifying the source of an upper GI bleed?

The skin examination can be quite helpful for suggesting a potential source if certain stigmata are present. Patients with cirrhosis may have spider angiomata on the anterior chest wall and face. Patients with underlying malignancy may have acanthosis nigricans or cutaneous Kaposi's sarcoma. Hereditary vascular anomalies seen on the skin may also be found within the GI tract. Lymphadenopathy or abdominal masses may suggest sources for intraabdominal pathology.

Peterson WL: Gastrointestinal bleeding. In Sleisenger MH, Fordtran JS (eds): Gastrointestinal Disease, 4th ed. Philadelphia, W.B. Saunders, 1989, pp 397–427.

5. When should endoscopy be performed in a patient with upper GI bleeding?

In the patient with active GI bleeding, endoscopy is the procedure of choice. Endoscopy allows clinical decisions to be made regarding further therapy of the bleeding lesion. Certain types of lesions may lend themselves to primary endoscopic therapy to stop bleeding. Endoscopy should usually be performed within the first 24 hours following admission to the hospital for major upper GI hemorrhage. The timing within that first 24 hours should depend in some respect on the stability of the patient and whether or not bleeding continues during the first several hours in the hospital. Patients who show evidence of ongoing bleeding during resuscitative efforts should have emergent endoscopy while resuscitation is occurring in order to define the source of bleeding and to attempt to institute some form of endoscopic therapy to halt the bleeding.

If it appears the bleeding has stopped, endoscopy can occur electively during more relaxed circumstances after full resuscitation has been achieved.

6. Which therapeutic modalities are available for use during endoscopy?

Endoscopic therapies available include thermal coagulation of bleeding ulcers, which has been shown to reduce the transfusion requirement and the need for emergent surgery, and injection sclerotherapy of esophageal varices and ulcers to stop acute bleeding.

7. What are the common causes of lower GI bleeding?

- **Diverticulosis** accounts for approximately 50% of all cases of lower GI bleeding severe enough to warrant angiographic examination.
- **Angiodysplasia** or **vascular ectasias** are increasingly well recognized causes of lower GI bleeding. They tend to occur most typically in older patients and are commonly found in the cecum and ascending colon.
- **Neoplasms** of the large bowel usually present with chronic occult bleeding but occasionally will acutely bleed.

- **Hemorrhoids** are the most common cause of lower GI bleeding but rarely present with massive bleeding to the point of hospitalization.
- Other less common causes of lower GI bleeding include Meckel's diverticulum, ischemic bowel disease, inflammatory bowel disease, solitary ulcers of the cecum and rectum, and arterial-enteric fistulae.

8. Describe the diagnostic approach to a patient with lower GI bleeding.

A complete history and physical examination may yield important information regarding the source of the bleeding. A history of hemorrhoids, inflammatory bowel disease, preceding crampy abdominal pain (suggesting ischemia), and painless faucet-like bleeding (suggesting a diverticular source) are important points.

The next step should be rigid proctoscopy. Proctoscopy will reveal obvious low-lying lesions such as bleeding hemorrhoids, anal fissures, rectal ulcers, colitis, or rectal tumors. If results are negative and it is clear the patient is bleeding from a lower tract source, the next stop should be colonoscopy, unless the bleeding is too massive to allow preparation and examination.

If the bleeding site is localized at colonoscopy, local endoscopic therapy may be undertaken to achieve hemostasis of certain lesions. If only diverticulosis is found, it is unlikely the endoscopist will be able to localize the specific diverticula that bled; however, the value of the procedure is in ruling out other lesions as the bleeding site.

If the patient is bleeding too rapidly to undergo colonoscopy, or if colonoscopy has been negative and brisk bleeding continues, arteriography should be the next step. With active bleeding, arteriography may reveal the site and localize it to the right or left colon or small bowel. This is extremely helpful in directing the surgeon to the correct location for resection. Additionally, the radiologist may be able to institute therapy by selective infusion of vasopressin or embolization of the bleeding vessel.

There are some circumstances in which the bleeding rate is too slow to yield a positive arteriogram but in which a radionuclide bleeding scan using technicum-99 sulfur colloid would be an effective means of detecting ongoing bleeding. The bleeding scan can be used as a good screen for active bleeding prior to angiography. If the bleeding scan is negative, the yield of arteriography will be low, since the blood pool scan can detect slower bleeding rates than can arteriography.

Any patient with a lower GI bleed in whom an obvious source has not been found should have a diagnostic upper endoscopy to rule out an upper-tract source as the cause of lower-tract bleeding. This should be done before any surgical procedure unless a definite source of the bleeding has been found.

Nath RL, et al: Lower gastrointestinal bleeding. Am J Surg 141:478, 1981.

Britt LG, et al: Selective management of lower gastrointestinal bleeding. Am Surgeon 49:121, 1983.

9. Does melena indicate a right-sided colonic source and hematochezia indicate a left-sided source?

Although right-sided lesions are usually associated with melena (dark, tarry stools) and left-sided lesions are usually associated with hematochezia (the passage of bright red blood per rectum), the opposite can also be seen. Therefore the evaluation of a patient with hematochezia must include examination of the proximal colon.

Fleischer DE, et al: Detection and surveillance of colorectal cancer. JAMA 261:580–586, 1989.

10. What are the possible causes of esophageal varices?

Elevation of pressure in the hepatic portal system leads to the development of varices. This may be due to diseases of the hepatic vasculature (i.e., Budd-Chiari syndrome), portal vein or splenic vein thrombosis, or intrinsic liver disease (i.e., cirrhosis).

11. Which two factors determine whether esophageal varices will develop and whether they will bleed?

Portal pressure and **variceal size** are the two factors that appear to be most important in determining whether varices will develop in the esophagus and whether or not they will bleed. It is known that portal pressure must reach an hepatic vein pressure gradient of approximately 12 mmHg (normal = 3 to 6 mmHg) for varices to develop. Beyond this level there is poor correlation between the portal pressure and the likelihood of bleeding. When varices reach a large size of over 5 mm in diameter, they are more likely to rupture and bleed. This relates to the wall tension of the varices, which is directly proportional to vessel radius and inversely proportional to wall thickness. Therefore, at any given pressure the wall of a large varix is under greater tension than that of a small varix and must be thicker to withstand the pressure.

12. What is the mortality rate of bleeding esophageal varices and the rebleeding rate during hospitalization? What percent will survive greater than 1 year after the index bleed?

The mortality rate for bleeding esophageal varices during the initial hospitalization approaches 30%. This is in part due to the fact that approximately 50 to 70% of patients admitted to the hospital with bleeding varices will experience a rebleeding episode during that hospitalization. At least one-third of patients will rebleed within 6 weeks after discharge from hospital and only one-third will survive beyond the first year following the index bleed.

13. What percentage of patients with upper GI bleeding and known esophageal varices will have a bleeding source other than varices at endoscopy?

In the patient with upper GI bleeding and a strong suspicion of esophageal varices, endoscopy must be performed to determine the site of bleeding, since up to one-third of these patients will be bleeding from a source other than varices. Other common causes of bleeding in patients with varices include Mallory-Weiss tears and peptic ulcers.

14. Describe the therapeutic approach to a patient with bleeding esophageal varices.

In patients with actively bleeding varices, the first line of therapy after volume resuscitation and blood transfusion should include some modality to stop the bleeding. Traditionally, this has included IV vasopressin to reduce splanchnic blood flow and portal venous system pressure, although controlled trials have not proven IV vasopressin's ability to stop the bleeding. Upper endoscopy should be done as soon as possible to document the site of bleeding and perform injection sclerotherapy to stop the bleeding. Using this technique, the endoscopist injects one of several different sclerosing solutions into and around the bleeding varix. This results in rapid occlusion of the varix by thrombus or perivariceal edema so that active bleeding ceases in 80–90% of patients.

If sclerotherapy is unsuccessful, the next step is surgery (either a portasystemic shunt or esophageal transection) or balloon tamponade of the bleeding varices using a Sengstaken-Blakemore tube.

Crotty B, et al: The management of acutely bleeding varices by injection sclerotherapy. Med J Aust 145:130, 1986.

15. How does the Sengstaken-Blakemore tube work?

This tube is a double-balloon system, one of which inflates in the stomach and the other in the esophagus to tamponade the bleeding site. Between 75–90% of patients will stop bleeding using this technique. However, there is a high incidence of complications related to balloon tamponade, including esophageal perforation and pulmonary aspiration. This technique should be reserved for the patient who fails to stop bleeding using standard measures.

16. Which two therapeutic procedures are available to prevent rebleeding in a patient who has bled from varices?

Surgical variceal systemic shunting is designed to divert blood away from the esophageal or gastric veins and from the high pressure portal circulation into the lower pressure systemic circulation. This can be accomplished in one of several ways, including portacaval, splenorenal, and mesocaval shunting.

The second method involves **endoscopic long-term repeated injection sclerotherapy.** This requires the patient to return for endoscopy every 3 to 4 weeks to undergo sclerotherapy of varices until they have been obliterated. Obliteration usually occurs after three to four sessions. Many studies have tried to evaluate the differences in these two therapies as related to mortality, and this remains a point of controversy and to some degree seems to depend upon the patient selected for entry into the study.

Cello JP, et al: Endoscopic sclerotherapy versus portacaval shunt in patients with severe cirrhosis and acute variceal hemorrhage. N Engl J Med 316:11, 1987.

HEPATITIS

17. What are the differences between hepatitis A, hepatitis B, and hepatitis C?

Hepatitis A is often called infectious hepatitis, because it is easily spread by the oral/fecal route. This virus causes a short-lived, benign, acute hepatitis that is not followed by chronic liver disease. IgG antibodies to hepatitis A remain positive for life. To determine if an acute viral hepatitis is hepatitis A, one must look for IgM antibodies in the serum.

Hepatitis B is often called serum hepatitis and is contracted by contact with blood or other bodily secretions from infected individuals, usually through a break in the skin or use of a contaminated needle. This type of hepatitis, unlike hepatitis A, may go on to cause chronic hepatitis and progress to cirrhosis. Hepatitis B infection also predisposes to hepatoma (liver cancer). Some patients may persist in demonstrating a positive hepatitis B surface antigenemia (HBsAg) but do not appear to have clinically evident disease. These patients are considered carriers and are able to transmit the viral disease.

Hepatitis C is the third viral hepatitis group, which has been previously included in non-A, non-B heptatitis and which includes all the viral hepatitides with no measurable serum antigenic markers. It is now known that the form of non-A, non-B hepatitis most commonly contracted from blood transfusion is hepatitis C. This form of hepatitis, similar to hepatitis B, can also cause a chronic disease.

Blood banks worldwide have been checking for hepatitis B markers in donor blood and discarding all units found to be positive. It will soon be feasible to check for hepatitis C markers in donor blood. Screening out blood donors who carry hepatitis C should greatly diminish the incidence of post-transfusion hepatitis.

18. How is hepatitis A viral infection transmitted?

Hepatitis A virus is typically transmitted through contaminated water supplies and is most common in developing countries where poor hygiene and inadequate sanitation are present. There has been no documentation of transplacental or perinatal transmission of the virus. Homosexual men have a higher prevalence of antibodies to hepatitis A, which suggests possible sexual transmission.

19. What are the symptoms and duration of illness in hepatitis A and how is it diagnosed and treated?

The symptoms of hepatitis A are relatively nonspecific and are similar to those due to any cause of hepatitis. These include anorexia, fatigue, malaise, right upper quadrant abdominal discomfort, and jaundice. The duration of illness tends to vary, but most patients recover within 4 weeks of the onset of clinical disease.

Hepatitis A can be diagnosed by the detection of hepatitis A specific IgM in the blood. This antibody is always present when symptoms from hepatitis A are present. Treatment of hepatitis A is purely supportive, and there has been no effective antiviral agent identified that will accelerate recovery.

Mijch AM, et al: Clinical, serologic, and epidemiologic aspects of hepatitis A virus infection. Semin Liver Dis 16:42–45, 1986.

20. How should you treat an adult exposed to hepatitis A at a day care center on the previous day?

After exposure to a person known to have acute hepatitis A, the adult plus his or her house-hold and sexual contacts, as well as other day care center exposures, should receive immunoglobulin for prevention of hepatitis A. This should be administered within 2 days after known contact. The adult dose is 0.02 mg/kg given in a single intramuscular (IM) dose.

Centers for Disease Control: Recommendations for protection against viral hepatitis. MMWR 34:313–335, 1985.

21. What is the incidence of chronic hepatitis following acute hepatitis A infection?

Chronic hepatitis has not been reported to result from acute hepatitis A viral infection. Occasionally, relapsing hepatitis, with recurrence of symptoms and biochemical abnormalities of liver function, may occur 1–4 months following the recovery from the initial infection.

22. What is the usual serologic response after naturally acquired hepatitis B virus infection?

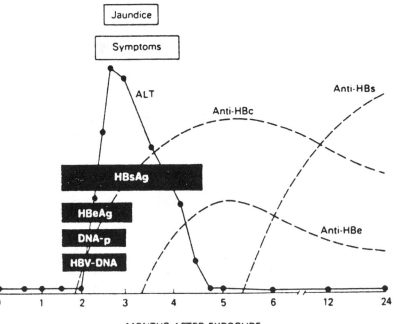

MONTHS AFTER EXPOSURE

The clinical and serologic course of a typical case of acute type B hepatitis. HBsAg: hepatitis B surface antigen; HBeAg: hepatitis B e antigen; DNA-p: DNA polymerase; HBV-DNA: hepatitis B virus DNA; ALT: alanine aminotransferase; Anti-HBc: antibody to hepatitis B core antigen; anti-HBe: antibody to HBeAg; anti-HBs: antibody to HBsAg. (From Hoofnagle JH: Acute viral hepatitis. In Mandell GL, et al (eds): Principles and Practice of Infectious Diseases, 3rd ed. New York, Churchill Livingstone, 1990, p 1007, with permission.)

23. What is the serologic profile of a person who has completed the hepatitis B vaccine protocol?

The currently available hepatitis B vaccine is composed only of hepatitis B surface antigen (HBsAg). The administration of this vaccine induces an antibody response only to HBsAg, and blood tests will reveal anti-HBsAg. The anti-HBsAg response correlates well with protection against hepatitis B virus infection. Of healthy persons vaccinated by the IM route, 95% will develop protection against hepatitis B virus.

Centers for Disease Control: Recommendations for protection against viral hepatitis. MMWR 34:313–335, 1985.

24. What are the differences between chronic active and chronic persistent hepatitis?

Differentiating Features in Chronic Hepatitis

FEATURES	CHRONIC ACTIVE HEPATITIS	CHRONIC PERSISTENT HEPATITIS
Clinical symptoms:		
Fatigue, malaise	Often marked	Mild
Jaundice	Common	Rare
Serum tests:		
Aminotransferases	Usually >60 IU/L; >400 IU/L common	Usually 40–200 IU/L
Bilirubin	Often >3.0 mg/dl, (occasionally >15.0)	<3.0 mg/dl
Gamma globulin	Often markedly elevated (3.0–7.0 g/dl)	Normally or mildly elevated (2.0 g/dl)
Flourescent anti-nuclear antibody	Frequently positive (LE cells in 10–20%)	Rarely positive
HB$_s$Ag	Positive in 10–20%	Positive in 10–20%
Prothrombin time	Often prolonged	Normal
Albumin	Often reduced	Normal
Liver biopsy:		
Spotty necrosis and inflammation	Mild to moderate	Mild
Portal inflammation	Moderate to marked	Mild to marked
Fibrotic septa	Present	Absent
Piecemeal necrosis	Often marked	Absent or minimal
Bridging and collapse	Often present	Absent

(From Rubenstein E, Federman D (eds): Scientific American Medicine. New York, Scientific American, Inc. Chapter 4 (Gastroenterology), Part VIII, Table 1, 1989, with permission.)

25. How should you treat a health care worker exposed to hepatitis B by a needle stick within the past 2 days?

Following accidental parental exposure to hepatitis B virus, the worker should receive hepatitis immunoglobulin (HBIg) at a dose of 0.06 ml/kg IM as soon as possible and within 7 days of exposure. If the subject has not been previously vaccinated for hepatitis B, it is recommended that the hepatitis B vaccination program be initiated with the usual three doses within 14 days after exposure and again at 1 and 6 months.

Centers for Disease Control: Recommendations for protection against viral hepatitis. MMWR 34:313–335, 1985.

26. What is non-A, non-B hepatitis? How is it transmitted and what are the possible sequelae of this disease? (See also hepatitis C on p. 145.)

Non-A, non-B hepatitis, particularly hepatitis C, is classically associated with and transmitted by blood transfusion. The exact virus or viruses responsible for non-A, non-B hepatitis have not been clearly identified. Approximately 10% of patients who have had multiple blood transfusions develop hepatitis, and more than 90% of these cases are due to non-A, non-B hepatitis. Additionally, almost a third of sporadic cases of viral hepatitis are due to non-A, non-B, and more than half of these have no documented blood exposure. Therefore, it does appear there may be a second major route of transmission through nonpercutaneous or covert percutaneous exposure. There have also been documented waterborne epidemics of non-A, non-B hepatitis. The long-term sequelae of this disease are more common than in hepatitis B. Almost 40% of patients with non-A, non-B hepatitis contracted after transfusion develop chronic liver disease, with many of these patients developing chronic active hepatitis that progresses to cirrhosis.

27. What is hepatitis D virus (delta virus) and how is it transmitted?
Hepatitis D virus is a very small RNA virus that contains a defective genome and requires HBsAg to become pathogenic. Transmission is closely linked with the transmission of hepatitis B virus, and in the U.S. is typically seen in parenteral drug abusers and high-risk HBsAg carriers (hemophiliacs, hemodialysis, and immunosuppressed patients).

28. What is required for infection by the hepatitis D virus?
Infection may occur under two circumstances, in conjunction with simultaneous infection with hepatitis B in the previously unexposed patient (co-infection) and in the chronic carrier of HBsAg (superinfection). Hepatitis D virus infection is diagnosed by detecting IgM antibody to the virus in the acute serum or an increase in IgG antibody to the virus in convalescent serum.

NUTRITION

29. What are the six common vitamins and trace minerals and what are the manifestations of their respective deficiency states on physical and laboratory examination?
a.	Thiamine	Beriberi, muscle weakness, tachycardia, heart failure
b.	Niacin	Pellagra, glossitis
c.	Vitamin A	Xerophthalmia, hyperkeratosis of skin
d.	Vitamin E	Cerebellar ataxia, areflexia
e.	Zinc	Hypogeusia, acrodermatitis
f.	Chromium	Glucose intolerance

30. What are the most common nutritional deficiencies in patients with intestinal disease?
The two most common nutritional deficiencies in patients with intestinal disease are folate and calcium. When the small bowel is diseased, intestinal loss of calcium is excessive and the rate of bone resorption is insufficient to maintain serum calcium. Calcium absorption in the healthy small bowel is about 33% of total available calcium. Therefore, small-bowel diseases that affect absorption, such as celiac sprue, will influence calcium absorption markedly.

Severe folate deficiency is found most often in association with chronic alcoholism, celiac sprue, tropical sprue, and in the blind loop syndrome. Minor deficiencies can be found in Crohn's disease and following partial gastrectomy. Since folate absorption is largely complete in the upper small intestine, malabsorption is worse in disorders that affect the upper gut. However, any intestinal disorder accompanied by a decrease in dietary intake or rapid transport may result in folate deficiency.

31. An elderly white male comes to the physician for evaluation of profound peripheral neuropathy. On routine screening he is found to have a markedly low serum B_{12}. Physical examination reveals only an abdominal scar consistent with previous laparotomy, but the patient doesn't remember what kind of surgery was done. What are two possible operations that would result in B_{12} deficiency and the mechanism responsible for the deficiency?

1. **Gastrectomy:** Vitamin B_{12} absorption starts in the stomach with binding of the vitamin to intrinsic factor and R-proteins (binding factors produced in the stomach). In the duodenum the R-proteins are hydrolyzed off of the vitamin B_{12} in the presence of an alkaline environment. This allows for further binding of vitamin B_{12} with intrinsic factor. Vitamin B_{12} cannot be absorbed unless bound to intrinsic factor. If the patient's stomach was completely or partially removed, the patient would have insufficient intrinsic factor to bind to vitamin B_{12}.

2. **Terminal ileal resection:** This patient may have had Crohn's disease and undergone resection of a large portion (greater than 100 cm) of terminal ileum. The terminal ileum is the site of vitamin B_{12}-intrinsic factor complex absorption. With surgical removal or advanced disease of the ileum, vitamin B_{12}-intrinsic factor will not be absorbed and a deficiency of vitamin B_{12} will result.

Both mechanisms of deficiency can be easily treated with supplemental IM vitamin B_{12} injections.

32. What is the most common disorder of carbohydrate digestion in humans?

Lactase deficiency. Lactase deficient adults retain 10% to 30% of intestinal lactase activity and develop symptoms (diarrhea and gas) only when they ingest sufficient lactose to overwhelm colonic conservation mechanisms. Although drinking one to two glasses of milk may induce symptoms, yogurt may be tolerated by lactase-deficient persons, because it has considerable bacterial lactase activity. The diagnosis may be made simply by advising the patient to avoid dairy products for 2 weeks to determine if the altered bowel habits reverse to normal.

33. What are medium-chain triglycerides and in which intestinal diseases are they used as therapy?

Medium-chain triglycerides are lipids containing only short and medium chain fatty acids (C6–C12) and are absorbed in a different manner from long-chain triglycerides, which are the more common form of triglycerides in the diet. Medium-chain triglycerides can be absorbed intact by enterocytes and pass directly into the portal circulation. Patients with a variety of small intestinal diseases, short bowel syndrome, biliary obstruction, and pancreatic insufficiency absorb medium-chain triglycerides more efficiently than long-chain triglycerides.

34. What are the fundamental principles of total parenteral nutrition (TPN)?

1. Patients will generally require 30 to 35 kcal/kg for maintenance.

2. The optimal calorie/nitrogen ratio appears to be about 160 calories per gram of nitrogen.

3. The average adult requires about 30 cc of water per kilogram of body weight per day.

4. IV lipid emulsions are a suitable source of nonprotein calories that contribute to conservation of body protein. A regimen in which calories are supplied by both dextrose solution and lipid emulsions, with fat providing 30% or more of the total calories, appears to be the most effective form of parenteral nutrition.

35. What are the most common complications of TPN and how are they treated?

1. The most common complications are those related to **catheter placement and management**. Complications can be minimized by maintaining strict and reproducible technique. The catheter should be placed by physicians or surgeons experienced in line insertion and managed by caretakers trained in meticulous line care.

2. In prolonged TPN, especially when excessive carbohydrate calories are given, patients frequently develop **liver tenderness** and **transaminase elevations.** These latter values are though to reflect hepatic steatosis. Liver function test abnormalities should return to normal when TPN is discontinued. If continuation of TPN is required, one should decrease the dextrose infusion and increase the amount of fat calories the patient is given.

3. A complication of long-term (home) TPN is **metabolic bone disease**. Bone biopsies have demonstrated changes similar to those in osteomalacia. It is thought that the addition of acetate or phosphate may offset the urinary calcium losses and restore positive calcium balance in these patients. In addition, an increased incidence of **cholecystitis** and **cholelithiasis** related to gallbladder stasis is seen in patients on TPN.

36. Which vitamin deficiencies might be expected to develop in a patient maintained on long term TPN (more than 6 months) containing only Na^+, K^+, Cl^-, HCO_3^-, glucose, and amino acids?

This TPN solution is clearly lacking in vitamins and trace minerals. In a matter of weeks, this patient would be expected to develop deficiencies in magnesium, zinc, essential fatty acids, and water-soluble vitamins, with the exception of vitamin B_{12}. Over several months vitamin K and copper deficiency would be encountered. Over a period of years deficiencies in the fat soluble vitamins A and D as well as selenium, chromium, and vitamin B_{12} would occur.

CANCER

37. A patient presents with an "apple core" lesion in the sigmoid colon which on biopsy is found to be adenocarcinoma. Which tests should be included in the routine preoperative evaluation for a patient with this disease?

If carcinoma is detected either radiographically or by sigmoidoscopy, a full colonoscopic examination should be done because of a high incidence of synchronous lesions. Up to half the patients with a single cancer of the colon have additional polyps that may required modification of the surgical procedure. The second test required is a preoperative serum carcinoembryonic antigen (CEA) level. The preoperative CEA, if elevated, in most cases will fall to a normal level if all tumor has been removed. This serves to help direct future therapy, since patients with a rising CEA level after total resection should be suspected of having a recurrence.

38. The primary therapy for colorectal carcinoma is surgical resection. However, radiation therapy may be useful for tumors arising in which part of the colon? Why?

Patients with rectal cancer who have lesions penetrating the bowel wall or who may have regional lymph nodes involved by tumor are at particularly high risk of recurrence following resection. Radiation therapy used either preoperatively or postoperatively in this disease may decrease the local recurrence rate. Although the recurrence rate may be decreased, it is uncertain whether pre- or postoperative radiation to the rectum prolongs survival.

39. What are the reasons for performing a total colonoscopy instead of flexible sigmoid-oscopy?

1. Surveillance for neoplasms (previous polyps or cancer, inflammatory bowel disease, or familial colon cancer syndromes).
2. Rectal bleeding with occult blood or acute severe hemorrhage.
3. Radiographic lesions above the sigmoid colon.
4. Mapping of inflammatory bowel disease.
5. Right-sided diverticular disease.
6. Miscellaneous conditions (volvulus, idiopathic pseudoobstruction, etc.)

40. Name the most common malignant neoplasms of the small intestine in decreasing order of frequency.

1. Adenocarcinoma 45%
2. Carcinoid. 34%
3. Sarcoma 18%
4. Lymphoma 3%

41. In decreasing order of frequency, what are the most common benign neoplasms of the small intestine?
1. Adenoma
2. Leiomyoma
3. Lipoma

42. What are adenomatous polyps and what is their significance?
Adenomatous polyps are neoplastic polyps found most often in the colon that give rise to symptoms only when they become large. They are more frequently detected incidentally on colonoscopic examination or barium enema. Their importance relates to the potential for their epithelium to progress through various degrees of dysplasia to frank carcinoma. Approximately 75% of all adenomatous polyps are tubular adenomas, 15% are termed tubulovillous adenomas, and the rest are villous tumors. It is well known that the potential for malignant transformation is related to morphology. Villous tumors are more likely to be malignant than tubular adenomas. Other factors that relate to malignant potential include tumor size, degree of cellular atypia, and number of polyps present. Patients who have had adenomatous polyps diagnosed usually have them removed with endoscopic polypectomy and should undergo colonoscopy at routine intervals so that additional polyps may be removed before they progress to malignancy.

INFLAMMATORY BOWEL DISEASE

43. Explain the differential diagnosis in a young patient with Crohn's disease of the ileum who presents with right upper quadrant (RUQ) discomfort and jaundice.
In the patient with inflammatory bowel disease who presents with jaundice, the diagnostic considerations should include pericholangitis, sclerosing cholangitis, choledocholithiasis, and primary hepatocellular disease. Pericholangitis is a histologic finding representing inflammatory changes of the small bile ductules and may be one end of the spectrum of sclerosing cholangitis. Sclerosing cholangitis is focal narrowing and inflammation of the intra- and extrahepatic biliary tree. These diseases have been reported only with inflammatory bowel disease affecting the colon and are much more common with ulcerative colitis than with Crohn's colitis.

A more likely consideration in this particular patient would be choledocholithiasis. Patients with longstanding ileal disease or patients who have had ileal resection are unable to reabsorb bile salts and therefore have a diminished bile salt pool. This results in supersaturation of bile with cholesterol and subsequent precipitation of cholesterol crystals and gallstone formation. With these possibilities in mind, this patient should be evaluated to determine whether there is extrahepatic duct obstruction or hepatocellular disease.

Vierling JN: Hepatobiliary complications of ulcerative colitis and Crohn's disease. In Zakim D, BoyerTA (eds): Hepatology: A Textbook of Liver Disease. Philadelphia, W.B. Saunders, 1990, pp 1126–1158.

44. What are the differences between Crohn's disease and ulcerative colitis?
Both Crohn's disease and ulcerative colitis are nonspecific inflammatory conditions of the bowel that lack a defined etiology.

Crohn's disease may involve any part of the gastrointestinal tract but most commonly involves the terminal ileum and colon. Crohn's disease may be associated with fistula formation. Its gross appearance is characterized by skip lesions (areas of normal mucosa between ulcers). On biopsy of the affected area of bowel, characteristic features of Crohn's disease include noncaseating granulomas.

Ulcerative colitis, as the name implies, is a disease limited to the colon. Features of the disease include universal involvement of the rectum with various degrees of proximal extension. Unlike Crohn's disease of the colon, ulcerative colitis is not characterized by skip lesions. An increased incidence of cancer of the colon has been associated with pancolitis of greater than 10 years' duration. A similar risk for colon cancer does not exist in the Crohn's patient. A characteristic finding on histologic examination of the biopsies from patients with ulcerative colitis is the presence of crypt abscesses. Total colectomy is curative but should be reserved for patients with severe disease or pancolitis of more than 10 years' duration.

45. What are the features associated with a fatal outcome in patients with their first attack of ulcerative colitis?

- Age greater than 60
- Pancolitis
- Toxic megacolon
- Hypoalbuminemia
- Hypokalemia

46. Which two colonic segments are most commonly involved in ischemic colitis? Why?

Ischemic colitis most commonly occurs in the regions lying in the "watershed" areas between two adjacent arterial supplies. These are the splenic flexure, which lies between the inferior and superior mesenteric arteries, and the rectosigmoid junction, which lies between the inferior mesenteric and interior iliac arteries.

ULCERS

47. What are the major functions of acid secretion in the stomach?

Acid activates the enzyme pepsin by converting pepsinogen to pepsin, thereby initiating the first stages of protein digestion. Acid also serves as an antibacterial barrier to protect the stomach from colonization.

48. Peptic ulcer disease is a term often used to describe both gastric and duodenal ulcer. What are the characteristic features of duodenal ulcer disease and gastric ulcer disease?

Duodenal ulcer disease has a peak incidence in the young adult. It is associated with *Helicobacter pylori* infection (see Q. 53) and excessive acid secretion. The disease is characterized by frequent recurrences, usually exacerbating and remitting over a period of 10 to 20 years.

Gastric ulcer disease is characteristically found in the elderly population. It is not associated with increased acid secretion but rather is more often associated with achlorhydria or hypochlorhydria.

Both types of ulcers are currently treated with H_2 antagonists such as cimetidine or ranitidine. Gastric ulcers, unlike duodenal ulcers, must be followed either endoscopically or radiographically until they are completely healed, since a small number of them are malignant. Duodenal ulcers are rarely malignant. Therefore, therapy and long-term follow-up are directed toward symptom relief alone.

49. What is the difference in pathogenesis of duodenal versus gastric ulcers?

The precise cause of duodenal ulcer disease is not completely understood, but its pathogenesis is associated with three factors:

1. Increased acid secretion that correlates with an increased number of parietal cells in the gastric mucosa.

2. Increased responsiveness of the parietal cells of the stomach to stimulation factors, such as food, gastrin, or histamine.

3. Increased vagal activity.

Gastric ulcers are not associated with these factors. As stated above, patients with gastric ulcers have normal or even decreased gastric acid secretion. Gastric ulcers probably develop because of a change in the mucosal resistance to the acid.

50. What are the five major indications for peptic ulcer surgery?

The five indications for ulcer surgery include:

1. **Intractability:** This relates to the symptoms and not to delayed ulcer healing. The diagnosis of intractability requires clinical confirmation that an ulcer is responsible for the patient's symptoms.

2. **Hemorrhage:** Surgery to control exsanguinating hemorrhage is occasionally necessary but carries a high mortality rate. It is more difficult to decide when elective surgery should be performed in the patient who has had a large bleed from a peptic ulcer. There are no clear-cut criteria for deciding when to operate. Surgery should be considered in patients who require a large volume (6 to 8 units) of blood transfusion to correct blood losses in 24 hours, who have one or more rebleeding episodes occurring in the hospital, or who have persistent bleeding requiring transfusion over 48 to 72 hours in the hospital.

3. **Perforation:** This requires immediate surgery.

4. **Penetration:** This represents erosion of an ulcer through the entire thickness of the wall of the stomach or the intestine without leakage of digestive contents into the peritoneal cavity. Penetration can be reliably diagnosed only at surgery or autopsy but clinically may be suspected by an alteration in the typical spectrum of symptoms experienced by the patient. This can occur gradually, with changes in the frequency, intensity, radiation and duration of pain. Diagnosis is usually made historically and treatment is surgical if complicated penetration exists.

5. **Obstruction:** Gastric outlet obstruction as a result of ulcer disease occurs in 2% of all ulcer patients. Standard therapy of outlet obstruction has been surgical. Endoscopic balloon dilatation of the stenotic pylorus has not been systematically compared with surgical treatment; therefore, it is not clear whether this is adequate therapy.

Graham DY: Complications of peptic ulcer disease and indications for surgery. In Sleisenger MH, Fordtran JS (eds): Gastrointestinal Disease, 4th ed. Philadelphia, W.B. Saunders, 1989, pp 925–938.

51. What are the reasons for recurrent ulcer in patients who have undergone previous ulcer surgery?

Primary factors that may contribute to recurrent ulcer disease following ulcer surgery include:

- Incomplete vagotomy.
- Adjacent nonabsorbable suture that acts as an irritant.
- "Retained antrum" syndrome, in which antral tissue left behind at surgery produces a continued source of gastrin production.
- Antral G-cell hyperplasia (a relatively uncommon entity).
- Zollinger-Ellison syndrome (gastrinoma).
- Gastric cancer.

Other factors that may contribute to recurrent ulcer but have not necessarily been implicated as primary causes include ulcerogenic drugs, smoking, enterogastric reflux (bile acid reflux), primary hyperparathyroidism, and gastric bezoar.

Cohen MM: Practical management of recurrent peptic ulcer. Can J Surg 21:21, 1978.

52. What is the most common presenting symptom of peptic ulcer disease in the elderly?

Melena is the most frequent presenting symptom of peptic ulcer disease in the elderly. Epigastric pain occurs in less than half of elderly patients, and many are asymptomatic. A fatal hemorrhagic event may be the first sign of an ulcer in the elderly.

Shamburek R, et al: Disorders of the digestive system in the elderly. N Engl J Med 322:438–443, 1990.

53. What is the relationship between *Helicobacter pylori* infection and duodenal ulcer disease?

It has been well established that patients with duodenal ulcer disease have an inflamed gastric mucosa. Recently, a spiral shaped bacteria called *Helicobacter pylori* has been found to be responsible for most cases of this inflammation (gastritis). It has been noted since the discovery of this bacterium that virtually 100% of patients with duodenal ulcer disease are infected with *Helicobacter pylori*. The incidence of infection for patients with gastric ulcer is 70 to 80%. New therapies directed to the treatment of *Helicobacter pylori* may result in a decreased recurrence rate of duodenal ulcer. Optimal therapy for *Helicobacter pylori* has not been well defined at this time. *Helicobacter pylori* infection alone does not invariably cause duodenal ulcer disease, because the majority of patients with *Helicobacter pylori* gastritis do not have duodenal ulcers. Other factors that may contribute to ulcer formation include cigarette smoking, hereditary tendency, and hypersecretion of acid.

Peterson WL: *Helicobacter pylori* and peptic ulcer disease. N Engl J Med 324:1043–1048, 1991.

54. What is the Zollinger-Ellison (ZE) syndrome?

The clinical triad characteristic of the ZE syndrome consists of gastric acid hypersecretion, severe ulcer disease of the upper intestinal tract as a direct result of acid hypersecretion, and a non-beta cell tumor of the pancreas that secretes the hormone gastrin (gastrinoma). The diagnosis should be suspected in patients with a compatible clinical history and gastric acid hypersecretion.

55. How do you make the diagnosis of the Zollinger-Ellison (ZE) syndrome?

This diagnosis can be made using a combination of several tests. The most sensitive and specific method for identifying the disease is demonstration of an increased serum gastrin level. Patients with ZE syndrome typically have fasting gastrin levels greater than 150 pg/ml and most commonly levels greater than 1000 pg/ml (vs. 20–50 pg/ml average in normal subjects). The elevation of serum gastrin must be accompanied by gastric acid hypersecretion (as measured by basal acid output studies) to be consistent with the diagnosis.

Further provocative tests utilizing IV secretin injection may be used to confirm the diagnosis. In a normal patient, IV secretin results in a slight lowering or no change in the serum gastrin level. A patient with the ZE syndrome will show a dramatic rise in the serum gastrin concentration following IV secretin. A rise in serum gastrin concentration by at least 200 pg/ml between 2 and 10 minutes after injection is considered a positive result.

Malagelada JR, et al: Medical and surgical options in the management of patients with gastrinoma. Gastroenterology 84:1524, 1983.

PANCREATITIS

56. What are the most common causes of acute pancreatitis in the U.S.?

Acute pancreatitis is caused by choledocholithiasis, ethanol abuse, or is idiopathic in 90% of cases in the U.S. In the private hospital setting, 50% of patients with acute pancreatitis are found to have gallstones (gallstone pancreatitis). In public hospitals up to 66% of first episodes of pancreatitis are caused by excessive alcohol consumption.

57. What drugs have a definite causative association with acute pancreatitis?

Drugs Causing Acute Pancreatitis

Ethanol and methanol	6-mercaptopurine
Hydrochlorothiazide	Furosemide
Sulfonamides	Tetracyclines
Estrogens	Valproic acid
L-asparaginase	

58. What are Ranson's criteria for the prognosis in acute pancreatitis?

Ranson et al, in 1974, published criteria that could be used to prognosticate in cases of acute pancreatitis. These are:

Prognostic Criteria in Acute Pancreatitis*

I. On Admission:	II. In Initial 48 Hours
• Age over 55	• Hematocrit decrease of more then 10%
• WBC > 16,000	• BUN rise of more than 5 mg/dl
• Serum LDH > 350 IU/l	• Serum calcium < 8 mg/dl
• Blood glucose > 200 mg/dl	• Arterial pO_2 < 60 mmHg
• SGOT > 250 IU/l	• Base deficit > 4 mEq/liter
	• Estimated fluid sequestration > 6 liters

*WBC = white blood count, BUN = blood urea nitrogen, LDH = lactate dehydrogenase, SGOT = serum glutamic-oxaloacetic transaminase, pO_2 = partial pressure of oxygen (arterial).
Ranson JH, et al: Prognostic signs and the role of operative management in acute pancreatitis. Surg Gynecol Obstet 139:69, 1974.

59. What are the causes of an increase in serum amylase?
There are several conditions that can cause an increase in serum amylase, **other than acute pancreatitis.** These include:

Macroamylasemia	Perforated peptic ulcer disease
Renal insufficiency	Ruptured ectopic pregnancy
Mesenteric infarction	Diabetic ketoacidosis
Parotitis	Peritonitis
Burns	Tumors of the pancreas, salivary glands, ovary,
Cholecystitis	lung, and prostate

60. What are Cullen's and Grey Turner's signs?
These signs are associated with acute hemorrhagic pancreatitis and are defined as follows:
1. *Cullen's sign:* ecchymotic discoloration in the umbilicus.
2. *Grey Turner's sign:* ecchymotic discoloration around the flanks.

61. Why is meperidine indicated for analgesia in acute pancreatitis?
Meperidine is indicated over other narcotic analgesic agents in acute pancreatitis because it has minimal effects on the ampulla of Vater. Other narcotic analgesics can cause increased ampullary pressure and may theoretically worsen pancreatitis.

VASCULAR DISEASE

62. What is intestinal angina?
When occlusive vascular disease, usually artherosclerosis, affects two of the three major arteries supplying the gut, it may be associated with a syndrome of intermittent, cramping, midabdominal pain commonly called intestinal angina. Patients usually report that symptoms are worse when eating. They may lose a great deal of weight simply because avoidance of pain can be achieved by avoiding meals or eating small meals. The diagnosis is facilitated by angiography, which documents significant stenosis of vessels. Treatment for patients with a significant gradient across the stenosis is surgical bypass, endarterectomy, or percutaneous translumenal angioplasty.

DIARRHEA

63. What differentiates osmotic from secretory diarrhea? Give examples of each.
Osmotic diarrhea is caused by ingestion of unusually large amounts of a poorly absorbable but osmotically active solute. This usually consists of a carbohydrate or a divalent ion (such as magnesium or sulfate). Clinically, osmotic diarrhea is characterized by diarrhea that

stops when the patient fasts (or stops ingesting the poorly absorbable solute). Commonly implicated causes include mannitol or sorbitol ingestion (seen in patients chewing large quantities of sugar-free gum), lactulose, magnesium sulfate (Epsom salt), sodium sulfate (Glauber's salt or Carlsbad salt), sodium phosphate, sodium citrate, and some magnesium-containing antacids. Additionally, carbohydrate malabsorption may cause osmotic diarrhea through the action of unabsorbed sugars.

Secretory diarrhea involves a disruption of normal bowel function. Normal small intestinal epithelial cells both secrete and absorb electrolytes and water. The secretion rate is less than the absorption rate and ultimately leads to a net absorption of fluid and electrolytes. If this normal process is interrupted by a pathologic process that either stimulates increased secretion or inhibits absorption, secretory diarrhea may occur. Causes of secretory diarrhea include enterotoxin-mediated secretion such as that seen with *Vibrio cholerae* and enterotoxigenic *E. coli* infection, tumor elaboration of hormones such as VIP (vasoactive intestinal peptide), calcitonin, serotonin, and laxatives containing phenolphthalein. Unabsorbed bile acids and fatty acids may also induce colonic secretion and diarrhea.

Fordtran JS: Speculations on the pathogenesis of diarrhea. Federation Proceedings 26:1405, 1967.

64. Which three diagnostic features can be used to distinguish secretory from osmotic diarrhea?

1. Stool osmolality in secretory diarrhea can be accounted for by the normal ionic constituents of stool, whereas osmotic diarrhea demonstrates an osmotic gap (see Q. 65).

2. Since secretory diarrhea is typically unrelated to ingested foods or solutes, it persists during 24 to 72 hour periods of fasting.

3. Patients with a pure secretory diarrhea do not have white blood cells, red blood cells, or fat in their stool.

65. What test can be used to differentiate secretory from osmotic diarrhea?

A pure osmotic or secretory diarrhea can be distinguished on the basis of stool analysis for electrolytes and osmolality. Normal fecal fluid osmolality is equal to that of plasma or approximately 290 milliosmoles per kilogram. Stool analysis in osmotic diarrhea typically reveals an osmolality $(2 \times [Na^+ + K^+])$ that is less than the measured osmolality of fecal fluid (osmotic gap). The size of the osmotic gap is approximately equivalent to the concentration of the poorly absorbed, unmeasured solute in the fecal water. An osmotic gap of less than 50 milliosmoles per kilogram is considered to be normal and gaps of over 50 are indicative of osmotic diarrhea. In cases of secretory diarrhea, the stool osmolality can be completely accounted for by the measured sodium and potassium.

66. What are the two basic mechanisms by which bacteria may cause infectious diarrhea at the cellular level? Give examples of each type.

Organisms that cause infectious diarrhea can be divided into two groups, based on the mechanism of diarrhea production: (1) those that adhere to the mucosa and subsequently secrete an enterotoxin that stimulates epithelial cell secretion, and (2) organisms that adhere to epithelial cells in preparation for invasion of the mucosa. Many of the invasive organisms also release toxins that stimulate secretion by the intestinal cell but by a mechanism that does not involve activation of adenylate cyclase.

The most common organism leading to enterotoxigenic diarrhea in the U.S. is the enterotoxigenic species of *Escherichia coli* (ETEC). *Vibrio cholerae* is a classic example of toxin-stimulated diarrhea. Organisms that invade the mucosa and result in diarrhea include *Salmonella, Shigella,* enteroinvasive *E. coli, Campylobacter,* and *Yersinia.*

The toxigenic bacteria do not induce visible changes in the intestinal mucosa during infection. In contrast, mucosal damage, inflammatory infiltrate, and ulceration are commonly seen in the intestinal tract of patients infected with invasive organisms. For this reason, fecal leukocytes are typically present in infections with invasive organisms, whereas few or no white cells are seen in the stool of patients infected with toxigenic organisms.

67. What is bacillary dysentery? What organisms are frequently responsible for this disease process?

The term dysentery refers to a diarrheal stool that contains inflammatory exudate (pus) and blood. Dysentery is a common term that refers to infectious diarrhea from invasive pathogens, most commonly, *Shigella* or *Salmonella*.

68. A 50-year-old woman complains of 6 to 8 loose stools per day for 1 month. The etiology is not immediately evident after a careful history and physical. What diagnostic tests should be performed at this stage?

There are certain diagnostic tests performed early in the evaluation that may help to delineate the most likely causes of diarrhea in this patient. A CBC, serum chemistry profile, and urinalysis may be helpful in pinpointing a source. For example, the patient who has an anemia with a very high MCV may be suspected of having malabsorption and diarrhea based on the presence of ileal disease and inability to absorb vitamin B_{12}.

Basic stool studies, including bacterial culture and sensitivity, Sudan stain for fat, Wright's stain for white blood cells, guaiac test for blood, and a phenolphthalein test for the presence of laxative ingestion are all simple and quickly obtainable tests that may give valuable results.

Proctosigmoidoscopy is a very important part of the examination in most patients with chronic and recurrent diarrhea. Examination of the rectal mucosa may reveal pseudomembranes seen with antibiotic-associated diarrhea, discreet ulceration typical of amoebiasis, or a diffusely inflamed granular mucosa seen in ulcerative colitis. Biopsy specimens can be obtained through the scope for histologic examination, and fresh stool samples can be collected for cultures.

Almy TP: Chronic and recurrent diarrhea. Disease-a-Month October, 1955.

69. A 28-year-old white male returned from a camping trip in the Rocky Mountains of Colorado complaining of cramping abdominal pain and diarrhea. On examination, the stool contains no red or white blood cells. What common parasitic infection could account for his symptoms and how would you treat it?

Giardia lamblia is a protozoan parasite found in water systems that fail to filter out the cysts (which resist chlorination). Although giardiasis can be contracted in any part of the country, it is most commonly associated with camping and backpacking in the mountainous west. Routine physical examination and laboratory findings are normal. Examination of the stools may reveal *Giardia* cysts or trophozoites. Duodenal aspiration and small bowel biopsy often show trophozoites. The majority of patients with giardiasis may be successfully treated with quinacrine (Atabrine) or metronidazole (Flagyl).

70. What is the pathogenesis of diverticulosis?

Diverticulosis increases with age, from an incidence of 5% in the fifth decade to 50% in the ninth. The exact pathogenesis of diverticulosis is not known. The low content of fiber in the Western diet may lead to decreased bulk of the colonic contents. This leads to a narrow colonic lumen with altered intraluminal pressures. A pseudodiverticula or herniation through the tunica muscularis can be formed.

Another theory speculates that normal intraluminal pressure is sufficient to allow herniation through a muscularis area whose fibrous tissue support has deteriorated with advancing age.

Shamburek R, et al: Disorders of the digestive system in the elderly. N Engl J Med 322:438–443, 1990.

71. What are the possible causes of diarrhea in a homosexual male with and without AIDS?

The evaluation of diarrhea in the homosexual population is complicated by the various enteric organisms to which they are frequently exposed. There are many organisms potentially carried by asymptomatic homosexual men that may not be involved in clinical illness (such as *Neisseria gonorrhoeae, Entamoeba histolytica,* and *Giardia lamblia*). In any event, organisms that must be considered in the differential diagnosis of a homosexual male who is HIV negative include amebiasis, giardiasis, shigellosis, *Campylobacter,* rectal syphilis, rectal spirochetes other than syphilis, rectal gonorrhea, *Chlamydia trachomatis* (lymphogranuloma venereum [LGV] infection), and *Herpes simplex* infection.

The immunocompromised patient with AIDS may have diarrhea secondary to the above-listed organisms in addition to others such as *Cryptosporidium, Candida albicans, Cryptococcus neoformans, Salmonella typhimurium, Mycobacterium avium-intracellulare,* cytomegalovirus (CMV), and *Isospora belli.* Many of the treatable causes of diarrhea can be diagnosed on historical and physical grounds, with the addition of stool culture for bacteria and ova and parasite examination. The addition of proctoscopy or flexible sigmoidoscopy may increase the diagnostic yield.

72. List the causative agents of food poisoning and the time of the onset of illness caused by these agents.

Though other syndromes may result from the ingestion of contaminated food, food poisoning is generally thought of as the onset of gastrointestinal or neurologic symptoms and signs following the ingestion of contaminated food. The causes may be characterized by the time to onset, clinical signs, and association with a microbial origin:

Onset Time	Symptoms and Signs	Agents
≤ 1 hour	Nausea, vomiting, and abdominal cramps	Heavy metal poisoning (copper, zinc, tin, cadmium)
≤ 1 hour	Paresthesias	Scombroid poisoning, shellfish poisoning, Chinese restaurant syndrome (excessive monosodium glutamate [MSG]), niacin poisoning
1–6 hours	Nausea and vomiting	Preformed toxins of *Staphylococcus aureus* and *Bacillus cereus*
≤ 2 hours	Delirium, parasympathetic hyperactivity, hallucinations, disulfiram reaction, or gastroenteritis	Toxic mushroom ingestion
8–16 hours	Abdominal cramps and diarrhea	In vivo production of enterotoxins by *Clostridium perfringens* and *B. cereus*
6–24 hours	Abdominal cramps, diarrhea, followed by hepatorenal failure	Toxic mushroom ingestion (*Amanita* sp.)
16–48 hours	Fever, abdominal cramps, and diarrhea	*Salmonella* sp., *Shigella* sp., *C. jejuni*, invasive *E. coli, Y. enterocolitica, V. parahemolyticus*
16–72 hours	Abdominal cramps and diarrhea	Norwalk agent and related viruses, enterotoxins produced by *Vibrio* sp., *E. coli*, and occasionally salmonellae, shigellae, and *C. jejuni*
18–36 hours	Nausea, vomiting, diarrhea, and paralysis	Food-borne botulism
72–100 hours	Bloody diarrhea without fever	Enterotoxigenic *E. coli*, most frequently serotype 0157:H7
1–3 weeks	Chronic diarrhea	Raw milk ingestion

Mandell GL, et al (eds): Principles and Practice of Infectious Diseases, 3rd ed. New York, Churchill Livingstone, 1990.

73. What is diabetic diarrhea?

"Diabetic diarrhea" is a chronic diarrhea that affects approximately 5% of type I diabetics. It is characterized by frequent (usually 10 to 30 per day) passages of watery brown stool that may occur during the daytime or at nighttime. Since diabetics are subject to all of the other causes of diarrhea, diabetic diarrhea is a diagnosis of exclusion. The cause of the diarrhea and steatorrhea is not clear in most patients. However, bacterial overgrowth may be the etiology in some patients, and treatment with broad-spectrum antibiotics often brings welcome relief. Chronic pancreatitis with exocrine pancreatic insufficiency is a disease that is more common in patients with longstanding diabetes. Steatorrhea due to exocrine pancreatic insufficiency may be relieved with pancreatic enzyme replacement therapy. Adult celiac disease is also more common in diabetics than in the general population.

LIVER DISEASE

74. What are the clinical manifestations of liver disease and their pathogenetic basis?

Clinical Manifestations of Liver Disease

SIGN/SYMPTOM	PATHOGENESIS	LIVER DISEASE
Constitutional		
Fatigue, anorexia, malaise, weight loss	Liver failure	Severe acute or chronic hepatitis Cirrhosis
Fever	Hepatic inflammation or infection	Liver abscess Alcoholic hepatitis Viral hepatitis
Fetor hepaticus	Abnormal methionine metabolism	Acute or chronic liver failure
Cutaneous		
Spider telangiectasias, palmar erythema	Altered estrogen and androgen metabolism	Cirrhosis
Jaundice	Diminished bilirubin excretion	Biliary obstruction Severe liver disease
Pruritus		Biliary obstruction
Xanthomas and xanthelasma	Increased serum lipids	Biliary obstruction/cholestasis
Endocrine		
Gynecomastia, testicular atrophy, diminished libido	Altered estrogen and androgen metabolism	Cirrhosis
Hypoglycemia	Decreased glycogen stores and gluconeogenesis	Liver failure
Gastrointestinal		
Right upper quadrant abdominal pain	Liver swelling, infection	Acute hepatitis Hepatocellular carcinoma Liver congestion (heart failure) Acute cholecystitis Liver abscess
Abdominal swelling	Ascites	Cirrhosis, portal hypertension
Gastrointestinal bleeding	Esophageal varices	Portal hypertension
Hematological		
Decreased red cells, white cells, and/or platelets	Hypersplenism	Cirrhosis, portal hypertension
Ecchymoses	Decreased synthesis of clotting factors	Liver failure
Neurological		
Altered sleep pattern, subtle behavioral changes, somnolence, confusion, ataxia, asterixis, obtundation	Hepatic encephalopathy	Liver failure, portosystemic shunting of blood

(From Andreoli TE, et al: Cecil Essentials of Medicine, 2nd ed. Philadelphia, W.B. Saunders, 1990, p 312, with permission.)

75. What are the two predominant forms of alcoholic liver injury? Which one may go on to cirrhosis?

Mild alcoholism impairs the excretion of triglyceride from hepatocytes. The typical "fatty liver" develops with fat globules in parenchymal cells. The fatty liver of alcoholism generally causes hepatomegaly and minimal changes in liver function tests. Jaundice is not seen.

The more severe form of alcoholic liver injury is alcoholic hepatitis, characterized by focal necrosis of liver cells. Clusters of neutrophils and Mallory bodies (clumps of hyaline) can be seen on liver biopsy. The lesions of alcoholic hepatitis are characteristically in the center of the lobule and accompanied by fibrosis. Alcoholic hepatitis in its severe clinical form is characterized by marked jaundice and transaminase elevations (up to 10 times normal), and may be accompanied by impaired synthesis of coagulation proteins leading to a prolonged prothrombin time. Typically in alcoholic hepatitis, unlike viral hepatitis, the SGOT is greater than the SGPT. Alcoholic hepatitis may progress to cirrhosis. Alcohol-induced cirrhosis is the most frequent cause of cirrhosis in the U.S.

76. Which drugs have been associated with the development of liver tumors?

Oral contraceptives have been associated with liver adenomas and vinyl chloride with angiosarcoma.

77. A patient with known cirrhosis of the liver presents to the hospital with massive swelling of his abdomen. A fluid wave may be elicited on examination of the abdomen by striking one flank and feeling the transmitted wave on the opposite flank. What is the appropriate diagnostic procedure at this point?

After the diagnosis of ascites is made by physical examination, all patients with new-onset ascites should undergo abdominal paracentesis and ascitic fluid analysis. A diagnostic paracentesis may be done at the bedside and provides valuable information with very little risk. A small amount of fluid is aspirated from the midline of the abdomen between the umbilicus and the pubis with a small-gauge needle.

The most important tests to order for fluid analysis include protein concentration and cell count. Fluids with protein concentration above 3 grams per deciliter are designated as **exudates.** Those with values below this are designated as **transudates.** Diseases usually associated with transudative ascites include congestive heart failure, cirrhosis, constrictive pericarditis, inferior vena cava obstruction, hypoalbuminemia, Meigs syndrome, and some cases of nephrotic syndrome. Exudates are more commonly seen with peritoneal neoplasms, pancreative ascites, myxedema, and tuberculous peritonitis.

A large number of red blood cells in the fluid or grossly bloody ascites suggests the diagnosis of neoplasm. An acidic fluid and leukocyte count of more than 500 per cubic millimeter is strongly suggestive of a peritoneal infection or inflammatory process. Other tests that should be ordered in the appropriate clinical setting include cytologic examination, lactic dehydrogenase (LDH), specific tumor markers, glucose, and cultures for bacteria, mycobacteria and fungi.

78. How should you manage a patient who presents within 4 hours of a 20-gram acetaminophen overdose?

Large doses of acetaminophen result in severe hepatotoxicity and ultimate death from acute liver failure. Ingestion of 15 grams or more is usually necessary to cause a severe or fatal reaction; however, lower doses have been shown to be severely hepatotoxic in certain patients. To be effective, treatment to prevent hepatotoxicity must be initiated early in the course of the injury. It is important to attempt to gain knowledge as to the timing and dose of ingestion. Since the dose ingested may not be reliably obtained from the suicidal or psychotic patient, determination of acetaminophen blood levels has been employed with some success and can be used to predict those patients in whom serious liver injury is likely to occur. The following graph can be used to determine the likelihood of hepatic toxicity based on the patient's acetaminophen plasma level and the time since ingestion:

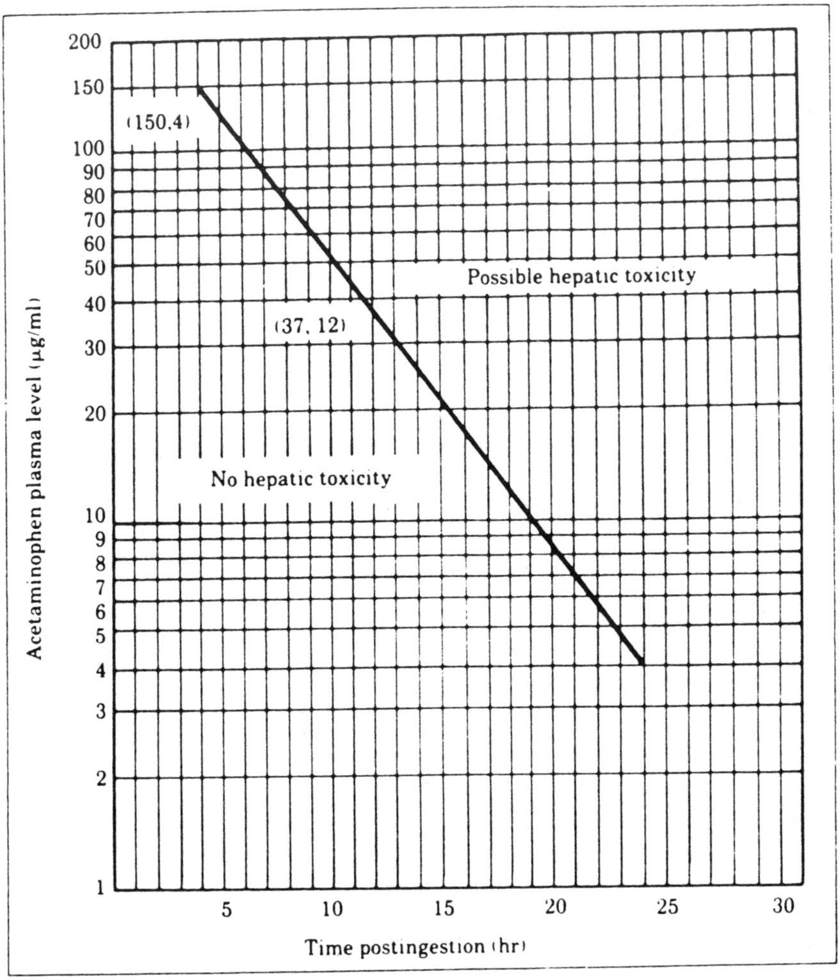

Nomogram for acetaminophen toxicity. (From Rumack BH, Matthew H: Acetaminophen poisoning and toxicity. Pediatrics 55:871, 1975, with permission.)

N-acetylcysteine (Mucomyst) is the drug of choice for treatment of acetaminophen overdose. It may be administered orally but has been shown to be effective only if treatment is initiated within the first 10 to 12 hours after ingestion. There are two clinical settings in which the drug should be used:

1. When the patient's parameters, fitted to the above curve, indicate the patient is at risk, or

2. When blood acetaminophen levels are not rapidly available but there is good reason to believe that a significant overdose has occurred.

The initial dose is 140 mg/kg orally, followed by maintenance doses of 70 mg/kg every 4 hours for a total of 72 hours. In addition, gastric contents should be lavaged free of any remaining pill fragments, and the patient should be monitored closely hemodynamically. Over 90% of patients may be expected to completely recover if treated in the early phases after ingestion.

Bass NM, Ockner RK: Drug-induced liver disease. In Zakim D, Boyer T (eds): Hepatology: A Textbook of Liver Disease, 2nd ed. Philadelphia, W.B. Saunders, 1990, pp 754–791.

79. What are the pathogenetic mechanisms responsible for ascites formation in patients with cirrhosis?

Ascites forms when there is a disturbance in the normal balance between the formation and reabsorption of peritoneal fluid in the direction of net formation. The factors that lead to this in cirrhotic patients are:

Pathogenetic Mechanisms of Ascites Formation in Cirrhosis

1. Increased hydrostatic pressure in the portal circulation due to increased resistance to flow through the cirrhotic liver favors net leakage of fluid into the extravascular space.
2. Increased renal sodium and water retention due to:
   a. Secondary hyperaldosteronism.
   b. Increased antidiuretic hormone (ADH) release.
3. Impaired hepatic and splanchnic removal of lymphatic fluid due to elevated hepatic sinusoidal pressure.
4. Decreased intravascular oncotic pressure due to decreased hepatic protein (albumin and others) synthesis.
5. Increased plasma vasopressin and epinephrine levels with resultant vasomotor changes.

80. What are the bedside history and physical examination findings for ascites?

In a study of 63 patients with ascites, Simel et al. noted the following history and physical examination findings, with the associated frequencies:

History	No.	Physical Examination	No.
Ankle swelling	(30)	Bulging flanks	(36)
Alcoholism	(29)	Flank dullness	(27)
Increased girth	(23)	Edema	(24)
Recent weight gain	(20)	Fluid wave	(16)
Heart failure	(18)	Shifting dullness	(14)
Jaundice	(10)	Flat or elevated navel	(11)
Carcinoma	(9)	Puddle sign	(9)
Hepatitis	(8)	Ballottable liver	(7)
Bleeding disorder	(8)	Telangiectasias	(4)
Previous ascites	(4)	Jaundice	(4)
Cirrhosis	(1)		
Nephrosis	(1)		

Simel DL, et al: Quantitating bedside diagnosis: Clinical evaluation of ascites. J Gen Intern Med 3:423–428, 1988.

81. What is the proper treatment for ascites?

The hallmarks of the treatment of ascites include:

1. **Removal by paracentesis:** Although an important diagnostic procedure, one can therapeutically remove 2–5 liters of ascitic fluid, usually with little risk. It is useful in cases of massive ascites or in the presence of complications (respiratory compromise).

2. **Sodium restriction:** Initially sodium intake should be restricted to less than 500 mg a day. This can be liberalized after diuresis so that the patient's diet will be both palatable and affordable in the ambulatory care setting.

3. **Fluid restriction:** Although not always necessary, it may used if dilutional hyponatremia occurs.

4. **Diuretic agents:** Used if dietary restriction does not suffice. They should be avoided in patients with renal insufficiency. A slow diuresis of less than 1 kilogram per day is the goal. Close monitoring of the patient's weight, electrolytes, and vital signs is required.

     a. *Potassium-sparing agents* such as spironolactone or triampterene are the initial choice.

     b. *Loop diuretics* (furosemide, ethacrynic acid, bumetanide) are used in patients who do not respond to potassium sparing diuretics.

5. **Peritoneovenous (LeVeen) shunts:** Used in patients resistant to maximal medical therapy (5–10% of patients).

ESOPHAGEAL DISEASE (see also GI Bleeding)

82. What is the approach to treatment of gastroesophageal reflux disease (GERD)?

Treatment of Gastroesophageal Reflux Disease

1. Dietary and lifestyle changes (Phase I)
    a. Limit intake of fatty foods, and acidic foods
    b. Discontinue intake of alcohol and caffeine
    c. Stop smoking
    d. Decrease the size of meals
    e. Weight reduction if obese
    f. Avoid tight-fitting garments around abdomen
    g. Postural therapy
       • Elevate head of bed 6–8 inches
       • Avoid lying down after eating
2. Medications (Phase II)
    a. Antacids and coating agents (postprandial antacids and sulcrafate to increase the pH of gastric contents and promote healing)
    b. Antisecretory agents (H_2 antagonists such as cimetidine or ranitidine, or omeprazole to decrease gastric acid secretion)
    c. Gastrokinetic agents (metaclopromide, bethanechol to increase lower esophageal sphincter pressure and promote esophageal and gastric emptying)
    d. Avoid anticholinergic agents (beta adrenergic agonists, tranquilizers, theophylline, nitrates, calcium channel blockers, and progesterone)
3. Surgery (Phase III)
    a. Procedures aimed to restoration of lower esophageal sphincter competence or prevention of reflux

83. What is pharyngeal or transfer dysphagia and what diseases may result in this problem?
Pharyngeal or transfer dysphagia is defined as the inability to initiate swallowing successfully. The patient may be able to move food around in the mouth but is unable to successfully transfer the bolus of food from the mouth into the esophagus. Liquids often cause the most severe symptoms and during the attempt to swallow the liquid is propelled into the larynx and trachea.

Patients with pharyngeal dysphagia may have a primary disease of the pharyngeal musculature or a neural disorder resulting in incoordination of swallowing. The patient with pharyngeal muscle weakness may be noted to have a nasal quality to the voice and report regurgitation of fluid into the nose during swallowing. These symptoms can be used to help distinguish pharyngeal or transfer dysphagia from esophageal dysphagia.

Pope CL: Heartburn, dysphagia, and other esophageal symptoms. In Sleisenger MH, Fordtran JS (eds): Gastrointestinal Disease, 4th ed. Philadelphia, W.B. Saunders, 1989, pp 200–203.

84. What are the two types of esophageal dysphagia? How can a patient's history be used to distinguish between the two?

True esophageal dysphagia may result from (1) **mechanical narrowing of the esophagus** or (2) **a motor disorder inhibiting normal peristalsis.** Narrowing of the lumen by a mechanical process may be due to intrinsic lesions such as peptic strictures, esophageal webs or carcinoma, or to extrinsic lesions such as mediastinal tumors resulting in compression of the esophagus. The second major cause of esophageal dysphagia is motor disorders in which the primary peristaltic pump of the esophagus fails. This is commonly seen in such entities as achalasia and scleroderma. Frequently, the history given by the patient can be used to help differentiate between a mechanical and motor disorder.

Mechanical obstruction typically presents with solid food dysphagia that may, over time, progress to include liquids. Motor disorders often begin with dysphagia to both solids and liquids. Solid food dysphagia associated with a long history of heartburn and regurgitation suggests a peptic stricture. Dysphagia that worsens upon ingesting cold liquids and improves with warm liquids suggests a motor disorder. Relief of obstruction by vomiting or regurgitation of the bolus suggests an organic narrowing. If the bolus can be dislodged by repeated swallowing or drinking water, a motor disorder is usually the cause.

85. What is presbyesophagus?

Presbyesophagus is a term that describes altered motor function of the esophagus as a result of degenerative changes in the elderly. It was coined by Soergel in a 1964 study. In fact, many of those patients had secondary illnesses that may have explained the abnormal manometric measurements. More recent studies have shown only mild manometric changes in elderly persons, who are usually asymptomatic.

Shamburek R, et al: Disorders of the digestive system in the elderly. N Engl J Med 322:438–443, 1990.

86. What is the most frequent cause of infectious esophagitis and how do patients with this disease present?

The most frequent cause of infectious esophagitis is candidal esophagitis. Most fungal infections occur in immunocompromised patients, especially patients with acquired immune deficiency syndrome. Patients with less obvious immune defects (diabetics, malnourished elderly, alcoholics, antibiotic- and steroid-treated patients) may also develop this disease. Patients will present with painful swallowing and retrosternal pain. They may also have dysphagia, fever, and bleeding. Physical examination of the patient may reveal oral thrush. Treatment of severely immunocompromised patients should begin with either ketoconazole or fluconazole, or IV amphotericin B. Less severely immunosuppressed patients may be treated with oral miconazole, nystatin, or clotrimazole. Ketoconazole is the drug of choice in patients with AIDS or when nystatin and clotrimazole have failed to eradicate the infection.

87. What drugs are commonly implicated as causes of pill-induced esophagitis?

Doxycycline, tetracycline, ascorbic acid, quinidine, and potassium chloride.

88. How can 24-hour pH monitoring, esophageal manometry, endoscopy, and an acid perfusion test (Bernstein test) be used to assess patients with suspected esophageal disease?

Twenty-four-hour ambulatory pH monitoring of the esophagus provides a temporal profile of acid reflux events and acid clearance and correlates these events with symptoms. Specific variables measured include the number of reflux episodes in 24 hours, acid clearance times from the esophagus, and esophageal exposure to acid. These values can be determined while the patient is in the upright or recumbent position. In general, patients with reflux disease show a higher rate of acid reflux into the esophagus and increased esophageal exposure time to acid as compared to normal subjects. Monitoring of pH can provide relevant information relating the patient's symptoms to the occurrence or nonoccurrence of reflux events. It is also useful in monitoring efficacy of medical or surgical therapy.

Esophageal manometry is useful in evaluating patients with noncardiac chest pain and a history suggestive of a possible esophageal motor disorder, achalasia, or esophageal reflux disease.

Endoscopy provides a direct view of the esophageal mucosa and allows directed biopsy when necessary. Visual inspection gives a gross anatomic examination of the interior lining of the esophagus. Endoscopy and biopsy are necessary to make a definitive diagnosis of many esophageal diseases.

The acid-perfusion or Bernstein test is a useful method for determining if chest pain is of esophageal origin. In this test, 0.1 N HCL is infused into the distal esophagus at a rate of about 1 ml per minute using saline infusion as a control. There appears to be good correlation between esophagitis symptoms and provocation of heartburn by the esophageal acid infusion test.

Chobanian SJ, et al: Systematic esophageal evaluation of patients with noncardiac chest pain. Arch Intern Med 146:1505–1508, 1986.

89. What is Barrett's esophagus and how should patients with this entity be managed and followed?

Barrett's esophagus is a complication that may develop in patients with longstanding reflux peptic esophagitis. It represents a unique reparative process whereby the original squamous epithelial cell lining of the esophagus is replaced by a metaplastic columnar-type epithelium. When the lower esophagus is lined by this columnar-type epithelium, it is termed Barrett's esophagus. The clinical significance of Barrett's esophagus lies primarily in its malignant potential. There is a risk of esophageal adenocarcinoma arising in the Barrett's epithelium and, although the actual incidence is unknown, the quoted average rate is approximately 10%. It has become clear that once Barrett's epithelium has developed, the process cannot be reversed by an antireflux operation or medical antireflux therapy. The optimal management of these patients has not been elucidated and the benefits of periodic endoscopic screening for dysplasia have not been shown. Yearly endoscopic surveillance and biopsy are advocated by some.

Spechler SJ, Goyal RK: Barrett's esophagus. N Engl J Med 315:362–371, 1986.

MALABSORPTION

90. What is Whipple's disease and how is it treated?

Whipple's disease, a traditional favorite for Grand Rounds, is a systemic disease that may affect almost any organ system of the body but in the majority of cases involves the small intestine. Patients present with intestinal malabsorption, weight loss, diarrhea, abdominal pain, fever, anemia, lymphadenopathy, and arthralgias. In addition, they may have nervous system symptoms, pericarditis, or endocarditis. The pathologic feature is infiltration of involved tissues with large glycoprotein-containing macrophages that stain strongly positive with a PAS stain. This diagnosis is most often made by biopsy of the small intestine. One can also see characteristic rod-shaped gram-positive bacilli that are not acid-fast. Effective treatment includes prolonged antibiotic therapy. Usually treatment with trimethoprim/sulfamethoxizole is instituted and continued for a minimum of 4 to 6 months. Repeat intestinal biopsy before discontinuing therapy should document disappearance of the Whipple bacillus.

91. A patient undergoes a small-bowel biopsy, and the mucosa shows flat villi and the crypts are markedly hyperplastic. How is this disease treated?

Celiac sprue, also called gluten enteropathy, is an allergic disease characterized by malabsorption of nutrients secondary to damaged small intestinal mucosa with the characteristic features described above. The responsible antigen is gluten, a water insoluble protein found in cereal grains such as wheat, barley, and rye. Withdrawal of gluten from the diet results in complete remission of both the clinical symptoms as well as the mucosal lesion. Although this disease is present worldwide, the distribution varies. The highest prevalence is in western Ireland.

92. What is dermatitis herpetiformis and how does this disease relate to celiac sprue?
Dermatitis herpetiformis is a skin condition that also may be reversed with dietary therapy (gluten restriction). Although the majority of patients with celiac sprue do not develop skin lesions of dermatitis herpetiformis, patients diagnosed with dermatitis herpetiformis will usually have the mucosal lesion in the small bowel consistent with sprue. The two diseases appear to be distinct entities that respond to the same dietary restrictions.

93. What is the blind-loop syndrome?
The blind-loop syndrome is a constellation of symptoms and laboratory abnormalities that include malabsorption of B_{12}, steatorrhea, hypoproteinemia, weight loss, and diarrhea. These symptoms are attributed to overgrowth of bacteria within the small intestine and have been associated with a number of diseases and surgical abnormalities. The common link between these associated conditions is abnormal motility of a segment of small intestine, resulting in stasis.

    The aim of therapy is reduction of bacterial overgrowth and consists of antibiotic administration and, when feasible, correction of the small intestinal abnormality that led to the condition.

94. What are the pathophysiologic mechanisms that can lead to fat malabsorption?
Normal fat absorption requires all phases of digestion to be intact. The process begins with secretion of pancreatic lipase and colipase. These enzymes are activated intraluminally and require an optimal pH of 6–8. Both enzymes are necessary for triglyceride hydrolysis in the duodenum. Any disorder that causes deficiencies of pancreatic enzyme secretion or leads to an acidic intraluminal environment that prevents proper enzyme activation could lead to fat malabsorption.

    The products of triglyceride hydrolysis, namely fatty acids and monoglycerides, must then be solubilized by bile salts to form micelles, and are subsequently absorbed by the small intestinal epithelium. Any disorder that interrupts the enterohepatic circulation or secretion of bile salts may lead to impaired micelle formation and therefore fat malabsorption.

    If the intestinal epithelial cell is in some way diseased, monoglyceride absorption and processing into chylomicrons for transport out of the small intestine may be impaired and lead to fat malabsorption. Disease of the intestinal lymphatics with impaired chylomicron transport has also been reported to result in fat malabsorption.

95. What diseases can affect fat absorption?
Diseases that may affect fat absorption include:
- Chronic pancreatitis
- Cystic fibrosis
- Pancreatic carcinoma
- Postgastrectomy syndrome
- Biliary tract obstruction
- Terminal ileal resection or disease
- Cholestatic liver disease
- Extensive small bowel destruction

- Intestinal epithelial disease, such as Whipple's disease, sprue, eosinophilic gastroenteritis
- Lymphatic disease, such as abetalipoproteinemia, intestinal lymphangiectasia, lymphoma, and tuberculous adenitis
- Small bowel bacterial overgrowth (bile salts are deconjugated and inactivated by bacteria)
- Zollinger-Ellison syndrome (in this disease pancreatic enzymes are inactivated by a low intraluminal pH).

Shiau YF: Lipid digestion and absorption. In Johnson LR (ed): Physiology of the Gastrointestinal Tract, 2nd ed. New York, Raven Press, 1987, pp 1527–1556.

96. Which conditions are associated with or may result in small bowel bacteria overgrowth?

Any abnormality of the small intestine that results in local stasis or recirculation of intestinal contents is likely to be associated with marked proliferation of intraluminal bacteria. The flora of the small intestine becomes predominantly anaerobic and closely resembles colonic flora. Disorders that are associated with malabsorption due to bacterial overgrowth include:

1. Gastric proliferation of bacteria as seen in hypochlorhydric or achlorhydric states, particularly when these are combined with motor or anatomic disturbances.

2. Small intestinal stagnation associated with anatomic alterations following surgery, such as afferent loop syndrome after a Billroth II procedure.

3. Duodenal and jejunal diverticulosis, particularly as seen in patients with scleroderma.

4. Surgically created blind loops, such as end-to-side anastomoses.

5. Chronic low-grade obstruction secondary to small intestinal strictures, adhesions, inflammation, or carcinoma may lead to proximal bacterial overgrowth.

6. Motor disturbances of the small intestine, such as scleroderma, idiopathic pseudo-obstruction, or diabetic neuropathy can result in stasis and bacterial overgrowth.

7. Abnormal communication between the proximal small intestine and the distal intestinal tract may result in bacterial colonization of the proximal region. This is seen in gastrocolic or jejunocolic fistulas and may follow resection of the ileocecal valve.

97. How does small bowel bacterial overgrowth result in fat malabsorption?

Small bowel bacterial overgrowth may lead to fat malabsorption because bacterial enzymes deconjugate intraluminal bile salts to free bile acids. Free bile acids are unable to solubilize monoglycerides and free fatty acids into micelles for absorption by the epithelial cells. The result is impaired absorption of fat and fat soluble vitamins.

98. What constitutes normal fecal fat concentration and what is steatorrhea? How is steatorrhea detected?

The typical U.S. diet consists of between 70 and 120 grams of fat per day. Fat absorption is extremely efficient and most of the ingested fat is absorbed with very little excretion into the stool. The average fecal fat concentration for the normal individual is between 4 and 6 grams per day. The upper limit of normal is approximately 9 grams in 24 hours. Patients with steatorrhea, or increased excretion of fecal fat, may have up to 10 times this amount in the stool. In order to detect steatorrhea, a 72-hour stool sample is collected while on a defined dietary fat intake ranging from 70 to 120 grams per day. The 3-day stool collection is taken to the lab where a chemical analysis measures the amount of fat present. This test is highly reliable but neither specific nor sensitive in determining the etiology of steatorrhea.

Shiau YF: Lipid digestion absorption. In Johnson LR (ed): Physiology of the Gastrointestinal Tract, 2nd ed. New York, Raven Press, 1987, pp 1527–1556.

99. Describe the proper evaluation of a patient with steatorrhea.

In evaluating a patient with steatorrhea (stool fat greater than or equal to 9 grams per 24 hours), the primary differential diagnosis consists of small intestinal disorders, pancreatic disorders, and biliary tract disorders. If the diagnosis is not obvious after a routine history and physical examination, a D-xylose absorption test should be done. If fat malabsorption is due to small intestinal disease, carbohydrate absorption as measured by D-xylose absorption is likely to be abnormally low. If the D-xylose test is normal, an abdominal radiograph or plain film should be done to look for evidence of chronic pancreatitis and pancreatic calcification.

Small intestinal barium x-ray studies may show evidence of previous intestinal surgery (e.g., subtotal gastrectomy or massive small bowel resection), or may reveal partial intestinal obstruction in a patient with unsuspected Crohn's disease or lymphoma.

A bentiromide test can be done as a noninvasive evaluation of pancreatic function. The underlying principle involved in this test is that adequate duodenal concentration of pancreatic chymotrypsin is necessary to cleave para-aminobenzoic acid (PABA) from the synthetic peptide N-benzoyl-L-tyrosyl-para-aminobenzoic acid (bentiromide). If adequate levels of chymotrypsin are present, bentiromide is hydrolyzed and free PABA is released into the duodenum, absorbed, conjugated in the liver, and subsequently excreted in urine, where it can be measured in a 6-hour urine collection test. If PABA excretion is reduced, severe pancreatic insufficiency should be expected.

If D-xylose absorption is abnormal, this suggests small intestinal disease resulting in fat malabsorption. The next step should be an endoscopic small intestinal biopsy to rule out intestinal sprue, Whipple's disease, and other specific mucosal entities that may lead to steatorrhea.

If the small intestinal biopsy is normal, a ^{14}C-D-xylose breath test may be used to rule out small bowel bacterial overgrowth. This test consists of the oral administration of a dose of ^{14}C-D-xylose and subsequent measuring of exhaled $^{14}CO_2$. In small intestinal bacterial overgrowth, gram-negative bacteria metabolize ^{14}C-D-xylose to $^{14}CO_2$, which is absorbed and exhaled in the breath. This breath test has been shown to be more reliable than quantitative bacterial culture of the small bowel for diagnosing bacterial overgrowth. If the test is abnormal, the patient should be treated for bacterial overgrowth with a course of broad-spectrum antibiotics, and the test should be repeated after therapy to confirm the response.

Yn NE, Olsen WA: A diagnostic approach to malabsorption syndromes. A pathophysiologic approach. Clin Gastroenterol 12:533, 1983.

100. What are the four stages of a Schilling test and what mechanisms of absorption does each stage test for?

The standard Schilling test measures vitamin B_{12} absorption and is used to detect intrinsic factor deficiency in patients with pernicious anemia. The test results are often abnormal in patients with genetic defects in vitamin B_{12} absorption; in bacterial overgrowth of the small bowel; following extensive destruction, resection, or bypass of the terminal ileum; and in pancreatic insufficiency.

Stage one of the standard Schilling test consists of an oral dose of radiolabeled vitamin B_{12} given simultaneously with an IM injection of 1 mg non-radiolabeled B_{12}. The urine is collected for 24 hours and the amount of radioactivity is measured. Patients with normal absorption of B_{12} and normal renal function will excrete greater than 7% of the radioactively labeled B_{12} in 24 hours.

In Stage two, the test is repeated following oral administration of 60 mg intrinsic factor. Patients with pernicious anemia normalize the level of urinary radiolabeled B_{12}.

Small intestinal bacterial overgrowth may cause B_{12} malabsorption and an abnormal result in stage one of the Schilling test due to bacterial utilization of the vitamin. This is not corrected with intrinsic factor in stage two. After 1 week of treatment with a broad-spectrum antibiotic (**stage three**) to eliminate the intestinal bacteria, stage one of the Schilling test should normalize.

Normal B_{12} absorption also requires normal pancreatic exocrine function. Pancreatic proteases are required for the cleavage of vitamin B_{12} from R-protein. If pancreatic insufficiency exists, B_{12} malabsorption may occur. Normalization of B_{12} absorption after administration of pancreatic enzyme therapy (**stage four**) suggests a pancreatic origin of B_{12} malabsorption.

OBSTRUCTION

101. What are the four most common causes of mechanical small bowel obstruction (SBO) in adults?
The four most common causes of mechanical SBO in adults are:
1. Adhesions, accounting for approximately 74%.
2. Hernias, which account for 8%.
3. Malignancies of the small bowel, which account for 8%.
4. Inflammatory bowel disease with stricture formation, which accounts for most of the remaining cases.

102. What historical and physical clues may be used to determine the location of the obstruction in a patient with SBO?
The patient with mechanical SBO typically presents with crampy intermittent abdominal pain occurring in paroxysms, 4 to 5 minutes apart. These symptoms are more indicative of proximal rather than distal obstruction. Certain clinical characteristics can be used to distinguish a proximal from a distal obstruction. A high obstruction presents in a more acute fashion, with vomiting as a very prominent complaint. The vomiting is typically bilious and nonfeculent and pain occurs at short-spaced intervals. Abdominal distention may be minimal or absent if the location is high in the small bowel.

Patients with distal SBO may have a more insidious onset of symptoms. Vomiting is often present but is a less prominent complaint. When present, the vomiting is often feculent. Pain occurs at longer spaced intervals compared with proximal SBO. The lower the blockage, the more likely there is to be abdominal distention resulting from accumulation of fluid and gas in the intestine.

103. What findings on the plain film x-ray would suggest a SBO?
Plain abdominal x-rays are quite useful in confirming SBO and usually reveal abnormally large quantities of gas in the bowel. This gas can be identified as small intestinal gas by the presence of the valvulae conniventes, which usually occupy the entire transverse diameter of the small bowel. This feature can be distinguished from colonic haustral markings, which occupy only a portion of the diameter of the bowel. Additionally, loops of small bowel are most commonly located in the more central portion of the abdomen, whereas colonic gas is usually seen in the periphery of the x-ray film. In the patient with classic mechanical SBO, there is minimal or no colonic gas. The upright or decubitus abdominal film will reveal multiple air-fluid levels with distended loops of small bowel resembling inverted U's.

104. Explain the appropriate management of a patient with SBO.
In the majority of circumstances, the most appropriate therapy for mechanical SBO is surgical relief of the obstruction. The three goals of management include (1) investigation of the cause and location of the obstruction, (2) resuscitation of the patient and preparing the patient for surgery, and (3) surgical correction of the problem.

The timing of the operation should depend upon the following three important factors:

1. The duration of obstruction as related to the severity of fluid, electrolyte, and acid base abnormalities.

2. The improvement of vital organ function (i.e., the management of concomitant cardiac and pulmonary disorders).

3. Consideration of the risk of strangulation.

Since the mortality rate of SBO associated with strangulation is quite high, early operative intervention should be performed. Surgical intervention can be postponed in lieu of a short trial of conservative nonoperative management if the patient has developed obstruction in the immediate postoperative period. These patients may respond to simple nasogastric (NG) suction. Similarly, the patient with obstruction caused by disseminated intra-abdominal carcinomatosis, Crohn's disease, radiation strictures, or adhesions following previous surgery may improve with simple management and NG suction. If conservative medical therapy is used, the patient should show continuous improvement during the first 12 to 24 hours of therapy. If not, surgical relief of the obstruction should be performed.

Stewardson RH, et al: Critical operative management of small bowel obstruction. Ann Surg 187–189, 1978.

105. What is ileus and what seven entities may cause small bowel ileus?

Paralytic ileus is a relatively common disorder and occurs when neural, humoral, and metabolic factors combine to stimulate reflexes that inhibit intestinal motility. The result is small bowel and/or colonic distention due to intestinal muscle paralysis. The seven common causes of paralytic ileus are (1) abdominal surgery, (2) peritonitis, (3) generalized sepsis, (4) electrolyte imbalance (particularly hypokalamia, which interferes with normal ionic movements and smooth muscle contraction), (5) retroperitoneal hemorrhage, and (6) spinal or (7) pelvic fractures. Drugs such as phenothiazines and narcotics inhibit small bowel motility and may contribute to paralysis. Treatment consists of NG suction to relieve distention and IV fluids to replace losses, followed by correction of the underlying disorder.

106. What conditions may aggravate or be associated with colonic pseudo-obstruction?

Conditions Associated with Colonic Pseudo-obstruction

1. Trauma (nonoperative) and surgery (gynecologic, orthopedic, urologic)
2. Inflammatory processes (pancreatitis, cholecystitis)
3. Infections
4. Malignancy
5. Radiation therapy
6. Drugs (narcotics, antidepressants, clonidine, anticholinergics)
7. Cardiovascular disease
8. Neurologic disease
9. Respiratory failure
10. Metabolic disease (diabetes, hypothyroidism, electrolyte imbalance, uremia)
11. Alcoholism

107. What is the most common cause of gastric outlet obstruction?

Peptic ulcer disease.

108. What is a bezoar and in what clinical setting are they likely to be seen?

Bezoars are clusters of food or foreign matter that have undergone partial digestion in the stomach, failed to pass through the pylorus into the small bowel, and formed a mass in the stomach. Substances that typically comprise bezoars include hair (trichobezoars) or plant matter (phytobezoars). Bezoars may become quite large and can present with abdominal mass, gastric outlet obstruction, attacks of nausea and vomiting, and peptic ulceration. The most common bezoar in current adult medicine is the phytobezoar. Factors important in the formation of bezoars include the amount of undigestible materials in the diet (pulpy, fibrous fruit or vegetables such as oranges), the quality of the chewing mechanism, and loss of pyloric function, which limits the size of food particles that may enter the duodenum.

The standard treatment of phytobezoars includes manual attempts at external disruption, a liquid diet, suction, and lavage. Endoscopic fragmentation using forceps and polypectomy snares or water pick devices may be used to break up the masses. Rarely, a patient requires gastrotomy to remove the bezoar.

BILIARY TRACT DISEASE

109. What is the prevalence of asymptomatic cholelithiasis in adult Americans over age 40? What percent of these will ultimately develop symptoms?
Forty percent of Americans over age 40 have gallstones and 10–30% of these will become symptomatic at some point.

110. Is surgery indicated for asymptomatic cholelithiasis?
Elective surgery is generally not indicated. It has been previously recommended that elective cholecystectomy be performed in diabetic patients with asymptomatic cholelithiasis, but there is evidence that they have a higher complication rate from elective cholecystectomy.

111. What ethnic groups have a higher prevalence of cholesterol gallstone formation?
American Indians and Mexican Americans have the highest prevalence of cholesterol gallstones.

112. What percent of gallstones is radiopaque?
Pigment gallstones, which account for 20–30% of gallstones in the U.S., are often radiopaque and can therefore can be seen on plain radiographs of the abdomen. Cholesterol gallstones, which account for 70–80% of gallstones, are radiolucent.

113. What is the therapeutic approach to the patient with suppurative cholangitis who has previously undergone cholecystectomy?
Suppurative cholangitis is a life-threatening illness that requires urgent intervention and immediate drainage of the common bile duct and relief of the obstruction. This can be performed via endoscopic retrograde cholangiopancreatography (ERCP) or by percutaneous transhepatic cholangiogram (PTC). The advantages of ERCP include the ability to treat the primary disease process utilizing papillotomy, with removal of common bile duct stones or placement of an internal drain, and avoiding the morbidity associated with percutaneous external drainage.

Nonoperative therapy utilizing ERCP and endoscopic drainage in the patient with cholangitis has a mortality rate of only 1–2%, in contrast to emergency surgery in this setting which has a mortality rate as high as 40%. Elective surgery can be done later, if needed, and is associated with a lower mortality than in the acute situation.

114. What is Charcot's triad?
Right upper quadrant (RUQ) pain, jaundice, and fever. This triad is present in 70% of

patients with bacterial cholangitis.

115. In the diagnostic evaluation of a patient with suspected obstructive jaundice, what diagnostic tests are available and how do they compare?

The cause of jaundice can be determined in many cases from clinical data and routine laboratory tests. The only special study that is routinely useful in the early evaluation of obstructive jaundice is an ultrasound scan of the gallbladder, bile ducts, and liver. Ultrasound is fairly specific for detecting gallbladder stones and ductal dilatation, the latter signifying ductal obstruction. However, a negative scan does not prove the absence of stones or obstruction, since the sensitivity of ultrasound in detecting obstruction is only about 85%.

Abdominal CT scan is fairly sensitive for detecting ductal dilatation and can be useful in estimating the site of ductal obstruction. A CT scan is less able to detect stones of the gallbladder and common bile duct than is ultrasound, but is better able to image mass lesions.

Liver biopsy in the patient with extrahepatic ductal obstruction is not routinely useful. It may reveal evidence of cholestasis and cholangitis but will not help to determine the cause. A liver scan using technetium sulfur colloid is of very little value in the jaundiced patient.

If the bile ducts are dilated on the sonogram or CT scan, the next step should be an evaluation to determine the cause of obstruction, and an attempt to relieve the obstruction and provide drainage should be made. The two modalities that can be used to obtain this information are endoscopic retrograde cholangiopancreatography (ERCP), and the percutaneous transhepatic cholangiogram (PTC). ERCP is a relatively simple procedure if a trained endoscopist is available. The common bile duct is cannulated endoscopically and cholangiograms obtained. If bile duct stones are seen, they can be removed at the time of ERCP and relief of the obstruction is obtained. If a bile duct or ampullary tumor is found, internal drainage can be established at the time of the procedure. PTC offers similar advantages; however, it adds the additional morbidity and discomfort of percutaneous needle-stick and the possibility of external biliary drainage following a procedure. The overall risk of both procedures is fairly low and they compare favorably to one another.

Thomas MJ, et al: Usefulness of diagnostic tests for biliary obstruction. Am J Surg 144:102, 1982.

BIBLIOGRAPHY

1 Fenoglio-Preiser CM, et al: Gastrointestinal Pathology: An Atlas and Text. New York, Raven Press, 1989.
2. Schiff L, Schiff ER (eds): Diseases of the Liver, 6th ed. Philadelphia, J.B. Lippincott, 1987.
3. Sleisenger MH, Fordtran JS (eds): Gastrointestinal Disease: Pathophysiology, Diagnosis, and Management, 4th ed. Philadelphia, W.B. Saunders, 1989.
4. Wyngaarden JB, Smith LH (eds): Cecil Textbook of Medicine, 18th ed. Philadelphia, W.B. Saunders, 1988.
5. Zakim D, Boyer TD (eds): Hepatology: A Textbook of Liver Disease, 2nd ed. Philadelphia, W.B. Saunders, 1990.

6. ONCOLOGY SECRETS

Mary Anne Zubler, M.D.

While there are several chronic diseases more destructive to life than cancer, none is more feared.

Charles H. Mayo (1865–1939)
Annals of Surgery 83:357, 1926

1. One of the risk factors for cancer is the genetic background of the patient. What are the known genetically related mechanisms of neoplasia?

Cancer may develop as a result of a single gene mutation or be the result of multiple mutations. It is theorized that there may be a genetic predisposition in some patients (initiation), which may not be expressed without a further environmental exposure (promoters). Disorders that have identified genetic predisposition include von Recklinghausen's neurofibromatosis, retinoblastoma, multiple endocrine neoplasia, and familial polyposis coli. Among the most common genetically transmitted cancers is breast cancer. "Site-specific aggregation" describes the phenomenon whereby relatives of patients with breast or large bowel cancer are at risk for developing these diseases. The pattern of frequency signifies the activity of the genetic factors.

2. Besides genetic predisposition, what are other risk factors for cancer?

Other risk factors for cancer include chemical exposure, parasites, radiation, and dietary factors. Benzopyrenes and nitrosamines (which may be formed endogenously from precursor nitrites or nitrates in food) are implicated in cancer production. Bile salts are thought to be promoters, acting to accelerate cancer growth. A high-fiber diet is theorized to reduce the risk for large bowel cancer. This may occur by increasing the bulk of the stool, thereby diluting the contents of the colon and promoting rapid emptying.

Chemicals that are felt to be carcinogenic react with oxygen and nitrogen atoms in DNA to form stable chemical adducts with guanine, adenine, and thymine. These adducts interrupt DNA-strand pairing or lead to a loss of base sequences, resulting in permanent alterations in the genome. They may transmit faulty information and/or produce abnormal protein products, which may abnormally regulate the growth of the cell.

Some substances may modify the effect of chemical carcinogenesis. The most well known are vitamin A (which promotes the differentiation of epithelial tissues), vitamin C (which blocks the formation of n-nitrosocarcinogens from nitrite and secondary amines), and vitamin E (which is a free-radical scavenger).

3. What are oncogenes and how do they function?

Oncogenes are genes in human and other animal tumors that have the capacity to transform normal cells into malignant cells. Some of these genes, acquired at conception, make the patient susceptible to cancer by virtue of altering or impairing the following processes:

1. The metabolism of potentially carcinogenic compounds
2. The ability to repair genetic damage
3. The growth regulation of specific cell types
4. The ability of the immune system to recognize and eradicate incipient tumors.

Other genes are acquired by somatic mutational mechanisms and these genes confer advantageous growth properties on the cells that express them, allowing these cells to proliferate more rapidly than their genetically normal counterparts.

4. How are tumor markers used in diagnosing and treating cancer?

Tumor markers are enzymes, hormones, and oncofetal antigens that are produced by some tumors. The markers reflect the presence of the tumor or the quantity of the tumor (tumor burden). Many common cancers do not produce these markers. Those tumors that are known to produce markers may sometimes fail to do so, particularly if they are very poorly differentiated. Some of the markers, such as prostatic acid phosphatase (PAP) and alphafetoprotein (AFP), are highly sensitive, highly specific, and of high predictive value. Others, such as lactic dehydrogenase (LDH), are quite nonspecific and are elevated in many conditions besides malignancies. The most important use of these markers is in following the effects of therapy on tumor burden and in detecting recurrent disease after initial therapy. Most markers have limited significance in the initial diagnostic evaluation.

5. Which are the three most common tumor markers? Identify their uses.

1. **Carcinoembryonic antigen (CEA).** CEA is a glycoprotein of 200,000 daltons that is found in gastrointestinal mucosal cells and the secretions of the pancreatobiliary system. Elevations occur with breaks in the mucosal basement membrane by a tumor, but can also occur in smokers, patients with cirrhosis, pancreatitis, inflammatory bowel disease, and rectal polyps. It is most useful in monitoring the activity of disease in recurrent colorectal cancer.

2. **Alphafetoprotein (AFP).** AFP is an alpha-globulin of 70,000 daltons that is made by the yolk sac and liver of the human fetus. It is elevated in hepatomas and certain germ cell neoplasms, and has been found to be a very sensitive marker for disease activity. However, it is rather nonspecific and can be elevated in acute viral and chronic active hepatitis.

3. **Human chorionic gonadotropin (HCG).** HCG is a glycoprotein normally secreted by the trophoblastic epithelium of the placenta. It is used as a sensitive and specific marker for germ cell tumors of the testes and ovary, and extragonadal presentations of these tumors.

6. List the principles used in formulating combination chemotherapy regimens.

Principles of Combination Chemotherapy

1. Drugs used should have activity against the tumor.
2. Drugs should be selected with dissimilar toxicities.
3. Drugs with different mechanisms of action should be used.
4. Several cycles of therapy, with adequate biological effect, should be used before determining efficacy.
5. Recovery time of normal tissues should be allowed before starting next cycle.

7. What are the mechanisms of drug resistance of tumors to chemotherapeutic agents?

Mechanisms of Drug Resistance in Chemotherapy

1. Intrinsic cytokinetic or biochemical resistance
2. Impaired transport of the drug
3. Altered drug affinity for the target enzyme
4. Amplification of genes
5. Membrane alterations from overproduction of high-weight glycoproteins

8. What are the toxic effects of chemotherapy?

The most common immediate effects are nausea and vomiting, which vary in presence and degree with the type of drug. Some, like cisplatin, are very emetogenic, whereas others, like methotrexate, are unlikely to cause emesis.

The most dangerous adverse effect is myelosuppression. Leukopenia predisposes to acute and serious infections; thrombocytopenia predisposes to bleeding; and anemia may worsen other problems, such as chronic obstructive pulmonary disease (COPD) and atherosclerotic cardiovascular disease (ASCVD).

Other adverse effects are drug-specific:

- Platinol and methotrexate are nephrotoxic.
- Cyclophosphamide can cause a hemorrhage cystitis. Long-term use has been associated with bladder cancer.
- Fluorouracil (5-FU) is associated with cerebellar ataxia, dacryocystitis, hand-foot syndrome, and light sensitivity.
- Fluorouracil and bleomycin can cause hyperpigmentation of the skin. With fluorouracil it is seen over the veins used for injection, and with bleomycin it is usually seen around the nail beds.
- Both fluorouracil and bleomycin have been associated with chest pain during infusion, possibly related to coronary artery spasm.
- Many agents cause mucositis, chief among them being methotrexate and adriamycin.
- Liver toxicity has been demonstrated with some drugs. Methotrexate, given chronically, has been associated with postnecrotic cirrhosis; fluorodeoxyuridine (FUDR), given by continuous infusion, is associated with chronic biliary sclerosis.
- Pulmonary toxicity (pulmonary fibrosis) has been described in conjunction with methotrexate, cyclophosphamide, and bleomycin.
- Cardiac toxicity is most frequently associated with doxorubicin (Adriamycin), which causes a progressive loss of cardiac muscle cells. In previously normal hearts, this toxicity is dose-related and does not become clinically important until a total dose of approximately 450 mg/m^2 is reached. Of course, in already compromised cardiac function, this toxicity may be seen at lower dosages. Cardiac radionuclide-gated wall-motion studies (multiple-gated acquisition [MUGA] scans) measuring ejection fraction are used to monitor changes in cardiac function.

9. Which tumors spread to bone most commonly? Are they osteoblastic or osteolytic?

Cancer of the lung, breast, kidney, prostate, and thyroid, as well as multiple myeloma and malignant melanoma, are the tumors that spread to bone most commonly. Renal cell carcinoma and multiple myeloma tend to be purely lytic, and prostate tends to be mainly blastic; the others are mixed. The most frequently involved bones are the spine, ribs, pelvis, and long bones. Those that are lytic are most often associated with hypercalcemia, whereas blastic metastases are rarely associated with this complication. The pain of these metastases is characterized by a dull, aching discomfort that is worse at night and improves with physical activity.

10. Which tumors metastasize to the lungs?

All tumors can metastasize to the lungs; therefore, the more common the tumor, the more commonly it is found to have spread to the lung (e.g., breast cancers). Although they can spread to the lungs, GI cancers tend to metastasize to the liver and locally before pulmonary involvement is seen. Those tumors that spread via the bloodstream, such as sarcomas, renal cell carcinoma, colon cancer, and thyroid cancers, tend to produce nodular lung lesions; those that spread via lymphatic routes, such as cancers of the breast, pancreas, stomach, and liver, manifest a pattern of lymphangitic spread.

11. What are the predisposing factors, organisms, and sources for infection in cancer patients?

Predisposing factors for infection in cancer patients include defects in cellular and humoral immunity, organ compromise due to tumor-related obstruction, granulocytopenia, disruption of mucosal (e.g., respiratory and alimentary tract) and integumental surfaces, iatrogenic procedures or placement of prosthetic devices, central nervous system dysfunction, and hyposplenic or postsplenectomy states.

Organisms accounting for the majority of infections in cancer patients are enterobacteriaceae (*Klebsiella, Enterobacter, E. coli*), *Staphylococcus* sp., *Streptococcus* sp., and *Pseudomonas* sp. Fungal organisms found in infected cancer patients include aspergillus, *Candida* sp., and cryptococcus. The most common viral infections found in cancer patients are herpes simplex and varicella-zoster.

Sources of infection in neutropenic cancer patients include the lungs, urinary tract, skin, upper aerodigestive tract (mouth, skin, teeth), central nervous system, rectum, perirectum, biopsy sites, and the GI tract (appendicitis, cholecystitis, perforations). The vast majority of infections originate from the patients' own endogenous flora. Cultures of the infected patient should include blood, urine, sputum, and, if appropriate, stool, pleural fluid, and peritoneal fluid.

12. How is the doubling time of tumors calculated from chest x-rays?

The doubling time of tumors can be roughly calculated from chest x-rays by measuring the diameter of the lesion, assuming it is approximately spherical, and calculating its volume. By calculating volume at two points in time, doubling time can be extracted from a plot of volume versus time.

This assumes very simple growth kinetics and the absence of other factors affecting the growth, which is rarely, if ever, the case. Tumor cell populations exhibit a reduction in net fractional growth rate with increasing population size. The Gompertz equation describes this slowing of growth with size and takes into account various other factors such as decreasing blood supply with increasing size of tumor. A graph showing Gompertzian tumor growth (curve C) as well as exponential tumor growth (curve A) and cube-root function growth (curve B) follows:

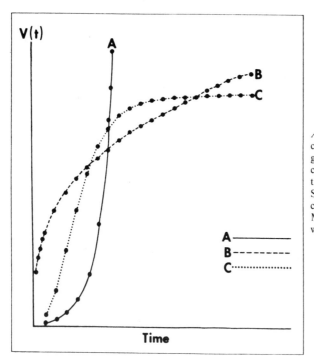

A, Exponential tumor growth curve; *B,* cube-root function growth curve; *C,* tumor growth curve from the Gompertz equation. (From Silver RT, et al: Some new aspects of modern cancer chemotherapy. Am J Med 63:772–787, 1977, p 774, with permission.)

13. Identify the characteristic lesions of melanoma in the small bowel.
Melanoma often metastasizes to the bowel, where it causes obstruction and bleeding. Lesions can be seen that are ulcerated with a central crater and a surrounding heaped-up border, causing the barium to pool in a "target" configuration.

14. Patients with melanoma have what typical physical characteristics?
Typical physical characteristics of patients with melanoma are fair skin, reddish hair, and freckles. Familial melanoma families have been described. In these families, more than 25% of the kindred are affected with a vertical distribution of disease. There is an early age of onset, from the third to fourth decades. The incidence of multiple primaries is increased, as is the presence of atypical nevi (B-K moles or familial atypical multiple melanoma [FAMM]) with melanocyte dysplasia. However, there is a superior overall survival, possibly related to earlier detection. Ocular melanoma is also seen in this group of patients.

15. What are the signs and symptoms of the syndrome of inappropriate anti-diuretic hormone (SIADH)?
Weakness, anorexia, nausea, and lethargy may be manifestations of hyponatremia, but they are so nonspecific that one must have an index of suspicion to include hyponatremia in the differential diagnosis. The most common cancer associated with SIADH is small cell carcinoma of the lung. It may also be seen with mesothelioma, increased intracranial pressure, and chronic lung diseases. Drugs that have been described in association with hyponatremia are diuretics, cyclophosphamide, vincristine, chlorpropamide, carbamazepine, amitriptyline and thioridazine.

Criteria for diagnosing SIADH include:
- Urine osmolality increased
- Urine sodium normal or increased
- Serum osmolality decreased
- Serum sodium decreased, with a low BUN (< 10 mg/dl)
- Normal intravascular volume
- No ascites or edema
- Normal renal function

Treatment of SIADH is dependent on the degree of hyponatremia and associated symptoms. If serum sodium is < 110 mmol/L and the patient is comatose or seizing, intravenous 3% sodium chloride is given with intravenous furosemide. This should only be done in an intensive care unit setting with appropriate monitoring.

If the serum sodium is > 110 mmol/L, and/or the patient is moderately symptomatic, fluid restriction to no more than 1000 cc per day should result in normal serum sodium in 3 to 5 days. Other therapies that may be used are demeclocycline 150–300 mg PO qid, or lithium 200 mg qid (levels must be monitored since lithium can be nephrotoxic).

16. What are the causes of anemia in cancer patients?
Anemia in patients with cancer may be secondary to blood loss due to bleeding from tumors or gastritis from the use of nonsteroidal anti-inflammatory agents such as aspirin. It may also be caused by hemolysis (which may be secondary to antibodies associated with the tumor), disseminated intravascular coagulation (DIC), sepsis, or related to a paraneoplastic syndrome in cases of cancer of the pancreas or prostate. Anemia can also be caused by bone marrow suppression by chemotherapy or marrow involvement by the tumor. Anemia of chronic disease is common in cancer patients, and the diagnosis is made when no other cause of anemia can be found and plasma iron is less than 60 μg/dl, total iron binding capacity (TIBC) is 100–250 μg/dl, and ferritin is greater than 60 ng/ml. The hematocrit is generally around 25%, although values as low as 16% are not uncommon in some patient populations. An inadequate erythropoietin response to the anemia has been

demonstrated in these patients. An inadequate response to treatment with recombinant human erythropoietin has also been demonstrated in some studies.

Miller CB, et al: Decreased erythropoietin response in patients with the anemia of cancer. New Engl J Med 322:1689–1692, 1990.

17. What are the presenting symptoms and signs of spinal cord compression?

Ninety-five percent of cancer patients with spinal cord compression present with back pain. One may also find lower extremity weakness, bowel or bladder incontinence, or increased deep tendon reflexes in the lower extremities. The diagnosis is made by myelogram (standard or computerized tomography [CT]), or by magnetic resonance imaging (MRI), which will demonstrate a blockage of the spinal canal. Treatment is directed first at relieving pain, using adequate pain medication and high dose steroids. However, definitive treatment must be carried out emergently to prevent further neurological deterioration, which may be irreversible. Radiotherapy and/or surgery should be initiated immediately.

The most common tumors causing cord compression are lung cancer, breast cancer, prostate cancer, carcinoma of unknown primary, lymphoma, and multiple myeloma. The most common site of cord compression is the thoracic spine, followed by the lumbosacral spine, and the cervical spine.

18. What are the symptoms of intracranial metastases?

Headache occurs in up to 50% of patients with intracranial metastases. It is classically described as occurring early in the morning, disappearing or decreasing after arising, and often associated with nausea and/or projectile vomiting. Other symptoms include focal signs, such as unilateral weakness, numbness, seizures, or cranial nerve abnormalities. Nonfocal complaints such as mental status changes or ataxia may be seen. The diagnosis is made by CT or MRI. Treatment consists of decreasing intracranial pressure with steroids, followed by radiotherapy. Surgery is sometimes used in patients with single intracranial lesions, no other sites of metastases, and a long time interval between the primary tumor and the intracranial metastasis.

19. What are the signs and symptoms of malignant pericardial effusion?

The presentation of malignant pericardial effusion can resemble heart failure, with dyspnea, peripheral edema, and an enlarged heart on chest x-ray. However, the dyspnea is often out of proportion to the degree of pulmonary congestion seen on the x-ray. Kussmaul's sign, or jugulovenous distention (JVD) with inspiration, and pulsus paradoxus of more than 10 mmHg with distant heart sounds are clues to the presence of a pericardial effusion.

Confirmation of the clinical diagnosis is made by echocardiogram, but may be made incidentally on a CT scan. Treatment is dependent on the degree of illness of the patient but should include drainage of the fluid for diagnostic as well as therapeutic reasons. Subxiphoid pericardial catheters, transthoracic catheters, pericardial windows, and pericardial stripping have all been used. Nonsurgical approaches often include sclerosis of the pericardium, most often with tetracycline.

The differential diagnosis includes superior vena cava syndrome, radiation pericarditis, myocardial infarction (MI), uremic pericarditis, and acute and chronic infections (such as bacterial and tuberculous pericarditis); also, connective tissue diseases, drugs such as hydralazine, hypothyroidism, and trauma.

Malignant effusions are usually exudates and are often hemorrhagic. Cytology is helpful if positive but does not exclude cancer if negative.

20. Which tumors are associated with nonbacterial thrombotic endocarditis?

This paraneoplastic syndrome is associated with mucinous adenocarcinomas, most commonly of the lung, stomach, or ovary, but has been described in other types as well. It is revealed by the appearance of embolic peripheral or cerebral vascular events causing arterial insufficiency, encephalopathy, or focal neurologic defects. Heart murmurs are often not present. Echocardiograms may often be negative, and the diagnosis is usually made post mortem. Treatment with anticoagulants or antiplatelet drugs has been tried with little success.

21. What is the tumor lysis syndrome?

When rapidly growing tumors are effectively treated with chemotherapy, breakdown products of tumor lysis are released into the vascular system in large amounts. This may cause hyperkalemia, hyperuricemia, hyperphosphatemia, and hypocalcemia. There may be renal failure from the hyperuricemia. This complication is usually seen within a few hours to days following the treatment of tumors such as acute leukemia, Burkitt's lymphoma, and occasionally other rapidly dividing lymphomas. It is rarely, if ever, seen with solid tumors, but has been described in small cell carcinoma of the lung.

Treatment is the same as for renal failure, with vigorous hydration, dialysis if necessary, and appropriate treatment of electrolyte disorders. Preventive treatment with allopurinol is effective in these patients.

22. What are the tumor-related causes of hypercalcemia?

Causes of increased calcium in cancer patients are:

1. **Lytic bone metastases,** which release calcium into the bloodstream. This is the most common cause in solid tumors with bony metastases.

2. **Humoral mediators** of hypercalcemia have been demonstrated in patients without bony metastases. Ectopic parathyroid hormone (PTH) and elevated prostaglandin activity have been described in the past, but the term humoral hypercalcemia of malignancy (HHM) is now used. This is a non-PTH substance with some PTH-like activity and is associated with squamous cell cancers of many origins, renal cell cancer, transitional cell carcinomas and ovarian carcinomas. Other mediators include interleukin 1, tumor necrosis factor, and prostaglandins.

3. **Osteoclast activating factor** has been shown to be the etiology of hypercalcemia in plasma cell dyscrasias.

4. **Vitamin D metabolites** are seen in some lymphomas. These promote intestinal calcium absorption.

23. Define the expression "tumor doubling time."

Tumor doubling time refers to the time required for the tumor to double in size. The doubling time of cancers varies greatly. Tumors may be ranked with respect to the doubling time. For some common cancers, both primary and metastatic, doubling times are as follows:

Tumor Type	Doubling Time (Weeks)
Primary lung cancer	
Adenocarcinoma	21
Squamous cell carcinoma	12
Anaplastic carcinoma (oat cell)	11
Breast cancer	
Primary	14
Lung metastases	11
Soft-tissue metastases	3
Colorectal cancer	
Primary	90
Lung metastases	14

(From Tannock IF, Hill RP (eds): The Basic Science of Oncology. Elmsford, NY, Pergamon Press, 1987, p 141, with permission.)

24. Summarize the epidemiology and list the risk factors for esophageal cancer.

Esophageal cancer occurs in the 40–60 year age group and is seen mainly in men. It is more common in the black race and in Far Eastern countries. Risk factors include:

- Geography: Africa, China, Russia, Japan, Scotland, and the Caspian region of Iran have an increased incidence
- Non-white male population
- Excessive alcohol use
- Excessive tobacco use
- Native Bantu beer
- Chronic hot beverage ingestion
- Lye ingestion: > 30% of cases develop esophageal cancer
- Tylosis: > 40% of cases develop esophageal cancer
- Achalasia
- Plummer-Vinson syndrome
- Nontropical sprue
- Oral and pharyngeal cancer
- Occupational: waiters, bartenders, metal workers, and construction workers

(From Livstone EM: Etiology, epidemiology, and diagnosis of esophageal and gastric cancer. Current Concepts in Oncology. Spring 1983, p 3, with permission.)

25. Esophageal cancer has what presenting symptoms?

The presenting signs and symptoms of esophageal cancer are:

Dysphagia: first with solids, then with liquids	Aspiration pneumonitis	Choking
	Hoarseness	Chest pain on swallowing
Weight loss	Cough	Gastroesophageal
Regurgitation	Fever	reflux

26. What is appropriate treatment for esophageal cancer?

This is greatly dependent on the patient and his physical condition at the time of presentation. The only curative procedure is surgery, but less than half of the patients are operable at the time of presentation, and of these only half to two-thirds of the tumors are resectable. Radical radiation therapy has been tried in selected patients, but the 5-year survival rates are less than 20%. Local recurrence is reported in about 50% of these patients, and toxicity is high, with complications of radiation pneumonitis, aspiration, tracheo-esophageal fistulas, mediastinal perforations, radiation myelitis, hemorrhage, and constrictive pericarditis reported. Chemotherapy has yet to play a major role in treatment of this disease, but several studies are investigating the use of chemotherapy in combination with radiotherapy, or prior to surgery. To date, encouraging responses have been noted, but no increase is seen in long-term survival.

27. List the risk factors, both accepted and proposed, for gastric cancer development.

Risk Factors for the Development of Gastric Cancer

Blood group A	Pernicious anemia *(Cont.)*
Loss of parietal cell mass	Gastric ulcer
Type B chronic atrophic gastritis	Achlorhydria
Intestinal metaplasia of mucosa	Acanthosis nigricans
Adenomatous polyps	Dermatomyositis
Pernicious anemia	"Cancer families"
Prior gastric resection	Barrett's esophagus
Prior vagotomy and gastroenterostomy	

28. List the risk factors for pancreatic cancer.

Risk Factors for the Development of Pancreatic Cancer

Males > females	Uterine myomas
Blacks > whites	History of oophorectomy
Black females > black males	History of spontaneous abortion
Jewish background	Occupational exposure to petroleum products
Diabets mellitus	(>10 yr increases risk to 5:1)
Smoking (2–3 times increased risk)	Elderly, heavy-smoking, alcoholic men
High calorie, high fat, and high protein diet	exposed to occupational carcinogens have
History of allergies	especially high risk
No tonsillectomy	

Three or more risk factors in men increases the risk by sixfold. A history of alcohol abuse or pancreatitis is *not* a proven risk factor for pancreatic cancer.

Lin RS, et al: A multifactorial model for pancreatic cancer in man—epidemiological evidence. JAMA 245:147, 1981.

29. What are the presenting symptoms and signs for patients with pancreatic cancer?

Signs and Symptoms of Pancreatic Cancer

	PERCENT OF PATIENTS WITH SELECTED SIGNS AND SYMPTOMS BASED ON THE TUMOR LOCATION	
Symptoms	*Head*	*Body/tail*
Weight loss	92%	100%
Jaundice	82%	7%
Pain	72%	87%
Anorexia	64%	33%
Nausea	45%	43%
Vomiting	37%	37%
Weakness	35%	43%
Signs		
Jaundice	87%	13%
Palpable liver	83%	—
Palpable gallbladder	29%	—
Tenderness	26%	27%
Ascites	14%	20%

(Adapted from Moossa AR, et al: Tumors of the pancreas. In Moossa AR, et al (eds): Comprehensive Textbook of Oncology, 2nd ed. Baltimore, Williams & Wilkins, 1991, p 964, with permission.)

30. Which tests are most useful in the diagnosis of pancreatic cancer?

In order of yield, the most useful tests are:

Test	*Diagnostic Yield (Various Series)*
CT scan of abdomen	94%
ERCP	94%
Angiography	90%
Ultrasound of abdomen	84%
MRI of abdomen	Data not available
Isotope scan	Data not available

After a radiographic diagnosis of a mass is made, percutaneous or open biopsy may be done. In various series, a positive cytologic diagnosis has been obtained in 87–100% of cases.

31. What are the risk factors for hepatocellular carcinoma?

The strongest evidence available indicates that chronic infection with hepatitis B virus is the major etiologic agent for human hepatocellular carcinoma. In addition, there are extensive studies of aflatoxins in human foods in Africa that suggest a quantitative relationship between average human aflatoxin consumption and the incidence of hepatocellular carcinoma around the world. Macronodular cirrhosis is found in 85% of patients with hepatocellular carcinoma, and it is theorized that this is a result of the chronic infection with the virus, which may occur as early as the perinatal stage. In a small proportion of hepatocellular carcinomas, the cause appears to be related to other factors, including other hepatotropic viruses, tobacco, alcohol, other chemicals, mycotoxins, and hepatic parasites. The relative importance of these factors seems to vary from one population to another.

32. List the common presenting features of primary tumors of the liver.

Common Presenting Features of Primary Liver Tumors

Asthenia	85–90%
Hepatomegaly	50–100%
Abdominal pain	50–70%
Jaundice	45–80%
Fever	9.5%

It is of interest that hepatomas can present in many unusual ways. Some of these are:
- Hemoptysis, secondary to pulmonary metastases
- Rib mass, secondary to bony metastasis
- Encephalitis-like picture, secondary to brain metastasis
- Heart failure, secondary to cardiac metastasis and thrombosis of the inferior vena cava
- Priapism, secondary to soft tissue metastasis
- Bone pain and pathological fractures, secondary to bony metastases.

33. What are the systemic manifestations of primary liver cell carcinoma?

Systemic Manifestations of Primary Liver Cell Carcinoma

A. Hepatoma
   Endocrine
      Erythrocytosis
      Hypercalcemia
   Nonendocrine
      Hypoglycemia
      Hyperlipidemia
      Porphyria cutanea tarda
      Dysfibrinogenemia
      Cryofibrinogenemia
      Alphafetoglobulin synthesis
      Osteoporosis
B. Hepatoblastoma
      Precocious puberty
      Hemihypertrophy
   Cystinuria

(From Margolis S, et al: Systemic manifestations of hepatoma. Medicine 51:381–390, 1972, with permission.)

34. Which environmental factors are thought to be related to the development of colon cancer?

There are abundant epidemiological data to support the link between environmental factors and colorectal cancer. The disease is more frequent among upper socioeconomic classes living in urban areas. There is a direct correlation with calorie consumption, dietary fat, oil, and meat protein. A direct correlation between mortality from coronary artery disease and mortality from colorectal cancer can be shown in epidemiological studies. Migrant groups tend to assume the incidence rates of their new environments. Burkitt noted many years ago that in South Africa the low incidence of large bowel cancer was correlated with a diet high in roughage. Others have correlated a diet high in cruciferous vegetables with a lower incidence of this cancer. Nevertheless, as with all epidemiologic data, confounding factors not identified may be significant.

35. In addition to those discussed in Question 34, what other risk factors are associated with the development of colon cancer?

Up to 25% of patients with colorectal cancer have a family history of the disease, suggesting the involvement of a genetic factor or factors. Two types are seen: (1) the uncommon hereditary polyposis syndrome, and (2) the more common nonpolyposis syndrome.

Polyposis coli is an autosomal dominant trait characterized by thousands of adenomatous polyps throughout the large bowel. If left untreated, cancer will develop in all patients with this syndrome. The cancer will usually manifest under the age of 40.

The more common nonpolyposis syndrome also appears to be an autosomal dominant trait. Most of these lesions involve the proximal large bowel. The median age at presentation is less than 50 years, and patients with a strong family history should be intensively screened.

Nonenvironmental Risk Factors in Colorectal Cancer

Age	>40 in asymptomatic patients
Associated disease	Ulcerative colitis
	Granulomatous colitis
	Peutz-Jeghers syndrome
	Familial polyposis syndrome
Past history	Colon cancer or polyps
	Female genital or breast cancer
Family history	Juvenile polyps
	Colon cancer or polyps
	Familial polyposis syndrome

(From Winawer S: Early diagnosis of colorectal cancer. Current Concepts in Oncology March/April 1981, p 8, with permission.)

36. What are the presenting symptoms of colon cancer?

The presenting symptoms of colon cancer depend on the location of the lesion. Lesions in the ascending colon, where the stool is still quite liquid, do not present with mass effects. However, these tumors frequently ulcerate, leading to chronic blood loss, and patients present with guaiac-positive stools on screening tests or with symptoms of anemia. In the transverse bowel the stool is more concentrated and formed, so that symptoms of obstruction such as abdominal cramping, abdominal pain, or perforation may bring the patient to the attention of the physician. Cancers in the rectosigmoid present with tenesmus, narrowing of the stool, and hematochezia. Anemia is unusual.

37. List the stages of colon cancer. What are the 5-year survival rates for each stage?

Staging and Prognosis of Colorectal Cancer

STAGE	DESCRIPTION	FIVE-YEAR SURVIVAL (%)	
		1940s AND 1950s	1960s AND 1970s
A	Infiltration no deeper than submucosa	80	> 90
B$_1$	Infiltration of muscularis; no penetration of wall; no lymph node involvement	60	85
B$_2$	Extension through colonic wall; no lymph node involvement	45	70–75
C$_1$	Infiltration of muscularis; no penetration of wall; lymph node involvement	15–30	35–65
C$_2$	Extension through colonic wall; lymph node involvement		
D	Distant mestastases	< 5	< 5

One staging classification that incorporates several modifications of the original Duke's system is useful for evaluating colorectal cancer. A tumor is classified according to the extent of infiltration of the bowel wall and by whether it has spread to lymph nodes or to distant organs such as the liver or lungs. Staging is significant for determining prognosis. (From Rubenstein E, Federman DD (eds): Scientific American Medicine. New York, Scientific American, Inc., 1986, Chapter 12 (Oncology), part VIII (Gastrointestinal Cancer), p 12, with permission.)

38. What are the uses and limitations for carcinoembryonic antigen (CEA) level testing?
CEA is an antigen produced by many colon cancers. It cannot be used for screening because it usually (in 85% of cases) is normal in patients with stage A disease (those who are most amenable to curative surgery). Testing should be done preoperatively in patients undergoing resection for colon cancer, so that the data can be used to follow the course of the disease and treatment. CEA returns to normal in 30–45 days after complete resection of tumors producing it. Thus, postoperative measurement should not be made prior to this time. If a preoperative elevated level, which returns to normal after surgery, subsequently becomes elevated, it is a very reliable indicator of tumor recurrence. False positive results have been associated with smoking and other types of cancer, so results must be interpreted in the context of the individual patient.

39. Chemotherapy plays what part in the treatment of colon cancer?
Chemotherapy has two roles in the treatment of colon cancer. The first, and broader, role is in the treatment of metastatic disease, where the agent most commonly used is 5-fluorouracil (5FU). Response rates to this drug in metastatic disease are only in the range of 15–20%. Many different schedules and combinations with other drugs such as methyl CCNU, levamisole, and leucovorin have been tried to improve this result, but with limited success. The second, more controversial, use of chemotherapy is that of adjuvant therapy. Several large cooperative groups have used 5FU with levamisole in early stage disease. Preliminary results indicate that an improvement in survival may be seen in selected stage C patients.

40. What is the mechanism of action of 5-fluorouracil (5FU), and what are its side-effects?
5FU is a potent inhibitor of thymidylate synthetase. Thymidylate synthetase binds strongly to 5-fluoro-deoxyuridylate, one of the endpoints of degradation of 5-fluorouracil.

Side-effects of 5FU include myelosuppression, cerebellar ataxia, dacryocystitis, angina, and hyperpigmentation.

41. What tests are available for the diagnosis and staging of prostate cancer, and how do they correlate with the stage?
See table on page 186.

42. What are the stages of prostate cancer and how do they correlate with overall survival?

Stages of Prostate Cancer and Survival

STAGE	SURVIVAL
A. No palpable lesion	
A1. Focal	No negative impact
A2. Diffuse	Lower than general population
B. Confined to prostate	**All Stage B:**
B1. Small discrete nodule or areas	5 yr, 75–55%; 10 yr, 57–61%;
B2. Large or multiple nodules or areas	15 yr, 28–40%
C. Localized to periprostatic area	**All Stage C:**
C1. No involvement of seminal vesicles, tumor 70 g or less	5 yr, 64%; 10 yr, 35%; 15 yr, 20%
C2. Involvement of seminal vesicles, tumor larger than 70 g	
D. Metastatic disease	**All Stage D:**
D1. Pelvic lymph node metastases or urethral obstruction causing hydronephrosis	Median survival, 2.5 yr
D2. Bone or distant lymph node organ or soft tissue metastases	

Diagnostic Evaluation and Staging of Prostate Cancer*

STAGE	HISTOLOGY OF PROSTATE BIOPSY SPECIMEN	URINARY SYMPTOMS	NONINVASIVE ASSESSMENT OF METASTATIC DISEASE					SURGICAL LYMPH NODE SAMPLING
			SERUM ACID PHOSPHATASE	PROSTATE-SPECIFIC ANTIGEN	CHEST X-RAY	BONE SCAN	PELVIC CT SCAN	
A1	Well-differentiated cancer present in fewer than 4 chips	Compatible with benign prostate hypertrophy	Normal	Sometimes elevated	Negative	Negative	Negative	Usually not performed
A2	Well-differentiated cancer present in 4 or more chips or cancer not well differentiated	Compatible with benign prostate hypertrophy	Normal	Often elevated	Negative	Negative	Negative	Positive in 25% of patients (indicating Stage D1 disease)
B	Well-differentiated nodule	Absent	Normal	Always elevated and proportional to tumor volume	Negative	Negative	Negative	Positive in 8% of patients (indicating Stage D1 disease)
	Nodule not well differentiated	Absent	Normal	Always elevated and proportional to tumor volume	Negative	Negative	Negative	Positive in 25% of patients (indicating Stage D1 disease)
C	Local, contiguously extended lesion that is not poorly differentiated	Present	Normal	Always elevated and proportional to tumor volume	Negative	Negative	Negative	Positive in 40–50% of patients (indicating Stage D1 disease)
	Local, contiguously extended lesion that is poorly differentiated	Present	Possibly elevated	Always elevated and proportional to tumor volume	Negative	Negative	Negative	Positive in 95% of patients who have elevated acid phosphatase
D1	Cancer present	Usually present	Often elevated	Always elevated and proportional to tumor volume	Negative	Negative	Negative or positive	Positive below the aortic bifurcation
D2	Cancer present	Usually present	Elevated in 80% of patients	Always elevated and proportional to tumor volume	Negative or positive	Usually positive	Negative or positive	Usually not performed

(From Rubenstein E, Federman DD (eds): Scientific American Medicine. New York, Scientific American, Inc., 1986, Chapter 12 (Oncology), part IX (Urologic Cancer) p 3, with permission.)

43. What is the use of acid phosphatase, prostatic acid phosphatase, and prostatic specific antigen in the treatment of prostate cancer?

Acid phosphatases are enzymes that hydrolyze esters of orthophosphoric acid in an acid milieu. One of these, the **prostatic acid phosphatase,** may be found to be elevated in the majority of patients with advanced or stage D prostatic cancer, and correlates with the activity of the disease. It may thus be used as a marker for treatment response. It has not been found to be useful, however, as a screening test in early-stage disease.

Prostatic specific antigen is a glycoprotein found in the ductular epithelium of normal and malignant prostate tissue. Serum levels reflect the volume of prostate; therefore, it may be elevated in large benign prostates as well as in tumors. It can be a useful immunohisto-chemical marker when the primary site of tumor is occult.

44. What are the effects and mechanisms of the various androgen-deprivation therapies for prostate cancer?

The various androgen and estrogen effects on the prostate are shown in the accompanying figure. The mechanisms and sites of blockage by various drugs are also noted.

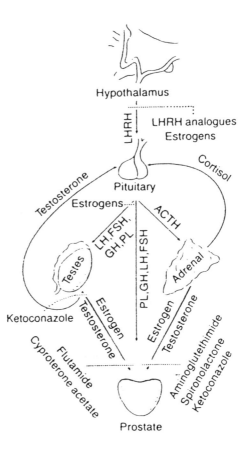

Various theoretical sites of activity of the agents used in blocking androgen effects on the prostate. (From Dawkins CA, et al: Newer treatment modalities for advanced prostate cancer. VA Practitioner 2(6):41–53, 1985, p 43, with permission.)

45. What is appropriate therapy for prostate cancer at each stage?

Therapy for Prostate Cancer by Stage

STAGE	THERAPY
A1	Transurethral resection followed by close observation
A2	Radiation therapy or radical prostatectomy
B	Radical prostatectomy or radiation therapy
C	Radiation therapy
D1	For urinary obstruction, transurethral prostatectomy (TURP) or radiation therapy
	For asymptomatic patients, endocrine manipulation or close observation
D2	Close observation for asymptomatic disease
	Hormonal therapy for symptomatic disease
	Chemotherapy for disease refractory to hormonal therapy
	Palliative radiation therapy for symptomatic areas

46. What are the risk factors for the development of bladder cancer?

Various epidemiological studies have identified the following as associated with the development of bladder cancer:

Environmental factors:

Occupational hazards
    Workers in dye industry
    Hairdressers
    Painters
    Leather workers
Geographic
    Endemic schistosomiasis

Self-ingested toxins
    Tobacco
    Phenacetin
    Artificial sweeteners (possibly)
Miscellaneous
    Alkylating agents—cyclophosphamide

Previous cancers, especially those of the uroepithelial tract.

47. What are the most common causes of isolated hematuria?

Major Causes of Isolated Hematuria

TYPE OF BLEEDING	CAUSES
Glomerular bleeding	Mild forms of glomerulonephritis:
	IgA nephropathy, hereditary nephritis, thin basement membrane disease, postinfectious glomerulonephritis
	Long-distance running
Extraglomerular renal bleeding	Pelvic calculi
	Hypercalciuria
	Carcinoma: renal cell, transitional cell (esp. with analgesic abuse)
	Sickle cell trait or disease
	Cystic diseases: polycystic kidney disease, medullary sponge kidney
	Coagulation disorders: hemophilia, anticoagulation therapy
	Trauma
	Vascular malformation
	Venereal diseases: emboli, vasculitis
Extrarenal bleeding	Ureters: calculi
	Bladder: catheterization, carcinoma, infection caused by common bacteria or *Mycobacterium tuberculosis*, cyclophosphamide
	Prostate: hypertrophy, carcinoma
	Urethra: trauma, urethritis

(From Rubenstein E, Federman DD (eds): Scientific American Medicine. New York, Scientific American, Inc., 1986, Chapter 10 (Nephrology), part III (Approach to Renal Disease) p 8, 1986, with permission.)

48. What are the presenting features of renal cell cancer?

The presenting features of renal cell cancer include:

Signs or Symptoms	Percent	Signs or Symptoms	Percent
Classic triad	9%	Anemia	21%
Gross hematuria		Tumor calcification on x-ray	13%
Abdominal mass		Symptoms from metastases	10%
Pain		Fever	7%
Hematuria	59%	Asymptomatic when diagnosed	7%
Abdominal mass	45%	Erythrocytosis	3%
Pain	41%	Hypercalcemia	3%
Weight loss	28%	Acute varicocele	2%

(From Skinner DG, et al: Diagnosis and management of renal cell carcinoma: A clinical and pathologic study of 309 cases. Cancer 28:1165, 1971, with permission.)

However, renal cell cancer has been called "the internist's tumor" and various unusual presentations have been reported. These include amyloidosis, hypercalcemia, hypertension, hepatopathy without liver metastases, enteropathy, heart failure, and immune complex glomerulonephritis, among others.

49. What are the currently used staging evaluations for renal cell cancer?

There are several staging systems for renal cell cancer, and it is important in evaluating data to compare staging categories from different systems correctly. Most systems have four stages, and the American Joint Commission for Cancer Staging and End-Results Reporting's TMN (Tumor, Metastases, Nodes) stages can be correlated with these. All systems require evaluation of the patient with history, physical, IVP, angiogram, venacavogram and/or CT scan of the abdomen. Additional studies may include lymphangiogram and ultrasound. In order to determine distant metastases, bone scans, x-rays, and routine hematological and biochemical studies are needed. Surgical staging includes laparotomy, with biopsy or resection of the primary tumor, and evaluation of the renal vein, Gerota's fascia, and other internal organs and nodes.

50. What is the prognosis for early-stage renal cell cancer?

Survival depends on stage as well as grade of the tumor:

Stage	5-year survival (%)
I: Confined to the renal parenchyma	76%
II: Confined to Gerota's fascia	65%
III. Involves the renal vein, inferior vena cava regional lymph nodes	35%
IV. Spread to adjacent organs or distant metastases	5%

Grade	5-year survival (%)
I: Highly differentiated tumors, sharply demarcated from surrounding tissue	100%
IIA: Moderately differentiated tumors, locally well circumscribed but not necessarily provided with capsule	59%
IIB: Moderately differentiated tumors, poorly circumscribed but not diffusely infiltrating or markedly polymorphous and mitotic	36%
III: Poorly differentiated, markedly polymorphous tumors that are diffusely infiltrating. Tumors with abundant growth in capillary vessels	0%

(From Bottiger LE: Prognosis in renal cell carcinoma. Cancer 26:780–787, 1970, with permission.)

51. What treatments are available for advanced stage renal cell cancer and how effective are they?

There are few effective therapies for advanced stage renal cell cancer. There are some data to suggest a hormonal influence in these tumors, theorized to be related to the embryonic origins of the tissue. Megestrol acetate has been used with variable success, mainly resulting in responses of 10–15%. A few chemotherapeutic agents have been slightly active, with response rates in the same range as the hormonal treatments. The most commonly used agent is vinblastine. Currently, biological response modifiers are being used, but no dramatic results have yet been reported.

The most effective therapy for renal cell carcinoma is early diagnosis and surgical therapy.

52. What is the incidence of testicular cancer in the U.S.?

The incidence of testicular cancer in the U.S. is approximately 2.2%. Only 1% of cancers in males are testicular cancers, but the majority of these are in patients 29 and 35 years of age, with 6000 new cases annually. The incidence of testicular cancer is higher in those patients with cryptorchidism, in Kleinfelter's syndrome, and in the testicular feminization syndrome. The etiology of this cancer is unknown, but age, genetic influences, repeated infection, radiation, and possible endocrine abnormalities have been suggested.

53. What are the presenting features of testicular cancer?

Tumors that present locally are brought to the physician's attention by a mass in the scrotum. It is often painless, although pain has been noted in about 25% of the reported cases. When the tumor has already spread (5–15%), symptoms of metastases to the lungs and liver are seen. Other diagnostic possibilities with a scrotal mass include epididymitis, hydrocele, inguinal hernia, hematocele, hematoma, torsion, spermatocele, varicocele, and gumma.

54. What are the pathological types of the most common testicular cancers?

Current Pathologic Classification of Germinal Tumors of the Testes

HISTOLOGY	FREQUENCY
Tumors of one histologic type	
Seminoma (germinoma)	
Typical	35%
Anaplastic	4%
Spermatocytic	1%
Embryonal carcinoma	20%
Teratoma	10%
Choriocarcinoma	1%
Tumors of more than one histologic type	
Embryonal carcinoma and teratoma (teratocarcinoma)	24%
Other combinations	5%

55. What are the stages of testicular cancer and their relation to overall survival?

Stages of Testicular Cancer

IA: tumor confined to the testes
IB: microscopic involvement of retroperitoneal lymph nodes
II: macroscopic involvement of retroperitoneal lymph nodes
III: extension beyond retroperitoneal lymph nodes

Survival can no longer be determined on the basis of stage, but is much more dependent on the response to therapy. In patients who respond, the survival curves plateau at about 90%.

56. What is the treatment of testicular cancer?

Transinguinal orchiectomy is performed in all patients with testicular carcinoma. This serves to make the pathologic diagnosis and is the treatment for stage A cancer.

For pure seminoma, in limited cases radiation is given to the retroperitoneal nodes. Disseminated disease is treated with combination chemotherapy.

For nonseminomatous tumors, retroperitoneal lymphadenectomy is most commonly done. If nodes are positive, the patients may be treated with two courses of adjuvant chemotherapy.

For patients with stage III disease, or earlier stage disease with bulky mediastinal or retroperitoneal masses, three to four courses of chemotherapy are given, followed by resection of any residual disease.

Tumor markers—alphafetoprotein (AFP) and human chorionic gonadotropin (HCG)—are followed for evidence of recurrent disease. They are quite sensitive for the presence of disease, although normal values do not rule out disease.

57. List the possible long-term effects of therapy for testicular cancer.

1. Impotence
2. Infertility
3. Renal dysfunction
4. Raynaud's phenomenon
5. Generalized vascular disorders (acute myocardial infarction [MI], deep venous thrombosis [DVT], and stroke)
6. Pulmonary fibrosis
7. Leukemia

58. Describe the extragonadal germ cell syndrome.

The extragonadal germ cell syndrome is a constellation of findings characterized by germ cell tumors found in relatively young males in the mediastinum, retroperitoneum, or pineal gland, with elevated human chorionic gonadotropin (HCG) or alphafetoprotein (AFP), and marked elevation of lactic dehydrogenase (LDH). These patients often respond to treatment with chemotherapy developed for testicular cancer.

It is very important that a careful search for an occult testicular primary be carried out, since the testes is thought to be a relative sanctuary from the effects of chemotherapy. Ultrasound evaluation is useful in this setting.

59. What is the most common cancer in the U.S. today, excluding skin cancer?

Lung cancer. See cancer incidence percentages in the figure on the next page.

1990 ESTIMATED CANCER INCIDENCE BY SITE AND SEX†

Cancer incidence by site and sex. (From American Cancer Society's Department of Epidemiology and Statistics: Ca—A Cancer Journal for Clinicians 40(1):9, 1990, with permission.)

	Male			Female	
MELANOMA OF SKIN	3%		3%	MELANOMA OF SKIN	
ORAL	4%		2%	ORAL	
LUNG	20%		29%	BREAST	
PANCREAS	3%		11%	LUNG	
STOMACH	3%		3%	PANCREAS	
COLON & RECTUM	15%		15%	COLON & RECTUM	
PROSTATE	20%		4%	OVARY	
URINARY	10%		9%	UTERUS	
LEUKEMIA & LYMPHOMAS	7%		4%	URINARY	
			6%	LEUKEMIA & LYMPHOMAS	
ALL OTHER	15%		14%	ALL OTHER	

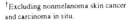

†Excluding nonmelanoma skin cancer and carcinoma in situ.

1990 ESTIMATED CANCER DEATHS BY SITE AND SEX

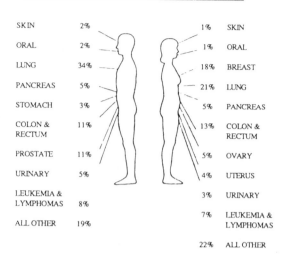

SKIN	2%		1%	SKIN
ORAL	2%		1%	ORAL
LUNG	34%		18%	BREAST
PANCREAS	5%		21%	LUNG
STOMACH	3%		5%	PANCREAS
COLON & RECTUM	11%		13%	COLON & RECTUM
PROSTATE	11%		5%	OVARY
URINARY	5%		4%	UTERUS
LEUKEMIA & LYMPHOMAS	8%		3%	URINARY
ALL OTHER	19%		7%	LEUKEMIA & LYMPHOMAS
			22%	ALL OTHER

Cancer deaths by site and sex. (From American Cancer Society's Department of Epidemiology and Statistics: Ca—A Cancer Journal for Clinicians 40(1):9, 1990, with permission.)

60. What are the common presenting signs and symptoms of lung cancer?

Common Signs and Symptoms of Lung Cancer

1. Symptoms secondary to central or endobronchial growth of the primary tumor:
   Cough
   Hemoptysis
   Wheeze and stridor
   Dyspnea from obstruction
   Pneumonitis from obstruction (fever, productive cough)
2. Symptoms secondary to peripheral growth of the primary tumor:
   Pain from pleural or chest wall involvement
   Cough
   Dyspnea on a restrictive basis
   Lung abscess syndrome from tumor cavitation
3. Symptoms related to regional spread of the tumor in the thorax by contiguity or by metastasis to regional lymph nodes:
   Tracheal obstruction
   Esophageal compression with dysphagia
   Recurrent laryngeal nerve paralysis with hoarseness
   Phrenic nerve paralysis with elevation of the hemidiaphragm and dyspnea
   Sympathetic nerve paralysis with Horner's syndrome
   Eighth cervical and first thoracic nerve compression with ulnar pain and Pancoast's syndrome
   Superior vena cava syndrome from vascular obstruction
   Pericardial and cardiac extension with resultant tamponade, arrhythmia, or cardiac failure
   Lymphatic obstruction with pleural effusion
   Lymphangitic spread through the lungs with hypoxemia and dyspnea

(From Cohen MH: Signs and symptoms of bronchogenic carcinoma. In Straus MJ: Lung Cancer: Clinical Diagnosis and Treatment, 2nd ed. New York, Grune & Stratton, 1983, pp 97–111, with permission.)

61. What are the accepted and proposed risk factors for lung cancer?

- **Cigarette smoking** is the cause of lung cancer in more than 80% of men who develop it. Lung cancer's incidence in women is increasing steadily and it will soon be the leading cause of cancer death in women as well. Passive smoking also increases the risk of lung cancer.

- **Radon exposure** increases the risk of lung cancer, especially in smokers, who have a tenfold higher risk. An estimated 25% of lung cancer in nonsmokers and 5% in smokers is attributed to radon daughter exposure in the home.
- **Smoking of marijuana** increases the risk of lung cancer in smokers.
- **Emphysema**, which develops in smokers, is associated with an increased risk.
- Other agents correlated with lung cancer include:

Bischloromethyl ether	Arsenic	Nickel
Ionizing radiation	Asbestos	Chromates
Mustard gas		

62. Which chromosomal defects are associated with lung cancer?

Deletion of 3p (usually 3p14–23) is found in virtually all cases (93%) of small cell lung cancer (SCLC) (both classic and variant), in 100% of bronchial carcinoids, and 25% of non-SCLC. Also seen are absent or reduced expression of the rb gene at 13q14, increased production of the c-jun oncogene product, and constitutive expression of c-raf-1 gene on 3p25.

63. Which paraneoplastic syndromes are associated with lung cancer?

Paraneoplastic Syndromes in Lung Cancer

1. Systemic symptoms
   Anorexia-cachexia (31%)
   Fever (21%)
   Suppressed immunity
2. Endocrine (12%)
   Ectopic parathyroid hormone: hyper-calcemia (epidermoid)
   Syndrome of inappropriate secretion of antidiuretic hormone (SIADH) (small cell)
   Ectopic secretion of ACTH: Cushing's syndrome (small cell)
3. Skeletal
   Clubbing (29%)
   Hypertrophic pulmonary osteo-arthropathy: periostitis (1–10%) (adenocarcinoma)
4. Neurologic-myopathic (%)
   Myasthenic syndrome: Eaton-Lambert syndrome (small cell)
   Peripheral neuropathy
   Subacute cerebellar degeneration
4. Neurologic-myopathic *(Cont.)*
   Cortical degeneration
   Polymyositis
   Retinal blindness
5. Coagulation-thrombotic
   Migratory thrombophlebitis, Trousseau's syndrome: venous thrombosis
   Nonbacterial thrombotic (marantic) endocarditis: arterial emboli
   Disseminated intravascular coagulation (DIC): hemorrhage
6. Cutaneous
   Dermatomyositis
   Acanthosis nigricans
7. Hematologic (8%)
   Anemia
   Granulocytosis
   Leukoerythroblastosis
8. Renal (<1%)
   Nephrotic syndrome
   Glomerulonephritis

(From Devita VT, et al (eds): Cancer: Principles and Practice of Oncology, 3rd ed. Philadelphia, J.B. Lippincott, 1989, with permission.)

64. Which tests are used for the evaluation of lung cancer?

The primary evaluation of lung cancer should include a chest x-ray and sputum cytology. If the expectorated sputum cytology is negative, bronchoscopy with biopsy or percutaneous biopsy may be done. Preoperative evaluation will include CT scan of chest and upper abdomen to evaluate for mediastinal and hilar nodes and for liver and/or adrenal metastases. Routine hematology and biochemical tests suggest the presence of bone marrow or liver metastases, and the presence of brain metastases can be screened for using a CT of the brain. Elevated alkaline phosphatase suggests bony metastases if the liver scan is normal, and a bone scan should be done.

65. What are the 5-year survival rates for the different pathological types of lung cancer?

Histological Type	5-year survival (%)
Epidermoid carcinoma	25%
Adenocarcinoma	12%
Large cell carcinoma	13%
Small cell carcinoma (oat cell)	1%

66. Describe the staging of small cell lung cancer.
After the diagnosis of small cell cancer is made, staging procedures should be completed. The staging system of small cell lung cancer is a simple one:
   1. **Limited:** defined as disease confined to one hemithorax with or without ipsilateral supraclavicular, hilar, and mediastinal lymphadenopathy.
   2. **Extensive:** defined as anything beyond limited disease. This also includes recurrent disease, wherever the location.
   The evaluation for staging consists of a chest x-ray with or without a CT scan of the chest to evaluate the intrathoracic nodes, and whatever scans are necessary to evaluate the presence of disease outside the chest (especially in the liver and brain). Since bone marrow metastasis is not uncommon in the presentation of this disease, a bone marrow exam is often done to evaluate this site. However, bone marrow involvement in the absence of other extensive disease is extremely rare.

67. Which drugs and other treatment modalities are used to manage small cell lung cancer?
After staging, patients are treated with chemotherapy consisting of combinations of cyclophosphamide, adriamycin, vincristine, etoposide, and platinum. Other agents have also been used, but mainly as second-line therapy. Treatment is continued for 6 to 12 months, depending on response. If limited disease responds completely, radiotherapy to the brain and mediastinum is used to prevent local recurrence. Extensive disease rarely responds completely, and treatment is continued until progression or resistance develops.

68. How effective is the treatment of small cell lung cancer?
Approximately 15–20% of limited disease patients will survive 3 years, but few patients with extensive disease reach this point. Median survival for patients with extensive disease, who respond to treatment, is 7 months. For patients with limited disease, the median survival is 14 months.

69. What are the appropriate treatments for non-small cell lung cancer?
The first decision to be made is whether or not the patient is a candidate for resection. If the patient is medically able to undergo resection, it should be performed if the following are *not* present:
   1. Distant metastases
   2. Pleural effusion
   3. Superior vena cava obstruction
   4. Involvement of the supraclavicular, cervical, contralateral mediastinal nodes
   5. Recurrent laryngeal nerve paralysis
   6. Involvement of the tracheal wall, or mainstem bronchus less than 2 cm from the carina
   7. Small cell carcinoma histology
If patients are not able to undergo surgery, and they do not have small cell cancer, then radiotherapy is indicated. The only contraindication is the presence of such bulky disease that treatment with radiotherapy would compromise remaining lung tissue.

70. What are the acute and long-term complications of chemotherapy and radiotherapy used in the treatment of lung cancer?

The adverse effects of treatment of lung cancer include:

Acute:
Tumor lysis syndrome
Myelosuppression predisposing to:
  Infection
  Bleeding
Hemorrhagic cystitis
  (cyclophosphamide)
Cardiotoxicity (adriamycin)
Renal toxicity (platinum)
Peripheral neuropathy (platinum,
  vincristine)
Radiation pneumonitis

Long-term:
Neurologic damage with resultant:
  Confusion
  Episodic hemiparesis
  Ataxia
  Progressive organic brain syndrome
Leukemia
Second primary carcinomas
  and sarcomas

71. What are the presenting symptoms of head and neck cancer, according to site?

Site	Symptoms

1. Oral Cavity
  Lips
  Buccal mucosa
  Alveolar ridge
  Retromolar trigone
  Floor of mouth
  Hard palate
  Anterior 2/3 of tongue
	1. Mass, ulcer, leukoplakia, bleeding, pain, loose teeth, earache, trismus, halitosis

2. Larynx
  Supraglottic
    False vocal cords
    Arytenoid
  Glottis
    True vocal cords
  Subglottic
	2. Hoarseness, bleeding, sore throat, thyroid cartilage pain

3. Pharynx
  Nasopharynx
  Oropharynx
  Soft palate
  Uvula
  Tonsil
  Base of tongue
  Hypopharynx
  Pyriform sinus
	3. Sore throat, earache, epistaxis, nasal voice, dysphagia, masses, hearing loss, blood-streaked saliva

4. Maxillary sinus cancer	4. Sinusitis, epistaxis, headache
5. All sites	5. Bleeding (oral or nasal), neck nodes, pain at the site of tumor or referred pain

72. What are the risk factors for squamous cell cancer of the head and neck area?

Tobacco is the most significant contributing factor to the development of head and neck cancers. Nine of ten patients with cancer in this area are smokers. Snuff dipping and tobacco chewing are also causally related to the development of oral cancer. Smoking increases the mortality related to head and neck cancer once it has been diagnosed. Several studies have shown a twofold increase in mortality for smokers over nonsmokers. Alcohol is also strongly correlated with the development of head and neck cancer. About half the patients with these cancers have cirrhosis and three quarters drink alcohol excessively. Another factor is poor dental hygiene. Woodworkers have an increased incidence of nasopharyngeal cancer. Syphilitic glossitis predisposes to tongue cancer and nickel compounds to nasal sinus cancer. The Epstein-Barr and herpes simplex type 1 viruses have been implicated in up to 15% of new cases.

73. How does one carry out an appropriate evaluation in the initial staging of patients with head and neck cancer?

Initial staging of head and neck cancer includes a thorough triple endoscopy of upper and lower airway and upper aerodigestive tract, with biopsy of any suspicious lesions. Measurement and biopsy, if indicated, of any cervical or supraclavicular nodes should be performed. A CT scan of the area is very helpful in determining the extent of disease. If elements of the routine blood counts and biochemical profile are abnormal, a bone scan and/or liver scan may be done. If there is a history of alcohol abuse, liver scans in the face of abnormal liver function tests are usually only useful if there is hepatomegaly. The most common sites of metastases of these tumors are local lymphatics, followed by lung metastases. Bone metastases occur in about 15% of the patients. Brain metastases are rare and are seen mainly in those patients with nasopharyngeal cancer. It is also important to remember that second primaries in the lung are not uncommon. Depending on tobacco and alcohol history, another cancer, usually of the esophagus or lung, may be seen in up to 20% of patients at some time in the course of their disease.

74. Currently, what is the most appropriate treatment of head and neck cancer?

Traditionally, head and neck cancers have been treated primarily with surgery. This has usually been extensive and radical, and often accompanied by postoperative radio-therapy. Radiotherapy was also used for recurrences that were no longer amenable to surgery. However, the current trend is to treat with "multimodality therapy," using chemotherapy, either in combination with radiotherapy or prior to surgery or radio-therapy. The optimum combination of these agents and modalities has not yet been deter-mined, and many trials are ongoing to answer these questions. The problem is complicated by the fact that the natural history of these tumors is quite divergent. This means that by treating and evaluating them as a group, results can be quite different, depending on the patient mix.

75. Which chemotherapeutic agents are used in the treatment of squamous cell cancers of the head and neck? How effective are they?

Several agents are effective, and include methotrexate, bleomycin, cisplatin, and 5-fluorouracil infusions. Response rates for these agents vary from 25–60%, depending on the agent, schedule, tumor type, previous treatment, and performance status. Combination chemo-therapy regimens have usually shown higher initial response rates, but have yet to show an increase in survival rates.

76. Define the expression "neoadjuvant therapy."

"Neoadjuvant therapy" means treatment with chemotherapy prior to definitive surgery or radiotherapy. It should not be confused with adjuvant therapy, which implies that the tumor has been grossly removed, and treatment is administered to prevent recur-rence. Patients with neoadjuvant therapy often have large tumors, and the idea is to shrink these tumors to make subsequent surgical removal or radiotherapy easier and more effective.

77. What are the neuromuscular complications of cancer?

Neuromuscular Complications of Malignant Disease

Neuromuscular disorder (common)
Myopathy
    Myositis and dermatomyositis
    Myasthenic syndrome (Eaton-Lambert syndrome)
    Carcinomatous myopathy
Neuropathy
    Distal sensorimotor polyneuropathy (common)
    Carcinomatous sensory neuropathy (rare)
Myelopathy
    Necrotizing myelopathy
    Subacute myelitis
Subacute cerebellar degeneration
Encephalopathy
    Limbic encephalopathy (very rare, ? viral)
    Progressive multifocal leukoencephalopathy (rare)

(From Rubenstein E, Federman DD (eds): Scientific American Medicine. New York, Scientific American, Inc., 1986, Chapter 12 (Oncology), part VIII p 5, with permission.)

78. What are the current recommendations for screening for breast cancer?

There are currently several sets of recommendations from the various specialty organizations whose members are engaged in breast cancer screening. These are as follows:

For women over 50 years of age:

1. The American Cancer Society (ACS) recommends an annual physical examination of the breast and mammogram.

2. The National Cancer Institute (NCI) recommends breast examinations at every periodic physical examination and mammography annually.

3. The American College of Obstetricians and Gynecologists (ACOG) recommends mammograms and physical examination of the breast at a frequency determined by a woman's physician.

4. The American College of Radiology (ACR) recommends annual mammograms and physical examination of the breast.

5. The American College of Physicians (ACP) recommends mammograms for women between the ages of 50 and 59 "on a routine basis." Mammograms are recommended for women 60 years of age and over, with the screening interval chosen by the physician and patient.

6. The U.S. Preventive Services Task Force (USPSTF) recommends annual mammograms and clinical breast examinations for women over 50 years of age.

For women less than 50 years of age:

1. The ACS recommends a baseline mammogram for women between the ages of 35 and 40, annual breast examination from age 40 to age 50, and a mammogram every 1 to 2 years from age 40 to age 50. Women who are 20 to 40 years of age are recommended to see their physicians every 3 years for breast examination.

2. The NCI recommends a breast examination at every periodic examination, encourages mammography every 1 to 2 years starting at age 40, and encourages annual mammograms for women with personal history of breast cancer.

3. The ACOG recommends a baseline mammogram for women between the ages of 35 and 50, and breast examinations in the same age group. At any age, mammograms are recommended if there are strong indications (such as a family or personal history) of breast cancer, breast augmentation implants, or first pregnancy after age 30.

4. The ACR recommends a baseline mammogram before the age of 40 years and subsequent mammograms every 1 to 2 years or more frequently based on the physician's assessment.

5. The ACP does not recommend mammography for women below 50 years of age.

6. The USPSTF recommends annual clinical breast examination for women 40 to 49 years of age but does not recommend mammograms for this age group.

79. How is the diagnosis of breast cancer established?

The diagnosis of breast cancer is made by tissue examination. This may be done by percutaneous fine needle aspirate, with or without x-ray direction, or by incisional or excisional biopsy. While mammograms are very helpful in screening and localizing tumors, the diagnosis cannot be definitively made without tissue confirmation.

80. At what age does the incidence rate of breast cancer peak?

Annual Age-specific Incidence Rates
of Breast Cancer (1983–1985)

AGE (years)	INCIDENCE (per 100,000 persons)
0–14	0.0
15–19	0.08
20–24	1.06
25–29	7.81
30–34	24.59
35–39	62.97
40–44	111.67
45–49	159.18
50–54	185.36
55–59	227.26
60–64	261.60
65–69	297.12
70–74	316.45
75–79	327.00
80–84	336.86
85 and older	312.48

(From Eddy DM: Screening for breast cancer. Ann Intern Med 111:389–399, 1989, p 390, with permission.)

81. What are the risk factors for breast cancer?

1. **High risk factors** (associated with a 3× or more increase)
   a. Age (more than 40 years old)
   b. Previous cancer in one breast
   c. Breast cancer in a first or second degree family member
   d. Gross cystic disease, multiple papillomatosis, and atypical hyperplasia, probably only if associated with family history
   e. Parity: Nulliparous, or first pregnancy after 31 years of age
   f. Lobular carcinoma in situ
2. **Intermediate risk** (1.2 to 1.5× risk)
   a. Early menarche or late menopause
   b. Oral estrogens
   c. History of cancer of the ovary, uterus, or colon
   d. Alcoholic beverages (possible)

82. What are the poor prognostic factors in primary breast cancer?

1. Estrogen receptors negative
2. Positive HER-2/neu oncogene
3. Premenopausal patient
4. Large tumor size

5. Positive nodes
6. Local skin involvement
7. Fixed axillary nodes
8. Presence of distant metastases

83. What is the appropriate treatment of local-regional breast cancer?

Although there is no single "right" way to treat localized breast cancer, and a great deal of controversy exists, the following guidelines are available:

Therapy for Breast Cancer

Stage I:	"Lumpectomy"[†] with axillary dissection and radiation **or** modified radical mastectomy.*
Stage II:	Modified radical mastectomy with postoperative chemotherapy for patients with positive nodes. The benefit of chemotherapy in node-negative patients is not clear at the present time. The value of postoperative hormonal therapy in postmenopausal patients is also being explored.
Stage III:	Preoperative radiation possibly with chemotherapy or hormonal therapy, followed by modified radical mastectomy and then chemotherapy; **or** simple mastectomy with postoperative radiotherapy and/or chemotherapy or hormonal therapy
Stage IV:	Systemic chemotherapy, reserving surgery and radiotherapy for local control.

* **Modified radical mastectomy is used if:** cosmesis is not important, **or** lesion size is large relative to breast size, **or** radiotherapy is not technically possible.
† **Lumpectomy/radiotherapy is used if:** cosmesis is important, **and** complete excision is possible, **and** >6000 rads can be delivered to the tumor bed.

84. What is the role of adjuvant therapy in the management of breast cancer?

Current Recommendations for the Use of Adjuvant Systemic Therapy in Breast Cancer*

	PREMENOPAUSAL	POSTMENOPAUSAL
Node positive:		
ERP negative	CMF × 6 months	None off study
ERP positive	CMF × 6 months	TAM × 2–5 years
Node negative:		
ERP negative	None[†]	None[†]
ERP positive	None[†]	None[†]

*ERP = estrogen receptor positive; CMF = cyclophosphamide, methotrexate & 5-fluorouracil; TAM = tamoxifen.
† None recommended unless as part of an experimental protocol.

In comparing four cooperative trials studying the place of adjuvant therapy in node-negative patients, it is noted that all were initiated at about the same time but are quite dissimilar in trial size, patient eligibility for enrollment, and therapeutic regimen. P values for overall survival differences between controls and treated patients were significant in only two of the studies. Therefore, it is felt that the answer to this question has not yet been determined and further long-term follow-up and study are necessary.

85. Which agents are used in the treatment of metastatic breast cancer? How effective are they?

The most commonly used agents with clinical activity in breast cancer are adriamycin, cyclophosphamide, methotrexate, fluorouracil, and prednisone. Various combinations of these agents are generally used in the treatment of advanced or metastatic breast cancer.

Overall induction response rates range from 55–65%. Median survival times are 14 to 18 months. The survival rates, however, depend more on the site of the metastatic disease than on the treatment. Most patients receive more than one treatment regimen, since the median time to failure of most programs is about 6 months.

86. What is the significance of estrogen receptors (ER) and progesterone receptors (PgR) in the management of breast cancer?
The response rates of metastatic breast cancer to hormonal treatment are related to the activities of estrogen and progesterone receptors in the tumor specimen as follows:

ER	PgR	Response Rate
Negative	Negative	5%
Positive	Negative	25%
Negative	Positive	35%
Positive	Positive	70%
Unknown	Unknown	30%

(From Casciato DA, Lowitz BB: Manual of Clinical Oncology, 2nd ed. Boston, Little, Brown, 1988, p 162, with permission.)

87. What are the current recommendations for screening for carcinoma of the cervix?
Recommendations concerning periodic screening of women in the U.S. using Pap* smears have been developed based on risk groups. Low risk groups are those women who have never had sexual activity, have had a hysterectomy for nonmalignant reasons, or have reached the age of 60 and have never had a positive Pap smear. High-risk patients are those who are sexually active early and with many partners.

The American Cancer Society recommends that asymptomatic women over 20 years of age and those under 20 years of age who are sexually active have cytologic screening for 2 consecutive years and at least one screening every 3 years until age 65. High-risk patients should be screened yearly.
   * From Papanicolaou-Traut smear.

88. What is the appropriate management of a patient with an abnormal Pap smear?
An abnormal Pap smear should lead to colposcopy and/or biopsy. If carcinoma in situ or dysplasia is found, cryotherapy, laser therapy, cone biopsy, or hysterectomy should be performed, depending on the size and extent of the lesion.

If invasive cancer is found on biopsy, a metastatic workup should be done. Stage I disease is treated with radical hysterectomy or radiation therapy, whereas all other stages are further evaluated with a CT scan. If the para-aortic nodes are enlarged, a needle biopsy should be done. Those with positive biopsy are treated with pelvic radiation therapy and chemotherapy and/or radiation therapy to para-aortic nodes. If nodes are found to be normal on the CT scan or if the needle biopsy is negative, then laparotomy with para-aortic node biopsies should be considered to determine the actual state of the nodes. If the biopsy is positive, then treatment should proceed as for other positive node biopsies. If it is negative, treatment is radiotherapy with two intracavitary radium implants.

89. Which studies are used in the staging of carcinoma of the cervix?

Pelvic exam	Barium enema, for advanced stage,
Biochemical profile	or age > 40 years
Chest x-ray	CT scan, to evaluate retroperitoneal nodes, or for
Cystoscopy	planning radiotherapy of bulky lesions
Proctosigmoidoscopy	Lymphangiograms and MRI may be useful in
Intravenous pyelogram (IVP)	selected cases

90. What are the 5-year survival rates, relative to stage, for carcinoma of the cervix?

Stage		5-year Survival
I:	Tumor strictly confined to the cervix.	80%
II:	Tumor extends beyond the cervix but has not extended on to the pelvic wall. The tumor involves the vagina but not the lower third.	55–60%
III:	Tumor extends to the pelvic wall. The tumor involves the lower third of the vagina. All cases with hydronephrosis or nonfunctioning kidney (unless known to be due to another cause).	30–32%
IV:	Tumor extends beyond the true pelvis or has involved the bladder or rectal mucosa.	8–10%

91. What is the treatment of carcinoma of the cervix relative to stage?

Stage	Treatment
IA	Simple hysterectomy or intracavitary radiation
IB, IIA	Radical abdominal hysterectomy with pelvic lymphadenopathy or radiation therapy
IIB, III	Radiation therapy
IVA	Pelvic exenteration ± radiation
IVB	Chemotherapy

92. Name the risk factors for carcinoma of the endometrium.

1. Infertility
2. Obesity
3. Failure of ovulation
4. Dysfunctional bleeding
5. Prolonged estrogen use

93. What are the 5-year survival rates for the various grades and stages of endometrial cancer?
Survival rates are related to both stage and grade, and both influence outcome. The treatment modalities used in various series also seem to affect outcome. It is difficult to compare results, as they vary from institution to institution. However, in general, they correspond to grade and stage:

Grades and Stages of Endometrial Cancer

Grade		5-year Survival
I:	Differentiated	81%
II:	Intermediate	74%
III:	Undifferentiated	50%

Stage		5-year Survival
I:	Tumor confined to the corpus	80%
II:	Tumor involves the corpus and cervix	70%
III:	Tumor extends outside the corpus, but not outside the true pelvis (it may involve the vaginal wall or the parametrium but not the bladder or rectum)	16%
IV:	Tumor involves the bladder or rectum or extends outside the pelvis	5%

94. Name the risk factors for ovarian cancer.
The risk factors for ovarian cancer include:

- Nulliparity or low parity
- Family history of ovarian cancer
- History of breast or colon cancer
- Presence of Peutz-Jeghers syndrome
- Presence of basal cell nevus syndrome
- Gonadal dysgenesis (46XY type)
- Asbestos exposure

95. List the paraneoplastic syndromes associated with ovarian cancer.

1. Neurologic:
   Peripheral neuropathy
   Organic brain syndrome
   AML-like syndrome
   Cerebellar ataxia
2. Blood antigens causing cross-matching problems
3. Cushing's syndrome
4. Hypercalcemia
5. Thrombophlebitis

96. What are the 5-year survival rates for the various stages of carcinoma of the ovary?

Stage		5-year Survival
I:	Growth limited to the ovaries.	80%
II:	Growth involving one or both ovaries with pelvic extension.	60%
III:	Tumor involving ovaries with peritoneal implants outside the pelvis and/or positive retroperitoneal or inguinal nodes. Patients with superficial liver metastases. Tumors limited to the true pelvis but with histologically verified malignant extension to small bowel or omentum.	30%
IV:	Tumor involving ovaries with distant metastases.	5%

97. Which viruses have been implicated in the development of lymphomas?

Human T-cell leukemia virus (HTLV) has been implicated in the development of adult T-cell lymphomas, whereas Epstein-Barr virus (EBV) has long been suspected to be associated with the cause of Hodgkin's disease.

98. What are some unusual epidemiological features of Hodgkin's disease?

The epidemiology of Hodgkin's disease is scientifically intriguing, suggesting an infective agent. It occurs more frequently in individuals from small families and in children raised in hygienic, isolated environments. Reports of epidemics of Hodgkin's disease in neighborhoods and among school classes are not completely convincing. Genetic predisposition, as well as infective agents, could explain the increased incidence in some families. Hodgkin's disease is more common in some tropical countries and in the Middle East in children younger than 10 years.

99. What is the differential diagnosis of lymphadenopathy?

Diseases Associated with Lymph Node Enlargement

1. Infectious diseases
   a. Viral infections: infectious hepatitis, infectious mononucleosis syndromes (cytomegalovirus, EB virus), AIDS, rubella, varicella-herpes zoster, vaccinia
   b. Bacterial infections: streptococci, staphylococci, salmonella, brucella, *Francisella tularensis, Listeria monocytogenes, Pasteurella pestis, Haemophilus ducreyi,* cat-scratch disease
   c. Fungal infections: coccidioidomycosis, histoplasmosis
   d. Chlamydial infections: Lymphogranuloma venereum, trachoma
   e. Mycobacterial infections: tuberculosis, leprosy
   f. Parasitic infections: trypanosomiasis, microfilariasis, toxoplasmosis
   g. Spirochetal diseases: syphilis, yaws, endemic syphilis (bejel), leptospirosis
2. Immunologic diseases
   a. Rheumatoid arthritis
   b. Systemic lupus erythematosus
   c. Dermatomyositis
   d. Serum sickness
   e. Drug reactions: phenytoin, hydralazine, allopurinol
   f. Angioimmunoblastic lymphadenopathy

Table continued on next page.

Diseases Associated with Lymph Node Enlargement (Continued)

3. Malignant diseases
   a. Hematologic: Hodgkin's lymphoma, acute and chronic T-, B-, myeloid, and monocytoid cell leukemias and lymphomas, malignant histiocytosis
   b. Metastatic tumors to lymph nodes: melanoma, Kaposi's sarcoma, neuroblastoma, seminoma, tumors of lung, breast, prostate, kidney, head and neck, gastrointestinal tract
4. Endocrine diseases: hyperthyroidism
5. Lipid storage diseases: Gaucher's and Niemann-Pick diseases
6. Miscellaneous diseases and diseases of unknown cause
   a. Giant follicular lymph node hyperplasia
   b. Sinus histiocytosis
   c. Dermatopathic lymphadenitis
   d. Sarcoidosis
   e. Amyloidosis
   f. Mucocutaneous lymph node syndrome
   g. Lymphomatoid granulomatosis
   h. Multifocal Langerhans cell (eosinophilic) granulomatosis

(From Wilson JD, et al (eds): Principles of Internal Medicine, 12th ed. New York, McGraw-Hill, 1991, p 355, with permission.)

100. Which are the "favorable" lymphomas?

The low-grade (or "favorable") lymphomas of the Rappaport classification are:

Diffuse, well-differentiated lymphocytic

Nodular, poorly differentiated lymphocytic

Nodular, mixed lymphocytic-histiocytic

They are described as favorable because their natural history is characterized by a relatively long survival, with an indolent course and easy response to minimal therapy.

101. Which are the "unfavorable" lymphomas, and what is their prognosis?

The unfavorable, or high grade, non-Hodgkin's lymphomas are:

Diffuse histiocytic

Lymphoblastic

Burkitt's

All the other types (nodular histiocytic, diffuse poorly differentiated lymphocytic, diffuse mixed lymphocytic and histiocytic, and diffuse large cell) are called intermediate grade, as their aggressiveness and responsiveness to treatment are intermediate between the other two groups.

102. Which cytogenetic abnormalities are associated with lymphomas?

Three recurrent chromosomal aberrations have been found to correlate with certain histological types of lymphoma:

1. A translocation between chromosome 18 and 14 in patients with follicular lymphoma (small cleaved cell, mixed cell, and large cell). If in addition, a deletion 13q32 is found, these patients have an accelerated course and a leukemic phase.

2. A translocation between chromosomes 8 and 14 in patients with small noncleaved cell (non-Burkitt's) or large cell immunoblastic lymphoma.

3. A trisomy 12 in patients with small cell lymphocytic lymphoma.

Other abnormalities have also been described:

A deletion 6q with a complete or partial trisomy 7 or trisomy 12 is associated with more aggressive follicular mixed small and large cell, or large cell histologic type.

A complete or partial trisomy 3, 18, or 21 with follicular large cell lymphoma. A trisomy 2 or duplication 2p in addition is indicative of an accelerated clinical course and a poor response to treatment.

103. What is the staging system for lymphomas?

Stage	Characteristics
I	Single node region or single extranodal site
II	Two or more node regions, same side of diaphragm
III	Nodal disease above and below diaphragm
IV	Disseminated extranodal disease

Additional designations
S	Splenic involvement
E	Localized extranodal involvement
A	Absence of constitutional symptoms
B	Presence of 10% or more weight loss in preceding 6 months, fever and/or night sweats
CS	Clinical stage
PS	Pathologic stage

104. Contrast the natural history of Hodgkin's disease with the non-Hodgkin's lymphomas.

	Hodgkin's Disease	Non-Hodgkin's Lymphomas
Age	Bimodal: 15–34 and over 50	Median age 50
Symptoms	B symptoms are more common in older age and higher stage; in mixed cellularity and lymphocyte depleted, may have severe symptoms with minimal nodes.	Less than 10% have B symptoms
Signs		
Nodes		
General	Seen in over 90% at presentation	Least common in histiocytic type
Waldeyer's	Uncommon	30% some series
Cervical	65%	10–20%
Mediastinal	10%	2–3%
Abdominal	Retroperitoneal	Mesenteric
Extranodal	3%	Up to 60% in histiocytic
GI	4%	20–40%
CNS	Uncommon except in immunocompromised	Common, esp. lymphocytic
Pleural effusion	From obstruction due to mediastinal nodes	Chylous

105. What are the 5-year survival rates relative to grade of the non-Hodgkin's lymphomas?

Grade	5-year Survival
Small lymphocytic	59%
Follicular, small cleaved cell	70%
Follicular mixed	50%
Follicular, large cell	45%
Diffuse, small cleaved cell	33%
Diffuse, mixed small and large cell	38%
Diffuse, large cell	35%
Immunoblastic	32%
Lymphoblastic	26%
Small, noncleaved cell	23%

106. What are the commonly used medications for mild to moderate cancer pain?

Oral Non-narcotic and Narcotic Analgesics for Mild to Moderate Pain

	EQUIANALGESIC DOSE (mg)*	DURATION (hr)	PLASMA HALF-LIFE (hr)	COMMENTS
Aspirin	650	4–6	3–5	Standard for nonnarcotic comparisons; gastrointestinal and hematologic effects limit use in patients with cancer
Acetaminophen	650	4–6	1–4	Weak antiinflammatory effects; safer than aspirin
Propoxyphene	65†	4–6	12	Biotransformed to potentially toxic metabolic norpropoxyphene; used in combinatin with non-narcotic analgesics
Codeine	32†	4–6	3	Biotransformed to morphine; available in combination with non-narcotic analgesics
Meperidine	50	4–6	3–4	Biotransformed to active toxic metabolite normeperidine; associated with myoclonus and seizures
Pentazocine	30	4–6	2–3	Psychotomimetic effects with escalation of dose; only available in combination with naloxone, aspirin, or acetaminophen (U.S.)

* Relative potency of drugs, as compared with that of aspirin, for mild to moderate pain.
† Some investigators have reported that a much larger dose (propoxyphene, 130 mg; codeine, 60 mg) is effective in patients with mild to moderate pain.
(From Foley KM: The treatment of cancer pain. N Engl J Med 313:89, 1985, with permission.)

107. What are some commonly used medications for severe cancer pain?

Oral and Parenteral Narcotic Analgesics for Severe Pain

	ROUTE*	EQUI-ANALGESIC DOSE (mg)†	DURATION (hr)	PLASMA HALF-LIFE (hr)	COMMENTS
Narcotic agonists					
Morphine	IM	10	4–6	2–3.5	Standard for comparison; also available in slow-release tablets
	PO	60	4–7		
Codeine	IM	130	4–6	3	Biotransformed to morphine; useful as initial narcotic analgesic
	PO	200	4–6		
Oxycodone	IM	15		—	Short acting; available alone or as 5-mg dose in combination with aspirin and acetaminophen
	PO	30	3–5		
Heroin	IM	5	4–5	0.5	Illegal in U.S.; high solubility for parenteral administration
	PO	60	4–5		
Levorphanol	IM	2	4–6	12–16	Good oral potency, requires careful titration in initial dosing because of drug accumulation
(Levo-Dromoran)	PO	4	4–7		
Hydromorphone	IM	1.5	4–5	2–3	Available in high-potency injectable form (10 mg/ml) for cachectic patients and as rectal suppositories; more soluble than morphine
(Dilaudid)	PO	7.5	4–6		

Table continued on next page.

Oral and Parenteral Narcotic Analgesics for Severe Pain (cont.)

	ROUTE*	EQUI-ANALGESIC DOSE (mg)†	DURATION (hr)	PLASMA HALF-LIFE (hr)	COMMENTS
Narcotic agonists *(cont.)*					
Oxymorphone	IM	1	4–6		Available in parenteral and
(Numorphan)	PR	10	4–6	2–3	rectal-suppository forms only
Meperidine	IM	75	4–5	3–4 norme-peridine	Contraindicated in patients with renal disease; accumulation of active toxic metabolite
(Demerol)					
	PO	300	4–6	12–16	normeperidine produces CNS excitation
Methadone	IM	10			Good oral potency; requires
(Dolophine)	PO	20		15–30	careful titration of the initial dose to avoid drug accumulation
Mixed agonist-antagonist drugs					
Pentazocine	IM	60	4–6		Limited use for cancer pain;
(Talwin)	PO	180	4–7	2–3	psychotomimetic effects with dose escalation; available only in combination with naloxone, aspirin, or acetaminophen; may precipitate withdrawal in physically dependent patients
Nalbuphine	IM	10	4–6		Not available orally; less severe
(Nubain)	PO	—		5	psychotomimetic effects than pentazocine; may precipitate withdrawal in physically dependent patients
Butorphanol	IM	2	4–6		Not available orally; produces
(Stadol)	PO	—		2.5–3.5	psychotomimetic effects; may precipitate withdrawal in physically dependent patients
Partial agonists					
Buprenorphine	IM	0.4	4–6		No psychotomimetic
(Temgesic)	SL	0.8	5–6	?	effects; may precipitate withdrawal in tolerant patients

*IM denotes intramuscular, PO oral, PR rectal, and SL sublingual.

† Based on single-dose studies in which an intramuscular dose of each drug listed was compared with morphine to establish the relative potency. Oral doses are those recommended when changing from a parenteral to an oral route. For patients without prior narcotic exposure, the recommended oral starting dose is 30 mg for morphine, 5 mg for methadone, 2 mg for levorphanol, and 4 mg for hydromorphone.

(From Foley KM: The treatment of cancer pain. N Engl J Med 313:90, 1985, with permission.)

108. What are radiosensitizers?

Radiosensitizers are chemical agents that have been reported to increase the sensitivity of cells in vitro to radiation and are usually classified as non-hypoxic cell sensitizers. This class of compounds includes drugs such as halogenated pyrimidine nucleoside analogs, 3-amino-benzamide, diamide, and various platinum compounds, among others. Radiosensitization by these compounds may be mediated by a variety of mechanisms, none of which is precisely known. However, it is often assumed that effects on the induction and/or repair of radiation-induced damage may be involved.

109. What is a molar pregnancy?

Molar pregnancies refer to a group of benign and malignant gestational trophoblastic neoplasms. The most malignant of these is choriocarcinoma, which was fatal within 1 to 2 years prior to the advent of chemotherapy. The most common variant, hydatidiform mole, occurs in only 1 in 2000 pregnancies in the U.S.

  Rutledge F, et al (eds): Gynecologic Oncology. New York, John Wiley, 1976.

110. What is the therapeutic classification of a molar pregnancy?
  1. Molar pregnancy
     a. Pre-evacuation
     b. Post-evacuation
  2. Persistent or retained mole (after 8 weeks)
  3. Nonmetastatic trophoblastic disease
     a. No histologic evidence of choriocarcinoma
     b. Choriocarcinoma
  4. Metastatic trophoblastic disease
     a. No histologic evidence of choriocarcinoma
     b. Choriocarcinoma (low risk)
     c. Choriocarcinoma (high risk)

(From Rutledge F, et al (eds): Gynecologic Oncology. New York, John Wiley, 1976, p 145, with permission.)

BIBLIOGRAPHY

1. Calabresi P, Schein PS, Rosenberg SA (eds): Basic Principles and Clinical Management of Cancer. New York, Macmillan, 1985.
2. Casciato DA, Lowitz BB (eds): Manual of Clinical Oncology, 2nd ed. Boston, Little, Brown, 1988.
3. DeVita T Jr, Hellman S, Rosenberg SA (eds): Principles and Practice of Oncology, 3rd ed. Philadelphia, J.B. Lippincott, 1989.
4. Moossa AR, Schimpff SC, Robson MC (eds): Comprehensive Textbook of Oncology, 2nd ed. Baltimore, Williams & Wilkins, 1991.
5. Tannock IF, Hill RP (eds): The Basic Science of Oncology. Canada, Pergamon Press, 1987.

7. NEPHROLOGY SECRETS

Donald E. Wesson, M.D. and Sangubhotla Prabhakar, M.D.

It is no exaggeration to say that the composition of the blood is determined not by what the mouth takes in but by what the kidneys keep.

Homer W. Smith (1895–1962)
From Fish to Philosopher, Ch. 1

Bones can break, muscles can atrophy, glands can loaf, even the brain can go to sleep, without immediately endangering our survival; but should the kidneys fail . . . neither bone, muscle, gland nor brain could carry on.

Idem

1. What is a drug?

A drug is a substance that when injected into a rat will produce a scientific report.

Matz R: Principles of medicine. NY State J Med 77:99–101, 1977.

ASSESSMENT OF RENAL FUNCTION

2. What is the glomerular filtration rate (GFR)?

The glomerular filtrate is the ultrafiltrate of plasma that exits from the glomerular capillary tuft and enters into Bowman's capsule to begin the journey along the tubule of the nephron. It is the initial step in the formation of urine and is basic to the function of the kidney. The volume of this filtrate formed per unit time is called the glomerular filtration rate (GFR) and is usually expressed in ml/min.

3. How is the GFR measured clinically?

The GFR is measured indirectly using a marker substance contained in glomerular filtrate, which is excreted in the urine. The marker substance is chosen such that its urinary mass excretion is equal to the mass of the substance that enters into Bowman's capsule per unit time. More simply put, the amount of this substance leaving the kidney is equal to the amount of substance entering the kidney as glomerular filtrate. This means that once having entered the kidney tubule, it must not be reabsorbed, secreted, or metabolized. The volume of glomerular filtrate represented by the urinary mass excretion of the marker substance can then be calculated by dividing the urinary mass excretion of the marker substance by the concentration of the substance in the glomerular filtrate.

The marker substance is chosen so that its concentration in the glomerular filtrate is equal to its concentration in the plasma, i.e., the substance is freely filterable across the glomerular capillary. Therefore, the amount of substance "X" entering the kidney equals the GFR multiplied by plasma concentration of the substance (P_x). Likewise, the amount of the substance leaving the kidney in the urine equals the urinary concentration of the substance (U_x) multiplied by the urine flow in ml/min (V). Therefore, the formula for calculating GFR using our marker substance "X" becomes:

$$GFR \times P_x = U_x \times V$$

or

$$GFR = \frac{U_x \times V}{P_x}$$

A stable plasma concentration of the substance (a steady-state situation) is required to make the above equation meaningful.

4. Name the marker substances used to measure GFR in the laboratory and in clinical settings.

To recapitulate, the marker substance chosen to measure GFR must have the following characteristics: (1) freely filterable, (2) stable plasma concentration, and (3) not reabsorbed, secreted, or metabolized. The polysaccharide **inulin** satisfies these criteria very well and is often used in laboratory determinations of GFR. It has little clinical usefulness because it requires constant intravenous infusion, making it somewhat impractical for routine use in patients. **Creatinine** is used as a marker substance in clinical settings.

5. Why is creatinine used as a marker substance for GFR determinations in clinical settings?

Creatinine is an endogenous substance, derived from the metabolism of creatine in skeletal muscle, that fulfills almost all of the requirements for a marker substance (as outlined above). It is freely filterable, is not metabolized, and is not reabsorbed once filtered. There is a small amount of tubular secretion that makes the creatinine clearance a slight overestimate of the GFR. This overestimate becomes quantitatively important only at low levels of GFR. Creatinine is released from muscle at a constant rate, resulting in a stable plasma concentration. The creatinine clearance is commonly determined from a 24-hour collection of urine. This time period is used to average out the sometimes variable creatinine excretion that may occur hour-to-hour. Creatinine is easily measured, making it a nearly ideal marker for GFR determination.

6. How can the completeness of a 24-hour urine collection be judged?

Since total creatinine excretion in the steady state is dependent on muscle mass, day-to-day creatinine excretion remains fairly constant for an individual and is related to lean body weight. In general, men excrete 20–25 mg of creatinine/kg of body weight/day, whereas women excrete 15–20 mg/kg/day. Therefore, a 70-kg man would be expected to excrete approximately 1400 mg of creatinine per day. Creatinine excretion levels measured on a 24-hour urine collection that are substantially less than the estimated value suggest an incomplete collection.

7. What is the relationship between plasma creatinine concentration and GFR?

Since creatinine production and excretion remain constant and equal, the amount of creatinine entering and leaving the kidney remains constant. Thus,

$$GFR \times P_{cr} = U_{cr} \times V = Constant$$
$$or$$
$$GFR = \frac{1}{P_{cr}} \times constant$$

This constant creatinine excretion continues as GFR declines and remains that way until the GFR reaches very low levels. Therefore, the GFR is a function of the reciprocal of the plasma creatinine concentration.

8. Does a given plasma creatinine concentration reflect the same level of renal function in different patients?

Not necessarily. Remember that creatinine production is directly proportional to muscle mass, and the plasma creatinine concentration is determined in part by creatinine production. Examination of the calculation of creatinine clearance for an 80-kg man compared to that of a 40-kg woman, assuming both individuals have plasma creatinine concentrations of 1.0 mg/dl (0.01 mg/ml), shows the following:

For the 80-kg man, creatinine excretion should be:

$$80 \text{ kg} \times 20 \text{ mg/kg/day} = 1600 \text{ mg/day} = 1.11 \text{ mg/min}$$

$$\text{GFR} = \frac{1.11 \text{ mg/min}}{0.01 \text{ mg/ml}}$$

or   111 ml/min

For the 40-kg woman, creatinine excretion should be:

$$40 \text{ kg} \times 15 \text{ mg/kg/day} = 600 \text{ mg/day} = 0.42 \text{ mg/min}$$

$$\text{GFR} = \frac{0.42 \text{ mg/min}}{0.01 \text{ mg/ml}}$$

or   42 ml/min

This demonstrates that the same plasma creatinine concentration can represent markedly different GFRs in different individuals. The difference in creatinine excretion is related to differences in muscle mass, which are related to lean body weight and age. The following formula was devised to provide a rough estimate of the GFR in situations where a measured creatinine clearance is not immediately available:

$$\text{Creatinine clearance} = \frac{140 - \text{Age} \times \text{Lean body wt in kg}}{\text{Plasma creatinine} \times 72}$$

If we use this formula to estimate the GFR of the above individuals and assume an age of 50 years for each, we get a GFR of 100 for the man and 50 for the woman. These estimates are in the range of those determined previously. They serve to illustrate the relative differences in the GFR calculated for these two individuals with the same P_{cr}. Recognizing this fact and using this formula to estimate GFR could prevent a serious error when selecting the dose of a drug that is excreted by the kidneys.

9. How does the blood urea nitrogen (BUN) relate to the GFR?

BUN is excreted primarily by glomerular filtration. Its level in the plasma tends to vary inversely with GFR. BUN, however, is a much less ideal marker of GFR than is creatinine. Its production may not be constant in that it varies with protein intake, liver function, and catabolic rate. In addition, urea can be reabsorbed once filtered into the kidney. This reabsorption increases in conditions with low urine flow, such as volume depletion. This latter circumstance is one cause of a high (greater than 15:1) BUN to creatinine ratio in the plasma. Thus, creatinine is the better marker for GFR, but the plasma level of BUN can be used along with the creatinine concentration as a clue to the presence of certain states, such as volume depletion.

10. What is clearance? What is the difference between clearance and excretion?

Urinary **excretion** of a substance is simply the mass amount of a substance excreted per unit time. It is usually expressed in mg/min. **Clearance** expresses the efficiency with which the kidney removes a substance from the plasma. It is the volume of plasma that would have to be completely cleared of a substance per unit time to account for the mass of that substance appearing in the urine per unit time. It is expressed in volume per unit time, usually ml/min. For example, a substance ("X") with the following measurements—

$$P_x = \text{Plasma concentration of "X"} = 1.0 \text{ mg/ml}$$
$$U_x = \text{Urine concentration of "X"} = 10 \text{ mg/ml}$$
$$V = \text{Urine flow} = 1.0 \text{ ml/min}$$

—has the following clearance:

$$\text{Clearance}_x = \frac{U_x \times V}{P_x} = \frac{10 \text{ mg/ml} \times 1.0 \text{ ml/min}}{1.0 \text{ mg/ml}}$$
$$= 10 \text{ ml/min}$$

The calculated clearance for substance "X" of 10 ml/min indicates that the amount of substance "X" appearing in the urine is the same as if 10 ml of plasma were completely cleared of the substance and excreted in the urine each minute. The urinary excretion of "X" is 10 mg/min, but this measurement does not indicate the efficiency with which the substance is removed from the plasma.

11. How does measurement of urinary protein excretion help in the evaluation of renal disease?

Normal urinary protein excretion is less than 150 mg/day. Failure of the tubules to reabsorb the normally filtered small-molecular-weight proteins leads to **tubular proteinuria.** This form of proteinuria occurs in diseases that affect tubular function, and the proteins are almost entirely of smaller molecular weight than albumin. **Glomerular proteinuria** occurs when the normal glomerular barrier to the passage of plasma proteins is disrupted. This results in variable quantities of albumin and sometimes larger molecular weight proteins spilling into the urine. Quantitatively, tubular proteinuria is usually less than 1 g/24 hr and glomerular proteinuria is usually greater than 1 g/24 hr. When the proteinuria is greater than 3.5 g/1.73 m^2 body surface area, it is said to be in the nephrotic range. Significant degrees of proteinuria (> 150 mg/day) usually indicate intrinsic renal disease. *Quantification and characterization of the proteinuria is useful in detecting not only the presence of renal disease but in determining involvement of the tubule, glomerulus, or both.*

12. What information can be gained from examination of the urine sediment?

Urine sediment is normally almost cell-free, usually crystal-free, and has a very low concentration of protein (less than 1+ by dipstick). Examination of this sediment is a very important part of the workup of any patient with renal disease. The examination should be performed by the physician prior to diagnostic or therapeutic decisions. The information obtained must be correlated with all other aspects of the patient's history, physical examination, and laboratory data base. The examination can provide evidence of many conditions, including renal inflammation (cells, protein), infection (white blood cells, bacteria), stone disease (crystals), and systemic diseases (bilirubin, myoglobin, hemoglobin, etc.).

ACUTE RENAL FAILURE

13. What is acute renal failure?

Acute renal failure (ARF) is a syndrome of many etiologies that is characterized by a sudden decrease in renal function leading to a compromise in the kidney's ability to regulate normal homeostasis. This inability is multifactorial. The kidney is unable to maintain the content and volume of the extracellular fluid or perform its routine endocrine functions. In most cases ARF is a potentially reversible process.

14. Why is it important to distinguish acute from chronic renal failure?

The clinical manifestations of ARF are generally more severe than those associated with chronic renal failure. Unlike chronic renal failure, the cause for ARF can usually be identified and must be addressed in an effort to prevent further insult to the kidney or other organ systems. Acute renal failure is a potentially reversible disorder if the causative factor or factors are identified and corrected. Appropriate supportive care must be given to optimize the chances for recovery of renal function.

15. What is meant by oliguria?

Oliguria refers to a urine volume that is inadequate for the normal excretion of the body's metabolic waste products. Since the daily load of metabolic waste products amounts to approximately 600 mOsm and the maximal urine concentrating ability of the human kidney is about 1200 mOsm/kg water, there is a minimal obligate urine volume of 500 ml/ day for most individuals. Therefore, a 24-hour urine volume less than 500 ml/day is said to represent oliguria. When associated with ARF, oliguria portends a poorer prognosis than does nonoliguric ARF.

16. What is anuria? Why is it important to distinguish it from oliguria?

Anuria refers to a 24-hour urine volume of less than 100 ml. It denotes a severe reduction in urine volume that is commonly associated with obstruction, renal cortical necrosis, or severe acute tubular necrosis. It is important to make the distinction between oliguria and anuria so that these diagnostic entities will be considered and appropriate therapy planned.

17. In approaching patients with ARF, it is recommended that an attempt be made to place patients into one of three diagnostic categories. What are these diagnostic categories and what is the importance of this diagnostic approach?

The categories are prerenal, renal and postrenal failure. This approach is important because pre- and postrenal causes of ARF can often be corrected rather quickly and, if corrected, further renal injury can frequently be avoided. Placement into the "renal" category should lead to a search for the agents, factors, or processes that may have resulted in renal injury (acute tubular necrosis or ATN). This approach not only aids in diagnosis but also leads to the appropriate therapy.

18. What are the most common causes of ARF in the U.S.?

A. **Prerenal causes:**
1. True volume depletion
    a. Gastrointestinal losses (vomiting, diarrhea, bleeding)
    b. Renal losses (diuretics, osmotic diuresis [glucose], hypoaldosteronism, salt-wasting nephropathy, diabetes insipidus [only if abnormal thirst prevents replacement of water losses])
    c. Skin or respiratory losses (insensible losses, sweat, burns)
    d. Third-space sequestration (intestinal obstruction, crush injury or skeletal fracture, acute pancreatitis)
2. Hypotension (shock)
3. Edematous states (heart failure, hepatic cirrhosis, nephrosis)
4. Selective renal ischemia (hepatorenal syndrome, nonsteroidal anti-inflammatory drugs [NSAIDs], bilateral renal artery stenosis [frequently made worse by angiotensin-converting enzyme inhibitors], calcium channel blockers)

B. **Renal causes (acute tubular necrosis [ATN])**
1. Postischemic (all causes of severe prerenal disease, particularly hypotension)
2. Nephrotoxins
    a. Drugs and exogenous toxins
       Common: Aminoglycoside antibiotics, radiocontrast media, cisplatin
       Rare: Cephalosporins, rifampin, amphotericin B, polymyxin B, methoxyflurane, acetaminophen overdose, heavy metals (mercury, arsenic, uranium), carbon tetrachloride, EDTA, tetracyclines
    b. Heme pigments:
       Rhabdomyolysis (myoglobinuria)
       Intravascular hemolysis (hemoglobinuria)

C. **Postrenal causes:**
1. Obstruction due to strictures, stones, malignancies, or prostatic enlargement.

19. What is meant by "prerenal failure"?

This syndrome refers to a decrease in renal function that results from a decrease in renal perfusion. The decrease in renal perfusion leads to functional changes within the kidney, which result in a compromise in the kidney's ability to perform its homeostatic functions. This disorder is potentially correctable by addressing the factors leading to renal hypoperfusion. In severe cases, renal hypoperfusion can be severe enough and prolonged enough to result in structural damage and hence the "renal" category of ARF. Therefore, it is important that the prerenal syndrome be identified and corrected promptly.

20. What is acute tubular necrosis (ATN)?

ATN is a nonspecific entity with multiple etiologies that is characterized by structural and functional damage of the renal tubules and a functional decrease of glomerular function. If the patient survives, ATN is self-limited, with most patients having recovered renal function within 8 weeks. It is most commonly caused by ischemia but there is a multitude of other causes.

21. How can the use of urinary indices help to distinguish prerenal failure from ATN?

Patients with prerenal azotemia have intact tubular function. The kidney, in this setting, is attempting to minimize solute and water excretion in an effort to preserve extracellular fluid volume. By contrast, the tubules of patients with ATN do not properly recover solutes and water that have been filtered into the kidney. Thus, the urine of patients with prerenal azotemia typically reveals:

1. Low urinary sodium concentration (< 20 meq/L)
2. Low fractional excretion of sodium ($< 1.0\%$), and
3. Low free-water excretion (high urine osmolality [> 500] and high urine specific gravity [≥ 1.015]).

By contrast, the urinary indices of patients with ATN reveal the kidney's relative inability to reabsorb sodium (urinary sodium concentration > 40 meq/L and fractional sodium excretion of $> 3.0\%$) and to reabsorb water (urine osmolality < 350 mOsm/L and urine specific gravity < 1.010). Remember that there is considerable crossover between renal and prerenal failure with regard to these indices and hence no value absolutely indicates one or the other diagnosis. The indices should be used along with other data (i.e., history, physical exam) to arrive at a clinical impression.

22. What is meant by the fractional excretion of sodium (FE_{Na})? What is its relevance to the diagnosis of ARF?

FE_{Na} is calculated by using the following equation:

$$FE_{Na^+} (\%) = \frac{U_{Na^+} \times P_{Cr}}{P_{Na^+} \times U_{Cr}} \times 100$$

FE_{Na^+} = fractional excretion of sodium
U_{Na^+} and P_{Na^+} = urinary and plasma sodium concentration in meq/L
U_{Cr} and P_{Cr} = urinary and plasma creatinine.

A FE_{Na^+} value below 1% favors prerenal states, whereas a value greater than 1% indicates intrarenal states or ATN. The test is more accurate than urinary sodium measurement in this differentiation. However, it should be noted that a FE_{Na^+} below 1% is occasionally reported for a variety of causes of ARF other than prerenal states.

It is also to be noted that an intact sodium reabsorptive capacity is necessary for the use of this test. Thus, in conditions such as underlying chronic renal disease, hypoaldosteronism, diuretic therapy, or metabolic alkalosis with bicarbonaturia, the FE_{Na^+} will be inappropriately high despite the presence of volume depletion.

23. List the four classic phases of ARF.

These phases are the initial, oliguric, diuretic, and recovery phases. The **initial stage** is usually not recognized clinically and represents the period of exposure to the insult. The classic **oliguric phase** is characterized by oliguria; however, patients in this phase are commonly nonoliguric. During this phase the deterioration in renal function becomes evident. The **diuretic phase** is characterized by a gradual increase in urine volume, often to very high levels. It is thought to represent movement of filtrate through tubules which have yet to completely recover their absorptive function. The **recovery phase** is characterized by the gradual return of glomerular function.

24. What are the indications for dialysis in ARF?

Definite Indications for Dialysis in ARF

1. Hyperkalemia uncontrollable by Kayexalate
2. Fluid overload with pulmonary edema
3. Uremic pericarditis
4. Uremic encephalopathy
5. Bleeding diathesis
6. Severe metabolic acidosis ($HCO_3^- <10$ mEq/L)

Rose BD (ed): Pathophysiology of Renal Disease, 2nd ed. New York, McGraw-Hill, 1980, p 101.

25. Is the mortality rate in ARF significant?

The overall mortality in ARF is very high (40–60%) despite the availability of dialysis. The mortality is worse in the subcategory of patients with a history of surgery or trauma. The prognosis is better in the absence of respiratory failure, bleeding, or infection, and also in patients with nonoliguric ATN. ARF occurring in the obstetrical setting also has a better prognosis, with only a 10–20% mortality rate.

26. How frequently does nephrotoxicity due to radiocontrast agents occur?

The incidence of contrast-induced renal failure is very variable. Most retrospective studies report an incidence of less than 1%, whereas the majority of prospective studies reported an incidence of 4–70%. In one of the more recent prospective studies, the frequency of this complication was 12%.

Hou SH, Bushinsky DA, Wish JB, et al: Hospital acquired renal insufficiency: A prospective study. Am J Med 74:243–248, 1983.

27. What are the important risk factors for radiocontrast-associated ARF?

Risk Factors and Prevalence in Contrast-induced ARF

1. Azotemia (Cr $>$ 1.5 mg/dl)	60%
2. Albuminuria $>$ 2+	56%
3. Hypertension	55%
4. Age $>$ 60 years	51%
5. Dehydration	41%
6. Uric acid $>$ 8.0 mg/dl	41%
7. Multiple studies	29%
8. Solitary kidney	13%
9. Contrast medium $>$ 2 ml/kg	11%
10. Multiple myeloma	2%

(From Berns AS: Nephrotoxicity of contrast media. Kidney Int 36:730–740, 1989, with permission.)

28. What are the pathogenetic factors responsible for ARF with contrast dyes?
Pathogenetic factors responsible for ARF are:

1. Hemodynamic changes   5. Allergic and immunologic reactions
2. Osmolality   6. Enzymuria
3. Proteinuria   7. Direct toxicity
4. Tubular obstruction   8. Altered glomerular permeability

(From Cronin RE: Southwestern Internal Medicine Conference: Renal failure following radiologic procedures. Am J Med Sci 298:342–356, 1989, with permission.)

29. Is there an increased risk of ARF with radiocontrast agents in patients with myeloma?
For several years multiple myeloma was believed to be an important risk factor for radiocontrast-agent-induced ARF. However, several large studies have noted a prevalence of less than 5%. In the absence of pre-existing renal failure or proteinuria, multiple myeloma by itself is unlikely to predispose to ARF following exposure to radiocontrast media. However, considering the high prevalence of renal disease in patients with myeloma, avoidance of radiocontrast agents in patients with myeloma is still recommended.

CHRONIC RENAL FAILURE

30. List in order the stages of progressive renal failure.
The stages, in order of progression, are (1) reduced renal reserve, (2) renal insufficiency, (3) renal failure, (4) uremic syndrome, and (5) end-stage renal disease (ESRD). Patients with normal renal function have nephron mass in excess of that necessary to maintain a normal GFR. Thus, with progressive loss of renal mass, that which is lost initially is the **renal reserve**, which is not reflected by a rise of BUN and creatinine or in a disturbance of homeostasis. If the progression continues, this stage is followed by **renal insufficiency,** which is associated with mild elevation of BUN and creatinine and very mild symptoms, including nocturia and easy fatigability. With further progression, **renal failure** ensues. This stage is characterized by apparent abnormalities of renal excretory function, including disturbances in water, electrolyte, and acid-base metabolism. Continued worsening of renal function is followed by the **uremic syndrome,** which includes multiple dysfunction of major organ systems in addition to the abnormalities of excretory function described. Finally, **ESRD** appears, at which time the remaining renal function is unable to sustain normal body function. Renal replacement therapy (dialysis or transplantation) is required at this time.

31. How do the remaining intact nephrons adapt in the diseased kidney?
When nephron mass is lost, the remaining intact (functioning) nephrons adjust their action in a compensatory effort to maintain the same excretory function performed by the kidney with a normal number of nephrons. The individual nephrons accomplish this task by increasing the glomerular filtration rate and excretory function of each of these individual nephrons. Thus, each individual functioning nephron now has a higher filtration rate and greater excretion of salt and water than it had when there was a full contingent of functioning nephrons. The increased excretory function is accomplished by reducing reabsorption of filtered salt and water. This reduced reabsorption often results in polyuria and nocturia.

32. The compensatory mechanisms described above can help to maintain near-normal excretory capacity for the diseased kidney with a reduced GFR. What is the major disadvantage these patients suffer with respect to excretory function when compared to patients with normal renal function?
Regarding excretory function, the patients with chronic renal insufficiency have a reduced ability to respond to changes in intake with appropriate changes in excretory function. For

example, if a person with normal renal function suddenly increases salt intake, the kidney will quickly adjust its function allowing for increased excretion of salt, which returns total body salt to or toward normal. The remaining functioning nephrons of persons with decreased GFR are chronically excreting a higher salt load and are thus much closer to their maximum salt-excreting ability. Hence, these patients are less able to adjust to an increased salt intake by increasing salt excretion. At the opposite extreme, the remaining nephrons of the patient with a decreased GFR are less able to reduce their high salt excretion to compensate for a reduction in salt intake. These patients are more at risk of becoming salt-depleted in response to salt restriction than are patients with normal renal function.

33. Explain the "trade-off" concept of progressive renal disease.
This concept refers to compensatory mechanisms intended to ameliorate the renal abnormalities resulting from compromised renal function, leading to adverse consequences in other organ systems. For example, the hyperphosphatemia and hypocalcemia occurring with progressive renal insufficiency result in stimulated parathyroid hormone secretion in an attempt to increase phosphate excretion and increase serum calcium levels. This secondary hyperparathyroidism has the desired effect on calcium and phosphate but leads to increased bone resorption and the bone disease called osteitis fibrosa cystica.

34. Why is renal potassium excretory ability usually well-maintained down to very low (10–15 ml/min) levels of GFR when the progression to this level of renal function has been chronic?
As is the case for sodium chloride excretion, the remaining intact nephrons significantly increase potassium excretion, such that the level of excretion per nephron is much higher than when there was a full contingent of nephrons. This allows for a total renal potassium excretion that is nearly normal. By this mechanism, patients with significant hyperkalemia, with only a moderate decrease in GFR, are unlikely to be hyperkalemic purely as a result of chronic renal insufficiency. In this clinical situation, consideration should be given to acute rather than chronic renal insufficiency, hormonal disorders (i.e., hyporenin hypoaldosteronism), or tubular disorders (i.e., obstructive uropathy).

35. What is the differential diagnosis of chronic renal failure (CRF)?

Differential Diagnosis of Chronic Renal Failure

All causes of acute renal failure	Amyloidosis
Hypertension	Polycystic kidney disease
Diabetes mellitus	Medullary cystic disease
Nephrotic syndrome	Medullary sponge disease
Glomerulonephritides	Chronic pyelonephritis
Collagen vascular diseases	Hypercalcemia
Papillary necrosis	Hyperuricemia
HIV infection	Heavy metal poisoning
Vasculitides	

Brenner BM, Rector FC (eds): The Kidney, 4th ed. Philadelphia, W.B. Saunders, 1991.

36. What are the postulated mechanisms of the hypertension commonly observed in patients with renal disease?
Most patients with renal disease have an expanded extracellular fluid volume that is felt to contribute to hypertension. Other contributing mechanisms that have been postulated include stimulation of the renin-angiotensin system and increased catecholamines.

37. What is meant by uremia?

Uremia refers to a symptom complex that results from severe renal insufficiency. It is characterized by some degree of dysfunction of most organ systems of the body. It is important to emphasize that this syndrome is a systemic process that involves more than just decreased renal excretory function.

DIALYSIS

38. What are the indications for dialysis in a patient with chronic renal failure (CRF)?

Dialytic therapy should be started when conservative management fails to maintain the patient in reasonable comfort. Usually dialysis will be required when GFR drops to 5–10 ml/min. It is both unnecessary and risky to adhere to strict biochemical indications. Broadly speaking, the development of uremic encephalopathy, neuropathy, pericarditis, and bleeding diathesis are indications to start dialysis immediately. Fluid overload, congestive heart failure, hyperkalemia, metabolic acidosis, and hypertension uncontrolled by conservative measures are the indications for starting patients on dialytic therapy.

39. What is "dialysis disequilibrium syndrome" and how do you prevent it?

Dialysis disequilibrium syndrome is a neurological complication that tends to occur during initiation of dialysis. It occurs in the first few dialyses and is characterized by nausea, vomiting, confusion, psychosis, and seizures. These symptoms occur toward the end of dialysis or afterward, when the dialysis has been particularly rapid. The syndrome is attributed to increased hydrogen ion concentration in the brain due to differential diffusion of CO_2 and HCO_3^- across the blood-brain barrier, leading to the generation of idiogenic osmoles and the development of cerebral edema. This complication is prevented by a gradual increase of dialysis time and blood flow rate, the use of slower dialyzers, and high dialysate sodium.

40. What are the clinical manifestations of chronic renal failure that can be improved with dialysis? What symptoms and manifestations worsen with dialysis?

The clinical manifestations of uremia that are improved with dialytic therapy include uremic encephalopathy, seizures, pericarditis, fluid overload, electrolyte imbalances, gastrointestinal symptoms, and metabolic acidosis. There are several uremic symptoms that tend to persist despite dialysis, including renal osteodystrophy, hypertriglyceridemia, amenorrhea and infertility, peripheral neuropathy, pruritus, and anemia. There are some symptoms that develop during chronic dialysis. These include dialysis dementia, nephrogenic ascites, dialysis pericarditis, dialysis bone disease, accelerated atherosclerosis, carpal tunnel syndrome (amyloid-related), and the risk of hepatitis.

41. What is the relationship of dialysis dementia and aluminum?

Dialysis dementia is a rare progressive neurological disorder first reported in the 1970s and seen in patients on chronic dialysis. The syndrome usually consists of disturbances of speech (apraxia, dysarthria) and memory, depression, myoclonus, and seizures. The disorder is progressive and death occurs in 6–15 months. One of the pathological hallmarks of the condition is a high level of aluminum in brain tissue derived mostly from ingestion of aluminum-containing phosphate binders. Use of reverse osmosis for dialysate treatment, careful monitoring of aluminum levels in dialysate water, and avoiding aluminum-containing antacids whenever possible reduces the incidence of this disorder.

42. Which poisons and toxins are dialyzable?

The toxins that can be removed by hemodialysis include alcohols (ethanol, methanol, ethylene glycol), salicylates, heavy metals (Hg, As, Pb), and halides. In addition, hemoperfusion successfully removes barbiturates, sedatives (meprobamate, methaqualone, and glutethimide), acetaminophen, digoxin, procainamide, quinidine, and theophylline.

43. What is the principle contraindication for chronic dialysis?

The most important contraindication for starting chronic hemodialysis is the presence of potentially reversible abnormalities. These include dehydration, urinary tract infection, urinary obstruction, hypercatabolic state, uncontrolled hypertension, hypercalcemia, nephrotoxic drugs, and low cardiac output state.

44. What are the different types of vascular accesses available for acute and chronic dialysis?

For acute dialysis, temporary catheters (single lumen, double lumen) are generally used in the subclavian and occasionally in the femoral vein. Sometimes arteriovenous shunts using silastic tubing and Teflon vessel tips are used in temporary dialysis. For chronic use, primary arteriovenous fistulae or arteriovenous graft fistulae (Goretex, Dacron, bovine grafts) are used.

45. What is chronic ambulatory peritoneal dialysis (CAPD)? What are the usual indications?

CAPD is a manual form of peritoneal dialysis, usually performed by the patient, in which 1-2 liters of dialysate fluid are infused into the peritoneal space through a Tenchkoff catheter, and then drained after a dwell time of 4-6 hours. The exchanges are repeated 4-5 times a day. CAPD began in the 1970s, and there are currently over 16,000 patients on CAPD worldwide. This form of dialysis is indicated in any patient with ESRD. However, it is the treatment of choice for diabetics with severe peripheral vascular disease, since they are at increased risk in hemodialysis. This method provides for more independence and motility, and it should be offered to all young patients leading active lives. The contraindications include blindness, severe disabling arthritis, colostomy, poor motivation, and quadriplegia.

46. What are the complications of CAPD?

1. Mechanical:
   Pain, bleeding, leakage, inadequate drainage, intraperitoneal catheter loss, abdominal wall edema, scrotal edema, incisional hernia, other hernia, intestinal hematoma, intestinal perforation
2. Infections, inflammation:
   Bacterial peritonitis, fungal peritonitis, tunnel infection, exit-site infection, diverticulitis, sterile peritonitis, eosinophilic peritonitis, sclerosing peritonitis, pancreatitis
3. Cardiovascular:
   Acute pulmonary edema, fluid overload, hypotension, arrhythmia, cardiac arrest, hypertension
4. Pulmonary:
   Basal atelectasis, aspiration, pneumonia, hydrothorax, respiratory arrest, decreased forced vital capacity
5. Neurologic:
   Convulsion, possible dialysis disequilibrium syndrome
6. Metabolic:
   Hyperglycemia, hyperosmolar nonketotic coma, postdialysis hypoglycemia, hyperkalemia, hypokalemia, hypernatremia, hyponatremia, metabolic alkalosis, protein depletion, hyperlipidemia, obesity

47. What are the common causes of death in dialysis patients?

Despite several important technical developments, the mortality in dialysis patients remains significant (about 15% in the first year). The commonest cause of death is cardiovascular failure, with hypertension and diabetes as important contributing factors. Sepsis is the next leading cause of death, followed by bleeding complications, cerebrovascular accidents, pericardial effusion with tamponade, trauma (accidents), suicides, and others.

48. What are the causes of peritonitis in a patient on peritoneal dialysis?
Peritonitis is an important complication of CAPD. The frequency of infection has decreased considerably since this dialysis method was introduced, to about one episode every 18–24 patient months. This result is mainly due to the addition of a Luer-Lock adapter between the catheter and tubing and institution of monthly tubing changes. Causative organisms include *Staphylococcus epidermidis* and *S. aureus* (70%), gram negative organisms (20%), and fungi and TB (5%). Aseptic peritonitis is found in 5% of cases.

49. What is the treatment of peritonitis in a patient on peritoneal dialysis?
The empiric treatment of acute peritonitis involves short lavage (two to three exchanges drained rapidly), followed by four exchanges of 2 liters per day containing antibiotic coverage for both the common gram positive and gram negative organisms discussed above, and 1000 units of heparin in each 2 liters. If the chosen antibiotic(s) is removed by peritoneal dialysis (i.e., aminoglycosides), the antibiotic must be added to the dialysate at a concentration comparable to the desired trough level in the serum to minimize removal of the drug(s). Appropriate changes in antibiotics can be made after sensitivity patterns are available. Treatment is stopped 1 week after the first negative culture.

50. Are there new developments in the treatment of anemia of chronic renal failure?
The most important development in the treatment of anemia of CRF is the use of recombinant human erythropoietin. Several studies since 1987 have documented the efficacy of this new agent in improving the anemia and minimizing the need for blood transfusion.

51. What is dialysis-induced hypoxemia? What is its pathogenesis?
A fall in P_aO_2 of 5–35 mmHg is a frequent and important complication of hemodialysis. It occurs in up to 90% of patients on dialysis and resolves within 1–2 hours after discontinuation of dialysis. This is clinically important in people with pre-existing respiratory compromise. The pathogenesis is multifactorial and depends in part on the type of hemodialysis (acetate versus bicarbonate). It is important to remember the CNS-controlled ventilation is normally inhibited by hypocarbia (decreased pCO_2) and alkalemia. Acetate dialysis removes CO_2 gas from the plasma, causing hypocarbia and depressed ventilation. Bicarbonate dialysis causes alkalemia due to diffusion of the bicarbonate into the patient and subsequent depressed ventilation. In addition, the cuprophan membrane of the artificial kidney can activate complement, leading to leukoagglutination in the pulmonary capillaries. This causes diffusion abnormalities, widening of the alveolar-arterial (A-a) oxygen gradient, and hypoxemia.

Ross E: Dialysis hypoxemia. In Nissenson AR, Fine RN (eds): Dialysis Therapy. Philadelphia, Hanley & Belfus, 1986, pp 98–99.

PROTEINURIA/NEPHROTIC SYNDROME

52. What are the factors that normally inhibit entry of plasma proteins into the glomerular ultrafiltrate?
The characteristics that determine entry of individual proteins into the glomerular ultra-filtrate are size, charge, and shape. The glomerular barrier is functionally a filter whose pores are of a given size and are lined by negatively charged proteins. Consequently, the

features of a given plasma protein that mitigate against entry into the glomerular ultrafiltrate include large size (as determined by molecular weight), negative charge, and a noncompact configuration.

53. What are the four general mechanisms by which greater than normal ($>$ 150 mg/day) urinary protein excretion occurs?

The four general mechanisms are glomerular, tubular, overflow, and secretory.

1. **Glomerular proteinuria** occurs as a result of damage to the glomerular filtration barrier (in glomerulonephritis), leading to excessive leakage of plasma proteins into the glomerular ultrafiltrate.

2. **Tubular proteinuria** occurs when there is suboptimal reabsorption of the normally filtered protein as a result of disease of the renal tubules. It is this recovery of the small amount of normally filtered protein (usually about 2 g/day) that allows for the normal urinary excretion of less than 150 mg/day of protein.

3. **Overflow proteinuria** results from disease states that lead to excessive levels of plasma proteins (such as in multiple myeloma); the proteins are filtered and overload the reabsorptive capacity of the renal tubules.

4. **Secretory proteinuria** describes the proteinuria that occurs because of the addition of protein to the urine after glomerular filtration. The protein may come from the renal tubules (as with Tamm-Horsfall protein from the ascending limb of the loop of Henle) or from the lower genitourinary tract.

54. What are the conditions associated with heavy proteinuria despite severe reduction in GFR?

Heavy proteinuria is generally indicative of glomerular disease. In the majority of glomerular diseases, proteinuria tends to decrease with diminishing GFR as the filtration of proteins also tends to decrease. However, in certain conditions, such as diabetic nephropathy, amyloidosis, focal glomerulosclerosis and probably reflux nephropathy, proteinuria (often in nephrotic range) persists despite severely diminished GFR.

55. A 23-year-old white male has 1.2 g of proteinuria in 24 hours. His urinalysis and other laboratory studies are otherwise normal. What is the differential diagnosis?

Significant (more than 0.5 g/24 hr) but nonnephrotic (less than 3.5 g/24 hr) proteinuria involves the following differential diagnosis.

1. Benign orthostatic proteinuria
2. Idiopathic glomerular disease (especially in early stages)
   - Focal glomerulosclerosis
   - IgA nephropathy
   - Membranous nephropathy
   - Amyloidosis
3. Systemic diseases
   - Diabetic nephropathy
   - Essential hypertension
   - Congestive heart failure
   - Febrile states

56. What is the most common mechanism for proteinuria in patients with renal disease?

Glomerular proteinuria is the most common mechanism for significant proteinuria in patients with renal disease.

57. The commonly available urinary dipstick is most sensitive to which urinary protein?

Albumin. Excretion of even large amounts of some nonalbumin proteins (such as Bence-Jones proteins) will not be evident using this screening test. A more sensitive quantitative test, such as sulfosalicylic acid must be employed to recognize the presence of nonalbumin urinary proteins. Electrophoresis can then be used to identify the specific protein(s).

58. At what age does orthostatic proteinuria most commonly occur and what is its prognosis?

This term refers to excessive urinary protein excretion that occurs only when standing and normalizes when recumbent. It occurs most commonly in adolescents and carries an excellent long-term prognosis. It usually resolves spontaneously.

59. Define nephrotic syndrome.

Nephrotic syndrome is generally defined as a "symptom complex" resulting from various etiologies and characterized by heavy proteinuria (usually > 3.5 g/day), generalized edema, and lipiduria with hyperlipidemia. Since all the other features are a consequence of marked proteinuria, some authorities restrict the definition of "nephrosis" to heavy proteinuria alone.

60. What is the nephritic syndrome?

The nephritic syndrome is a renal disorder that results from diffuse glomerular inflammation. It is characterized by the sudden onset of gross hematuria, decreased glomerular filtration rate, low urine output (oliguria), hypertension, and edema. It can result from many different etiologies but is traditionally represented by postinfectious glomerulonephritis following infections with certain strains of group A beta hemolytic streptococci.

61. What are the various causes of an acute nephritic syndrome?

1. Post infectious glomerulonephritis (PSGN)
   a. Poststreptococcal glomerulonephritis
   b. Postinfectious (nonstreptococcal) glomerulonephritis
      • Bacterial: pneumococci, *Klebsiella,* staphylococci, gram negative rods, meningococci, secondary syphilis, brucellosis, leptospira, mycoplasma, salmonella
      • Viral: Varicella, infectious mononucleosis, mumps, measles, hepatitis B, coxsackie virus
      • Rickettsial: Rocky Mountain spotted fever, typhus
      • Parasitic: Falciparum malaria, toxoplasmosis, trichinosis
2. Idiopathic glomerular diseases
   a. Membranoproliferative glomerulonephritis
   b. Mesangial proliferative glomerulonephritis
   c. IgA nephropathy
3. Multi-system diseases
   a. Systemic lupus erythematosus (SLE)
   b. Henoch-Schonlein purpura
   c. Essential mixed cryoglobulinemia
   d. Infective endocarditis
4. Miscellaneous
   a. Guillain-Barré syndrome
   b. Postirradiation of renal tumors.

62. Which four general categories of renal diseases cause the idiopathic nephrotic syndrome?

The four general categories are minimal change disease, focal and segmental glomerulosclerosis, membranous nephropathy, and proliferative glomerulonephritides.

63. What is the most common cause of nephrotic syndrome in children? In adults?

The most common cause of nephrotic syndrome in children is minimal change disease (also called lipoid nephrosis or nil lesion). The most common cause of nephrotic syndrome in adults is membranous nephropathy.

64. In evaluating patients with nephrotic syndrome, what other categories of disease must be ruled out before considering the syndrome to be due to a primary renal disease? Why is this distinction important?

The general disease categories to be ruled out include:

- Drugs that may result in excessive urinary protein excretion (gold and penicillamine)
- Systemic infections
- Neoplasia (lymphomas)
- Multisystem collagen vascular diseases (systemic lupus erythematosus)
- Diabetes (its nephropathy is classically associated with nephrotic syndrome)
- Heredofamilial diseases such as Alport's syndrome.

It is important that the distinction between the above causes and primary renal disease be made for a number of reasons. Therapeutically, treatment of the disorder may involve simple discontinuation of the offending agent (such as a drug). In addition, management may need to be directed at the systemic disease (infection) rather than at the renal lesion itself. Diagnostically, identification of some of these processes may lead to identification of the renal lesion without the need for a renal biopsy (as in diabetes).

65. What are some common complications of the nephrotic syndrome?

1. **Edema**
2. **Hypovolemia** with acute prerenal and/or parenchymal renal disease. The nephrotic syndrome is a state of decreased effective arterial blood volume that can lead to various degrees of renal underperfusion. In severe cases, the renal underperfusion can lead to renal failure.
3. **Protein malnutrition** can occur because of the massive protein losses in excess of dietary replacement.
4. **Hyperlipidemia,** which raises the risk of atherosclerotic cardiovascular disease.
5. **Increased susceptibility to bacterial infection,** which occurs most frequently in the lungs, meninges (meningitis), and peritoneum. Common organisms include streptococcus species (including *Strep. pneumoniae), Hemophilus influenzae,* and *Klebsiella* sp.
6. **Proximal tubular dysfunction,** which may lead to the Fanconi syndrome with urinary wasting of glucose, phosphate, amino acids, uric acid, potassium, and bicarbonate.
7. **Hypercoagulable state** manifested by an increased incidence of venous thrombosis, particularly in the renal vein. The precise mechanism is not clear, but it appears to be partially due to the urinary loss of factors that normally inhibit clotting.

66. A 62-year-old male with nephrotic syndrome is found to have "nil lesion" on biopsy. What is the differential diagnosis?

As opposed to children, minimal lesion on renal biopsy in an elderly patient warrants extensive search to rule out underlying malignancy, especially lymphomas (both Hodgkin's and non-Hodgkin's) and other solid tumors, such as renal cell carcinoma.

NEPHROLITHIASIS

67. Which three major mechanisms are felt to be important in determining the presence of nephrolithiasis?

Urinary tract stones occur in a wide variety of disease states and as a consequence of a variety of physiological and pathological processes. The three mechanisms currently felt to contribute to the development of urinary stones are (1) precipitation-crystallization from super-saturated solutions, (2) the absence of inhibitors to stone formation normally present in the urine, and (3) the presence of a macromolecular matrix.

Precipitation of a substance to form stones depends on many factors, including solubility, concentration, and urine characteristics (i.e., pH). Normal constituents of urine that inhibit stone formation include citrate, pyrophosphate, and magnesium. Reduced concentrations of these substances are felt to contribute to stone formation. Protein matrix contributes to the formation, growth, and/or aggregation of stones. This matrix derives in part from renal tubular epithelial cells and from the uroepithelium.

68. What are the common components of urinary stones in the U.S.?
Calcium is present in approximately 80% of urinary stones recovered in the U.S. Calcium oxalate is the most common pure-substance stone and accounts for 35%. An additional 35% of stones also contain calcium apatite. Magnesium ammonium phosphate (struvite) containing stones comprise 18% of the total, uric acid stones about 6%, and cystine 3%.

69. How does urine pH affect urinary stone formation?
In general, an alkaline urine pH favors precipitation of inorganic stones and an acid pH favors precipitation of organic stones. However, urine pH has little effect on calcium oxalate solubility and therefore little influence on the formation of these stones. Alkaline pH favors precipitation of calcium phosphate (which can then undergo rearrangement into hydroxyapatite) and magnesium ammonium phosphate (struvite). Acid pH favors precipitation of uric acid and cystine.

70. Which factors predispose to the formation of magnesium ammonium phosphate (or struvite) stones?
Alkaline urine pH and high concentrations of urinary ammonia contribute to supersaturation of this substance. This environment is created by the presence of urea-splitting bacteria (commonly *Proteus*, *Pseudomonas*, *Klebsiella*, and *Staphylococcus*) that contain the enzyme urease and convert urea to ammonia and CO_2.

71. Which common metabolic conditions predispose to the formation of urinary stones?
Many different metabolic conditions predispose to the formation of urinary stones, and more than one of these conditions are commonly present in a typical stone-forming patient.
- **Idiopathic hypercalciuria** is present in approximately 50% of stone-forming patients in the U.S. It is divided into absorptive (felt to be due to excessive GI absorption of calcium) and renal (due to renal leak of calcium).
- **Hyperuricosuria** (with and without gout) is present in approximately 30% of stone-formers. Increased uric acid excretion can also contribute to the formation of calcium-containing stones.
- **Hyperoxaluria** of various causes is present in about 15% of patients with nephrolithiasis.
- **Low urinary citrate excretion** is present in about 50% of stone-forming individuals and can contribute to stone formation in most states as described above.
- Other less common causes include chronic urinary tract infection, primary hyperparathyroidism, cystinuria, and distal renal tubular acidosis.

72. What are the three common anatomic sites of the genitourinary tract where urinary stones are retained and obstruct urine flow?
Stones commonly lodge at the ureteropelvic junction, the midureter as it crosses the iliac artery, and at the ureterovesical junction.

73. What are the consequences of urinary obstruction by a stone?
A stone acutely lodged in the genitourinary tract can cause severe, colicky pain that radiates toward the lower abdomen and genital area. In women who have children, the pain is often

described as more severe than the pain of labor. The increased pressure inside the collecting system decreases the net pressure for glomerular filtration, resulting in a decrease in the GFR. The resulting urinary stasis predisposes to infection. All of these problems correct toward normal if the stone passes or is removed from the urinary tract within a few days. If the obstruction becomes chronic, permanent renal injury can ensue, with an irreversible reduction in GFR and chronic dilatation of the collection system. This dilated collecting system is less efficient in delivering urine to the bladder (because of compromised peristalsis), predisposing to urinary stasis and infection.

74. How should you manage the patient with acute urinary tract obstruction due to a stone?

Most stones pass spontaneously in hours to a few days. Supportive management with analgesics and oral fluids will usually suffice. Such patients should have serum chemistries done to document the degree of renal dysfunction (if any) and a radiological procedure (IVP, renal ultrasound, etc.) to locate the stone and to estimate its size in order to help determine the possible need for surgical intervention. Once the acute phase ends with exit of the stone from the urinary tract, attention should be aimed at identifying the condition that led to the formation of the stone. Identification of the underlying condition will allow for designing a protocol for long-term management.

75. Are patients often successful in recovering stones that are passed at home?

A reasonable percentage of patients will successfully screen stone material from their urine. However, laboratory analysis is usually not readily available, and the approach to management is more often empirical than based on recovery and analysis of stones.

76. What long-term, nonsurgical management is recommended for patients with a propensity to form renal stones?

In general, such patients should maintain a dilute urine, which can be accomplished by a high intake of hypotonic fluids. Recovery and characterization of stones, if possible, helps in the diagnosis of the predisposing condition and in guiding management.

Except for the oxalate stones, whose formation is not much influenced by urine pH, maintenance of an acid urine inhibits the formation of inorganic stones (calcium apatite, struvite) and maintenance of an alkaline urine inhibits formation of organic stones (uric acid, cysteine). Increasing the urinary concentration of natural inhibitors that limit aggregation and growth of crystals is also helpful. These inhibitors include citrate, pyrophosphate, and magnesium.

More specific management depends on the predisposing condition. Absorptive hypercalciuria can be managed by reducing dietary calcium (type 2 only); by use of cellulose sodium phosphate, which binds intestinal calcium and prevents its absorption (type 1); and by use of the diuretic thiazide, which promotes renal calcium absorption. Renal hypercalciuria can also be treated with thiazides. Primary hyperparathyroidism should be treated with parathyroidectomy. Uricosuric states resulting from the overproduction of uric acid should be treated with allopurinol. Potassium citrate is an effective alternative to allopurinol for patients with hyperuricosuria associated with calcium oxalate stones. States associated with excessive intestinal oxalate absorption can be treated with a low oxalate diet and use of magnesium or calcium salts, which bind oxalate and inhibit its reabsorption. Cystinuria can be managed conservatively with the above measures (dilute and alkaline urine) and with penicillamine (increases the solubility of cystine) if the conservative measures are ineffective. Patients with struvite stones must have their urinary tract infections treated and may also be additionally managed using the urease inhibitor acetohydroxamic acid.

77. What is lithotripsy and what three forms are now available as alternatives to operation or cystoscopy for the removal of stones in the kidney and urinary tract?
Litho- (stone or calculus) -tripsy (crushing) is a way of breaking up stones by use of shock waves or ultrasound. The three forms now available clinically are:
1. Extracorporeal shock-wave lithotripsy
2. Percutaneous ultrasonic lithotripsy
3. Endoscopic ultrasonic lithotripsy

URINARY TRACT OBSTRUCTION

78. What are the common causes of ureteric obstruction in adults?
The major causes of ureteric obstruction in adults include:
- Renal stones
- Prostatic, bladder, or pelvic malignancy
- Retroperitoneal lymphoma, metastasis, or fibrosis
- Accidental surgical ligation
- Blood clot
- Pregnancy
- Stricture

79. How do unilateral and bilateral obstruction differ in their effects on GFR?
Unilateral obstruction does not necessarily lead to a clinically measurable decrease in GFR, but bilateral obstruction consistently does decrease the GFR. Patients with normal renal function and normal nephron reserve have an excess of nephron mass necessary to maintain what would be called a "normal" GFR. Unilateral obstruction with complete obliteration of ipsilateral function will force recruitment of the nephron reserve of the contralateral kidney. In an attempt to maintain the baseline GFR, and as a compensatory response to the loss of functioning nephron mass, the individual nephrons of the contralateral kidney will increase their filtration rate ("hyperfiltration"). These compensatory changes commonly result in no changes, or only small changes, in total GFR. Relatively large reductions in functioning nephron mass (about 40%) are necessary to elicit an appreciable rise in the plasma creatinine concentration when baseline renal function is normal (plasma creatinine 0.8 to 1.2 mg/dl). The relatively small change in GFR, described to occur in patients with normal baseline renal function who are subjected to unilateral obstruction, will very likely not be reflected by a rise in plasma creatinine.

The response would be different for patients with baseline renal insufficiency. Such patients have already lost their reserve nephron mass and are likely using compensatory mechanisms to maintain their GFR at the compromised level. Unilateral obstruction in such a patient may result in a significant fall in GFR and is more likely to be associated with a rise in plasma creatinine.

Bilateral obstruction leads to a decreased GFR in patients with both normal and abnormal renal function.

80. What are the differences in clinical presentation between acute compared to chronic obstruction of the urinary tract?
Partial or complete obstruction of the urinary tract compromises urine passage whether it is acute or chronic. Nevertheless, the urinary findings and clinical consequences are different, depending on the length of time the urinary tract was obstructed. After release of acute (less than 24 hours) obstruction, there is commonly a decrease in excretion of sodium, potassium, and water. This results in excretion of a urine low in sodium concentration and with increased osmolarity, a situation also seen with volume depletion. By contrast, release of chronic obstruction commonly results in *increased* excretion of sodium and water and decreased excretion of acid (with urinary loss of bicarbonate) and potassium. These abnormalities can lead to volume depletion, free-water deficit (reflected by hypernatremia), and hyperkalemic, non-anion-gap metabolic acidosis.

81. What are the abnormalities of tubular function that can occur with chronic obstruction?

Chronic obstruction affects primarily distal rather than proximal nephron functions. These functions include reabsorption of sodium and water and secretion of acid and potassium. The decreased water reabsorption results from decreased responsiveness of the collecting tubule to ADH, yielding a form of nephrogenic diabetes insipidus. The acid secretory defect results in incomplete bicarbonate recovery from the urine and a non-anion-gap metabolic acidosis. The potassium secretory defect results in potassium retention and hyperkalemia. Therefore, obstructive nephropathy is a common cause of hyperkalemic, hyperchloremic, non-anion-gap metabolic acidosis. These abnormalities usually resolve after correction of the obstruction but may require weeks or even months to do so.

82. Which components of the polyuria (postobstructive diuresis) are seen immediately after correction of chronic obstruction?

The patient with urinary tract obstruction and compromised renal function accumulates solute and water that are ordinarily excreted by the normally functioning kidney. Correction of the obstruction results in appropriate excretion of the accumulated urea, NaCl, and water in an effort to return to normal the volume and content of the extracellular fluid. This polyuria is physiologic. However, a minority of such patients will have a pathologic polyuria, resulting from poor salt and/or water reabsorption. These abnormalities commonly resolve within a few hours but may last for days.

Note that the pathologic polyuria may occur because of either salt or water loss (or both). Pathologic salt loss will be reflected by continued excretion of a large amount of urinary sodium in the setting of volume depletion. Pathologic water loss will be reflected by excretion of large volumes of dilute urine in the face of rising serum osmolality. Therefore, patients undergoing postobstructive polyuria should be observed to determine whether the polyuria is physiologic (as is usually the case) or pathologic. In the case of pathologic polyuria, appropriate fluid replacement therapy should be instituted. If such fluid replacement is instituted during the physiologic polyuria, one will "chase" the patient's volume status such that the polyuria will continue as a result of the fluids being administered.

83. What are some complications of urinary tract obstruction?

In addition to the decrease in GFR and the potential tubular abnormalities, the resulting urinary stasis can predispose to infection, renal stones, and papillary necrosis. Furthermore, the salt and water retention can lead to hypertension.

84. What is "functional" obstruction of the urinary tract?

This refers to abnormalities that compromise the exit of urine from the kidney in the absence of anatomic obstruction of the outflow tract. Two examples are atonic bladder and vesicoureteral reflux. An **atonic bladder** is unable to completely empty itself and hence contains urine continuously yielding a higher than normal hydrostatic pressure. This high bladder pressure is transmitted via the ureters and may cause the abnormalities described above. Patients with **vesicoureteral reflux** have retrograde flow of urine into the ureter and/or kidney during voiding. This occurs because of an incompetent vesicoureteral valve. The transmitted pressure is felt to contribute to the renal abnormalities. Both of these conditions also predispose to urinary tract infections.

85. How is the diagnosis of urinary tract obstruction made?

The history, clinical setting, and the laboratory findings provide important clues. A palpable urinary bladder on exam is strong evidence for lower tract obstruction or atonic bladder. The distended bladder as well as hypertrophied kidneys can sometimes be demonstrated on plain abdominal x-rays. A post-void residual urine of greater than 100 ml obtained upon Foley catheter insertion is supportive of lower tract obstruction. A large volume of urine return in response to Foley catheter insertion also strongly favors lower tract obstruction. Renal ultrasound is a relatively sensitive, noninvasive procedure that is commonly used to investigate the possibility of urinary tract obstruction. Intravenous pyelograms (IVPs) should be avoided due to the risk of additional renal injury from the contrast dye. Retrograde pyelography (selective catheterization and insertion of contrast dye into both ureters via cystoscopy) is occasionally necessary when the above studies do not yield a diagnosis and clinical suspicion remains strong for obstruction. Abdominal CAT scan is also helpful but is more expensive than ultrasound. Finally, radionuclide renal scans suggest obstruction when there is prompt uptake of the dye with prolonged excretion.

PRIMARY GLOMERULAR DISORDERS

86. What is a primary glomerulopathy?
The term primary glomerular disease (or primary glomerulopathy) is used to denote a heterogenous group of diseases in which the glomeruli are the predominantly involved elements. Extrarenal involvement, if present, is usually secondary to consequences of the glomerular insult. The majority of these disorders are idiopathic. The cardinal manifestations of the primary glomerular disorders are proteinuria, hematuria, alterations in GFR, and salt retention leading to edema, hypertension, and pulmonary congestion.

87. Which clinical entities are encompassed by the primary glomerulopathies?
The clinical features of the primary glomerulopathies appear in various combinations in any given glomerular disorder and present as one of the following clinical syndromes.

1. **Acute glomerulonephritis (AGN):** An acute illness of abrupt onset characterized by variable degrees of hematuria, proteinuria, decreased GFR, and fluid and salt retention. It is usually associated with an infectious agent and tends to resolve spontaneously.

2. **Nephrotic syndrome:** An illness of insidious onset characterized primarily by heavy proteinuria of usually more than 3.5 g per day in an adult and usually associated with hypoalbuminemia, lipidemia, and anasarca.

3. **Chronic glomerulonephritis:** A vague illness of insidious onset characterized primarily by progressive renal insufficiency, with a protracted downhill course of 5 to 10 years duration. Varying degrees of proteinuria, hematuria, and hypertension accompany the illness.

4. **Rapidly progressive glomerulonephritis (RPGN):** A clinical disorder of rather subacute onset but with rapid progression to renal failure and no tendency towards spontaneous recovery. Patients are usually hypertensive, hematuric, and oliguric.

5. **Asymptomatic urinary abnormalities:** Patients have microscopic hematuria and/or proteinuria (usually less than 3 g/day) but with no clinical symptoms.

88. Which nephritogenic strains of streptococci cause poststreptococcal glomerulonephritis (PSGN)? What factors determine the nephritogenicity?
It should be noted that only certain serotypes of group A (beta hemolytic) streptococci are nephritogenic. In addition to type 12, which is the most common, types 1, 2, 3, 18, 25, 49, 55, 57, and 60 are also nephritogenic. In contrast, all strains of streptococci can cause acute rheumatic fever, which is why the incidence of nephritis differs from rheumatic fever in outbreaks of streptococcal infection.

The M-protein in streptococci is poorly linked to nephritogenicity. Recent evidence indicates that nephritogenicity is more closely related to endostreptosin, which is a cell membrane antigen. Other streptococcal cytoplasmic antigens and autologous antigens have also been implicated.

89. What is the typical urine sediment from a patient with poststreptococcal glomerulonephritis (PSGN)? Does a normal urinalysis rule out this diagnosis?

The urinalysis in PSGN is characterized by a nephritic sediment (see Q. 93), high specific gravity, and nonselective proteinuria. The proteinuria is less than 3 g/day in over 75% of patients, although proteinuria in the nephrotic range is occasionally seen. Pyuria is often noted, indicating glomerulitis. Hematuria is almost always present in either gross (smoky urine) or microscopic form. Red cell casts, if present, are very diagnostic. Dysmorphic erythrocytes are found in abundance. However, a benign urinary sediment does not rule out acute poststreptococcal nephritis if clinical features are suggestive. In some cases biopsy studies have confirmed PSGN.

90. What are the prognosis and the poor prognostic signs in acute PSGN?

In children the immediate and late prognosis is quite favorable in both epidemic and sporadic cases. A diuresis occurs in 1 week and serum creatinine returns to normal in 3–4 weeks. The mortality in acute cases is less than 1% and chronic sequelae are very uncommon. Microscopic hematuria may last 6 months and proteinuria may persist for as long as 3 years in 15% of patients. The factors that indicate poor prognosis include persistent heavy proteinuria, extensive crescents or atypical humps in initial biopsy, and severe disease in the acute phase needing hospitalization. In adults the prognosis is good in epidemic forms. However, in sporadic cases the prognosis is less predictable than in children. Severe impairment of renal function at the onset, persistent proteinuria, elderly age, and crescentic formation on biopsy are, in general, poor prognostic factors.

91. How do you treat hypertension associated with acute PSGN?

Fluid and salt retention are the basis of development of hypertension in PSGN. Therefore loop diuretics, like furosemide, are very useful. Potassium-sparing diuretics are to be avoided. Other antihypertensives are rarely indicated. When needed, vasodilators like hydralazine, diazoxide, and nitroprusside are most useful. Plasma renin activity levels are often decreased and hence beta blockers and angiotensin-converting enzyme (ACE) inhibitors are less useful alone but may be used in conjunction with vasodilators. Clonidine, methyldopa, or nifedepine can also be used.

92. What is rapidly progressive glomerulonephritis (RPGN)? Is it synonymous with crescentic nephritis?

The term RPGN is used to denote the clinical syndrome associated with rapid and progressive deterioration of renal function, often terminating, if untreated, in end stage renal disease in a matter of weeks to months. Histologically, it is characterized by extensive glomerular crescent formation, in most cases involving over 75% of glomeruli. The cells of the crescents are now thought to be derived from blood-borne monocytes. RPGN is strictly a clinical expression, whereas crescentic nephritis denotes the histological picture in such patients.

93. How does routine urinalysis help in the evaluation of a primary glomerular disease?

In glomerular disease, the urinary sediment usually conforms to one of three different forms.

Nephrotic	Nephritic	Chronic
Heavy proteinuria	Red cells	Less proteinuria and hematuria
Free fat droplets	Red cell casts	Broad, waxy casts
Oval fat bodies	Variable proteinuria	Pigmented granular casts
Fatty casts	Frequent white cell and granular cells	
Variable hematuria		

(From Schreiner GE: The identification and clinical significance of casts. Arch Intern Med 99:356–369, 1957, p 366, with permission.)

RENAL BONE DISEASE

94. What is Bricker's "trade-off" hypothesis?

Early in the course of renal failure, the kidney fails to excrete phosphorus, leading to a transient and often undetectable rise in serum phosphorus. This tends to lower the serum ionized calcium temporarily, leading to stimulation of parathyroid hormone (PTH) secretion. The increased levels of PTH reduce tubular reabsorption of phosphate, leading to phosphate excretion and thereby tending to normalize the serum calcium and phosphorus levels. However, this is occurring at the expense of an elevated PTH level. With further declines in renal function, the serum phosphorus tends to rise, and the whole cycle is repeated. With advancing renal failure, the changes just described tend to keep serum calcium and phosphorus levels below normal at the expense of increasing serum PTH levels. The serum level of PTH is increased in an attempt to normalize serum phosphate and calcium levels, but the "trade-off" is the bone disease caused by the elevated PTH levels (osteitis fibrosa cystica). This is the so-called "trade-off" hypothesis propounded by Neil S. Bricker, a well-known American nephrologist, and is the basis for the secondary hyperparathyroidism seen in renal failure.

95. Name the earliest biochemical change in renal bone disease.

The earliest detectable change is elevated serum PTH level, although in a very small number of patients with chronic renal failure, PTH levels may be normal. Changes in serum phosphorous and calcium are seen in more advanced stages of renal failure.

96. Which bone histological subtypes are found in renal osteodystrophy?

There are three histological pictures in patients with renal osteodystrophy. The common types are **osteitis fibrosa cystica** (bone changes due to secondary hyperparathyroidism) and **osteomalacia.** Occasionally a picture of **osteosclerosis** is seen for reasons that are not clear.

97. What is the role of aluminum in renal bone disease?

Recent evidence has shown that aluminum accumulation in the bone is a major factor in causing osteomalacia, encephalopathy, and anemia in patients with chronic renal failure and those on dialysis. After the dialysate concentration of aluminum was lowered to insignificant amounts, it became obvious that oral ingestion of aluminum in the form of aluminum-containing phosphate binders was an important cause of aluminum-related bone disease. Orally ingested aluminum can accumulate over the course of time to levels significant enough to cause aluminum bone disease. The mechanism of the aluminum effect on bone is felt to be due to deposition of the metal along the mineralization front, leading to interference with mineralization. In addition, aluminum may impair the function of osteoblast.

98. Why will a patient with chronic renal failure and marked hypocalcemia often fail to manifest tetany?

Tetany is a clinical manifestation of severe hypocalcemia in adults. Ionized calcium is decreased in the presence of alkalemia, so that tetany usually manifests only in the presence of an alkalemic pH. The degree of ionization is favorably increased by the acidemia seen in chronic renal failure, the result being that the ionic calcium is usually not reduced enough to cause tetany. However, if the acidosis is excessively treated with alkalizing agents, tetany may become manifest.

99. Is bone disease improved with dialysis or renal transplantation?

Renal osteodystrophy is not always improved with dialytic therapy. The symptoms may indeed worsen or progress because a number of additional factors are introduced that either directly or indirectly influence the severity of renal bone disease. These include the aluminum content of dialysate, heparin administration, and administration of large amounts of acetate.

In patients who undergo renal transplantation, the uremic bone disease improves to a great extent. Increased osteoclastic and osteoblastic activity are noted within a few weeks following transplantation. However, in some patients osteoporosis and effects of secondary hyperparathyroidism may persist as long as 1–2 years. In addition, steroid therapy may be responsible for osteoporosis and osteonecrosis that complicate the later phases of the post-transplant period. Another abnormality that may develop in the post-transplant phase is a renal phosphate leak, which if severe may contribute to osseous abnormalities.

RENAL TRANSPLANTATION

100. When should renal transplantation be considered? What are some important contraindications?

Renal transplantation is indicated in all patients with end stage renal disease (ESRD) who need some form of renal replacement therapy. Nevertheless, there are contraindications to the procedure.

1. **Absolute contraindications:**

    Reversible renal disease   Active infection
    Recent malignant disease   Active glomerulonephritis
    Presensitization to donor Class I major
       transplantation antigens

2. **Relative contraindications:**

    Fabry's disease   Oxalosis
    Advanced age   Psychiatric problems
    Presence of anatomic urologic   Iliofemoral occlusion
       abnormality   Chronic active hepatitis

101. What is the role of blood transfusion prior to kidney transplantation?

It is now generally agreed that blood transfusion before renal transplantation significantly improves graft survival. More than 5 units of blood are considered optimal. The nontransfused recipient is at a higher risk. It is believed that blood transfusions affect the enhancement of graft survival by inducing a state of specific suppression. Alternatively, it may involve a selection process that screens out responders to certain HLA+ antigens.

102. What are the donor criteria in living related transplantation?

Donors for "living related donor kidney transplantation" should have a normal physical examination, be under the age of 50 years, and have the same ABO blood group as the recipient (or be type O, the "universal donor"). An angiogram is necessary to exclude the presence of multiple or abnormal renal arteries, because such abnormalities make the surgery prolonged and difficult. In general, the left kidney is preferred because of the long renal vein.

103. What factors are considered important in evaluating suitability of a cadaver kidney?

In the case of cadaveric kidneys, the donor should have been free of neoplastic or infectious disease, preferably under 60 years of age, and have had good urine output before death and a normal serum creatinine. Urinalysis should be normal and urine cultures should be negative. The kidney should be transplanted as early after harvesting as possible. The graft function tends to be worse after 24 hours following harvesting. Of course, the donor should be free of infection with the hepatitis B virus and the human immunodeficiency virus (HIV).

104. What are the current survival figures for a renal transplant in the U.S.
The 1-year patient survival rate with living related renal transplantation is now around 95–100% and cadaveric transplantation about 90%. With the advent of cyclosporine therapy, graft survivals are 95% and 80%, respectively.

DIABETIC RENAL DISEASE

105. What is the incidence of renal involvement in diabetes mellitus?
Chronic renal failure is the most common cause of death in insulin dependent diabetes and is an important cause of morbidity and mortality in all diabetes. Diabetes contributes up to 50% of all cases of end-stage renal failure (ESRD) in this country. Of type I diabetics, 40–60% develop renal failure between 10–30 years of onset of diabetes. Although about one-third of type II diabetics develop proteinuria, only 4% develop nephrotic syndrome and 6% develop ESRD. The difference between the behavior of type I and II diabetics is probably dependent on the age of onset of diabetes.

106. What is the earliest evidence of renal involvement due to diabetes mellitus?
The earliest renal changes in diabetes manifest as an increase in GFR of 25–50% and a slight enlargement of the kidney that persists for 5–10 years. At this stage, there may be a slight increase in albumin excretion, but the total protein excretion remains in the normal range.

107. Why is diabetic nephropathy associated with large kidneys?
Diabetic nephropathy is one of the causes of CRF associated with normal size or large kidneys. Renal size is increased early in the course of diabetic renal disease and involves hypertrophy and hyperplasia. Elevated levels of growth hormone, often seen with uncontrolled hyperglycemia, are incriminated in this renal hypertrophy. However, the exact etiology still remains unknown.

108. Do patients with microalbuminuria develop overt renal disease more often than others?
The natural course of diabetic nephropathy is characterized by a preclinical phase, followed by a clinical phase. The clinical phases start with the appearance of proteinuria on urine dipstick. Even in the preclinical phase, there is an increased amount of albumin excretion over the normal (20–40 μg/min) measurable by sensitive radioimmunoassays. Studies indicate that patients with this "microalbuminuria" are more likely to develop overt diabetic nephropathy than those who do not exhibit microalbuminuria.

109. What is the most important factor that influences the course of diabetic nephropathy?
Hypertension is the most important factor that affects the course of diabetic renal failure. In the proteinuria phase, 50–75% of all diabetics tend to develop hypertension, and by the time they reach end-stage renal disease, almost all diabetics have hypertension. By controlling hypertension, the rate of decline of GFR can be decreased from 1 ml/min/month to 0.4 ml/min/month in the proteinuric phase.

Parving et al: Early aggressive anti-hypertensive treatment in diabetic nephropathy. Lancet i:1175, 1983.

110. How do diabetics with renal failure fare on dialysis compared to nondiabetics?
Several years ago it was thought that diabetics were not good candidates for dialytic therapy, because about 80% of diabetics with end-stage renal disease placed on hemodialysis died within the first year. Over the last 15 years the results have shown significant improvement. One of the recent reports indicates a 1-year survival of 85% and a 3-year

survival of 60% in diabetics on hemodialysis. It is to be noted that even today diabetics tend to do poorly compared to nondiabetics. Their 3-year survival is 20–30% less and their mortality is 2.25 times higher than nondiabetics. Atherosclerotic cardiac disease is the commonest cause of death, with infections a close second.

111. Does diabetic nephropathy recur following renal transplantation?
Histological lesions typical of diabetic renal disease appear in kidneys transplanted into diabetics in as little as a year. However, clinical deterioration of kidney function attributable to these lesions is very uncommon.

112. What is "pseudodiabetes of uremia"?
In nondiabetics with chronic renal failure, there is a peripheral resistance to the action of endogenous insulin, resulting in hyperglycemia. If a glucose tolerance test is performed, the resulting curve resembles that of diabetics. This phenomenon is called "pseudodiabetes of uremia." The absence of fasting hyperglycemia and the typical changes of diabetic retinopathy distinguish this pseudodiabetes from diabetic uremic patients.

113. Does meticulous control of blood sugar level prevent diabetic renal disease?
The hyperfiltration and hypertrophy seen early in the course of diabetic renal disease can be corrected with insulin treatment. Therefore, strict euglycemic control can reverse the elevated GFR and renal hypertrophy and also can decrease the spontaneous or exercise-induced microalbuminuria that is seen in the preclinical phase. However, strict glycemic control is not beneficial once overt proteinuria (> 500 mg/day) or renal insufficiency starts.

MISCELLANEOUS RENAL DISORDERS

114. What are the risk factors associated with aminoglycoside nephrotoxicity?

Risk Factors for Aminoglycoside Nephrotoxicity

1. Dose and duration of drug therapy
2. Recent aminoglycoside therapy
3. Pre-existent renal or liver failure
4. Elderly age
5. Volume depletion
6. Concurrent nephrotoxin administration
7. Potassium and/or magnesium depletion

Humes D: Aminoglycoside nephrotoxicity. Kidney Int 33: 900–911, 1988.

115. What is a simple renal cyst? How do you distinguish it from a malignant cyst?
Simple cysts represent 60–70% of renal masses. They are common after the age of 50 and are most often asymptomatic. Usually they are detected as incidental findings in radiological procedures done for other reasons. On sonography a simple cyst has smooth, sharply delineated margins, has no echoes within the mass, and has a strong posterior wall echo indicating good transmission through the cyst. These features generally exclude the possibility of malignancy. However, if there is any further suspicion, a CT scan should be done. CT findings consistent with a simple cyst include fluid that is homogenous with a density of 0–20 Hounsfield units and no enhancement of the cyst fluid following the administration of radiocontrast media.

116. What are the renal manifestations of sickle cell disease?

1. Hematuria
2. Renal infarction and papillary necrosis, which may predispose to urinary tract infection
3. Abnormal tubular function:
   a. Reduced concentrating ability
   b. Reduced acid and potassium secretion
   c. Increased uric acid and creatinine secretion
   d. Increased phosphate reabsorption
4. Nephrotic syndrome which may progress to renal failure

117. What are the causes of papillary necrosis?

Renal papillary necrosis is one of the most common renal complications of sickle cell anemia. The other common conditions in which this renal complication is observed include analgesic nephropathy and diabetes mellitus.

118. What are the renal manifestations of infective endocarditis? What is the pathogenesis of these lesions?

Renal manifestations in infective endocarditis include incidental microscopic or gross hematuria and proteinuria. Renal failure is usually mild or absent. The histology in these cases reveals focal proliferative glomerulonephritis. Rarely, a rapidly progressive renal failure with extensive crescent formation is reported. Nephrotic syndrome is rare. Serum IgG and C3 levels are often decreased and immunofluorescence often demonstrates IgG, IgM, and C3 in subendothelial and subepithelial deposits, suggesting an immune-complex etiology.

119. What is the "internist's tumor"?

Renal cell carcinoma is often referred to as the "internist's tumor" because the condition is often diagnosed by its systemic, rather than urological, manifestations. These systemic effects include fever, anemia, hypercalcemia, galactorrhea, feminization or masculinization, and Cushing's syndrome (see also pp 189–190).

120. What are the major differences between fibromuscular dysplasia and atherosclerotic renal artery stenosis?

	Fibromuscular Dysplasia	Atherosclerosis
Age at onset	<40	>45
Gender	80% female	Primarily males
Distribution of lesion	Distal main renal artery and intrarenal branches	Aortic orifice and proximal main renal artery
Progression	Uncommon	Common, may progress to complete occlusion

121. Describe the screening tests for renovascular hypertension.

Screening Tests for Renovascular Hypertension

Radiologic evaluation:	Medical evaluation:
Rapid-sequence intravenous pyelogram	Plasma renin activity
	Both at baseline and after converting-enzyme inhibition
Intravenous digital subtraction angiogram	
Sequential radioisotope scan	Hypotensive response to saralasin or
Renal arteriogram (the definitive test)	angiotensin-converting enzyme (ACE) inhibition

(From Rose BD: Pathophysiology of Renal Disease, 2nd ed. New York, McGraw-Hill, 1987, p 560, with permission.)

122. How do you diagnose acute renal failure secondary to rhabdomyolysis? What are the peculiarities of this form of ARF?

Rhabdomyolysis can cause ARF due to acute tubular necrosis (ATN). It occurs in various clinical conditions, including trauma, ischemic tissue damage following a drug overdose, alcoholism, seizures, and heat stroke (especially in untrained subjects or those with sickle cell trait). Hypokalemia and severe hypophosphatemia can also precipitate rhabdomyolysis. Typically these patients have pigmented granular casts in urine sediment, a positive orthotolidine test in the urine supernatant (indicating the presence of heme), and markedly elevated plasma creatine phosphokinase (CPK) and other muscle enzymes, owing to their release from damaged muscle tissue. The other characteristics of ARF due to rhabdomyolysis include hyperphosphatemia, hyperkalemia, and a disproportionate increase in plasma creatinine (all these being due to release of cellular constituents). A high anion gap metabolic acidosis and severe hyperuricemia are also characteristic of this entity. Oliguria or anuria is also common. The mechanism of renal failure is not completely understood. Although myoglobin is not directly nephrotoxic, concurrent vasoconstriction or volume depletion decreases the renal perfusion and rate of urine flow in tubules, thereby promoting the precipitation of these pigment casts.

BIBLIOGRAPHY

1. Brenner BM, Rector FC (eds): The Kidney, 4th ed. Philadelphia, W.B. Saunders, 1991.
2. Frommer JP, Wesson DE, Eknoyan G: Side effects and complications of diuretics. In Eknoyan G, Martinez-Maldonado M (eds): The Physiological Basis of Diuretic Therapy. New York, Grune & Stratton, 1986.
3. Rose BF: Pathophysiology of Renal disease, 2nd ed. New York, McGraw-Hill, 1987.
4. Schrier RW (ed): Manual of Nephrology, 3rd ed. Boston, Little, Brown, 1990.
5. Suki WN, Massry SG (eds): Therapy of Renal Diseases and Related Disorders. Boston, Martinus Nijhoff, 1984.
6. Wyngaarden JB, Smith LH (eds): Cecil Textbook of Medicine, 18th ed. Philadelphia, W.B. Saunders, 1988.

8. ACID/BASE AND ELECTROLYTE SECRETS

Donald E. Wesson, M.D., Sangubhotla Prabhakar, M.D., and Anthony J. Zollo, Jr., M.D.

In all things you shall find everywhere the Acid and the Alcaly.
Otto Tachenius (1670)
Hyppocrates Chymacus, Ch. 21.

Hence if too much salt is used in food, the pulse hardens.
Huang Ti (The Yellow Emperor) (2697–2597 B.C.)
Nei Chung Su Wen, Bk. 3, Sect. 10, tr. by Ilza Veith,
in The Yellow Emperor's Classic of Internal Medicine.

REGULATION OF SODIUM, WATER AND VOLUME STATUS

1. List the osmolality and electrolyte concentrations of serum and commonly used intravenous (IV) solutions.

Serum and Solutions	Osmolality (mOsm/kg)	Glucose (g/L)	Sodium (mEq/L)	Chloride (mEq/L)
Serum	285–295	65–110	135–145	97–110
5% D/W	252	50	0	0
10% D/W	505	100	0	0
50% D/W	2520	500	0	0
½ NS* (0.45% NaCl)	154	0	77	77
NS (0.9% NaCl)	308	0	154	154
3% NS	1026	0	513	513
Ringer's lactate**	272	0	130	109

* NS = normal saline
** Ringer's lactate also contains 28 mEq/L lactate, 4 mEq/L K^+, 4.5 mEq/L Ca^{++}.

2. How can you estimate a patient's serum osmolality?
A close estimate of a patient's serum osmolality can be derived from measurements of the serum sodium, glucose, and blood urea nitrogen (BUN). The following equation can be used in the estimation:

$$Osmolality = 1.86 \times [Na^+] + \frac{Glucose}{18} + \frac{BUN}{2.8} + 9$$

3. What percentage of the adult human body is made of water? What percentage of the water content is intracellular versus extracellular?
Approximately 60% of the adult man and 50% of the adult woman are made of water. Approximately two-thirds of this volume is intracellular and one-third is extracellular. About 20% of the extracellular fluid volume is plasma water.

4. What are the sources and daily amounts of water gain and loss?
The average adult male gains and loses 2600 ml of water each day. The gains occur from direct fluid ingestion (1400 ml/day), the fluid content of ingested food (850 ml/day), and as a product of water produced by oxidation reactions (350 ml/day). The water losses occur through the urine (1500 ml/day), perspiration (500 ml/day), respiration (400 ml/day), and feces (200 ml/day.) (Of course, these values are only averages and subject to a great deal of variation.)

5. What are the necessary factors that allow the kidney to adequately excrete free water?
The required factors are:

1. GFR: There must be a filtrate formed to allow for renal excretion of free water. The lower the GFR, the lower the kidney's ability to rapidly respond to a free-water challenge with excretion of free water.

2. Glomerular filtrate must escape reabsorption in the proximal tubule to get to the diluting segment (ascending limb of the loop of Henle). This is where free water is created as described above. Pathologic states in which there is vigorous fluid reabsorption in the proximal tubule are associated with a compromised ability to excrete free water. Examples include true volume depletion and states of decreased effective arterial blood volume, such as congestive heart failure (CHF), cirrhosis, and nephrotic syndrome.

3. An adequately functioning diluting segment must be present. Intrinsic disorders of function of this segment are unusual. Endogenous prostaglandin E_2 and loop diuretics inhibit NaCl transport in this segment and can thereby limit formation of free water.

4. The free water formed by the diluting segment must leave the nephron without being reabsorbed by the collecting tubule. This nephron segment is intrinsically impermeable to water but is made permeable by antidiuretic hormone (ADH). In the presence of this hormone, water is reabsorbed from the collecting tubule into the hypertonic interstitium instead of being excreted.

6. Explain the meaning of "serum sodium concentration" with respect to sodium balance and water balance.
Serum sodium concentration (mEq/L) reflects the concentration of this cation in the extra-cellular fluid. Since its units are mass per unit volume, it indicates the relative relationship between sodium and water in the body. It is not indicative of total body sodium content but is more an indication of the water status (hydration) of the body. Serum sodium concentration may be low, normal, or increased with any given perturbation of total body sodium content.

Alterations of the serum sodium concentration reflect alterations in free-water balance. Therefore, a true low serum sodium indicates a free-water excess compared to sodium content, and a high serum sodium indicates a relative free-water deficit.

7. What happens to serum sodium concentration in response to loss of isotonic fluid, as would occur with hemorrhage?
Isotonic fluid losses in and of themselves cause a decrease in extracellular fluid volume with no change in serum sodium concentration. If, however, these losses are replaced with hypotonic fluids, dilutional hyponatremia will result.

8. What is meant by a state of "decreased effective arterial blood volume"?
The extracellular space is dynamic, with an ongoing balance between its capacity and its actual volume. Both of these parameters are biologically monitored and normally coordinated to maintain optimal tissue perfusion. A state of "decreased effective arterial blood volume" occurs when there is a large capacity combined with a smaller volume. This is seen most commonly with CHF, cirrhosis, and the nephrotic syndrome.

9. Why is it that sodium has an effective distribution in total body water despite being confined largely to the extracellular space?
Sodium is the major determinant of serum osmolality, and changes in its concentration lead to water shifts between the extracellular and intracellular compartments. This osmotic shift of water gives sodium an effective distribution greater than its chemical distribution and equivalent to that for the total body water.

10. What is the "diluting segment" of the nephron?

The diluting segment is the thick ascending limb of the loop of Henle. This segment actively reabsorbs sodium chloride without water. This process leads to urine that is hyposmotic compared to plasma, creating free water for excretion.

11. How can patients with hyponatremia be categorized according to history and physical examination findings, thereby allowing an initial diagnostic and therapeutic approach?

Patients with hyponatremia can be categorized according to their volume status as estimated from physical examination and historical data. An attempt is made to determine whether the volume status is grossly low, normal, or high.

1. **Patients with low volume status:** This is supported by a history of volume loss or decreased intake, and orthostatic blood pressure changes on examination. These patients need to have the lost volume replaced to turn off the factors that limit the kidney's ability to excrete free water.

2. **Patients with expanded volume:** This is supported by a history of a condition with decreased effective arterial blood volume and an examination showing edema. These patients must have therapeutic attention directed to their underlying disorder. If the hyponatremia is mild and asymptomatic, free-water restriction, in addition to specific treatment of the underlying disorder, would be the suggested initial therapeutic approach. If the hyponatremia is severe and symptomatic, more aggressive treatment with hypertonic saline and furosemide may be required.

3. **Patients with an apparently normal volume status:** In these patients a wide variety of pathologic processes must be considered in the diagnostic evaluation. These include the syndrome of inappropriate ADH (SIADH) production and drugs that can limit free-water excretion in some patients, such as chlorpropamide.

12. What are "pseudo-" and "spurious" hyponatremia? Why is it important to distinguish these kinds of hyponatremia from true hyponatremia?

These terms refer to two categories of hyponatremia that should be distinguished from true hyponatremia associated with hyposmolality.

"Pseudo"-hyponatremia occurs when quantitative serum sodium measurement is performed on a given volume of plasma that contains a greater than normal amount of water-excluding particles, such as lipid or protein. In this setting, plasma water (which contains the sodium) comprises a smaller fraction of the plasma volume, which leads to a factitiously low serum sodium concentration when the quantitative sodium measurement is expressed in mEq/L. The sodium concentration in plasma water is normal in this setting; therefore these patients are asymptomatic. Attention should be directed to hyperlipidemia or hyperproteinemia.

"Spurious" hyponatremia results from hyperosmolality of the serum (i.e., from hyperglycemia), resulting in movement of intracellular water to the extracellular space and subsequent dilution of the sodium in the extracellular space. These patients are not symptomatic from hyposmolality (as are patients with true hyponatremia). If they are symptomatic at all, it is due to their hyperosmolar state. In this setting, attention should be directed to correcting the hyperosmolar state.

It is important to distinguish these conditions from true hyponatremia, because the diagnostic workup and therapeutic management are different.

13. How do you correct the serum sodium for a given level of hyperglycemia?

Hyperglycemia, one of the causes of spurious hyponatremia, causes a decrease in the measured serum sodium concentration. For each increase in the serum glucose of 100 mg/dl above normal, the serum sodium will decrease by 1.6 mEq/L. For example, if a patient's serum glucose increases from a normal value of 100 mg/dl to 600 mg/dl (an increase of

500, or 5 × 100 mg/dl), the serum sodium would be expected to decrease by 8.0 mEq/L
(5 × 1.6 mEq/L).

14. What is essential hyponatremia?

Essential hyponatremia or "sick cell syndrome" is a term used to denote hyponatremia in
the absence of a water diuresis defect. One of the hypotheses is that the osmoreceptor cells
in the hypothalamus are reset so that they maintain a lower plasma osmolality. Essential
hyponatremia is seen in several conditions such as CHF, cirrhosis of the liver, and
pulmonary tuberculosis. The condition is diagnosed by demonstration of normal urinary
concentration and dilution in the face of hyponatremia. Generally, this entity does not
require treatment.

15. What causes the signs and symptoms of hyponatremia?

The manifestations of hyponatremia are mainly attributable to central nervous system
(CNS) edema, which is usually not seen until the serum sodium falls to 120 mEq/L or less.
The symptoms range from mild lethargy to seizure, coma, and death.

16. Why is it that two patients with the same degree of hyponatremia can have dramatically different signs and symptoms?

The signs and symptoms of hyponatremia are more a function of the rapidity of the drop
in serum sodium than the absolute level. In patients with chronic hyponatremia, there has
been time for solute equilibration, resulting in less CNS edema and less severe manifestations.
In acute hyponatremia, there is no time for equilibration, so smaller changes in serum
sodium are accompanied by larger degrees of CNS edema and more severe manifestations.

17. How do you approach hyponatremia in edematous states?

Treatment of hyponatremia depends on the underlying etiology, the presence or absence of
symptoms attributable to hyponatremia, and the rapidity of its development. In general,
patients with edematous states such as the nephrotic syndrome, who have extracellular fluid
(ECF) expansion, will have some degree of hyponatremia unless water-restricted. Generally
this condition is asymptomatic and requires no treatment. Treatment is required only if the
hyponatremia is severe (less than 125 mEq/L), and especially if there are symptoms such as
lethargy, confusion, stupor, and coma.

18. A 41-year-old black male is in the hospital with acute bacterial meningitis. His chemistries show a blood urea nitrogen (BUN) and creatinine of 11 and 1.2 mg/dl, respectively, but his serum sodium is 130 mEq/L. How do you evaluate his hyponatremia and correct it?

Hyponatremia in the setting of bacterial meningitis (or any pathologic CNS process)
requires evaluation to rule out the syndrome of inappropriate ADH (SIADH) secretion.
SIADH is a form of hyponatremia in which there are sustained or intermittently elevated
levels of ADH. These levels are inappropriate for the osmotic or volume stimuli that
normally affect ADH secretion. The essential points in the diagnosis of SIADH are:
  1. The presence of hypotonic hyponatremia
  2. Inappropriate antidiuresis (urine osmolality higher than expected for the degree of
     hyponatremia)
  3. Significant sodium excretion when the patient is normovolemic
  4. Normal renal, thyroid, and adrenal function
  5. Absence of other causes of hyponatremia, volume depletion, or edematous states.
Thus, the workup includes measurement of serum and urine sodium concentrations, and
osmolality. In the majority of cases, urinary osmolality exceeds plasma osmolality, often by
more than 100 mOsm/L. Urinary sodium excretion exceeds 20 mEq/L unless the patient is
salt-restricted. The hypotonic hyponatremia, as well as the tendency to urinary sodium

wasting, improves with fluid restriction. In the majority of cases, restriction of fluids to 1000–1200 ml per day is all that is needed. Occasionally patients with symptomatic and marked hyponatremia may require demeclocycline therapy and/or hypertonic saline.

19. What is the differential diagnosis of SIADH?

Differential Diagnosis of SIADH

1. Malignant neoplasia
  a. Carcinoma (bronchogenic, duodenal, pancreatic, ureteral, prostatic, bladder)
  b. Lymphoma and leukemia
  c. Thymoma, mesothelioma, and Ewing's sarcoma
 	
2. CNS disorders
  a. Trauma, subarachnoid hemorrhage, subdural hematoma, Rocky Mountain spotted fever
  b. Infection (encephalitis, meningitis, brain abscess)
  c. Tumors
  d. Porphyria
  e. Guillain-Barré syndrome
  f. Psychosis, delirium tremens
  g. Stroke
  h. Multiple sclerosis
	3. Pulmonary disorders
	  a. Tuberculosis
	  b. Pneumonia
	  c. Mechanical ventilators with positive pressure
	  d. Pneumonia (bacterial, viral, mycobacterial, fungal)
	  e. Asthma and cystic fibrosis
	  f. Pneumothorax
	  g. Lung abscess
	
	4. Drugs (including vasopressin, chlorpropamide, thiazide diuretics, oxytocin, vincristine, haloperidol, nicotine, phenothiazines, tricyclic antidepressants)
	
	5. Others
	  a. "Idiopathic" SIADH
	  b. Hypothyroidism

20. How does one estimate the free-water deficit in a patient with hypernatremia?
It is important to estimate this deficit so that one can determine how much free-water replacement will be necessary to correct the hypernatremia. To calculate the deficit, it can be assumed that the patient has lost free water without salt. Thus, the patient has reduced total body water (TBW) but maintains the same total body sodium content. This change results in an increase in the serum sodium concentration that is proportional to the decrease in TBW. In other words, the ratio of the initial serum sodium concentration (which is assumed to be normal) to the current serum sodium concentration (which is higher than normal) is equal to the ratio of the present TBW (which is less than normal) to the initial TBW (which is assumed to have been normal).

$$\frac{\text{Current TBW}}{\text{Initial TBW}} = \frac{\text{Initial serum sodium}}{\text{Current serum sodium}}$$

This relationship can be used to calculate the current TBW. Subtracting this value from the initial (normal) TBW yields the estimated free-water deficit. For example, let us assume that a 70-kg patient with a history of a stroke, who does not drink and cannot ask for water, is found to have a serum sodium of 160 mEq/L. His normal TBW should be 60% of his body weight (or 0.6 × 70 kg = 42 L), and we will assume that his initial serum sodium concentration was 140 mEq/L. Using our formula from above,

$$\text{Current TBW} = \frac{\text{Initial serum sodium} \times \text{Initial TBW}}{\text{Current serum sodium}} = 36.8 \text{ liters}$$

This analysis demonstrates that the increase in his serum sodium from 140 to 160 mEq/L by free-water loss without sodium loss requires that his TBW decrease from 42 to 36.8 liters. Thus, his calculated free-water deficit is 5.2 liters. This deficit must be replaced with fluids containing no salt.

21. What are the manifestations of hypernatremia?

The manifestations of hypernatremia are basically those of hyperosmolality and are similar to the symptoms manifested by other causes of hyperosmolality (such as hyperglycemia). These are mainly produced by fluid shifts from the CNS and increased CNS osmolality, resulting in "shrinking" of the brain. The symptoms range from lethargy to seizures, coma, and death. The severity of the symptoms is dependent on the severity of the hyperosmolality and the speed with which it develops.

22. What are some common causes of hypernatremia?

Hypernatremia is seen in diabetes insipidus, severe dehydration due to extrarenal fluid losses (e.g., burns, excessive sweating, etc.), and hypothalamic disorders (e.g., tumors, granulomas, cerebrovascular accidents) leading to defective thirst and vasopressin regulation.

23. How do you correct hypernatremia?

Once the free-water deficit is calculated, hypernatremia is usually corrected by its replacement. In mild cases this can be accomplished orally, simply by having the patient drink. If IV fluids are to be used to replace the deficit, dextrose in water can be used. If salt-containing fluids are deemed necessary, the equivalent free-water volume must be given. For example, if half-normal saline is used (one liter of which can be viewed as containing 500 ml of normal saline and 500 ml of free water), twice the amount of the estimated free-water deficit is needed to correct the free-water deficit.

This volume deficit is replaced slowly. The first half is given over 24 hours. If the patient is hemodynamically unstable, with signs of severe extracellular fluid (ECF) volume depletion, therapy with 0.9% normal saline (NS) is warranted before dextrose infusion is started.

POTASSIUM BALANCE

24. How is potassium distributed between intracellular and extracellular fluid compartments?

A 70-kg man contains approximately 3500 mEq of potassium (about 50 mEq/kg body weight). The vast majority of this (98%) is in the intracellular space. Therefore, the amount in the extracellular compartment (the portion that we routinely measure) represents only a small percentage of the total body potassium.

25. How is the large chemical gradient between intracellular and extracellular potassium concentration maintained?

The Na^+, K^+ ATPase pump actively extrudes sodium from the cell and pumps potassium into the cell. This pump is present in all cells of the body. In addition, the cell is electrically negative compared to the exterior, which serves to keep potassium inside the cell.

26. Given the relatively small extracellular compared to intracellular concentration of potassium, why are some electrical processes in the body (cardiac conduction, skeletal and smooth muscle contraction) sensitive to changes in the extracellular potassium concentration?

It is the ratio of the extracellular to intracellular potassium concentration more than the absolute level of either that determines the sensitivity of these electrical processes. Since the extracellular concentration of potassium is small compared to the intracellular concentration, a small absolute change in extracellular potassium concentration results in a large change in the ratio of extracellular to intracellular potassium concentration.

27. What are some common factors that influence the movement of potassium between the intracellular and extracellular compartments?

Some common factors are:

1. **Acid-base changes:** Acidemia (increased concentration of hydrogen ion in the serum) leads to intracellular buffering of the hydrogen ion, with subsequent extrusion of potassium into the extracellular space, increasing the concentration of potassium in this compartment.

2. **Hormones:** Insulin, epinephrine (beta-2 mediated), growth hormone, and androgens all promote net movement of potassium into cells.

3. **Cellular metabolism:** Synthesis of protein and glycogen is associated with intracellular potassium binding.

4. **Extracellular concentration:** All other things being equal, potassium tends to enter the cell when its extracellular concentration is high and vice versa.

28. How is potassium handled by the kidney?

Most of the filtered potassium is reabsorbed in the proximal tubule, and there is net secretion or net reabsorption in the distal nephron, depending on the body's potassium needs. Under most conditions we are in potassium excess, and the kidney is required to excrete potassium in order to maintain whole-body potassium balance. Potassium restriction leads to renal potassium conservation, but this conservation process for potassium is not as rapid nor efficient as is that for sodium.

29. How does aldosterone influence potassium metabolism?

Aldosterone is the main regulatory hormone for potassium metabolism. It promotes sodium reabsorption and potassium secretion in the distal nephron, the gut, and the sweat glands. Quantitatively, its greatest effect is in the kidney. Its secretion is increased by increasing potassium concentration in the extracellular fluid and is decreased by low potassium concentrations.

30. What are some factors that can lead to increased renal potassium excretion?

These factors include:

1. Increased dietary potassium intake.
2. Increased aldosterone secretion (as in volume depletion).
3. Alkalosis.
4. Increased flow rate in the distal tubule.
5. Increased sodium delivery to the distal nephron—this promotes sodium reabsorption in exchange for potassium secretion in the distal nephron. The process is accelerated in the presence of aldosterone.
6. Decreased chloride concentration in tubular fluid in the distal nephron. This allows for sodium to be reabsorbed with a less-permeable ion (like bicarbonate or sulfate) that increases the negativity of the tubular lumen in the distal nephron. The increased negativity of the tubular lumen promotes potassium secretion.
7. Natriuretic agents—drugs like the loop diuretics, thiazides, and acetazolamide—lead to increased sodium delivery to the distal nephron, volume depletion with increased aldosterone secretion, and subsequent increased renal potassium excretion, as described above. Some natriuretic agents are "potassium sparing" in that they inhibit potassium secretion in the distal nephron. These agents include spironolactone, triamterene, and amiloride.

31. In addition to the kidney, what is the other major route of potassium loss?

The GI tract and the kidney make up the major routes of potassium loss. Fluids in the lower GI tract, particularly those of the small bowel, are high in potassium. Therefore, diarrhea can result in significant losses of potassium. However, upper GI losses such as vomiting or nasogastric suction cause *renal* potassium loss. This is multifactorial and includes the following:

- **Alkalosis**
- **Volume depletion,** which leads to increased aldosterone secretion.
- **Chloride depletion** from the loss of hydrochloric acid in the gastric fluid. This leads to a high tubular concentration of bicarbonate, which is a relatively nonreabsorbable anion.

All of these factors combine to increase renal potassium losses according to the mechanisms described above.

32. What are the causes of a spuriously elevated serum potassium determination?

1. **Hemolysis,** with the release of intra-erythrocytic potassium.
2. **Pseudohyperkalemia,** seen in marked thrombocytosis or leukocytosis. It is due to the disproportionately increased amounts of the normally released potassium that occurs with clotting. This can be corrected by inhibiting clotting and measuring plasma potassium concentration.

33. What are the common causes of hyperkalemia?

Causes of Hyperkalemia

1. **Inadequate excretion**
   a. Renal failure
      i. Acute renal failure
      ii. Severe chronic renal failure
      iii. Tubular disorders
   b. Adrenal insufficiency
      i. Hypoaldosteronism
      ii. Addison's disease
   c. Diuretics that inhibit potassium secretion (spironolactone, triamterine, amiloride)

2. **Shift of potassium from tissues**
   a. Tissue damage (muscle crush, hemolysis, internal bleeding)
   b. Drugs (succinylcholine, arginine, digitalis poisoning, beta-adrenergic antagonists)
   c. Acidosis
   d. Hyperosmolality
   e. Insulin deficiency
   f. Hyperkalemia periodic paralysis

3. **Excessive intake**

4. **Pseudohyperkalemia**
   a. Thrombocytosis
   b. Leukocytosis
   c. Poor venipuncture technique
   d. In vitro hemolysis

(From Levinksy N: Fluids and electrolytes. In Wilson JD, et al (eds): Harrison's Principles of Internal Medicine, 12th ed. New York, McGraw-Hill, 1991, p 287, with permission.)

34. Which electrocardiographic (ECG) changes are associated with hypo- and hyperkalemia?

The common ECG changes seen with hypokalemia of increasing severity are depressed ST segment, appearance of u waves, and lowering and inversion of the T wave. The changes seen with hyperkalemia of increasing severity are tall, peaked T waves, decreasing amplitude and eventual disappearance of the P wave, widening of the QRS complex with eventual spread to include the T wave, biphasic (sine wave) curve, and eventual cardiac standstill or ventricular fibrillation.

35. Describe the general diagnostic approach to patients with disturbances in serum potassium concentration.

In the initial approach to such patients, it is important to determine whether the disturbance results from (1) abnormal potassium intake or metabolism (excessive catabolism or anabolism); (2) from intracellular and extracellular compartmental shifts; or (3) from disturbances in renal excretion or extrarenal loss. After placing the patient in one of these three categories, it is possible to narrow the differential diagnosis, order appropriate diagnostic tests, and decide on the appropriate management. Disturbances of intake can be investigated by history and physical examination. The possibility of cellular shifts can be investigated by looking for any of the disturbances described above that result in compartmental movement of this cation. Determination of the urinary potassium concentration can help in distinguishing renal from nonrenal causes of perturbations of serum potassium. High urinary potassium excretion in the setting of hypokalemia is compatible with a renal cause for potassium deficiency. By contrast, an appropriately low urinary potassium excretion in the setting of hypokalemia suggests extrarenal (possibly GI) losses of potassium.

36. Other than the ECG changes, what are the other manifestations of hypokalemia?

The major manifestations of hypokalemia are seen in the neuromuscular system. When the potassium falls to between 2.0 and 2.5, muscular weakness and lethargy are seen. With further decreases, the patient will manifest paralysis with eventual respiratory muscle involvement and death. Hypokalemia can also cause rhabdomyolysis, myoglobinuria, paralytic ileus, and prolonged hypokalemia, which can lead to renal tubular damage (called hypokalemic nephropathy).

37. What is the management of hypokalemia?

Management must be directed at the disturbance that led to the abnormal potassium concentration. If hypokalemia is associated with alkalosis, then the alkalosis should be corrected in addition to providing potassium supplements.

In general, patients with potassium depletion should be given supplements slowly to replace the deficit. The oral route is the preferred one because of its safety as well as its efficacy. Some instances require more rapid repletion with intravenous supplements. This intravenous supplementation should not exceed 20 mEq/hr. It is unwise to administer more than 40 mEq of potassium intravenously per hour. Cardiac monitoring should accompany infusions of greater than 10 mEq/hr.

38. Other than the ECG changes, what are the other manifestations of hyperkalemia?

The most important manifestation of hyperkalemia is the increased excitability of cardiac muscle. With severe elevations in potassium, a patient can suffer diastolic cardiac arrest. Skeletal muscle paralysis can also be seen. Again, the symptoms produced by hyperkalemia are dependent on the rapidity of the change. Patients with chronically elevated serum potassium levels can tolerate higher levels, with fewer symptoms than patients with acute hyperkalemia.

39. What is the management of hyperkalemia?

The treatment depends on the patient's serum potassium level and the clinical setting. Mild levels of hyperkalemia (5.0–5.5 mEq/L) associated with the hyporenin, hypoaldosterone syndrome are tolerated well and usually require no treatment. Higher levels not associated with ECG changes may require treatment with a synthetic mineralocorticoid.

Hyperkalemia occasionally presents as a medical emergency with very high levels (>7.0 mEq/L) and cardiac conduction system abnormalities as determined by the ECG changes described above. In this emergent setting, intravenous calcium must be administered to counteract immediately the effect of the hyperkalemia on the conduction system. This must be followed by maneuvers intended to shift potassium into cells, thereby decreasing the ratio of extracellular to intracellular potassium concentration, as described above. This can be accomplished by administering glucose with insulin and/or bicarbonate administration to increase serum pH. Finally, a maneuver to remove potassium from the body must be instituted. This can be accomplished by use of a cation exchange resin (Kayexalate) and/or by dialysis (hemodialysis or peritoneal dialysis).

40. A 61-year-old female with end-stage renal disease (ESRD) missed her dialysis twice and is in the ER with a serum potassium of 6.4 mEq/L. How would you proceed to manage this patient?

The severity of hyperkalemia is assessed by both serum K^+ level as well as ECG changes. If the ECG shows only tall T waves, and serum K^+ is less than 6.5 mEq/L, the hyperkalemia is mild, whereas K^+ levels of 6.5–8 mEq/L are associated with more severe ECG changes, including absent P waves and wide QRS complexes. At higher K^+ levels, ventricular arrhythmias tend to appear and prognosis is grave unless treated promptly.

The first step in the management of this patient is obtaining an ECG or observing the cardiac monitor. If the latter shows tall T waves only (which is likely to be the case in this situation), the patient can be treated with:

1. Hypertonic glucose infusion, along with 10 units insulin (e.g., 200–500 ml of 10% glucose in 30 minutes followed by 1 liter of the same in the next 4–6 hours).
2. Sodium bicarbonate, 50–150 mEq given intravenously (if the patient is not in fluid overload).

Both of these maneuvers shift K^+ into cells and start acting within an hour. Total body K^+ can be decreased by using cation exchange resins such as sodium polysterone sulfonate. Usually 20 g with 20 ml of 70% sorbitol solution is started every 4–6 hours. If the ECG shows more advanced changes of hyperkalemia (including absent P waves, wide QRS complexes, or ventricular arrhythmias), intravenous 10% calcium gluconate (10–30 ml) is given first, while the patient is monitored. At the same time arrangements must be made to dialyze the patient as soon as possible, since dialysis effectively corrects hyperkalemia.

41. A 71-year-old diabetic with a nonhealing foot ulcer is on tobramycin and piperacillin. This patient has a resistant hypokalemia. How will you approach this problem?

Aminoglycosides and penicillin are both known to deplete serum K^+. The former do this by defective proximal tubular K^+ reabsorption and the latter by increased renal K^+ excretion induced by the poorly reabsorbable anion (penicillin). With aminoglycosides, magnesium wasting is another complication. Hence, in addition to K^+ repletion, correction of hypomagnesemia is important, since hypokalemia is often resistant to correction unless the magnesium deficit is also corrected.

42. A 67-year-old white male with CHF treated with furosemide has a serum potassium of 2.4 mEq/L. How would you correct this K^+ deficit?

Hypokalemia is an important complication of diuretic therapy (except with K^+-sparing diuretics). It is important to monitor serum K^+ periodically in these patients, especially in patients with cardiac illness who are likely to be on digoxin, because hypokalemia can exacerbate digitalis toxicity. The potassium deficit requires replacement (except in patients who are on minimal doses of diuretics), especially if serum K^+ is less than 3 mEq/L. Potassium chloride elixir or tablets are the treatment of choice. Enteric-coated potassium supplements are known to cause gastric ulceration.

ACID/BASE REGULATION

43. What is the Henderson-Hasselbalch equation? What is its significance?

An acid-base disorder is suspected on a clinical basis and confirmed on arterial blood gas (ABG) analysis of the pH, P_aCO_2 or bicarbonate concentration ($[HCO_3^-]$). It is useful to be able to confirm that a given set of these parameters are mutually compatible. The relationship between these parameters is described in the Henderson-Hasselbalch equation:

$$pH = pKa + \log \frac{[HCO_3^-]}{\alpha CO_2 \times P_aCO_2} = 6.1 + \log \frac{[HCO_3^-]}{0.03 \times P_aCO_2}$$

The value of pKa, the negative logarithm of the equilibrium constant K, and the CO_2 solubility coefficient (αCO_2) are constant at any given set of temperature and osmolality. In plasma, at $37°C$, the pKa is 6.1 and the αCO_2 is 0.03. This equation describes the relationship of the pH, P_aCO_2, and bicarbonate concentration as measured in blood gas analysis.

It can be seen from the Henderson-Hasselbalch equation that the pH is dependent on the ratio of the bicarbonate concentration to the P_aCO_2 and not on the absolute individual values alone. A primary change in one of the values will usually lead to a compensatory change in the other value. This serves to limit the degree of the resulting acidosis or alkalosis.

44. The integrated action of which three organs is involved in acid-base homeostasis?

The liver, lungs, and kidneys cooperate to maintain acid-base balance. The liver metabolizes protein contained in the standard North American diet such that net acid (protons) is produced. Hepatic metabolism of organic acids (lactate) can consume acid, which is the equivalent of producing bicarbonate. Acid released into the extracellular fluid titrates bicarbonate to H_2O and CO_2, and the CO_2 is excreted by the lungs. In addition, CO_2 produced from cellular metabolism is excreted by the lungs. The kidney reclaims the filtered bicarbonate and excretes the accumulated net acid. The integrated action of all three organs is required to maintain acid-base balance.

45. What is the fate of a load of nonvolatile acid administered to the body?

The acid load is initially buffered by extracellular (40%) and intracellular (60%) buffers. These buffers minimize the decrease in pH that would otherwise occur in response to the acid load. The major extracellular fluid buffer is the bicarbonate system, and most intracellular buffering is provided by histidine-containing proteins. The administered acid reduces extracellular fluid bicarbonate concentration, and new bicarbonate is then regenerated by the kidney during the process of proton (acid) secretion. Therefore, the administered acid is initially buffered as described and eventually excreted by the kidney.

46. State the two major roles of the kidney in monitoring acid-base balance.

The kidney must *reclaim* the filtered bicarbonate and *regenerate* the bicarbonate lost by acid titration. This latter process is equivalent to acid excretion. Reclamation of bicarbonate is quantitatively a more important process than regeneration (4500 mEq/day versus 70 mEq/day). Nevertheless, without regeneration of new bicarbonate (excretion of acid), plasma bicarbonate concentration could not be maintained and net acid retention would result.

47. Which two principal urinary buffers allow for net acid excretion (new bicarbonate regeneration)?

Dibasic phosphate and ammonia are the major urinary buffers allowing for net acid excretion (equivalent to new bicarbonate regeneration). By accepting a proton, they respectively become monobasic phosphate and ammonium ions and are excreted in the urine. The phosphate is measured as titratable acid, and the ammonium is measured directly. Urinary excretion of these two substances minus urinary bicarbonate excretion constitutes net acid excretion.

48. What are the four primary acid-base disturbances and how are they characterized?

They are **metabolic acidosis** and **metabolic alkalosis**, and **respiratory acidosis** and **respiratory alkalosis**. In the steady-state maintenance of normal acid-base balance, the addition of hydrogen ions to the body fluids is balanced by their excretion, such that the hydrogen ion concentration [H^+] of the extracellular fluid remains relatively constant at 40 nM (40×10^{-9} M or pH = 7.40). An imbalance in this process that leads to a net increase in [H^+] is called acidosis. Alkalosis refers to an imbalance that leads to a net decrease in [H^+]. Metabolic versus respiratory are terms used to describe how the imbalance occurred.

Describing a disorder as *metabolic* infers that the imbalance leading to the change in [H+] occurred either because of addition of nonvolatile acid or base or because of a gain or loss of available buffer (bicarbonate). Bicarbonate as a buffer reduces the concentration of free hydrogen ions in solution. Referring to an acid-base disorder as *respiratory* infers that the net change in [H+] occurred secondary to a disturbance in ventilation that resulted in either a net increase or decrease in CO_2 gas in the ECF.

The phrase "metabolic acidosis" means there has been a net increase in [H+] as a result of a net gain in nonvolatile acid or from a net loss of bicarbonate buffer. Respiratory acidosis means that there has been a net increase in [H+] as a result of decreased ventilation, leading to CO_2 retention. Metabolic alkalosis denotes a net decrease in [H+] that occurs as a result of gain of bicarbonate or loss of acid. Respiratory alkalosis means that there has been a net decrease in [H+] because of increased ventilation leading to decreased CO_2. Note that these disorders refer to the imbalance that leads to the directional change in [H+] and do not denote what the final [H+], PCO_2, and [HCO_3] will be. This should remind us of two important facts: (1) there are compensatory changes that occur in response to these disorders, and (2) more than one acid-base disturbance may occur simultaneously, such that the final parameters measured depend not only on the algebraic sum of the different disorders but also on their respective compensatory responses.

49. How do you diagnose the four primary acid-base disorders?

The following table illustrates the expected compensations seen in simple acid-base disorders and the expected compensatory responses:

Relationships Between HCO_3^- and PCO_2 in Simple Acid-Base Disorders

CONDITION	PRIMARY DISTURBANCE	PREDICTED RESPONSE
Metabolic acidosis	↓ HCO_3^-	ΔPCO_2 (↓) = 1–1.4ΔHCO_3^-*
Metabolic alkalosis	↑ HCO_3^-	ΔPCO_2 (↑) = 0.4–0.9ΔHCO_3^-*
Respiratory acidosis	↑ PCO_2	Acute: ΔHCO_3^- (↑) = 0.1ΔPCO_2 Chronic: ΔHCO_3^- (↑) = 0.25–0.55ΔPCO_2
Respiratory alkalosis	↓ PCO_2	Acute: ΔHCO_3^- (↓) = 0.2–0.25ΔPCO_2 Chronic: ΔHCO_3^- (↓) = 0.4–0.5ΔPCO_2

* After at least 12 to 24 hours.
(From Hamm L, Jacobsen HR: Mixed acid-base disorders. In Kokko JP, Tannen RL (eds): Fluids and Electrolytes, 2nd ed. Philadelphia, W.B. Saunders, 1990, p 487, with permission.)

50. What are secondary acid-base disturbances?

The phrase "secondary acid-base disturbance" is actually a misnomer. More correctly stated, these are physiologic responses ("compensatory responses," if you will) to the cardinal acid-base disturbances. They usually ameliorate the change in hydrogen ion concentration ([H+]), and therefore the pH that would otherwise occur. This can be seen more clearly by examining the mass-action equation defining the relationship of [H+], [HCO_3^-], and the PCO_2:

$$[H^+] = \frac{PCO_2}{[HCO_3^-]} \times 24$$

This equation is derived from the more familiar Henderson-Hasselbalch equation. One can see that in the setting of metabolic acidosis, in which there is a primary decrease in [HCO_3^-], the [H+] will increase (defining a metabolic acidosis as discussed above). It is also evident that the increase in [H+] in this setting can be ameliorated by concomitantly decreasing the PCO_2. This is exactly what occurs as a result of a *physiologic* increase in ventilation. This situation is properly described as metabolic acidosis with a directionally appropriate respiratory response. It is incorrect to describe the condition as primary metabolic acidosis with secondary respiratory alkalosis. To say that a patient has respiratory alkalosis is to say that a patient has *pathologic* hypoventilation, which is not the case in the situation described above. There are tables and formulas that can be used to calculate the expected respiratory response to a given degree of metabolic acidosis.

If the decrease in PCO_2 in response to the degree of metabolic acidosis is exactly what we would have predicted from the formulas, then the patient is said to have one acid-base disorder: metabolic acidosis. By contrast, if the measured decrease in PCO_2 is more than what would be predicted for the degree of metabolic acidosis, then we can say that the patient has an *additional* (not secondary) acid-base disorder: respiratory alkalosis in addition to metabolic acidosis. In other words, the patient would have a **mixed disorder**, which, incidentally, is very common. If the measured PCO_2 is higher than predicted, then one could say that the patient has an additional respiratory acidosis. Therefore, one should not think in terms of "secondary" acid-base disorders but instead should consider whether there is an entirely appropriate and physiologic response and/or whether there are additional acid-base disorders present.

51. What is a respiratory acidosis?

Respiratory acidosis is a drop in the pH (acidosis) caused by alveolar hypoventilation. The alveolar hypoventilation leads to a rate of secretion of CO_2 that is less than its metabolic production. This net gain in CO_2 causes a rise in the P_aCO_2. The lungs may be subject to diffuse hypoventilation (global alveolar hypoventilation) or only parts of the lungs may be involved (regional alveolar hypoventilation). As can be seen in the Henderson-Hasselbalch equation, any increase in the P_aCO_2, if not accompanied by an increase in $[HCO_3^-]$, will lead to a measurable drop in the pH.

52. How do you treat respiratory acidosis?

The treatment of respiratory acidosis is aimed at the correction of the cause of the hypoventilation. This may involve the treatment of airway obstruction or, in respiratory failure, even mechanical ventilation.

53. What is a respiratory alkalosis?

Respiratory alkalosis, the opposite of respiratory acidosis, is a rise in pH (alkalosis). It is due to alveolar hyperventilation, which in turn leads to an increase in the excretion of CO_2 and a drop in the P_aCO_2.

54. What are the causes of respiratory alkalosis?

Causes of Respiratory Alkalosis

1. Central nervous system stimulation of ventilation:
   a. Physiologic (voluntary, anxiety, fear, fever, pregnancy)
   b. Pathologic (intracranial hemorrhage, cerebrovascular accidents, tumors, brainstem lesions, salicylates)

2. Peripheral stimulation of ventilation:
   a. Reflex hyperventilation due to abnormal lung or chest wall mechanics (pulmonary emboli, myopathies, interstitial lung diseases)
   b. Arterial hypoxemia, high altitudes
   c. Pain
   d. Congestive heart failure, shock of any etiology
   e. Hypothermia

3. Hyperventilation with mechanical ventilation

4. Others:
   a. Severe liver disease
   b. Uremia

55. Are the plasma electrolytes alone (Na⁺, K⁺, Cl⁻, and HCO₃⁻) sufficient to determine a patient's acid-base status?

No. Remember that the regulatory systems of the body work to maintain the pH (or hydrogen ion concentration [H⁺]), and that pH is a function of the ratio of PCO_2 and bicarbonate concentration ([HCO₃⁻]). The pH is not determined by the absolute value of either PCO_2 or [HCO₃⁻] alone. Thus a set of plasma electrolytes demonstrating a normal [HCO₃⁻] does not necessarily indicate a normal acid-base status. Furthermore, a low [HCO₃⁻] and high [Cl⁻] could represent either a metabolic acidosis (probably a nonanion gap acidosis) or a chronic respiratory alkalosis with an appropriate metabolic response (renal lowering of [HCO₃⁻] as a response to the chronically low PCO_2). This is an attempt to maintain a more normal pH. Likewise, a high [HCO₃⁻] with low [Cl⁻] may represent a metabolic alkalosis or a chronic respiratory acidosis with an appropriate metabolic response (renal increase in [HCO₃⁻] in response to chronically high PCO_2) in an attempt to maintain a more normal pH. Note that without an accompanying pH and PCO_2, one cannot tell if an abnormal [HCO₃⁻] is due to a metabolic cause (a metabolic acidosis or alkalosis) or to a metabolic response to a primary respiratory disorder. This illustrates the importance of obtaining arterial blood gases (with a pH and PCO_2) in addition to a [HCO₃⁻] to properly assess a patient's acid-base status.

56. What is meant by the anion gap?

The anion gap represents the difference between the routinely measured cations and anions in the plasma. It is usually calculated as follows: ([Na⁺]) – ([Cl⁻] + [HCO₃⁻]). Since electroneutrality is always maintained in solution, there is no actual anion "gap." This "gap" is composed predominantly of negatively charged proteins in plasma and averages 12 (±3) mEq/L. An increase in this quantity is most commonly caused by addition of an acid salt (H⁺A⁻), which reduces plasma bicarbonate concentration by titration. Electroneutrality is maintained in the face of the reduced plasma bicarbonate concentration by the accompanying anion. Since the anion is not measured routinely in the electrolyte profile, the routine measurement would reveal only decreased bicarbonate concentration. With plasma sodium and chloride remaining unchanged, this reduced bicarbonate concentration leads to an increased anion gap. Note that the anion gap would not change if the added acid were HCl. Other circumstances that can increase the anion gap include increased protein concentration and alkalemia, which increase the net negative charge on plasma proteins. The presence of a large quantity of cationic (positively charged) proteins, as with multiple myeloma, can reduce the anion gap.

57. What is the conceptual difference between an anion gap and a non-anion gap metabolic acidosis?

An anion gap acidosis is caused by the addition of a nonvolatile acid to the extracellular fluid. Examples include diabetic ketoacidosis, lactic acidosis, and uremic acidosis. A non-anion gap acidosis commonly (but not exclusively) represents a loss of bicarbonate. Examples include lower GI losses from diarrhea and urinary losses due to renal tubular acidosis. Therefore, when approaching a patient with an anion gap acidosis one should look for the source and identity of the acid gained. By contrast, when evaluating a patient with a non-anion gap metabolic acidosis, one should begin by looking for the source of bicarbonate loss.

58. What are the causes of anion gap metabolic acidosis?

Causes of an Increased Anion Gap Metabolic Acidosis

Ketoacidosis	Uremia	Paraldehyde
Diabetes	Lactic acidosis	Ethylene glycol
Alcoholism	Toxins	Methanol
Starvation	Salicylates	

59. What is the differential diagnosis of metabolic acidosis?

The mnemonic "KUSMAL" can be used to remember the differential diagnosis of metabolic acidosis. It stands for the following:

Ketones (diabetic, alcohol, starvation)
Uremia
Salicylates
Methyl alcohol
Acid poisoning (ethylene glycol, paraldehyde)
Lactate (circulatory/respiratory failure, sepsis, liver disease, tumors, toxins)

Morganroth ML: An analytical approach to the diagnosis of acid-base disorders. J Crit Illness 5:138–150, 1990.

60. What are the common causes of a normal anion gap metabolic acidosis?

Causes of a Non-anion Gap Metabolic Acidosis

Associated with K⁺ loss:	**Drugs:**
Diarrhea	Acetazolamide
Renal tubular acidosis	Amphotericin B
Proximal	Amiloride
Distal	Spironolactone
Interstitial nephritis	Toluene ingestion
Early renal failure	**Ureteral diversions:**
Urinary tract obstruction	Ureterosigmoidostomy
Post-hypocapnia	Dual bladder
Infusions of HCl	Ileal ureter
HCl	
Arginine HCl	
Lysine HCl	

(Adapted from Toto RD: Metabolic acid-base disorders. In Kokko UP, Tannen RL (eds): Fluids and Electrolytes, 2nd ed. Philadelphia, W.B. Saunders, 1990, p 326, with permission.)

61. What causes decreased anion gap?

There are certain disorders that are associated with an anion gap lower than normal. This can be due to an increase in **unmeasured cations** like K^+, Ca^{++}, or Mg^{++}, the addition of **abnormal cations** (lithium), or an increase in **cationic immunoglobulins** (plasma cell dyscrasias). It can also be decreased by loss of unmeasured anions like albumin (serum hypoalbuminemia) or if the effective negative charge (on albumin) is decreased by severe acidosis.

62. What is renal tubular acidosis (RTA)?

This term refers to a disorder of tubular function in which the kidney has a compromised ability to excrete acid and/or recover filtered bicarbonate in the setting of higher than normal $[H^+]$ in the ECF. The laboratory presentation is that of a non-anion gap metabolic acidosis. Traditionally, RTA is classified as types I, II, and IV.

Type I or distal (so-called classic) RTA is characterized by reduced net proton secretion by the distal nephron in the setting of systemic acidemia. Since the distal nephron is largely responsible for net acid excretion, patients with this disorder have continuous net acid retention (they have less net acid excretion than net acid production) and are therefore *not* in net acid balance. The diagnosis is made by demonstrating an inappropriately alkaline urine (pH > 5.5) in the setting of an acidemic serum (pH < 7.36) and excluding the presence of drugs that alkalinize the urine (acetazolamide) or urea-splitting bacteria in the urine that can increase the urinary pH.

Type II or proximal RTA is characterized by a reduced capacity for bicarbonate recovery by the proximal tubule but intact distal nephron function. These patients waste bicarbonate in the urine until the ECF concentration of bicarbonate is reduced to a level such that the reduced filtered load of bicarbonate (GFR × plasma bicarbonate concentration) can now be more completely reabsorbed and the urine becomes nearly bicarbonate-free. The reduction in plasma bicarbonate concentration results in an increase in [H+], but in the steady-state condition of the low plasma bicarbonate concentration (as described above) these patients can excrete an appropriately acid urine (pH < 5.5) because distal nephron function is intact. In addition, because of the intact distal nephron function, these patients are able to excrete the acid load produced from metabolism and are thus in acid balance (the amount of acid excreted = amount of acid produced), unlike the situation described for type I.

Type III RTA represents a variant of type I, so the term has been abandoned.

Type IV RTA is characterized by reduced aldosterone effect on the renal tubules, which may result in insufficient secretion of acid necessary to maintain normal acid-base status. These patients nevertheless can excrete an appropriately acid urine in the face of acidemic stress. Unlike the prior disorders described, type IV RTA is commonly associated with hyperkalemia due to a coexisting reduction in potassium secretion. This disorder is commonly seen in patients with hyporenin-hypoaldosteronism but is also seen in isolated aldosterone deficiency and resistance.

63. How are the common types of renal tubular acidosis managed?

Type I (distal) RTA is treated with alkali in amounts necessary to correct the acidosis and to buffer the acid being retained. Potassium supplements are commonly required at the initiation of treatment but are less commonly required in the steady-state treatment once the acidosis has been corrected.

Type II (proximal) RTA does not usually require alkali treatment in adult patients, because they do not have net acid retention and have only mild acidemia. The chronic acidemia inhibits bone growth in children and so type II RTA must be treated with alkali in children with this disorder. Large amounts of alkali are required as well as large potassium supplements (the increased urinary bicarbonate losses are accompanied by accelerated urinary potassium losses).

Type IV RTA is usually characterized by mild, clinically less important degrees of acidemia and therefore rarely requires alkali treatment. It is the associated hyperkalemia that is more commonly a clinical concern and dictates whether mineralocorticoid replacements with synthetic steroids are required.

64. What is lactic acidosis and what are its causes?

Lactic acidosis is due to the accumulation of lactic acid, the end product of glycolysis. This accumulation leads to a depletion of the body's buffers and a drop in the pH. Lactate, being an unmeasured anion, makes this one of the causes of an increased anion gap acidosis.

Lactic acidosis results from the following basic mechanisms:

1. **Cellular hypoxia:** Oxygen is required for the oxidative phosphorylation of the lactic acid produced by glycolysis. Anything that interferes with the available cellular supply of oxygen, or its utilization, will lead to the accumulation of lactic acid. This category includes respiratory failure, circulatory failure, and carbon monoxide poisoning.

2. **Decreased hepatic utilization of lactic acid:** This is seen in advanced hepatocellular insufficiency of any cause.

3. **Cyanide poisoning:** Cyanide causes increased lactic acid production because it blocks oxidative phosphorylation, leading to increased glycolysis, decreased utilization of lactic acid, and therefore lactic acid accumulation.

4. **Alcohol consumption:** Alcohol causes a modest increase in the production of lactic acid. In association with caloric depletion, the lactic acidosis can be severe.

5. **Neoplasms with a large tumor burden:** Neoplasms can lead to increased production of lactic acid, even with sufficient oxygen, since the tumor cells can have higher rates of glycolysis than normal cells.

6. **Diabetic ketoacidosis (DKA):** is associated with increased lactic acid levels even in the absence of shock or other etiologies.

7. **Lactic acidosis X:** This is a condition in which severe lactic acidosis occurs without obvious cause.

8. **Factitious lactic acidosis:** This occurs when blood is drawn and then stored for prolonged periods of time. The red and white cells generate the lactic acid in the tube as it is stored. It is most commonly seen in patients with high white blood cell counts.

65. What is metabolic alkalosis?

Metabolic alkalosis is a disorder characterized by a directional decrease in $[H^+]$ from metabolic causes. It results from addition of excess bicarbonate or alkali, or loss of acid. Note that a low chloride and a high bicarbonate concentration can result from both metabolic alkalosis as well as from a metabolic response to a respiratory acidosis (as noted above). However, the pH and P_aCO_2 help to differentiate these two disorders.

66. What are the common causes of metabolic alkalosis?

The following classification not only lists causes of metabolic alkalosis but also encompasses some diagnostic and therapeutic implications. Those forms of alkalosis responsive to chloride salt administration are generally associated with extracellular fluid volume depletion and low urinary chloride concentration in spot urine tests, whereas the chloride-unresponsive alkaloses are associated with ECF volume expansion and urine $[Cl^-] > 20$ mEq/L.

Causes of Metabolic Alkalosis

CHLORIDE RESPONSIVE (Urine $[Cl^-] < 10$ mEq/L)	CHLORIDE RESISTANT (Urine $[Cl^-] > 20$ mEq/L)
Gastric fluid loss	Primary aldosteronism
Postdiuretic therapy	Primary reninism
Posthypercapnia	Hyperglucocorticoidism
Congenital chloride diarrhea	Hypercalcemia
	Potassium depletion
	Liddle's syndrome
	Bartter's syndrome
	Chloruretic diuretics

(From Toto RD: Metabolic acid-base disorders. In Kokko UP, Tannen RL (eds): Fluids and Electrolytes, 2nd ed. Philadelphia, W.B. Saunders, 1990, p 356, with permission.)

67. What is the commonest acid-base disturbance in cirrhosis of the liver?

Primary respiratory alkalosis due to centrally mediated hyperventilation is the most common acid-base disturbance in patients with severe hepatic disease, especially with superimposed encephalopathy. The exact etiology is unclear but may be related to the hormonal imbalance associated with liver failure. Estrogens and progesterone have been implicated, a situation somewhat similar to that seen in pregnancy.

CALCIUM, PHOSPHATE, AND MAGNESIUM METABOLISM

68. How is calcium distributed in the body?

A 70-kg man has approximately 1000 grams of calcium in his body. Of this, bone contains 99% of the total calcium, whereas only 1% is in the extracellular and intracellular fluid. Furthermore, only about 1% of skeletal calcium is freely exchangeable with extracellular fluid calcium.

69. How is calcium distributed in the serum?

The routine measurement for serum calcium (normal = 9–10 mg/ml = 4.5–5.0 mEq/L = 2.25–2.5 mM/L) measures total calcium. Approximately 40% of this is protein-bound, 5–10% is complexed to other substances (like phosphate and sulfate), and 50% is ionized.

70. Why is it important to recognize the differences between ionized and protein-bound calcium?

It is the ionized fraction of calcium that determines the activity of this electrolyte with respect to cellular and membrane function. It is possible to vary the concentration of total calcium without changing the ionized fraction by changing the protein concentration. By contrast, it is also possible to vary the ionized fraction without changing the total concentration by changing serum pH. Increasing serum pH decreases the ionized fraction of calcium and vice versa.

71. What are the major sites of calcium reabsorption in the nephron?

About 50% of the filtered calcium is reabsorbed in the proximal tubule and most of the remainder (about 40% of the total) is reabsorbed in the loop of Henle. An important site of loop reabsorption is the ascending limb of the loop of Henle. A small amount of calcium is reabsorbed in the distal convoluted tubule and an even smaller amount in the collecting tubule.

72. What are the major hormones involved in calcium metabolism?

These hormones are parathyroid hormone (PTH), vitamin D, and calcitonin. PTH is secreted in response to a decrease in serum calcium and promotes calcium reabsorption from bone, because it enhances renal reabsorption of calcium and excretion of phosphate. Low serum calcium concentration stimulates 1-hydroxylation of 25–hydroxy-vitmanin D by the kidney to form 1,25-dihydroxy-vitamin D (the active form of vitamin D). This hormone promotes calcium reabsorption from the gut and mineralization of bone. Increases in serum calcium lead to increased secretion of calcitonin. This hormone inhibits bone reabsorption and 1–hydroxylation of 25–hydroxy-vitamin D, and thereby ameliorates hypercalcemia.

73. What are some factors that affect renal calcium excretion?

With some exceptions, renal calcium handling varies directly with renal sodium handling. Therefore, renal calcium excretion is increased by saline diuresis, loop diuretics, and volume expansion. In contrast, renal calcium excretion is decreased in volume depletion and other states associated with renal salt retention. One notable exception to this general rule is that the natriuresis associated with thiazide diuretics is accompanied by decreased rather than increased urinary calcium excretion.

74. What is meant by pseudohypocalcemia or pseudohypercalcemia?

These terms refer to an alteration of the total calcium concentration in the setting of a normal ionized fraction. Since the ionized fraction is normal, these patients are asymptomatic. Abnormalities in the concentration of serum proteins are a common cause of these disorders.

75. How do you correct the total serum calcium level for changes in the serum albumin?
Hypoalbuminemia will cause a decrease in the total serum calcium level without a change in the level of ionized calcium. For each decrease of 1.0 g/dl in serum albumin, one should expect a drop in the total serum calcium of approximately 0.8 mg/dl.

76. What are some common causes of true hypocalcemia?
Common causes of true hypocalcemia include hypoparathyroidism (usually following thyroid or parathyroid surgery), vitamin D deficiency, magnesium depletion (usually at levels less than 0.8 mEq/L), liver disease (decreased synthesis of 25–hydroxy-vitamin D), renal disease (hyperphosphatemia and decreased synthesis of 1,25-dihydroxy-vitamin D), acute pancreatitis, the tumor lysis syndrome, and rhabdomyolysis.

77. What are some common causes of true hypercalcemia?
Common causes of true hypercalcemia include primary hyperparathyroidism (approximately 50% of cases), malignancy, use of thiazide diuretics, vitamin D excess, hyper- and hypo-thyroidism, granulomatous disorders, immobilization, and milk-alkali syndrome.

78. What are the signs and symptoms of hypocalcemia?
The symptoms of hypocalcemia are dependent on the severity of the decrease in serum calcium, the rate of the drop, and its duration. The symptoms of hypocalcemia are due to the resultant decrease in the excitation threshold of neural tissue. This causes an increase in excitability, repetitive responses to a single stimulus, reduced accommodation, or even continuous activity of neural tissue. The varied symptoms and signs include:

Signs and Symptoms of Hypocalcemia

Tetany and paresthesias	QT interval prolongation on the ECG
Altered mental status (lethargy to coma)	Increased intracranial pressure
Seizures	Lenticular cataracts

79. What are Trousseau's sign and Chevostek's sign seen in hypocalcemia?
Both of these signs are indications of the latent tetany caused by hypocalcemia. Of the two signs, Trousseau's is more specific and reliable. They are demonstrated as follows:
   1. **Trousseau's sign:** A sphygmomanometer is placed on the arm and inflated to greater than systolic blood pressure, and left in place for at least 2 minutes. A positive response is carpal spasm of the ipsilateral arm. Relaxation will take 5–10 seconds after the pressure is released.
   2. **Chevostek's sign:** Tap the facial nerve between the corner of the mouth and the zygomatic arch. A positive response is twitching of the ipsilateral facial muscle, especially the angle of the mouth. This sign may be seen in 10–25% of normal adult patients.

80. What are the symptoms and signs of hypercalcemia?
Symptoms of hypercalcemia include weakness, constipation, nausea, anorexia, polyuria, polydipsia, and pruritus. Severe hypercalcemia may present with progressive CNS symptoms of lethargy, depression, obtundation, coma, and seizures. Rapid onset of a high calcium level is more likely to be symptomatic than a slowly progressive level, regardless of the ultimate level at presentation.

81. Describe the appropriate treatment for hypercalcemia.
The treatment of hypercalcemia depends on the level of calcium and the symptoms of the patient. Acute, symptomatic hypercalcemia should be treated aggressively, first with saline infusion to expedite calcium excretion. Most patients with hypercalcemia are significantly volume-depleted as a result of the osmotic diuresis related to the hypercalciuria.

1. **Normal saline** should be given at a rapid rate, 300 or more ml/hr, with KCL and possibly magnesium added to the solution, depending on measured blood values. After the patient is adequately volume repleted, furosemide may be given to promote calciuresis. Care must be taken to keep input equal to or greater than output, to avoid making the patient hypovolemic again.

2. **Mithramycin** is effective when the patient cannot tolerate large fluid loads due to congestive heart failure or third-space losses, or if there is an inadequate response to IV volume replacement. It should be given at a dose of $15\mu g/kg$ (i.e., 1–2 mg) IVSS for one dose. The dose can be repeated if necessary, but doses more frequent than once every 3 to 7 days have been associated with renal and hepatic toxicity. Mithramycin can also cause a coagulopathy, which can lead to serious bleeding complications.

3. **Calcitonin** is a useful agent for decreasing serum calcium and has the added advantage of rapid onset of action. It may be given in the presence of renal insufficiency, thrombocytopenia, or when mithramycin is contraindicated. Its disadvantage is that rapid resistance to the drug is often encountered, probably related to the development of antibodies. This resistance can sometimes be delayed by concomitant administration of prednisone, given either as an IV infusion over 24 hours or subcutaneously.

4. **Diphosphonates** inhibit osteoclast activity and are effective with those cancers in which this mechanism is present. They are given as an IV infusion over 5 days and are now available as an oral tablet. Less significant levels of hypercalcemia can be treated with other agents, such as glucocorticoids (prednisone 20–40 mg/d), phosphates (1–6 g/d), prostaglandin inhibitors (aspirin and nonsteroidal anti-inflammatory drugs [NSAIDs]), or oral diphosphonates. All of these agents are less effective but may suffice for chronic maintenance.

82. What are the major sites of phosphate reabsorption in the nephron?
Phosphate is reabsorbed predominantly in the proximal tubule with small amounts being absorbed in the distal tubule.

83. What are some factors that can increase urinary phosphate excretion?
PTH, alkalosis, saline diuresis, ketoacidosis, and increased dietary phosphate intake.

84. What are some factors that can lower serum phosphate concentration by shifting this ion into cells?
Some of these factors include insulin, glucose (by stimulating insulin secretion), and alkalosis.

85. In which clinical situations can you see hypophosphatemia?
The clinical circumstances of hypophosphatemia are listed below:

1. **Decreased dietary intake:**
   a. Decreased intestinal absorption due to vitamin D deficiency, malabsorption, steatorrhea, secretory diarrhea, vomiting, or phosphate-binders
   b. Alcoholism
2. **Shifts from serum into cells:**
   a. Respiratory alkalosis as seen in sepsis, heat stroke, hepatic coma, salicylate poisoning, gout, etc.
   b. Recovery from hypothermia
   c. Hormonal effects of insulin, glucagon, androgens, etc. (recovery from diabetic ketoacidosis)
   d. Carbohydrate administration (hyperalimentation, fructose or glucose infusions)
3. **Increased excretion into the urine:**
   a. Hyperparathyroidism

    b. Renal tubule defects as in aldosteronism, inappropriate secretion of ADH, mineralocorticoid hormone administration, diuretics, corticosteroids

    c. Hypomagnesemia

4. **Spurious**

    a. Mannitol infusion

86. What are the main disturbances thought to be responsible for the abnormalities of calcium and phosphate metabolism seen with progressive renal disease?

Patients with progressive renal disease develop hyperphosphatemia, hypocalcemia, and secondary hyperparathyroidism. They are also at risk of developing at least two kinds of bone disease. The main disturbances that contribute to these abnormalities are:

    1. A rise in inorganic phosphate concentration in the serum due to poor renal excretion. This leads to a decrease in serum calcium concentration and stimulation of PTH secretion. The increased PTH secretion leads to increased bone resorption and osteitis fibrosa cystica.

    2. Resistance to the action of vitamin D. One function of this hormone is to promote calcium reabsorption from the gut. Decreased gut reabsorption of calcium exacerbates the hypocalcemia and reduces available calcium for bone mineralization.

    3. Defective synthesis of 1,25 dihydroxy-vitamin D, the active form of this hormone. Reduced levels of 1,25 dihydroxy-vitamin D results in defective bone mineralization (osteomalacia in adults, rickets in children).

87. How does magnesium depletion affect calcium and phosphate metabolism?

Magnesium depletion results in decreased secretion and end-organ responsiveness of PTH. This leads to functional hypoparathyroidism and the resultant effects on the serum level and urinary excretion of calcium and phosphate. This disorder can be corrected with magnesium repletion.

88. What are the major nephron sites for magnesium reabsorption?

Magnesium is reabsorbed predominantly in the thick ascending limb of the loop of Henle with a smaller amount being reabsorbed in the proximal tubule.

89. What are some common causes of magnesium deficiency?

Some common causes of significant magnesium deficiency include:

- Dietary insufficiency (decreased intake, protein-caloric malnutrition, and prolonged intravenous feeding)
- Intestinal malabsorption
- Chronic loss of GI fluids
- Diuretics
- Other drugs (gentamicin, cisplatin, pentamidine, cyclosporin)
- Alcoholism
- Hyperparathyroidism
- Lactation

90. What is the milk-alkali syndrome?

The milk-alkali syndrome is the presence of hypercalcemia, increased BUN and serum creatinine, increased serum phosphate, and metabolic alkalosis in a patient ingesting large quantities of milk and calcium-carbonate-containing antacids. The patients usually present with nausea, vomiting, anorexia, weakness, polydipsia, and polyuria. If it continues, metastatic calcification can occur, leading to mental status changes, nephrocalcinosis, band keratopathy, pruritus, and myalgias. The treatment is withdrawal of the milk and antacid.

BIBLIOGRAPHY

1. Brenner BM, Rector FC (eds): The Kidney. 4th ed. Philadelphia, W.B. Saunders, 1991.
2. Haperin ML, Goldstein M: Acid-Base, Fluid and Electrolyte Emergencies. Philadelphia, W.B. Saunders, 1986.
3. Seldin DW, Giebisch G (eds): The Regulation of Acid-Base Balance. New York, Raven Press, 1989.
4. Suki WN, Massry SG (eds): Therapy of Renal Diseases and Related Disorders. Boston, Martinus Nijhoff, 1984.
5. Wyngaarden JB, Smith LH (eds): Cecil Textbook of Medicine, 18th ed. Philadelphia, W.B. Saunders, 1988.

9. HEMATOLOGY SECRETS

Mark M. Udden, M.D.

Blood is the originating cause of all men's diseases.

The Talmud
Baba Nathra, III.58a

The blood is the life.

The Bible
Deuteronomy 12:23

HYPOPROLIFERATIVE ANEMIAS

1. What are the two most helpful laboratory investigations in the initial evaluation of anemia?

The **reticulocyte count** and review of the **peripheral blood film** are the basis of a methodical approach to anemia. The peripheral blood film will demonstrate whether or not important abnormalities of red blood cell (RBC) shape, size, or hemoglobinization exist. In addition, an impression of the white blood cell (WBC) count and platelet count can be obtained. RBCs must also be examined for the presence of inclusions (such as Howell-Jolly bodies).

2. What are reticulocytes and why is their count important?

Reticulocytes are young RBCs newly released from the marrow that are detected by their lacy network of RNA, which can be precipitated by basic dyes such as new methylene blue. If the reticulocyte count is high, then blood loss or hemolysis is likely to be the cause of anemia. If the reticulocyte count is low, a primary marrow disorder (hypoproliferative anemia) should be considered. Thus, the reticulocyte count helps to determine whether or not the bone marrow's response to anemia is appropriate. The reticulocyte count is usually reported as a percentage of 1000 cells counted. This may be adjusted to reflect the degree of anemia and length of time a reticulocyte matures. In severe anemia reticulocytes are released early and circulate longer.

Physiologic Classification of Anemia

RETICULOCYTE COUNT LOW	RETICULOCYTE COUNT HIGH
Hypoproliferative anemia	Blood loss
	Response to treatment of iron, folate, or B_{12} deficiency
	Hemolysis

Perrotta AL, Finch CA: The polychromatophilic erythrocyte. Am J Clin Path 57:471–477, 1972.

3. How are the mean cell volume (MCV) and the red cell distribution width (RDW) used in the evaluation of anemias?

The complete blood count (CBC) now includes the MCV, and many clinical laboratories also determine an index of the heterogeneity of cell size, the RDW. In iron deficiency anemia (IDA), for example, RBCs have been produced during periods of iron sufficiency and varying degrees of deficiency, so cell size in IDA is more heterogenous than that of a person with thalassemia minor whose cells are all small. This results in a larger RDW for IDA and a normal RDW for thalassemia.

A classification scheme of anemias based on the MCV and RDW has been developed by Bessman:

Classification of Anemias Based on MCV and RDW

MCV LOW		MCV NORMAL		MCV HIGH	
RDW NORMAL	RDW HIGH	RDW NORMAL	RDW HIGH	RDW NORMAL	RDW HIGH
Chronic disease	Iron deficiency	Normal	Early or mixed nutritional deficiency	Aplastic anemia	Folate or vitamin B$_{12}$ deficiency
Nonanemic heterozygous thalassemia	Hb S-α or β thalassemia	Chronic disease	Anemic abnormal hemoglobin		Sickle cell anemia ($^1/_3$ of cases)
Children	Hb H	Nonanemic hemoglobin or enzyme abnormality	Myelofibrosis		Immune hemolytic anemia
		Splenectomy	Sideroblastic		Cold agglutinins
		CLL (except extreme high lymphocyte number)	Myelodysplasia		Preleukemia
		Acute blood loss			Newborn

Note: Chronic liver disease, chronic myelogenous leukemia, and cytotoxic chemotherapy may be associated with high or normal MCV, and high or normal RDW.
(From Bessman JD: Automated Blood Counts and Differentials: A Practical Guide. Baltimore, Johns Hopkins University Press, 1986, p 11, with permission.)

4. What are the causes of hypochromic, microcytic anemias, and how are iron studies used in their differentiation?

Hypochromic, microcytic anemias are the most frequently encountered anemias in hospitalized and ambulatory patients. A working knowledge of these anemias and their laboratory diagnosis is essential to avoid wasting time and resources.

Causes of Hypochromic, Microcytic Anemias

	NORMAL	IDA*	ANEMIA OF CHRONIC DISEASE	SIDERO-BLASTIC ANEMIA	THALASSEMIA
Serum iron (μg/dl)	115 (70–180)	<30	30 (15–65)	>180	Normal or elevated
TIBC* (μg/ml)	340	>400	200	250	250
Transferrin saturation (%)	35 (25–50)	<16	15 (10–40)	80 (60–100)	Normal or elevated
Marrow hemosiderin	2+	0	3+	4+	2+ to 4+
Serum ferritin	Normal	Decreased	Slightly elevated	Elevated	Normal or elevated

*IDA = iron deficiency anemia; TIBC = total iron-binding capacity.

Note that a bone marrow examination in sideroblastic anemia shows increased iron stores and abnormal iron distribution in ringed sideroblasts. Both IDA and anemia of chronic disease (ACD) have a low transferrin saturation. In IDA the TIBC is often increased, whereas ACD is marked by an unusually low TIBC. Iron stores are usually normal in thalassemia-minor, although beta-thalassemia major may be a disorder complicated by iron overload.

Beutler E: The common anemias. JAMA 259:2433, 1988.

5. Summarize the symptoms and signs of iron deficiency.

Patients may have the symptoms of **anemia:** fatigue, dyspnea on exertion, and, in certain cases in which underlying cardiac disease exists, signs of congestive heart failure (CHF) or angina. However, in many cases the anemia develops insidiously and is well tolerated. Iron deficiency is associated with **pica.** Adults may crave ice, starch, or even dirt. Iron-deficient children in older neighborhoods may eat lead-containing paint chips, leading to the association of iron deficiency and **plumbism.** Iron deficiency is also associated with **esophageal webs** (sometimes causing dysphagia), **painless stomatitis,** and **spooning of the fingernails** (koilonychia).

6. In the treatment of IDA, how much iron should be administered, in what form, and for how long?

Iron is best given as ferrous sulfate in a formulation that does not include enteric coating. Typically, patients take 325 mg PO TID until the anemia corrects and for several months thereafter. This provides 60 mg of elemental iron per tablet, or 180 mg per day. Of this, 18–36 mg can be absorbed and utilized by an otherwise unimpaired marrow. When a low serum ferritin value is used to make the diagnosis of iron deficiency, the ferritin can be checked to verify that iron stores have increased with therapy. In some instances patients improve but do not fully correct their anemia. If the ferritin has normalized, another cause of anemia (i.e., coexistent thalassemia minor) should be sought. A useful guide to success is the occurrence of reticulocytosis about 10 days after initiation of iron therapy.

7. What are common causes of iron deficiency?

Iron deficiency results from dietary causes, malabsorption, chronic blood loss, and chronic intravascular hemolysis. The last-mentioned is usually seen in the rare stem cell disorder **paroxysmal nocturnal hemoglobinuria** (PNH) or in patients with malfunctioning cardiac valves. Examination of a urine sediment stained for iron discloses iron-laden tubular cells **(hemosiderosis).**

Common Causes of Iron Deficiency

1. Chronic blood loss
    Gastrointestinal (GI): gastritis, peptic ulcer disease (PUD), GI varices,
        GI malignancy, polyps, diverticulosis, telangiectasia (Osler-Weber-Rendu
        disease, scleroderma), angiodysplasia
    Menstrual loss and pregnancy
2. Dietary deficiency (infants)
3. Malabsorption: sprue, postgastrectomy patients
4. Other: chronic intravascular hemolysis, idiopathic pulmonary hemosiderosis

8. What are the causes and consequences of iron overload?

Iron overload results from chronic administration of iron to non-iron deficient persons, chronic transfusion therapy, hemochromatosis, and in patients with thalassemia major and certain refractory anemias such as sideroblastic anemia.

Iron overload has many effects: including:
1. Cardiomyopathy, arrhythmias
2. Hepatic dysfunction and cirrhosis
3. Hepatoma
4. Endocrine dysfunction (hypothyroidism, hypogonadotrophic hypogonadism, hyperpigmentation, diabetes mellitus)
5. Arthropathy (chondrocalcinosis, synovial fluid containing calcium pyrophosphate or hydroxyapatite crystals)
6. Osteopenia and subcortical cysts
7. Peripheral neuropathy

When hereditary hemochromatosis is identified, screening of relatives can detect young individuals at risk, who may then be saved considerable morbidity.

Basset ML, et al: Diagnosis of hemochromatosis in young subjects: Predictive accuracy of biochemical screening tests. Gastroenterology 87:628, 1984.

9. When is it appropriate to order a hemoglobin electrophoresis to evaluate hypochromic, microcytic anemia?

This is best done when iron stores are established as being normal. The microcytic disorders that may be detected are beta-thalassemia minor and the so-called thalassemic hemoglobinopathies (including hemoglobin E in Asians). Beta-thalassemia minor is marked by an increased hemoglobin A2 and sometimes increased fetal hemoglobin. Iron deficiency results in a decreased pool of alpha chains for which the beta chain of hemoglobin A and the gamma chain of hemoglobin A2 must compete. The beta chains are more successful, resulting in diminished hemoglobin A2 during iron deficiency. For this reason a search for β-thalassemia may be thwarted when patients are also iron deficient.

10. Which diseases are usually associated with "the anemia of chronic disorders (ACD)"?

The ACD is typified by a low serum iron, low TIBC, low % saturation, but increased iron stores, as evidenced by an increased ferritin. Traditionally, ACD is associated with inflammatory states, including malignancy, rheumatologic disease, and infection. However, a recent study of hospitalized patients shows that the laboratory pattern of ACD occurs in a significant number of anemic patients who do not have inflammatory conditions. These patients were severely ill with complications of diabetes, renal failure, and hypertension.

Cash JM, Sears DA: The anemia of chronic disease: Spectrum of associated disease in a series of unselected hospitalized patients. Am J Med 87:638, 1989.

11. What are the causes of macrocytosis, or a large mean cell volume (MCV)?

Macrocytosis is not always associated with folate or vitamin B_{12} deficiency. Macro-ovalocytic RBCs are much more specific for folate or vitamin B_{12} deficiency.

Causes of Macrocytosis

Megaloblastic anemia (macro-ovalocytosis)	Sideroblastic anemia*
Alcoholism	Chronic obstructive pulmonary disease
Malignancy	(COPD)
Hemolysis (usually poorly compensated)	Artifacts and idiopathic
Aplastic anemia	Pregnancy
Hypothyroidism	Liver disease
Refractory anemias (myelodysplasia)	

*Often marked by dual populations of RBCs—one hypochromic, microcytic and the other macrocytic.

12. How are folate and vitamin B_{12} deficiency states recognized? How do they differ?

Common features of B_{12} and folate deficiency are those of megaloblastic anemia:

1. **Marrow:** A hyperplastic marrow demonstrating a markedly ineffective erythropoiesis is usually seen. Megaloblastic RBCs with open, granular nuclei, and mature cytoplasm or nuclear-cytoplasmic asynchrony are also evident. Giant metamyelocytes are also found.

2. **Peripheral blood:** Macro-ovalocytosis with occasional Howell-Jolly bodies and basophilic stippling are present. Hypersegmented neutrophils and a variable degree of neutropenia and thrombocytopenia may also be present.

3. **Megaloblastic changes:** These changes occur in rapidly proliferative cells of the mouth, gut, small intestine, and cervix. They may show immature-looking nuclei (indeed, some cervical Pap smears are mistakenly read as atypical or malignant).

Distinguishing Features of Folate vs B₁₂ (Cobalamin) Deficiency

FEATURE	B_{12}	FOLATE
Neurologic disease	Subacute, combined systems	None, or associated with alcohol
Diet	Normal	Alcoholism, junk food, "tea and toast"; no green, leafy vegetables
Serum folate level	Normal	Low
RBC folate level	Low or normal	Low
Response to physiologic dose of folate (200 μg/d)	Absent*	Present
Urine formiminoglutamic acid	Absent	Increased
Serum methylmalonic acid and homocysteine levels	Increased	Absent

*Pharmacologic dose of folate (1 mg/d) can correct the anemia, but may exacerbate the neurological symptoms.
Babior BM: The megaloblastic anemias. In Williams WJ, et al (eds): Hematology, 4th ed. New York, McGraw-Hill, 1990.

13. How is B₁₂ absorbed from the diet?

The absorption of cobalamins (B₁₂) is described in the figure below:

Cobalamins are released from food into the gastric lumen, where they are taken up by R binder. In the duodenum, the R binder-Cbl complexes are digested by pancreatic proteases, once again liberating the cobalamins, which this time are taken up by protease-resistant IF molecules originally secreted by the gastric parietal cells. The IF-Cbl complexes migrate down the small intestine until they reach the ileum, where they are transported into the epithelial cells by means of specific receptors. After several hours' sojourn in the epithelial cells, the cobalamins, now complexed to TC II, are delivered into the portal circulation. (From Babior, BM: Metabolic aspects of folic acid and cobalamin. In Williams WJ, et al (eds): Hematology, 4th ed. New York, McGraw-Hill, 1990, p 349, with permission.)

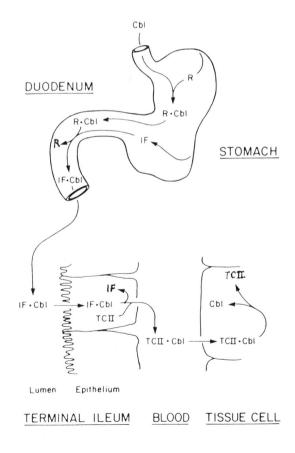

14. What processes may interrupt B_{12} absorption?

Causes of B_{12} Deficiency

1. Pernicious anemia associated with gastric atrophy and loss of intrinsic factor due to an autoimmune-mediated attack on the gastric mucosa.
2. Postgastrectomy: after total gastrectomy, megaloblastic anemia develops 5–6 years later.
3. Disorders of the small intestine: ileal resection, Crohn's disease, sprue.
4. Competition with intestinal flora: blind-loop syndrome, tapeworm (*Diphyllobothrium latum*).
5. Pancreatic disease: deficiency of R-binders with chronic pancreatitis.
6. Dietary: strict vegetarians (no meat or eggs or milk), breast-fed infants of strict vegetarians.

15. What is the pattern of neurologic disease associated with B_{12} deficiency? Is the severity of anemia a good predictor of neurologic involvement?

B_{12} deficiency is associated with the findings of combined systems disease:

1. Posterior column (paresthesias, disturbed vibratory sense, loss of proprioception)
2. Pyramidal (spastic weakness, hyperactive reflexes)
3. Cerebral (dementia, psychosis [megaloblastic madness], optic atrophy)

Folate deficiency may be associated with peripheral neuropathy in alcoholics. Of interest is the lack of correlation between severity of anemia and neurologic manifestations of B_{12} deficiency. A recent study suggests that a significant minority of patients with peripheral neuropathy or other neurological manifestations of B_{12} deficiency have a normal hematocrit and MCV, but low or low-normal B_{12} levels. It is possible that serum methylmalonic acidemia and homocystinemia are better indicators.

Lindebaum J, et al: Neuropsychiatric disorders caused by cobalamin deficiency in the absence of anemia or macrocytosis. N Engl J Med 318:1720, 1988.

16. When are a bone marrow biopsy and aspirate indicated?

Bone marrow biopsy and aspiration are a safe and easily performed procedure and are particularly helpful in the evaluation of pancytopenia, thrombocytopenia, neutropenia, and in the evaluation of hypoproliferative anemia. Because of the high prevalence of IDA and anemia of chronic disease, a hypoproliferative (low reticulocyte count) anemia need not always require bone marrow biopsy if iron studies are consistent. The diagnosis of a sideroblastic anemia requires a bone marrow study to demonstrate the presence of ringed sideroblasts. Other common reasons are outlined below.

Indications for Bone Marrow Biopsy and Aspirate

1. Pancytopenia: myelodysplasia, aplastic anemia, myelophthistic states, hypersplenism, megaloblastic anemia	4. Thrombocytopenia: evaluation of ITP
	5. Neutropenia
2. Anemia: sideroblastic anemia, refractory anemia, pure red cell aplasia	6. Infectious diseases: typhoid, tuberculosis, pancytopenia seen in AIDS, brucellosis
3. Staging of malignancy: Hodgkin's disease, leukemias, non-Hodgkin's lymphoma, small cell carcinoma of the lung, multiple myeloma	7. Lipid storage diseases

17. What are the diagnostic criteria for severe aplastic anemia?

Aplastic anemia is marked by peripheral pancytopenia and a hypocellular bone marrow aspirate. Commonly used criteria for severe aplastic anemia are:

1. Marrow biopsy cellularity less than 25%.
2. Neutrophil counts less than 0.5×10^9/liter.
3. Platelet counts less than 20×10^9/liter.
4. Corrected reticulocyte count less than 1%.

Patients meeting these criteria have a median survival of less than 6 months, with only 20% surviving a year.

Camitta BM, et al: Severe aplastic anemia: A prospective study of the effect of early marrow transplantation on acute morbidity. Blood 46:63, 1976.

18. What is the best therapy for aplastic anemia in a young person?

For patients who are less than age 40, a bone marrow transplantation from an HLA identical sibling is the current standard of care. Increasingly, HLA identical but nonrelated donors may be used for such patients. For nontransfused patients, 80% long-term survival rates have been achieved with transplantation, although this is accompanied in some cases (10–20%) by disabling graft-versus-host disease (GvHD).

19. What alternative treatment is available for aplastic anemia?

Patients who do not have donors or who are otherwise unsuitable bone marrow transplant candidates have been successfully treated with a number of immunosuppressive regimens. The most effective of these has been **antithymocyte globulin** (ATG), which produces remission rates of 40–60%. ATG or **antilymphocyte globulin** (ALG) is administered via a central line in daily doses of 15 to 40 mg/kg for 4 to 10 days. Severe serum sickness and thrombocytopenia are consequences. Patients frequently have partial responses, freeing them from infections or the need for transfusions. Unfortunately, relapses occur in 10% and some patients, although clinically improved at first, develop myelodysplastic syndromes later. Recently, **cyclosporine A** has been employed in the treatment of aplastic anemia with good results.

20. How aggressively should transfusions be employed in the management of young patients with aplastic anemia?

Transfusions of platelets or RBCs are needed when there is life-threatening bleeding in a patient with aplastic anemia. Caution must be exercised in the use of transfusions because they may sensitize the recipient to HLA antigens and reduce dramatically the results of bone marrow transplantation. Thus, transfusions should be limited and relatives should not be used as donors. Because CMV-related disease in the post-transplant period may be lethal, candidates should receive CMV-negative blood products until their CMV status and the status of the donor are known.

Storb R, et al: Marrow transplantation with or without donor buffy coat cells for 65 transfused aplastic anemia patients. Blood 59:236, 1982.

21. Alcoholics admitted to the hospital are frequently anemic. Why?

Causes of Anemia in Alcoholics

Primary bone marrow toxicity of alcohol	Hemolytic anemia
Vacuolated marrow erythroid cells	Hypersplenism
Megaloblastic erythropoiesis due to folate deficiency	Spur cell anemia
	Transient hemolysis with hyperlipemia
Iron deficiency due to hemorrhage	(Zieve's syndrome)
Sideroblastic anemia	Hypophosphatemia

22. How should you carry out an evaluation of anemia in the alcoholic?

Savage and Lindenbaum surveyed alcoholics and found that megaloblastic changes in the marrow were not usually associated with disorderly iron accumulation in the macrophages as is seen in anemia of chronic disorders. They emphasize the multifactorial nature of anemia and offer the following guide to workup:

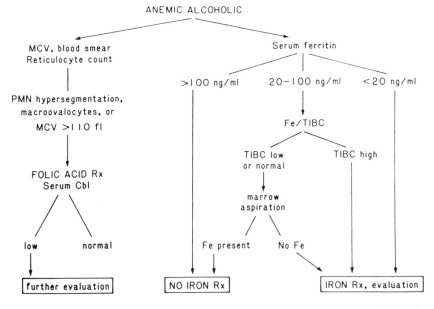

Diagnostic and therapeutic approach to anemia in alcoholics (cbl = cobalamin, Fe = iron, fl = femtoliters, MCV = mean corpuscular volume; PMN = polymorphonuclear leukocytes, Rx = therapy, TIBC = total iron binding capacity). (From Savage D, Lindenbaum J: Anemia in alcoholics. Medicine 65:322, 1986, with permission.)

HEMOLYTIC ANEMIAS

23. Patients with hemolytic anemia have a shortened RBC survival. What are the laboratory features of hemolysis and how is intravascular hemolysis distinguished from extravascular?
During hemolysis the bone marrow responds to the premature destruction of the RBCs by increasing its production of RBCs 7- or 8-fold. This expansion is marked by reticulocytosis. Other clues to accelerated RBC destruction are:

1. Indirect hyperbilirubinemia—acholuric jaundice (unconjugated bilirubin is not excreted in the urine)
2. Hemoglobinuria
3. Fall of hemoglobin greater than 1 g/7 days in the absence of GI bleeding or massive hematoma.

Laboratory Studies in Hemolysis

INTRAVASCULAR	EXTRA- AND INTRAVASCULAR
Hemoglobinemia	Increased reticulocyte count
Hemoglobinuria	Indirect, unconjugated bilirubin increased
Hemosiderinuria	Increased urobilinogen
Low serum haptoglobin	
Methemalbumin	
Low serum hemopexin	
Increased LDH	

Examples of intravascular hemolytic disorders are hemolytic transfusion reactions, paroxysmal nocturnal hemoglobinuria, paroxysmal cold hemoglobinuria, march hemoglobinuria, and RBC fragmentation syndromes.

24. What are the three basic types of RBC defects that lead to hemolysis in the hereditary hemolytic anemias? Cite some examples of each.

The RBC is extraordinarily well adapted to a circulatory system that requires resistance to shear stresses in the arterioles and suppleness to negotiate small orifices in the spleen and in capillaries.

Hereditary Red Cell Defects Resulting in Hemolysis

MEMBRANE DISORDERS		HEMOGLOBIN ABNORMALITIES	ENZYMATIC DEFECTS
Spherocytosis	Cation transport	Sickle cell anemia	G6PD deficiency
Elliptocytosis	Xerocytosis	Unstable hemoglobins	Pyruvate kinase
	Stomatocytosis	Thalassemia	5' Nucleotidase

These hereditary disorders are examples of intracorpuscular defects. Acquired hemolytic disorders typically result from extracorpuscular defects. These include autoimmune hemolytic anemia, fragmentation syndromes, malaria, hypersplenism, and physical agents such as heat, copper, and certain oxidants.

25. A patient presenting with lifelong anemia and spherocytosis on the peripheral blood film probably has hereditary spherocytosis (HS). How do you confirm the diagnosis?

Patients with HS, usually an autosomal-dominant disorder, may have affected siblings as well as an affected parent. As in other autosomal-dominant disorders, there is a significant (10%) spontaneous mutation rate, so paternity need not be questioned when neither parent is affected. A confirmatory test frequently obtained is the **osmotic fragility test** (see figure). The patient's blood is incubated in a series of tubes containing decreasing amounts of saline. In increasingly hypotonic media, RBCs swell until a critical hemolytic volume is reached, beyond which the RBC membrane ruptures. Since the RBC in HS is already a sphere, lysis occurs in media of relatively high osmotic strength. Osmotic fragility is therefore increased. Normal RBCs are under-filled spheres and can accommodate a lot of water before they reach their critical hemolytic volume.

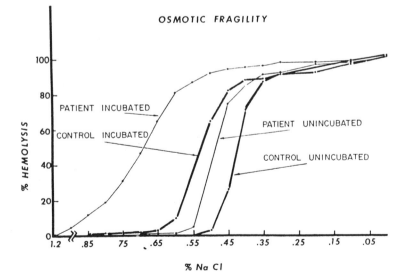

Osmotic fragility of unincubated and incubated RBCs from a normal individual and from a patient with hereditary spherocytosis. The striking increase in fragility produced by incubation of hereditary spherocytosis RBCs is obvious. (From Rappaport S: Introduction to Hematology, 2nd ed. Philadelphia, J.B. Lippincott, 1987, with permission.)

26. What should you tell the patient with HS to expect in the way of complications?

Complications of Hereditary Spherocytosis

Aplastic crises (associated with parvovirus B19)	Pigment gallstones
Hemolytic crises	Splenomegaly
Megaloblastic anemia (increased demand for folate)	Stasis ulcers

27. What therapeutic interventions can be made in HS?

1. **Dietary:** Patients should receive dietary supplementation with folate and counseling that their children may have this disorder.

2. **Splenectomy:** Older children and adults who have symptomatic anemia with ordinary viral illness or who have troublesome splenomegaly usually undergo splenectomy. Splenectomy prevents aplastic crises and gallstone formation. Many people who have adapted to mild anemia feel better. After splenectomy there is increased risk for overwhelming pneumococcal bacteremia and greater morbidity and mortality from this and other encapsulated organisms. Risks are lessened by administration of pneumococcal vaccine. Decisions about attempts to cure HS by splenectomy should be individualized.

28. What are the underlying membrane structural defects associated with HS?

HS is marked by decreased amounts of spectrin, the principal membrane protein found in erythrocytes. Spectrin has self-associative properties and forms a lattice with other RBC membrane proteins and actin. This supportive lattice on the inner aspect of the lipid bilayer gives the RBC its unique properties of strength and suppleness. In HS the deficiency of spectrin is not readily explained. In some kindreds an abnormal spectrin exists with defective binding to another membrane protein identified as band 4.1. New studies suggest the possible role of another protein, ankyrin, which anchors the spectrin lattice to the transmembrane anion transporter Band III protein. A deficiency of ankyrin may result in loss of spectrin, decreased membrane surface area and spherocytosis.

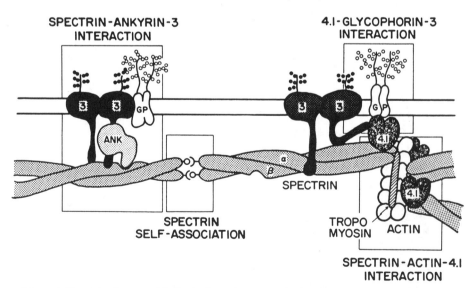

Schematic illustration (not to scale) of red cell membrane organization. GP, glycophorin; Ank, ankyrin. (From Lux SE: Disorders of the red cell membrane. In Nathan DG, Oski FA (eds): Hematology of Infancy & Childhood, 3rd ed. Philadelphia, W.B. Saunders, 1987, p 462, with permission.)

29. What is hereditary elliptocytosis (HE) and what are its most important subsets?

HE includes a broad spectrum of disorders that result in an elliptical RBC shape and hemolysis. Some families possess a mild variant—a normal hematocrit and a mild reticulocytosis. Others have a more striking degree of hemolysis, anemia, and more bizarre morphology. Infants who subsequently are shown to have hemolytic HE at birth may have striking hemolysis with bizarre RBCs and jaundice (infantile poikilocytosis).

Other HE variants are shown in the accompanying figure and table.

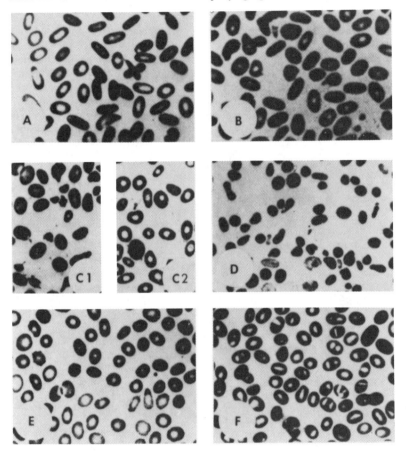

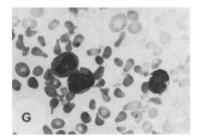

Peripheral blood morphology in the various types of hereditary elliptocytosis. *A,* Mild common HE; *B,* Mild common HE with chronic hemolysis; *C,* Mild common HE with poikilocytosis in infancy; C1 = at birth, C2 = at 1 year; *D,* Homozygous mild common HE; *E,* Spherocytic HE; *F,* Melanesian (stomatocytic) HE; *G,* Hereditary pyropoikilocytosis. (*A* from Wintrobe MM, et al: Clinical Hematology, 7th ed., Philadephia, Lea & Febiger, 1974, p 760; *B* from Jensson O, et al: Br J Haematol 13:844, 1967; *C* from Austin RF, Desforges JF: Pediatrics 44: 196, 1969; *D* from Lipton EL: Pediatrics 15:67, 1955; *E* from Dacie JV: Hemolytic Anemias, Congenital and Acquired, Part I: The Congenital Anemias, 2nd ed., New York, Grune & Stratton, 1960, p 151; *F* from Booth PB, et al: Vox Sang 32:99, 1977.)

Clinical Subtypes of Hereditary Elliptocytosis

PHENOTYPE	HEMOLYSIS	RED CELL MORPHOLOGY	OF*	FAMILY HISTORY	COMMENT
Common HE (HE_c) *One Abnormal Gene*					
Silent carrier	None	Normal	Normal	One parent a silent carrier or has HE[Spα^{174}–Sp]	—
Mild HE$_C$	Mild or none	Elliptocytes, rod forms	Normal	All races, one parent with mile HE$_C$	Significant hemolysis with diseases producing splenomegaly
HE$_C$ with chronic hemolysis	Mild– moderate	Elliptocytes, rod forms, variable poikilocytes and fragments	Normal	Sporadic in families with mild HE$_C$	Responds well to splenectomy
HE$_C$ with infantile poikilocytosis	Moderate	Budding, frag- ments, bizarre poikilocytes, some elliptocytes	Normal	Especially in blacks; one parent with mild HE$_C$	Neonatal juandice; disease converts to mild HE$_C$ during first year of life
HE$_C$ with dys- erythropoiesis	Mild– moderate	Rounded ellipto- cytes	Normal	Sporadic in some Italian families with mild HE$_C$	Gradual onset of erythroid dys- plasia and ineffective erythropoiesis; incomplete response to splenectomy
Two Abnormal Genes					
Homozygous HE$_C$	Severe	Elliptocytes, budding, frag- ments, bizarre poikilocytes, ± spherocytes	↑↑	Both parents with HE$_C$	Low MCV; good response to splenectomy
Hereditary pyro- poikilocytosis	Severe	Budding, frag- ments, sphero- cytes, bizarre poikilocytes, ± elliptocytes	↑↑	Usually both parents asymptomatic; sometimes one with mild HE$_C$	Low MCV; all patients with abnormal spectrin; partial response to splenectomy
Spherocyte HE (HE_S) *One Abnormal Gene*					
HE$_S$ with chronic hemolysis	Mild– moderate	Rounded ellipto- cytes, sphero- cytes, variable morphology within kindred	↑	One parent with HE$_S$; especially N. Europeans	↑ Glucose- responsive autohemolysis; responds well to splenectomy
Melanesian (Stomato- cytic) HE					
? One or ? Two *Abnormal Genes*	Mild or none	Rounded ellipto- cytes, some with transverse bars (stomatocytic elliptocytes) or knizocytic, elliptocytic macrocytes	Normal	Inheritance uncertain; especially Melanesians and Malay- sians	↓ Expression of blood groups; rigid RBCs; protection against all forms of malaria

*OF = osmotic fragility.
(From Lux SE: Disorders of the red cell membrane. In Nathan DG, Oski FA (eds): Hematology of Infancy & Childhood, 3rd ed. Philadelphia, W.B. Saunders, 1987, p 492, with permission.)

30. What is the most common enzymatic defect in RBCs leading to hemolysis and how is it diagnosed?

Glucose-6-phosphate dehydrogenase (G6PD) deficiency is the most common enzymatic defect of RBCs. There are hundreds of variants of this x-linked enzyme that have been characterized. Because this is the first enzyme in the hexose monophosphate pathway, deficiency compromises the RBC's ability to regenerate NADPH from NADP+. NADPH is necessary for the reduction of glutathione-containing disulfides (GSSG to GSH). The RBC as a carrier of oxygen is very vulnerable to oxidative attack when GSH is depleted. Oxidation results in precipitation of hemoglobin, which can be detected as Heinz bodies by supravital staining with crystal violet.

The diagnosis is established by measuring the enzymatic activity of G6PD.

31. How do patients with G6PD deficiency present?

Most patients are well until they come into contact with an oxidant drug. Some experience hemolysis with infections. Hepatitis in G6PD-deficient persons can result in spectacular jaundice. In the Mediterranean region, ingestion of the fava bean results in a severe hemolytic episode. American blacks have an increased prevalence of the A-type, which is unstable, losing G6PD activity as the red cell ages. During a hemolytic episode, the G6PD activity is normal because of the young RBCs present. The deficiency is therefore not recognized until months later when the patients no longer have a reticulocytosis.

32. What is the most common enzymatic defect in the erythrocyte Embden-Meyerhof pathway?

Pyruvate kinase deficiency is the most common of these uncommon deficiencies. It follows an autosomal recessive pattern of inheritance and results in an impressive peripheral blood picture of echinocytes and spheroechinocytes.

33. Many abnormal hemoglobins with single amino acid changes are known. Of these, which sickle or participate in the sickling process during deoxygenation?

Sickle hemoglobin coexists with other β-chain variants to produce clinically significant disease or clinically mild, insignificant disease.

Sickle Syndromes

SICKLE CELL DISEASE	SICKLE CELL TRAIT
SS (homozygous)	AS
Sβ-thalassemia	S-hereditary persistence
SC	of fetal hemoglobin
SD Los Angeles	
SO Arab	

34. What is the incidence of sickle hemoglobinopathies in births among black Americans?

Black Americans Affected by Sickle Cell Disorders

AS	8.0%	(1 of 12)
SS	0.16%	
AC	3.00%	
SC	0.12%	
SBo	0.03%	

Note that SBo + SC $\cong$ SS. In adults, as many patients with sickle β-thalassemia or SC will be seen as there are homozygous S patients. Although SBo is clinically very similar to SS disease, SBo and SC patients are more likely to have palpable spleens and may experience splenic sequestration/infarctive crises as adults rather than in early childhood, as is the case in SS disease. Also, SC patients tend to have higher hematocrits. These patients may present with blindness due to retinopathy or aseptic necrosis of the hip.

35. Are any other ethnic groups at risk for sickle cell disease?

Sickle cell disease is usually thought of as a disease of blacks, but other ethnic groups originating from areas where malaria is or was prevalent also have the sickle gene. Consequently, Hispanics, Greeks, Turks, Arabs, and Veddoid Indians have an increased incidence of sickle cell disease. In many of these groups, hemoglobin S is inherited with beta-thalassemia to produce Sβ-thal. Interestingly, Arabs and Veddoid Indians have an increased proportion of F (fetal) hemoglobin that seems to ameliorate the course of their disease.

36. What are the main clinical manifestations of sickle hemoglobinopathies?

Manifestations of Sickle Cell Disease

Hemolytic anemia:	**Chronic end organ damage:**
Gallstones	Retinopathy
Increased folate needs	Aseptic necrosis of the hip
Aplastic crises	Osteomyelitis
Indirect hyperbilirubinemia	Isosthenuria, hematuria, chronic
Increased LDH	renal failure
Periodic vaso-occlusive disease ("crises"):	Nephrotic syndrome
Pain crises	**Hyposplenism:**
Chest syndrome	Pneumococcal septicemia
Abdominal pain	Increased morbidity with other
Stroke	encapsulated organisms
Splenic infarct	**Reproductive:**
Splenic sequestration syndrome	High-risk pregnancy
Priapism	Impotence

37. Is there any morbidity truly associated with sickle trait?

Since 8% of American blacks are heterozygous for sickle trait, this is an important question. The following abnormalities have been associated with sickle trait:

Abnormalities Reported in Association with the Sickle Trait

Association with sickle cell trait very likely:	Association with sickle trait possible:
Splenic infarction at high altitude (over 10,000 feet)	Complications induced by prolonged use of tourniquet
Hyposthenuria	Renal papillary necrosis
Hematuria	Proliferative retinopathy
Bacteriuria and pyelonephritis in pregnancy	Avascular necrosis of bone
Reduced mortality from *Plasmodium falciparum* infection	Intravascular sickling with strenuous exertion

Sears DA: The morbidity of sickle cell trait. Am J Med 64:1021, 1978.

38. What are sickle crises?

Patients with sickle cell disease are susceptible to sudden unheralded vaso-occlusive events that are called crises. The most common event is a simple pain crisis during which pain is experienced in the limbs, low back, chest, or abdomen. Sometimes specific organs are affected by definite infarcts so that patients may experience bone infarcts, splenic infarcts (if splenic tissue has been preserved), or what is called the "chest syndrome." These events are marked by dyspnea, fever, pain, and the sudden appearance of an infiltrate on chest x-ray consistent with pneumonia. Often as not, no infection exists. Instead there is probably a sickle vaso-occlusion.

39. How are patients in a sickle crisis managed? How often do crises occur?

Patients with the chest syndrome often receive antibiotics and require oxygen. When hypoxemia continues despite oxygen therapy, exchange transfusions are helpful. The pathophysiology of the pain crisis is not well understood. It is interesting to note that most patients experience pain relatively infrequently—once a year or every 2 years. About 20% of patients, however, are troubled by crises more frequently and may be seen in the emergency room or hospitalized monthly. Why some homozygotes do poorly while others do relatively well is one of the mysteries of sickle cell disease. Similarly, it is not known what initiates crises or what mechanisms of spontaneous recovery act to terminate crises while patients are receiving only supportive care. The severity and duration of crises are variable. Stays for patients requiring hospitalization vary from 3–10 days.

40. What are the routine health maintenance measures employed in patients with sickle cell anemia?

Routine health maintenance in sickle cell disease includes genetic counseling about the risk of sickle cell disease in relatives or children. Patients are given folate supplementation, and periodic ophthalmoscopic examinations should also be undertaken. All patients should receive pneumococcal vaccine if they have not already been vaccinated. As patients get older, periodic review of renal function seems prudent.

41. How should women with sickle cell anemia be counseled about pregnancy?

With modern obstetrical care the risk of pregnancy for a woman with sickle cell disease has been greatly reduced. However, most obstetricians consider these pregnancies to be high risk and advocate close follow-up. Even so, the maternal mortality is less than 2% and the incidence of stillbirths and neonatal deaths is less than 15%. There is some controversy over the appropriate use of blood transfusions. A recent study suggests that patients who receive prophylactic transfusions during pregnancy do no better than those who are transfused only when symptomatic. Many women with sickle cell disease are successful mothers. However, women who are often ill and who require frequent hospitalizations for control of pain may require a great deal of support from other family members if they are to have children. Women who do not wish to become pregnant can be placed on oral contraceptives.

Koshy M, et al: Prophylactic red cell transfusions in pregnant patients with sickle cell disease. N Engl J Med 319:1447, 1988.

42. Under what circumstances should RBC transfusion be considered in the treatment of sickle cell disease? What are the hazards of RBC transfusions in such patients?

Indications for Transfusion in Sickle Cell Anemia

1. Strong indications	2. Relative indications
Aplastic crises	Before general anesthesia
Hypoxemia and chest syndrome	During pregnancy
	Priapism
CNS events, stroke	Prior to arteriography
Sequestration crises	3. Not indicated
	Management of typical pain crises

The hazards of transfusion include transmission of hepatitis, iron overload, and sensitization. The last-mentioned can be a significant problem. Delayed transfusion reactions occur in patients with a history of transfusions but with a negative crossmatch. After a few days, an anamnestic response occurs that results in hemolysis due to the sudden appearance of an IgG antibody. Delayed transfusion reactions usually involve Kidd, Kell, or Duffy antigens. In homozygous sickle cell disease, delayed transfusion reactions can mimic a crisis and may result in death.

Milner P, et al: Post transfusion crises in sickle cell anemia. South Med J 78:1462, 1985.

43. When a patient with sickle cell disease presents with a history of a viral syndrome followed by dramatic worsening of the anemia, what entity needs to be strongly considered?

Aplastic crisis needs to be considered. Typically, patients have a flu-like illness with or without an evanescent rash, fever, and myalgias, followed 5–10 days later by weakness and dyspnea. The patient presents with a sharply reduced hematocrit. A key finding is the nearly absolute absence of reticulocytes. This disorder is really a transient pure red cell aplasia. The platelet count and white count are usually unaffected. The bone marrow shows the absence of erythroid progenitors except for a few "giant pronormoblasts." This syndrome is most often caused by parvovirus B19, which seems to have a unique tropism for erythroid progenitors. In patients with hemolysis, parvovirus-induced aplasia is significant, because the duration of aplasia (5–10 days) coincides with the half-life of RBCs. Thus, cessation of RBC production for 10 days in a patient with a hematocrit of 22% and erythrocyte life span of 9 days spells trouble. In these individuals, transfusions of packed RBCs are lifesaving. The 10-day cessation of erythropoiesis caused by the parvovirus goes unnoticed in a normal person with a hematocrit of 40% and an RBC life span of 120 days. The parvovirus may be the cause of fifth disease, arthritis, and spontaneous abortions.

Saarinen UM, et al: Human parvovirus B19-induced epidemic acute red cell aplasia in patients with hereditary hemolytic anemia. Blood 67:1411, 1986.

44. What are the disorders resulting in decreased alpha-chain production and why are they less severe than disorders of beta-chain production?

Thalassemia minor is a frequent cause of microcytic, hypochromic anemia. It is due to an imbalance of alpha- and beta-chain production. The genetic information for the alpha chain of hemoglobin is organized as two adjacent genes on chromosome 16. Thus, normal individuals have four copies of the gene for alpha hemoglobin. In alpha-thalassemias, deletions of one or more of these genes are present and result in a deficiency of alpha chains and an excess of beta chains.

Deletion of a single gene is silent, but deletion of two genes is noticed as a microcytic, mild anemia, with a normal hemoglobin electrophoresis. About 30% of American blacks are heterozygous for a single-gene deletion, so that alpha thalassemia is found in about 2.0% of individuals. Asians have a much higher incidence of a chromosome 16 with two deleted alpha genes. Asians, therefore, are at risk for bearing children with only one or without any functional alpha genes. Those with only one functional alpha gene have a mild hemolytic anemia (hemoglobin H disease). Hemolysis results from oxidative attack on the $\beta 4$ tetramers present in the red cells of affected individuals.

Hydrops fetalis in association with a tetramer of gamma chains (hemoglobin Bart's) is the unfortunate cause of death at birth of a fetus with four alpha gene deletions.

In beta-thalassemia, the absence of beta chains results in the presence of alpha 4, a tetrameric alpha-chain protein that is highly toxic to the RBC membrane. Developing RBCs perish in the marrow or limp out to live a short, withered existence in the circulation.

45. What treatment now allows children with beta-thalassemia major to survive into adulthood?

In the modern era, aggressive transfusion therapy has greatly improved the outlook for these children. However, iron overload and the expense and aggravation (to patients) of chelation therapy are burdensome to these individuals when they reach young adulthood.

46. What are the consequences of beta-thalassemia major?

Clinical Manifestations of Beta-Thalassemia

Hypochromic microcytic anemia
Transfusion dependence
If not transfused aggressively:
  Hepatosplenomegaly
  Frontal bossing of the skull
  Pathological fractures
  Gallstones, ischemic ulcers
  Infections
  Pericarditis
  Growth retardation
  Delayed or absent sexual maturity
Transfused patients:
  Iron overload

47. A young man presents with asymptomatic cyanosis. What is the most likely hematologic cause and how is it evaluated?

There are two likely possibilities. The first is a **congenital methemoglobinemia** due to an abnormal hemoglobin, M-hemoglobinopathy. These patients have congenital cyanosis that is transmitted as an autosomal dominant disorder. The M-hemoglobins are among the 400 or more human hemoglobin variants that have been reported in various parts of the world and are generally known by place names of first discovery, such as M-Boston, Saskatoon, Milwaukee, and Kochikuro. M-hemoglobins have been only rarely identified in blacks. These hemoglobins stabilize iron in its oxidized (Fe^{+3}) state and have a muddy brown appearance.

The second possibility is **methemoglobin reductase** (cytochrome b_5 reductase) deficiency, which is an autosomal recessive disorder. Cyanosis caused by hypoxemia requires at least 5 g/dl of deoxyhemoglobin to be noticeable, whereas only 1.5 g/dl of methemoglobin will be recognized.

Differential Diagnosis of Cyanosis

1. Hypoxemia
   a. Pulmonary disease
   b. Cardiac right to left shunting
   c. Shock, congestive heart failure
   d. Low oxygen affinity hemoglobin
2. Methemoglobinemia
   a. Congenital
      i. M-hemoglobin
      ii. Cytochrome b_5 reductase
   b. Acquired
      i. Drugs (dapsone)
      ii. Chemicals (well-water nitrates)
3. Sulfhemoglobinemia

48. A 20-year-old woman with a history of two previous laparotomies for abdominal pain presents to you with confusion, fever, tachycardia, abdominal pain, and peripheral neuropathy. Her mother had a similar history and died at a young age. What disorder do you suspect? How do you make a diagnosis?

The history is strongly suggestive of **porphyria, acute intermittent type** (AIP). Porphyria is a diagnosis that sends even the most knowledgeable physicians to the textbooks for help.

Who can remember that AIP results from a deficiency of porphobilinogen deaminase? The inexperienced physician must be aware of two unfortunate facts about porphyria. Many people carry a diagnosis that is not founded upon adequate testing; many others with the disease are unrecognized. Hence, before embarking on specific therapy, laboratory studies must be obtained to confirm the diagnosis.

The clinical features of AIP include:

Clinical Features of AIP

Autosomal dominant inheritance
Urine: 8-aminolevulinic acid, porphobilinogen, uroporphyrin
Symptoms:
    Abdominal pain: fever, leukocytosis, vomiting, constipation are common.
    Neurologic manifestations: peripheral neuropathy, paraplegia, Guillian-Barré,
        respiratory arrest, cranial nerve findings, psychosis, seizure, coma.
    Other: hyponatremia, hypertension, tachycardia.

49. In the above case, how should you manage the patient based on your presumptive diagnosis?

Treatment should include carbohydrate infusions, hematin, beta blockers, and observation for respiratory compromise while obtaining appropriate lab studies to confirm the diagnosis. The patient should avoid barbiturates, anticonvulsants, estrogens, oral contraceptives, and alcohol.

50. What are the different laboratory and clinical features of warm and cold antibody-mediated immune hemolytic anemias?

Warm vs. Cold Antibody Autoimmune Hemolytic Anemia

	Warm	Cold
Antibody	IgG	IgM
Complement	±	+
Spontaneous agglutination	–	+++
Active temperature	37°	4°
Antigen	Rh (pan)	I, i
Response to therapy with:		
Steroids	Good	Poor
Splenectomy	Good	Poor
Gloves, warmth	None	Good

Note that cold agglutinin disease may be a self-limited disorder brought on by mycoplasma infection (usually anti-I) or infectious mononucleosis (usually anti-i). Chronic cold agglutination disease may be an idiopathic syndrome or associated with a lymphoproliferative disorder. Warm autoimmune hemolytic anemia is associated with lupus, chronic lymphocytic leukemia (CLL), Hodgkin's disease, non-Hodgkin's lymphomas, and certain drugs.

51. How is the Coombs' test used to evaluate autoimmune hemolytic anemia?

The Coombs' test is used to detect antibodies present on RBCs (direct Coombs' or direct antiglobulin test positive) or in the plasma. In the direct test, the patient's RBCs are washed and incubated with an antiglobulin serum (rabbit or other species), and then examined for agglutination. In the indirect test, the patient's serum is reacted with a "panel" of RBCs bearing antigens of interest. Antibodies, if present in the patient's sera, bind to the RBCs bearing the relevant antigen. The panel cells are washed to reduce nonspecific binding, then incubated with an antiglobulin serum to detect agglutination. The antiglobulin reagent is necessary because antibodies attached to RBCs are usually IgG in low numbers and cannot ordinarily cross-link to agglutinate. The antiglobulin serum bridges these antibodies, favoring agglutination.

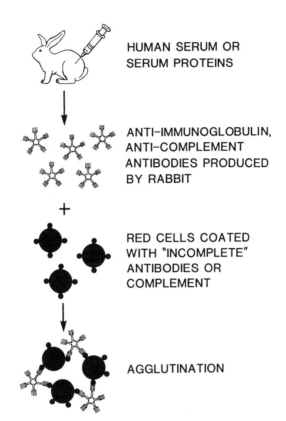

HUMAN SERUM OR
SERUM PROTEINS

ANTI-IMMUNOGLOBULIN,
ANTI-COMPLEMENT
ANTIBODIES PRODUCED
BY RABBIT

+

RED CELLS COATED
WITH "INCOMPLETE"
ANTIBODIES OR
COMPLEMENT

AGGLUTINATION

Direct antiglobulin test. Rabbits or goats are immunized with human serum or serum components. The resulting sera containing anti-gamma globulin or anti-complement antibodies are then added to test samples of red cells. If human gamma globulins and/or complement components are bound to the cell surface, agglutination occurs. (From Wintrobe MM, et al: Clinical Hematology, 8th ed. Philadelphia, Lea & Febiger, 1981, p 909, with permission.)

In autoimmune hemolytic anemia the direct test is usually positive, indicating the presence of an autoantibody on the RBCs. The indirect test, indicating the presence of that same antibody in the serum, may also be positive. Persons who have been exposed to blood, or who have had a miscarriage or an abortion, may develop antibodies to certain antigens present on the transfused RBCs that do not exist on their native RBCs. Later these individuals will have a positive indirect Coombs' test and negative direct Coombs' test.

52. What are the possible causes of fragmented RBCs on a peripheral smear of a patient with a hemolytic anemia?
Fragmentation hemolysis is characterized by the appearance of schistocytes, helmet cells, burr cells (echinocytes), and spherocytes. The hemolysis is intravascular and associated with a wide variety of conditions.

Fragmentation Syndromes

Macroangiopathic:	Microangiopathic*:
Valve hemolysis	Cavernous hemangiomas
Endocardial cushion defect repair	Thrombotic thrombocytopenic purpura (TTP)
Extracorporeal circulation	Hemolytic uremic syndrome
	Eclampsia/pre-eclampsia
	Malignant hypertension
	Scleroderma
	Disseminated carcinomatosis
	Disseminated intravascular coagulation (DIC)

*Thrombocytopenia often present.

53. What important syndrome is characterized by the triad of thrombocytopenia, fragmentation hemolysis, and fluctuating neurological signs? (Hint: Sometimes a pentad, including fever and renal disease, is present in this disorder.)

This is **thrombotic thrombocytopenic purpura** or TTP. This disorder is perhaps the most spectacular of the fragmentation syndromes. Patients may present with seizures, coma, paresis, or more subtle neurologic signs and thrombocytopenia. Although the cause(s) are unknown, treatment with steroids, plasma exchange, or plasma infusion appears to be effective. The mortality is 20–50%. Some patients (20–30%) pursue a relapsing course. During remissions of their illness, unusually large multimers of von Willebrand factor have been found in the plasma, which disappear during relapse.

Moake JL, et al: Unusually large plasma factor VIII: von Willebrand multimers in chronic relapsing thrombotic thrombocytopenic purpura. N Engl J Med 307:1433, 1982.

WHITE BLOOD CELLS (WBCs)

54. What constitutes the lower limit for the absolute neutrophil count? What ethnic group may have lower counts without any clinical disorder?

For adults, the level below which neutropenia is a consideration is 1.8×10^9/liter. Black Americans have a lower mean neutrophil count, which may be encountered during routine examinations. These persons do not have an increased incidence of infections nor do they have increased severity of infectious disease. When the neutrophil count is below 0.5×10^9/liter, neutropenia is severe and there is a greater propensity for compromised response to infection.

Shaper AG, Lewis P: Genetic neutropenia in people of African origin. Lancet ii:1021, 1971.

55. What are the causes of neutropenia?

There are a number of interesting congenital causes of neutropenia. Acquired neutropenia may occur in the setting of autoimmune disease, ingestion of certain drugs, folate or B_{12} deficiency, and myelodysplastic syndromes. Of interest is the association between rheumatoid arthritis, splenomegaly, and neutropenia or Felty syndrome. Some of the patients have been recognized to have a proliferation of lymphocytes with large granules and immunologic characteristics of natural killer cells. Certain infections are commonly associated with neutropenia. These include Rickettsia, gram-negative septicemia, measles, dengue, mono-nucleosis, and of course human immunodeficiency virus.

56. What drugs commonly cause neutropenia?

Drugs such as phenothiazines, antithyroid drugs, or chloramphenicol may cause neutropenia in a dose-dependent fashion by inhibiting cell replication. Immune-related neutropenia may be seen with penicillins, cephalosporins, and other agents. A table of the more common agents associated with idiosyncratic neutropenia is shown:

Drugs That Commonly Cause Neutropenia

Analgesics/anti-inflammatory agents	Antibiotics	Others
Indomethacin	Chloramphenicol	Phenytoin
Para-aminophenol derivatives	Penicillins	Cimetidine
Acetaminophen	Sulfonamides	Captopril
Phenacetin	Cephalosporins	Chlorpropamide
Pyrazolon derivatives	Phenothiazines	
Aminopyrine	Antithyroid drugs	
Dipyrone		
Oxyphenbutazone		
Phenylbutazone		

The International Agranulocytosis and Aplastic Anemia Study: Risks of agranulocytosis and aplastic anemia. JAMA 256:1749, 1986.

57. What is the significance of finding myelocytes, metamyelocytes, and nucleated RBCs in the peripheral blood?

Leukoerythroblastosis, or the presence of immature WBCs and nucleated RBCs, is often associated with a malignancy that has metastases to the bone marrow. Numerous other, less serious conditions are also associated with leukoerythroblastosis, albeit sometimes transiently.

Conditions Associated with Leukoerythroblastosis

MALIGNANCIES	NONMALIGNANT CONDITIONS
Solid tumors	Hemolysis—including sickle cell disease
Prostate	Thrombocytopenic purpura
Breast	Infancy
GI	GI bleeding
Lymphoma	Renal transplants
Myelofibrosis	Septicemia
Leukemia	Chronic lung disease
Preleukemia	Myocardial infarction
	Liver disease

Weick JH, Hagedorn AB, Linman JW: Leukoerythroblastosis: Diagnostic and prognostic significance. Mayo Clin Proc 49:110, 1974.

58. What are the features of lymphocytosis caused by infections?

When infections (usually viral) cause lymphocytosis, the lymphocyte morphology is unusual or atypical. Thus infection with the Epstein-Barr virus (EBV) or cytomegalovirus (CMV) can cause an infectious mononucleosis syndrome of fever, sore throat, lymphadenopathy, hepatosplenomegaly, and in the case of EBV an increased titer of the heterophile antibody (see table). An acute lymphocytosis may be associated with primary infection with HIV-1. In EBV infection, B-cells are penetrated by the virus, eliciting a polyclonal T-cell response manifested in the peripheral blood as atypical lymphocytosis. Cold agglutinin disease may also occur in EBV virus disease. These IgM antibodies are usually directed against the i antigen. These disorders are usually self-limited. CMV, toxoplasmosis, or less commonly, EBV infection during the first trimester of pregnancy has been associated with serious developmental defects in the newborn.

Causes of Heterophile-negative Mononucleosis

Cytomegalovirus	Epstein-Barr virus
HIV-1	Toxoplasma
Adenovirus	Rubella
Herpes simplex II	

MYELOPROLIFERATIVE DISORDERS

59. Polycythemia is a frequent problem encountered by internists. Before embarking on a long and expensive workup, what two steps are necessary?

There is really no point in pursuing a workup of polycythemia without demonstrating that (1) the red cell mass is increased and that (2) hypoxemia is not present as a cause of secondary erythrocytosis. Many patients who are receiving diuretics have an increased hematocrit, but typically they also have a decreased plasma volume and a normal red cell mass. Some patients who are not on diuretics (usually smokers) have so-called "stress erythrocytosis" and normal red cell mass and reduced plasma volume. Patients with chronic lung disease or congenital heart disease resulting in significant left-to-right shunts are also polycythemic.

60. What are the major and minor criteria widely used to diagnose polycythemia vera (PCV)?

The Polycythemia Study Group has developed the following guidelines to establish a diagnosis of PCV:

    Category A (major criteria)
        1. Increased red cell mass ($\geq$ 36 ml/kg men, $\geq$ 32 ml/kg women)
        2. Normal arterial oxygen saturation ($\geq$ 90%)
        3. Splenomegaly
    Category B (minor criteria)
        1. Thrombocytosis: platelets $\geq 400 \times 10^9$/liter
        2. Leukocytosis: WBC $\geq 12 \times 10^9$/liter
        3. Elevated leukocyte alkaline phosphatase (LAP)
        4. Elevated B_{12} level (> 900 pg/ml) or unbound B_{12}-binding capacity (≥ 2200 pg/ml)

A diagnosis of PCV is supported by either (1) all three of category A or (2) increased red cell mass, normal arterial saturation, and two of the criteria in category B. Although these criteria are useful, important causes of secondary polycythemia need to be considered. Carboxyhemoglobin should be measured if the patient is a heavy smoker, and in certain families a high affinity hemoglobin may be identified by determining the P50 (oxygen half-saturation pressure). A neoplasm producing ectopic erythropoietin also may result in erythrocytosis. Typically, these are obvious, but CT scans or liver scans may be necessary to evaluate the possibility of an occult neoplasm of the kidney or liver. In PCV the erythropoietin level is usually low or normal, whereas in secondary conditions erythropoietin levels are increased.

61. What establishes PCV as a clonal stem cell disorder?

The clonal nature of the proliferation that results in striking erythrocytosis and sometimes thrombocytosis and leukocytosis has been clearly shown in studies of women heterozygous for X-linked G6PD. Because of inactivation of one of the X-chromosomes during embryonic development, these women are essentially mosaics in which half of the somatic cells express one isoenzyme and the other half express the other. In such women who also had PCV, only one isotype was found in their erythrocytes, neutrophils, B-lymphocytes, and platelets. Fibroblasts from the bone marrow showed the characteristic mixture of two isoenzymes. Thus the disorder we recognize as PCV is clonal and probably originates in a stem cell.

    Adamson JW, et al: Polycythemia vera: Stem cell and probable clonal origin of the disease. N Engl J Med 295:913, 1976.

62. Once the diagnosis of PCV is established, how are patients treated and what are the expected complications of therapy?

Treatment of PCV is important, since untreated patients are uncomfortable and at risk for life-threatening thrombotic events. Initially, phlebotomy of 500 ml of blood every other day as tolerated is undertaken until the hematocrit is reduced to a normal range. Some patients are not well-controlled and require myelosuppressive therapy with hydroxyurea, alkylating agents, or ablation with the isotope P[32]. As phlebotomy proceeds, patients develop iron deficiency, which reduces the rate at which phlebotomy is necessary for control of the disease. In an important Polycythemia Vera Study Group publication, treatment with phlebotomy, P[32], or chlorambucil was compared. Treatment with phlebotomy alone was associated with an increased incidence of stroke and other thrombotic events, whereas treatment with chlorambucil or P[32] was associated with a high incidence of transformation into acute leukemia. Therefore, patients who are over age 70, or those who have had previous thrombotic events, may do better with hydroxyurea and occasional phlebotomy, whereas phlebotomy alone usually suffices for younger patients.

Berk PD, et al: Therapeutic recommendations in polycythemia vera based on Polycythemia Study Group protocols. Semin Hematol 23:132, 1984.

63. What is the typical cytogenetic abnormality found in chronic myelogenous leukemia (CML) and are there any other hematologic malignancies that share this finding?

The cytogenetic marker of CML is the 9:22 translocation in which portions of the long arms of chromosomes 9 and 22 are exchanged, resulting in a shortened 22 or Philadelphia chromosome (Ph[1]). This balanced translocation is now known to result in the juxtaposition of an oncogene C-abl originating on 9 with genes in the breakpoint cluster region (bcr) of 22. Cell lines established from CML cells express a new messenger RNA (mRNA), which reflects the chimeric gene produced by the fusion of the bcr and c-abl genes. From this mRNA a unique tyrosine phosphoprotein kinase, P210 bcr-abl, is translated. This enzyme may act to phosphorylate tyrosine residues in important cellular proteins. A small minority of CML patients have normal cytogenetics but have the C-abl, bcr translocation when studied at the molecular level. Some patients with acute lymphoblastic leukemia (ALL) also have 9:22 translocations. Although some of these may have been lymphoblastic transformations of CML, most are thought to be de novo leukemias with subtle differences in the location of the c-abl translocation into the bcr region of 22.

64. How is CML differentiated from a leukemoid reaction?

Occasionally patients who have an inflammatory disease, infection, or cancer will have a leukocytosis up to, but not frequently over, 50×10^9/liter. In some instances the cause may not be apparent and CML is a consideration. These two entities may be differentiated by considering the characteristics outlined below.

CML Compared to Leukemoid Reaction

	CML*	LEUKEMOID REACTION
Juvenile neutrophils (metamyelocytes, myelocytes, etc.)	+	---
Basophilia	+	---
Eosinophilia	+	---
Marrow fibrosis	+/-	---
Splenomegaly	+/-	---
Leukocyte alkaline phosphatase (LAP)	Low	Increased
Philadelphia chromosome	+	---

*+ = present, – = absent.

65. What is the natural history of CML and its acceleration into blast phase? What are the clinical and laboratory features of acceleration?

Despite control of symptoms with agents like hydroxyurea or busulfan, patients with CML uniformly transform into an acute leukemia that is typically poorly responsive to chemotherapy. The median survival of patients ranges from 39–47 months. After the first year, the risk of transformation into blast phase is about 20% per year. Thus a minority of patients enjoy long survivals of 10–25 years with CML. Experience has taught us that certain clinical events herald the transformation from chronic to blast phase. These include enlarging spleen (with splenic infarcts), increased basophilia and eosinophilia, fever, fibrosis in the marrow, and resistance to alkylators or hydroxyurea. In many instances an accelerated phase (marked by an increased percentage of blasts and promyelocytes) occurs before frank leukemia. In about two-thirds of cases of transformation into acute leukemia there is the appearance of a new cytogenic abnormality in addition to the Philadelphia chromosome. These new cytogenetic abnormalities suggest that the Ph[1]-positive clone has undergone evolution into a more malignant cell. Four typical chromosomal changes in the setting of transformation are: (1) a second Ph[1] chromosome, (2) trisomy 8, (3) isochromosome 17, (4) trisomy 19. Interestingly, the phenotype of a leukemic cell in the blast crisis of CML is variable. While most patients have blasts with the characteristics of myeloid cells, about a third have cells that are lymphoid in character. Less often the cells have features of erythroblastic leukemia or megakaryocytic leukemia.

Rosenthal S, et al: Characteristics of blast crisis in chronic granulocytic leukemia. Blood 49:705, 1977.

66. What are the roles of interferon and bone marrow transplantation in the treatment of CML?

Recent studies have demonstrated the usefulness of alpha-interferon in the treatment of CML in the chronic phase. Interferon seems to be a particularly good agent for the control of those patients who have thrombocytosis as a manifestation of CML. An exciting aspect of treatment with alpha-interferon is the observation of loss of the cytogenic abnormality. A significant number of patients receiving alpha-interferon had no Ph[1] chromosomes detected in mitotic figures obtained from bone marrow aspirate. Whether or not this form of therapy will delay the onset of blast crises is not known.

Bone marrow transplantation is the only therapy at present that offers a hope of cure for CML. Although the peritransplant mortality is significant, the long-term outlook is better for young patients who have CML and an HLA-identical sibling. The outlook is better for those patients who undergo transplantation during chronic phase. Once patients reach blast crises, their outlook is poorer.

Champlin RE, et al: Bone marrow transplantation in chronic myelogenous leukemia. Semin Hematol 25:74, 1988.

67. Patients presenting with large spleens, fibrotic marrows, and the presence of teardrop shaped erythrocytes on the peripheral blood film have what myeloproliferative disorder?

Myelofibrosis or agnogenic myeloid metaplasia is a myeloproliferative disease marked by splenomegaly, tear-dropped RBCs, fibrotic marrow, and immature erythroid and myeloid cells in peripheral blood (leukoerythroblastic blood picture). Extramedullary hematopoiesis is usually present in the liver and spleen of affected individuals. Patients may have neutrophilia, thrombocytosis, and anemia. Other patients, typically with massively enlarged spleens, may be cytopenic instead. Patients with enlarged spleens and neutrophilia resemble patients with CML. Determination of the presence of Ph[1] chromosome may distinguish the two. The fibroblast proliferation that is typically present in the marrows of these patients is polyclonal and appears to be fostered by fibroblast growth factors released by abnormal megakaryocytes. Patients may be troubled by bone pain and often have radiographic evidence of osteosclerosis. Massive splenomegaly may lead to portal hypertension and varices. Treatment is largely supportive and ineffective. As in other myeloproliferative diseases, transformation into acute leukemia has been observed in some patients.

68. Patients without massive splenomegaly may have platelet counts above 1,000,000/μl ("platelet millionaires"). What myeloproliferative disease do these patients have?

Patients may become platelet millionaires for a variety of reasons. Occasionally patients with severe iron deficiency and concurrent hemorrhage or inflammatory disease have platelet counts of over 1,000,000/μl. Once iron deficiency is corrected or the inflammatory disorder resolves, platelet counts return to normal levels. Another myeloproliferative disorder, essential thrombocythemia (also referred to as "primary thrombocythemia" or "primary hemorrhagic thrombocythemia") needs to be considered when the platelet count rises above 600,000/μl, although a count over 1,000,000/μl is the rule. In this disorder, there is also evidence for clonal proliferation. During physical exam, modest splenic enlargement and purpura may be evident. Patients are often troubled by hemorrhage due to poorly functioning platelets. Purpura, epistaxis, and gingival bleeding are typical manifestations. These may be exacerbated by aspirin use. Erythromelalgia, characterized by a localized burning pain and warmth of the distal extremities, is commonly seen. Dramatic relief is obtained after taking small doses of aspirin. Also seen are neurologic manifestations such as dizziness, seizures, and transient ischemic attacks.

69. What are the causes of thrombocytosis?

The disorders that must be considered in the differential diagnosis of essential thrombocythemia are summarized in the following table.

Causes of Thrombocytosis

REACTIVE	MYELOPROLIFERATIVE DISORDERS
Malignancy	Essential thrombocythemia
Iron deficiency	Polycythemia vera (PCV)
Splenectomy	Chronic myelogenous leukemia (Ph^1 present)
Inflammatory bowel disease	Myelofibrosis
Infection	Myelodysplastic syndromes
Collagen-vascular diseases	

Iron studies, collagen vascular screen, and cytogenetics of the bone marrow aspirate are helpful in differentiating these disorders. PCV may present as essential thrombocythemia and iron deficiency with chronic GI blood loss. When the iron deficiency is corrected, the erythrocytosis of PCV will be manifest.

70. What is the most likely finding in patients suffering from a myeloproliferative disease who present with a swollen, hot ankle?

Patients with myeloproliferative syndromes (PCV, CML, myelofibrosis, essential thrombocythemia) may develop hyperuricemia and gout. Thus, arthritis in such patients should be investigated thoroughly, including arthrocenteses and examination for intracellular positively birefringent crystals under polarized light.

ACUTE MYELOGENOUS LEUKEMIA (AML)

71. How is AML classified and how do the subtypes differ in natural history and complications?

The French American British (FAB) classification system sorts AML into seven categories (M1–M7). The approach to the analysis of a bone marrow and the essentials of the classification are shown in the accompanying table.

The diagnosis of AML M1–M5 requires a cellular bone marrow aspirate with blasts representing > 30% of all nucleated RBCs. If erythroblasts comprise > 50% of the

nucleated bone marrow cells, erythroleukemia (M6) is present. If the marrow is cellular but
blasts account for $< 30\%$ of the nucleated RBCs, myelodysplasia is present. Peroxidase
stain is important in the definition of AML. In practice, the blasts are peroxidase- (or
Sudan black) positive in AML and peroxidase-negative in acute lymphoblastic leukemia
(ALL).

FAB Classification of AML

TYPE	DESCRIPTION	CRITERIA
M1	Myeloblastic leukemia without maturation	$>3\%$ of blasts are peroxidase positive. A few granules, Auer rods, or both; one or more distinct nucleoli; no further maturation
M2	Myeloblastic leukemia with maturation	$>50\%$ of marrow cells are myelocytes and promyelocytes. Myelocytes, metamyelocytes, and mature granulocytes are seen. Eosinophilia may predominate in some cases
M3	Hypergranular promyelocytic leukemia	Majority of cells are abnormal promyelocytes, reniform (kidney-shaped) nuclei, bundles of Auer rods; also some have closely packed bright pink or purple granules.
M4	Myelomonocytic leukemia	$>20\%$ of bone marrow, peripheral blood nucleated cells, or both are promonocytes and monocytes. An eosinophilic variant is also recognized.
M5	Monocytic leukemia (M5a = poorly differentiated) (M5b = differentiated)	Granulocyte component $< 10\%$ of marrow cells. Monocytoid cells have a fluoride-sensitive esterase reaction cytochemically
M6	Erythroleukemia	$>50\%$ of cells are erythroblasts. Myeloblasts represent $>30\%$ of nonerythroid nucleated cells.
M7	Megakaryoblastic	$>30\%$ of marrow cells are blasts. Platelet peroxidase is positive on electron microscopy, or blasts react with antiplatelet monoclonal antibodies. Marrow fibrosis is prominent. Cytoplasmic budding is also a feature.

Bennett JM, et al: Proposal for the classification of the acute leukemias. Br J Hematol 33:451, 1976.

72. Which cytogenetic abnormalities have been described in AML? What is their significance?

At least 90% of patients with AML have cytogenetic abnormalities. Some of these, when
detected, indicate a relatively good prognosis and others bode ill for the patient.
Interestingly, specific morphological variants of AML have been linked to characteristic
cytogenetic abnormalities. These are shown in the table below.

Cytogenetics in AML

CYTOGENETIC ABNORMALITY	LEUKEMIA TYPE	PROGNOSIS
Trisomy 8	M2	Average
t(8;21) (translocation 8;21)	M2 with splenomegaly, chloromas, Auer rods	Good
t(15;17)	M3, many promyelocytes, DIC	Average
Inv 16 (inversion of 16)	FAB M4 with abnormal eosinophils	Good
t(9;11)	M5, monocytic leukemia	Average
t(6;9)	M2 with increased basophils	Average
t(4;11)	Biphenotypic leukemia lymphoid and monocytic phenotype	Poor
5q–, 7q–, 5–, 7–	Therapy-related leukemia	Poor

Yunis JJ, et al: High resolution chromosomes as an independent prognostic indicator in adult acute
non-lymphocytic leukemia. N Engl J Med 311:812–818, 1984.
Koeffler HP: Syndromes of acute nonlymphocytic leukemia. Ann Intern Med 107:748–758, 1987.

73. How do patients with AML typically present?

Patients with AML typically present with malaise, pallor, weight loss, fever, and bleeding. Bleeding may be manifested by nosebleeds, melena, hematuria, or purpura. Patients may also experience bone pain and may have sternal tenderness. Abdominal fullness, early satiety, and left upper quadrant pain radiating to the shoulder may be seen in those patients with splenic enlargement. Occasionally, there may be skin involvement or gum involvement, particularly in monocytic leukemia. Acute leukemia may present as arthritis or may be associated with gout. Headache, nausea, and vomiting may be a sign of CNS bleeding in the thrombocytopenic patient. CNS meningeal involvement (more often seen in acute lymphoblastic leukemia [ALL]) may produce stiff neck, papilledema, and cranial nerve palsies. Examination of the peripheral blood smear discloses the abnormal myeloid cells. *Interestingly, only half of patients presenting with leukemia have an elevated white count, so careful attention to leukocyte morphology is paramount in making a diagnosis.*

74. What are the main causes of death in AML?

Death in patients with treated AML is usually due to infection (70%) or to hemorrhage from thrombocytopenia (10%).

75. What are the most frequent organisms causing infection during induction-chemotherapy-induced bone marrow aplasia?

Patients receiving induction chemotherapy usually endure a period of absolute granulocytopenia (leukocyte nadir) at a time when there have been breakdowns of important barriers to infection. These breakdowns include mucositis throughout the GI tract and the presence of chronic indwelling venous catheters.

Organisms Causing Infection in AML

BACTERIAL	FUNGI
Pseudomonas aeruginosa	*Candida* sp.
Escherichia coli	*Aspergillus*
Staphylococcus aureus	*Phycomycetes*
Klebsiella aerobacter	
Proteus vulgaris	
Bacteroides sp.	
Staphylococcus epidermidis	

Antibiotic therapy is usually designed to meet the challenges posed by the bacterial pathogens on the list. If after a period of adequate treatment the patient remains febrile, amphotericin is usually begun. Controversy still rages over the need for reverse isolation, enteric sterilization with antibiotics, or other prophylactic measures that could be taken to reduce infection.

76. What proportion of AML patients attain complete remission and how many of these have a survival of 5 years or more?

This is, of course, *the* question from the patient's point of view. "What are my chances, Doctor?" An interesting response to this question can be found in the clinical studies of the Toronto Leukemia Study Group. In their analysis of 272 patients, the complete remission rate of AML ranged from 43.8 to 85.3%, depending on the exclusion criteria used. The lower remission rate can be accounted for by patients who were elderly (over age 70), having an antecedent myelodysplastic syndrome, or partial treatment. Hence, a younger patient with no previous hematologic disorder has between 70–85% chance of attaining a complete remission, which may last for 11–16 months on the average. Of those who attain a complete remission, in some series 20% have a remission that is durable, (i.e., greater than 5 years).

The Toronto Leukemia Study Group: Results of chemotherapy for unselected patients with acute myeloblastic leukemia. Lancet i:788, 1986.

77. Young patients with AML in first remission are usually evaluated or considered for bone marrow transplantation (BMT). Do syngeneic (identical twin) transplants or allogeneic (HLA-identical) transplants fare better after BMT?

Patients in remission who are age 40 or younger and have HLA-identical siblings are usually evaluated for BMT. In BMT, marrow cells are obtained by multiple aspirations from the posterior iliac crest of an anesthetized donor. The marrow cells are collected and filtered. The recipient must be "conditioned" with cytotoxic and immunosuppressive therapy to ablate his or her own marrow and immune system, so that the donor graft will be tolerated. RBCs are often removed, and then the remaining marrow cells are infused into the donor. In comparisons of BMT versus maintenance or other forms of post-induction chemotherapy, there seems to be an advantage for patients receiving transplants. This may be due to the intensity of the preparative regimen for BMT, which includes lethal doses of chemotherapy often in conjunction with total body irradiation. However, studies of identical twin donor recipient pairs indicate that the recipients have a higher relapse rate than HLA-identical sibling transplants. These studies indicate that there is an important "graft-versus-leukemia" effect of allogeneic bone marrow transplantation.

Champlin R, Gale RP: Bone marrow transplantation for acute leukemia: Recent advances and comparison with alternative therapies. Semin Hematol 24:55–67, 1987.

78. What are the most important causes of death in patients undergoing bone marrow transplantation (BMT)?

BMT is a challenging mode of therapy. After conditioning, patients become pancytopenic during the 3 weeks or so that is required for engraftment. During that time they are prone to infectious complications similar to those experienced by patients undergoing remission-induction chemotherapy for AML. These patients are treated with antibiotics and transfusions of RBCs and platelets. Blood products must be irradiated to prevent graft-versus-host disease (GvHD) from lymphocytes in the donor units. After engraftment, interstitial pneumonitis is a frequent complication, with a high mortality rate. Some of these deaths are due to infectious agents such as CMV.

Another consequence of engraftment is the potential for GvHD, which is caused by T-cells from the donor. GvHD may be either acute or chronic. Acute GvHD arises during the first 100 days after transplant. The targets for donor T-lymphocytes are skin, liver, and GI tract. Patients may have mild skin rashes or more severe disease resulting in toxic epidermal necrolysis. Diarrhea and transient elevation of liver function may occur, and in some patients are more severe, resulting in massive diarrhea and liver failure. Immunologic competence is also delayed by GvHD, so that patients are susceptible to new infections, including those mediated by encapsulated organisms like the pneumococcus.

Chronic GvHD results in the same organ involvement but in addition there are features of a scleroderma-like illness. Dry eyes, dry mouth, myasthenia, bronchiolitis, and infections are also observed.

ACUTE LYMPHOBLASTIC LEUKEMIA (ALL)

79. How reliably can ALL be differentiated from AML (M1) by examination of the peripheral blood smear only?

Although hematologists can sometimes distinguish these two entities by looking at the morphology of the blasts, there is a very high rate of discordance with the results of special studies. Flow cytometry is now frequently used to show typical lymphoid markers in ALL and myeloid markers in AML. Some patients with leukemia show evidence of both types of markers and are called "biphenotypic."

Distinguishing Features of ALL and AML

WRIGHT'S STAIN MORPHOLOGY	AML	ALL
Cytoplasm	More abundant	Scanty
Granules	Sometimes present	Absent
Nucleoli	3–5 distinct	1–3, often indistinct
Auer rods	May be present	Absent
STAINING CHARACTERISTICS		
Peroxidase or Sudan black	+	–
PAS	+/–	+

80. What are the indicators of a poor prognosis in adult patients with ALL?

ALL has a 50% cure rate in young children, but in adults the outlook is much worse. Certain features at presentation of ALL in adults confer a worse prognosis and may suggest the desirability of very aggressive therapy. Interestingly, adult T-cell ALL may have a better outlook than common ALL (pre-B). This is the reverse of the situation found in childhood ALL, in which T-cell disease heralds a worse outcome. In adults, B-cell disease (Burkitt's, or L3 subtype of the FAB system) has the worst outlook. Older patients, those presenting with a white count greater than 25–35 × 10⁹/liter, and cytogenetic abnormalities do less well. One of the differences between adult and childhood ALL is the greater frequency of t(9,22) (Philadelphia chromosome) in adults.

Hoelzer D, Gale RP: Acute lymphoblastic leukemia in adults, recent progress, future directions. Semin Hematol 24:27–39, 1987.

LYMPHOPROLIFERATIVE DISEASE

81. What is the most common leukemia of adults?

Chronic lymphocytic leukemia (CLL) is the most common form of leukemia seen in adults. This disorder is a neoplastic growth of lymphocytes, most often B-lymphocytes. Patients are often elderly and CLL is detected during examination for other problems. Lymphadenopathy and splenomegaly are also relatively frequent. Some patients present only with an elevated WBC count, made up of lymphocytes with a normal morphology.

82. What are the diagnostic criteria for CLL?

A recent proposal made by the International Workshop on CLL suggests the following criteria:

1. Sustained lymphocyte count equal to or greater than 10 × 10⁹/liter. Morphology should be "typical."

2. Bone marrow involvement (greater than 30% lymphocytes).

3. B-cell immunophenotypes (typically weak expression of membrane immunoglobulin, CD5 expression, and rosette formation with mouse erythrocytes).

To make a diagnosis of CLL, criterion **1** should be satisfied along with either criterion **2** or **3**. If criterion **1** is not satisfied (the lymphocyte count is less than 10 × 10⁹/liter), then criteria **2** and **3** must be present.

International Workshop on Chronic Lymphocytic Leukemia: Chronic lymphocytic leukemia: Recommendations for diagnosis, staging, and response criteria. Ann Intern Med 110:236–238, 1989.

83. Patients with CLL are typically staged to determine prognosis and to consider therapy. What are the current staging systems?

Many patients with CLL present with limited disease and live without trouble from their leukemia. Since most are elderly, death from other causes is most likely. Patients with more advanced disease, however, do less well. Unfortunately, chemotherapy used to treat this disorder has not improved survival. Treatment is usually given to patients who have anemia or thrombocytopenia, or bulky lymphadenopathy. Two staging systems have been in use for CLL. They are summarized in the accompanying tables.

Rai Staging System for Chronic Lymphocytic Leukemia

STAGE	CLINICAL FEATURES	SURVIVAL* (mo.)
0	Lymphocytosis in blood and bone marrow only	>120
I	Lymphoctyosis and enlarged lymph nodes	95
II	Lymphocytosis plus hepatomegaly, or splenomegaly, or both	72
III	Lymphocytosis and anemia (hemoglobin, < 110 g/L)	30
IV	Lymphocytosis and thrombocytopenia (platelets <100 × 10^9/L)	30

*Weighted median survival was derived from eight different series that involved a total of 952 patients. (From International Workshop on Chronic Lymphocytic Leukemia: Chronic lymphocytic leukemia: Recommendations for diagnosis, staging, and response criteria. Ann Intern Med 110:236–238, 1989, Appendix with permission.)

Binet Staging System for Chronic Lymphocytic Leukemia

STAGE	CLINICAL FEATURES	SURVIVAL* (mo.)
A	Hemoglobin, ≥ 100 g/L; platelets, ≥ 100 × 10^9/L; and < three areas[†] involved	>120
B	Hemoglobin, ≥ 100 g/L; platelets, ≥ 100 × 10^9/L; and ≥ three areas involved	61
C	Hemoglobin, < 100 g/L or platelets, < 100 × 10^9/L, or both (independently of the areas involved)	32

*Weighted median survival was derived from eight different series that involved a total of 1117 patients.
[†] The three areas include the cervical, axillary, and inguinal lymph notes (whether unilateral or bilateral), the spleen, and the liver.
(From International Workshop on Chronic Lymphocytic Leukemia: Chronic lymphocytic leukemia: Recommendations for diagnosis, staging, and response criteria. Ann Intern Med 110:236–238, 1989, Appendix with permission.)

84. What are the autoimmune complications of CLL?

Autoimmune phenomena are commonplace in CLL. Of these, warm antibody autoimmune hemolytic anemia is the most frequent, occurring in 15–35% of patients during the course of their illness. Immune thrombocytopenia or neutropenia is also seen in association with CLL. Pure red cell aplasia has also been observed.

Gale RP, Foon KA: Chronic lymphocytic leukemia. Ann Intern Med 103:101–120, 1985.

85. What lymphoproliferative disorder is associated with pancytopenia, splenomegaly, absence of lymphadenopathy, and circulating lymphoid cells with multiple projections?

Hairy cell leukemia (HCL) is the disorder described. Although an uncommon malignancy, accounting for 2% of all leukemias, HCL receives a lot of attention because of the advances that have been made in its treatment and in part because of the unusual infections observed in the course of the disease. HCL is an important consideration in the workup of individuals who present with pancytopenia. Although the bone marrow aspirate is often scanty, characteristic "hairy" lymphs may be observed. The biopsy may show a diffusely involved marrow with mononuclear cells situated in a network of fibrosis. Some patients have had presentations as aplastic anemia. Although hairy cells may be present in the marrow, the biopsy picture is one of profound hypocellularity. The hairy cell is a B-lymphocyte with an immunophenotype consistent with a cell between a CLL-lymphocyte and a plasma cell. Hairy cells also possess the Tac antigen, a receptor for interleukin-2, usually seen on activated T-cells. The distinctive cytochemical feature of the hairy cell is a tartrate-resistant acid phosphatase activity. Many patients improve after splenectomy. Interferon has been used successfully in ameliorating this disorder.

86. What are the infectious complications of HCL?

The course of HCL is marked by increased incidence of infections with atypical mycobacteria or fungi, such as histoplasmosis and cryptococcus. There may also be an increased incidence of bacterial infections and perhaps legionellosis. Factors in the occurrence of atypical mycobacterial and fungal infections in these patients may be (1) decreased neutrophils, (2) absolute monocytopenia, and (3) inability to form granuloma normally.

Westbrook CA, Golde DW: Clinical problems in hairy cell leukemia: Diagnosis and management. Semin Oncology 11:514, 1984.

HODGKIN'S AND NON-HODGKIN'S LYMPHOMAS

87. What are the common presentations of Hodgkin's disease?

Patients most often present with lymphadenopathy, usually in the neck or axilla, with lymph nodes that are usually nontender, rubbery, and discrete. Sometimes these nodes wax and wane in size until attention is sought. Important symptoms that figure into the staging of Hodgkin's disease are (1) fever, (2) weight loss ($> 10\%$ of body weight), and (3) night sweats. Some patients are troubled by pruritus. Hodgkin's disease tends to originate in central lymph nodes so that some patients present with mediastinal lymphadenopathy.

88. How does Hodgkin's disease spread and how does this pattern affect the staging of Hodgkin's disease?

Hodgkin's disease is thought to spread from a unifocal site to contiguous lymph nodes. There may be early hematogenous dissemination to the spleen, with subsequent spread to the splenic hilar and retroperitoneal nodes as well as the liver. With development of large tumor masses, there may be extension into adjacent organs. It is important to remember that the spleen is often significantly involved in the absence of palpable splenomegaly. Hence, many centers recommend staging laparotomy to avoid missing splenic and hepatic disease. The importance of staging in Hodgkin's disease is to determine the extent of disease and thereby decide on therapy.

A summary of the Ann Arbor classification system for Hodgkin's disease is shown below:

Ann Arbor Staging of Hodgkin's Disease

STAGE		INVOLVEMENT
I:	I	Single lymph node
	IE	Single extralymphatic organ
II:	II	Two or more lymph nodes on same side of the diaphragm
	IIE	With localized extralymphatic site
III:	III	Lymph nodes above and below the diaphragm
	IIIE	With localized extralymphatic site
	IIIS	With isolated splenic site
	IIISE	With both extralymphatic and splenic sites
IV:	IV	Disseminated or diffuse involvement or one or more extralymphatic sites
Substage A:	Asymptomatic	
Substage B:	Fever, sweats, weight loss $> 10\%$ of body weight	

Aisenberg A: The staging and treatment of Hodgkin's disease. N Engl J Med 299:1228, 1978.

89. What are the histological subtypes of Hodgkin's disease? Which carry the worst prognosis and why?

Histological Subtypes of Hodgkin's Disease

Nodular sclerosis   (35%)
Mixed cellularity   (33%)
Lymphocyte predominant   (16%)
Lymphocyte depletion   (16%)

Nodular sclerosis more frequently affects women, whereas the other three types more often affect males. While staging generally determines the outlook, histologic subtype is also important. Nodular sclerosing and lymphocyte predominant disease tend to present with limited disease. Lymphocyte depletion is associated with more advanced disease, retroperitoneal involvement, and presentation in older adults.

90. What is the classic cell seen in the lymph node of patients with Hodgkin's disease?

The salient feature of lymph node pathologic change in Hodgkin's disease is the Reed-Sternberg cell. This is a large cell with two nuclei, each possessing a distinct nucleolus. Reed-Sternberg cells are plentiful in mixed cellularity and lymphocyte depletion Hodgkin's disease. In nodular sclerosis and lymphocyte predominant disease, Reed-Sternberg cells may be rare, being overwhelmed by reactive lymphocytes, polys, and eosinophils. In nodular sclerosis there is retraction of the cells surrounding the Reed-Sternberg cell during fixation, producing the "lacunar cell." Also present are bands of fibrosis.

91. Under what circumstances should patients with Hodgkin's disease undergo staging laparotomy?

Patients must first undergo a comprehensive clinical staging evaluation before surgical staging is contemplated. The key elements in the clinical staging are as follows:

Clinical Staging of Hodgkin's Disease

Detailed history	Radiology: PA and lateral of the chest,
Detailed physical exam, with attention to	abdominal and chest CT, bilateral
lymph node areas, spleen, and liver	lower extremity lymphangiogram
Laboratory: CBC, erythrocyte sedimentation	Bone marrow aspirate and biopsy
rate, alkaline phosphastase, renal and	
liver function tests	

Once this evaluation is complete, the need for surgical staging with laparotomy can be considered. If disseminated or diffuse extralymphatic involvement is found, there is no need for staging laparotomy. Generally speaking, there is no need for staging laparotomy if the results of this would not change therapy. In centers where treatment includes chemotherapy for limited disease, then the need for laparotomy is less apparent. Unfortunately, staging laparotomy carries a high morbidity from pulmonary emboli, subphrenic abscesses, stress ulcers, and wound infections.

92. In patients cured of Hodgkin's disease, what are the late sequelae of therapy?

The treatment of Hodgkin's disease is so successful that there exists an excellent opportunity to see late effects of radiation and chemotherapy that we do not see in disorders where such therapy provides only a temporary remission. The most important of these sequelae is the occurrence of leukemia and non-Hodgkin's lymphoma 3–10 years after therapy. Certain complications of the high-dose irradiation given to patients are also evident: acute radiation pneumonitis with fever, cough, and shortness of breath. Cardiac effects of irradiation include pericarditis, pericardial effusions, and pericardial fibrosis. There may be an acceleration of coronary artery disease. Neurologic effects of irradiation include Lhermitte's syndrome (paresthesias produced by flexion of the neck).

93. How does the pattern of lymph node involvement (diffuse versus nodular) correlate with the pace of disease progression?
In nodular lymphomas, the neoplastic lymphocytes congregate into aggregates that superficially resemble germinal centers. Lymphomas of this type generally pursue an indolent course. Diffuse lymphomas tend to behave in a more aggressive manner.

94. How often do lymphoma patients have bone marrow involvement?
Bone marrow involvement is extremely common in non-Hodgkin's lymphoma, whereas it is relatively uncommon in Hodgkin's disease. Diffuse well-differentiated lymphocytic lymphoma is associated with bone marrow involvement 100% of the time. Small, cleaved-cell lymphomas, follicular and diffuse types, are associated with bone marrow involvement 40–50% of the time. Large-cell or histiocytic lymphomas are less likely to spread to the marrow (15% incidence of involvement).

95. In Africa, Denis P. Burkitt (b. 1911) described an aggressive neoplasm that bears his name. What are the salient features of this lymphoma and what are its characteristic cytogenetic abnormalities?
Burkitt's lymphoma results from a proliferation of B-lymphocytes with a striking appearance. They present as round or oval cells with abundant basophilic cytoplasm-containing vacuoles that stain positively for fat. The tissue is replaced with a monotonous infiltrate of cells with interspersed macrophages giving a "starry sky" appearance. When the presentation is that of a leukemia, it is classified as L3 in the FAB scheme. These cells proliferate rapidly and have a potential doubling time of 24 hours. In African Burkitt's, patients present with large extranodal tumors of the jaws, abdominal viscera including kidney, and ovaries and retroperitoneum. In American Burkitt's, patients present with intra-abdominal tumors arising from the ileocecal region or mesenteric lymph nodes. In Africa, the disease is associated with Epstein-Barr virus, this this is less often true in American cases. A t(8;14) translocation is recognized in all cases. The proto-oncogene C-myc is located on 8 and usually becomes translocated to the locus of the heavy-chain immunoglobulin gene. This results in the activation of C-myc.
    Ziegler J: Burkitt's lymphoma. N Engl J Med 305:735, 1981.

96. Should all patients with non-Hodgkin's lymphoma receive chemotherapy or radiotherapy?
In an evaluation of patients with favorable histology and Stage III or IV disease, it was found that deferral of treatment until patients became symptomatic did not adversely affect survival. In fact, during the course of nontreatment, spontaneous regression was frequently observed. In such patients the median time to treatment was 31 months. In the absence of curative chemotherapy for indolent lymphomas, deferral of treatment is a reasonable course, provided patients are followed closely.
    Portlock CS, Rosenberg SA: No initial therapy for Stage III and IV non-Hodgkin's lymphoma of favorable histologic types. Ann Intern Med 90:10, 1979.

PLASMA CELL DYSCRASIAS

97. What disorders are associated with the presence of a serum monoclonal immunoglobulin paraprotein?
See table on next page.

Disorders Associated with Monoclonal Gammopathy

Collagen-vascular diseases (SLE, scleroderma, Sjögren's disease, rheumatoid arthritis)	Hepatitis, cirrhosis
Crohn's disease	Infectious disease (TB, SBE, AIDS, purpura fulminans)
Skin disease (pyoderma gangrenosum, psoriasis, scleromyxedema, urticaria)	Myeloproliferative diseases
	Post bone marrow transplantation
Gaucher's disease	Cryoglobulinemia

Lichtman MA: Essential and secondary monoclonal gammopathies. In Williams WJ, et al (eds): Hematology, 4th ed. New York, McGraw-Hill, 1990, pp 1109–1114.

98. How do you differentiate multiple myeloma (MM) from benign monoclonal gammopathy (BMG)?

The discovery of a monoclonal protein on serum protein electrophoresis should be followed by a careful workup to determine if MM is present. The features distinguishing MM from BMG are outlined below. Patients who have a small serum spike, normal CBC, no proteinuria, and no lytic lesions, hypercalcemia or renal dysfunction are usually followed with periodic serum protein electrophoresis. Patients meeting some of the criteria for MM, but showing no progression with follow-up, are described as having indolent MM. These patients generally do not have anemia or lytic bone lesions.

Differentiation of Multiple Myeloma from Monoclonal Gammopathy

	MM	BMG
M-protein	>3.5 g/dl	<3.5 g/dl
Anemia or other cytopenia	Usually present	Absent
Urine protein	>500 mg/24 h	<500 mg/24 hr
Bones	Lytic lesions or osteoporosis	Normal
Marrow plasma cells	>10%	<10%
Serum B_2 microglobulin (mg/L)	>3.0	<3.0
Calcium	Elevated in 30%	Normal
Creatinine	± elevation	Normal
Change in monoclonal protein with time	Increases	No change

99. What are the common complications of multiple myeloma?

The effects of the proliferation of plasma cells that results in MM are many:

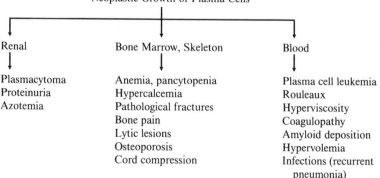

Proliferation of plasma cells, resulting in multiple myeloma.

100. What are the renal manifestations of multiple myeloma?

Renal Disease in Multiple Myeloma

Myeloma kidney	Glomerulonephritis
Dense tubular casts and progressive azotemia	Urate nephropathy
Hyperviscosity	Pyelonephritis
Renal tubular dysfunction	Dye-nephropathy
Isosthenuria	Hypercalcemia renal damage
Renal tubular acidosis	Plasma cell infiltration
Adult Fanconi syndrome	Amyloid kidney
	Nephrotic syndrome

DeFranzo RA, et al: Renal function in patients with multiple myeloma. Medicine 57:151, 1978.

101. What are the clinical manifestations of Waldenstrom's macroglobulinemia? What treatment modality is often effective in rapidly reversing these manifestations?

Waldenstrom's macroglobulinemia is a B-cell disorder of proliferating plasmacytoid lymphs that produce an IgM monoclonal protein. Patients frequently have hepatosplenomegaly, lymphadenopathy, and bone marrow involvement. Elderly people are affected most often. Neurologic disease, including peripheral neuropathy and cerebellar dysfunction, is also seen. A prominent feature is retinopathy with large sausage-shaped, dilated retinal veins. Bleeding and purpura are also commonly seen. Of particular importance is the recognition of the hyperviscosity syndrome, which can also occur in MM. This syndrome can respond dramatically to plasmapheresis, because IgM does not have a large extravascular distribution.

102. What are the manifestations of the hyperviscosity syndrome?

Hyperviscosity Syndrome

Global CNS dysfunction and stupor
Retinopathy
   Retinal hemorrhages
   Papilledema
Hypervolemia, congestive heart failure (CHF)
Headache, vertigo, ataxia
Stroke
Coagulopathy

103. Patients with the lambda-light-chain type of MM are prone to developing amyloidosis. What are the clinical and laboratory clues to the presence of this systemic disorder?

Amyloid is a lardaceous substance that accumulates in the tissue of patients with a variety of disorders, including myeloma. In myeloma the amyloid is comprised of light chains, most often lambda, arranged in a B-pleated sheet. When stained with Congo red and viewed under polarized light, amyloid shows an apple-green birefringence. Patients may develop purpura from skin involvement, hepatosplenomegaly, macroglossia, orthostatic hypotension, CHF, malabsorption, nephrotic syndrome, peripheral neuropathy, and carpal tunnel syndrome. Interestingly, the consequences of amyloid include an acquired factor X deficiency, resulting in a prolonged PT and PTT and functional hyposplenism. The latter results in the presence of Howell-Jolly bodies, even though the spleen is present.

Kyle RA, Griepp PR: Amyloidosis (AL): Clinical and laboratory features in 229 cases. Mayo Clin Proc 58:665–683, 1983.

HEMOSTASIS

104. How do you define the primary and secondary phases of hemostasis? How does the clinical presentation differ?

The patient with abnormal bleeding challenges our ability to diagnose and treat effectively. Hemostasis is a complicated process with several components, all of which must work well, for normal hemostasis. Two overlapping phases of the formation of a clot or hemostatic plug are: (1) **primary hemostasis**—the ruptured vessel wall interacts with platelets that must adhere and aggregate to form the basis of the clot; (2) **secondary hemostasis**—the clotting factors circulating in the blood activate each other in a cascade that results in the activation of thrombin and the deposition of fibrin around the platelet plug. Bleeding disorders may be roughly classified into disorders of primary or secondary hemostasis, with certain shared characteristics.

Bleeding Disorders

	PRIMARY	SECONDARY
Onset	Immediate	Delayed, hours after trauma
Sites, type of lesion	Mucosa, skin, GI, GU, purpura	Joints, retroperitoneum, muscles, hematuria
Components involved	Vessel wall, platelet adhesion	Generation of fibrin from fibrinogen
Typical disorder	von Willebrand disease	Hemophilia A (factor VIII:C deficiency)

105. What conditions are associated with immune thrombocytopenias?

Immune thrombocytopenias occur in many situations. In idiopathic thrombocytopenic purpura (ITP), an autoantibody arises (usually IgG) that interacts with the patient's own platelets. Sometimes these antibodies interact with specific antigens related to functional proteins. Platelets coated with the auto-IgG are then sequestered and removed by macrophages in the spleen, liver, and bone marrow. Production of megakaryocytes as judged by a bone marrow aspirate appears to be normal. However, recent studies indicate that megakaryocytopoiesis is in fact suboptimal for the degree of peripheral destruction. Thus, megakaryocytes may be affected by the autoantibody of ITP. ITP implies no known cause and is a diagnosis of exclusion. The typical patient used to be a young woman, often a young pregnant woman. HIV infection results in a typical ITP-like illness as well. As a result of the epidemic of HIV-related disease in urban centers, the typical patient may be a young man with a positive serology for HIV virus. Some of the conditions associated with immune thrombocytopenia are outlined below.

Disorders Associated with Immune Thrombocytopenia

1. Collagen-vascular diseases (SLE)
2. Impaired immunity (Bruton's agammaglobulinemia, IV drug users, HIV-1 infection)
3. Lymphoid neoplasias (Hodgkin's disease, non-Hodgkin's lymphoma, CLL)
4. Drug-induced (quinine, quinidine, hydrochlorothiazide, gold, heparin)
5. Others (thyrotoxicosis, sarcoidosis, antithymocyte globulin, solid tumors, anaphylaxis)
6. Iso-immune (post-transfusion purpura, fetal-maternal isoimmunization)

106. What disorders are associated with nonimmune destruction of platelets?

Thrombocytopenia can occur with a wide variety of disorders of hematopoiesis. What is of concern here are those situations that result in the increased peripheral destruction of platelets. Some of these conditions listed below may have immune components.

Increased Platelet Destruction

Infections	Microangiopathic disease
Sepsis, gram negative or gram positive	Disseminated intravascular coagulation
Viral, rickettsial	Thrombotic thrombocytopenic purpura
Histoplasmosis	Eclampsia, pre-eclampsia
Malaria	Burns
Typhoid, brucella	Cavernous hemangiomas
Hypersplenism	Kasabach-Merritt
	Extra-corporeal circulation, hypothermia
	Massive transfusion

107. What disorder results in a prolonged bleeding time and decreased factor VIII coagulant activity (VIII:C)?

An autosomal dominant disorder, von Willebrand's disease, results from several abnormalities in the production of a large, multimeric adhesive protein, von Willebrand factor (VIII:vWF). Classic vWF (type I) disease results from decreased release of vWF from the endothelial cell. von Willebrand factor is also synthesized by megakaryocytes and is a constituent of the alpha granules of platelets. Decreased presence of vWF at the site of endothelial damage results in impairment of platelet adhesion and consequently poor primary hemostasis. Patients with von Willebrand's disease have problems with epistaxis, hematuria, menorrhagia, GI bleeding, and bleeding after trauma. In classic type I vWF disease, the platelet count is normal, the bleeding time is prolonged. Factor VIII:C is also reduced in the plasma of patients with von Willebrand's disease. The reduction of factor VIII:vWF seems to shorten the circulating life of factor VIII:C.

108. What are the hereditary disorders of platelet function?

Since von Willebrand disease is associated with platelet dysfunction, it is often considered with disorders resulting from congenital structural abnormalities of the platelet. These bleeding disorders are identified by a prolonged bleeding time and abnormal functional behavior in platelet aggregation tests. Three of these disorders are described below.

Hereditary Disorders Resulting in Platelet Dysfunction

	VON WILLEBRAND'S DISEASE	BERNARD-SOULIER SYNDROME	GLANZMANN'S THROMBASTHENIA
Defect	Reduced or abnormal factor VIII:vWF	Absence of platelet glycoprotein Ib, a receptor for vWF	Absence of platelet glycoprotein IIb/IIIa, a receptor for vWF and fibrinogen
Inheritance	Autosomal dominant	Autosomal recessive	Autosomal recessive
Platelet appearance	Normal	Macrothrombocytes	Normal
Aggregometry:			
Ristocetin	Decreased	Decreased	Normal
ADP	Normal	Normal	Decreased
Collagen	Normal	Normal	Decreased

109. What conditions result in an acquired platelet defect?

The biggest offender in this category is aspirin. Platelet cyclooxygenase is irreversibly inhibited by low doses of aspirin. As a result, the platelet has lifelong impaired function. Aspirin will exacerbate the bleeding tendencies associated with von Willebrand's disease and other platelet disorders and by itself can produce prolongation of the bleeding time. The potential benefit of this aspirin effect is to reduce platelet activity in critical areas—

such as a stenosed coronary artery. The typical finding in platelet aggregometry with aspirin-treated platelets is the absence of the secondary wave of aggregation produced by ADP. Another important acquired disorder of platelet function is that associated with uremia. Although the pathogenesis of this mild hemostatic defect is poorly understood, it appears that the administration of the vasopressin analog DDAVP increases factor VIII:vWF and shortens the bleeding time.

110. What two factor deficiencies result in hemophilia? What is their pattern of inheritance?
Hemophilia results from deficiency of factor VIII:C (hemophilia A) or factor IX (hemophilia B). These are X-linked disorders. The family history of an affected boy reveals affected maternal uncles and cousins. Patients may have mild or severe disease. Patients with severe hemophilia require frequent administration of factor VIII or IX concentrates. Hemophilia care is optimal if it is organized around a hemophilia center and home care. In the past, hemophilia was a crippling disorder because of the frequency of hemarthroses and arthritis that ensued. Prophylactic administration of factor VIII concentrate after trauma has reduced the incidence of complications dramatically. The tragedy of hemophilia care has been the acquisition of HIV-1 viral infection from the factor VIII and IX concentrates pooled from thousands of donors. Now safeguards against donation by HIV-positive individuals are in place. A variety of pasteurization and purification processes are now utilized to make these products safer. The availability of factors produced by recombinant DNA technology may eliminate blood-borne viral disease altogether.

111. How necessary is a preoperative measurement of the PT and PTT in a patient without a history of bleeding? What questions need to be asked in such a history?
Although physicians order a preop or prebiopsy PT and PTT by reflex, the value of these tests as screens for coagulation defects has been disputed. In recent studies, no advantage was seen in performing these tests on the asymptomatic patient. The low prevalence of clinically important, yet unsuspected bleeding disorders, results in more false-positive tests than true positives. However, both tests are indicated in the symptomatic patient and in the monitoring of warfarin (via the PT) or heparin (via the PTT) administration.

The patient interview should include questions regarding personal or family history of bleeding problems, including prolonged bleeding after dental extraction, injury, or surgical procedure. Patients should be asked about frequent nose bleeds, menorrhagia, melena, and bruising. A history of liver disease, obvious malnutrition, or malabsorption syndrome should also be sought. Although irrelevant to the PT and PTT, a recent history of aspirin ingestion needs to be sought. The physical exam should include an inspection of the skin and mucosa for purpura or petechiae, hematomas, and ecchymotic lesions.

Suchman AL, Griner PA: Diagnostic uses of the activated partial thromboplastin time and prothrombin time. Ann Intern Med 104:810–816, 1986.

112. What hereditary disorders and what common acquired disorder result in a prolonged PTT without bleeding?
When routine preoperative screening PT and PTT tests are obtained, occasional patients will have a dramatic, reproducible prolongation of the PTT, but no history or physical findings to suggest a hemostatic disorder. Familial disorders causing this phenomenon are (1) hereditary deficiency of factor XII (Hageman factor) and (2) deficiency of factors in the contact activation system that activates XII. Fletcher factor (pre-kallikrein) and Fitzgerald factor (high molecular weight kininogen) are two proteins in the contact activation pathway that have been identified as rare deficiencies in individuals. These disorders produce an interesting in-vitro phenomenon that does not seem to result in any hemorrhagic tendency. In fact, Mr. Hageman, the first person recognized to be deficient in factor XII, died of pulmonary embolism.

When a prolonged PTT is identified, a mixing study is usually done to determine if normal plasma will correct it. If correctable, then a deficiency in the intrinsic pathway is suggested. If not corrected, an inhibitor may be present in the plasma. Spontaneous production of antibodies against factor VIII has been well-documented. Such individuals with acquired hemophilia typically bleed. Another more common inhibitor is the lupus anticoagulant, which is usually an IgG directed against phospholipid moieties. This acquired inhibitor is also seen frequently in patients without lupus. Although it most often causes a prolongation of the PTT, the PT may also be slightly prolonged. Several tests now exist to identify the lupus anticoagulant activity. Patients with this disorder do not usually bleed. Often the prolonged PTT is accompanied by mild thrombocytopenia, a false-positive VDRL, and anticardiolipin antibodies. When the latter are present in pregnancy, there may be associated with them an increased frequency of spontaneous abortions. The lupus anticoagulant may also be associated with stroke or other thrombotic disease.

Patients who have severe bleeding and a prolonged PTT typically have deficiencies of factor VIII:C or factor IX (hemophilia A, B, respectively). Mild bleeding and prolongation of the PTT may be caused by factor XI deficiency. Bleeding and a normal PTT, but a prolonged PT, are caused by factor VII deficiency, or initiation of coumarin anticoagulation.

Espinoza LR, Hartman RC: Significance of the lupus anticoagulant. Am J Hematol 22:231, 1986.

113. What are the causes of disseminated intravascular coagulation (DIC)?

Causes of DIC

Infections	Collagen-vascular disease
Viral (epidemic hemorrhagic fevers,	Vasculitis
herpes, rubella)	Polyarteritis
Rickettsial (Rocky Mountain spotted fever)	SLE
Bacterial (gram-negative sepsis,	Obstetric complications
meningococcemia)	Abruptio placentae
Fungal (histoplasmosis)	Septic abortion
Protozoan (malaria)	Amniotic fluid embolism
Neoplasms	Intrauterine fetal death
Carcinomas (prostate, pancreas, breast,	Saline-, urea-induced abortions
lung, ovary)	Eclampsia
Acute promyelocytic leukemia	Hemolytic transfusion reactions
Vascular disease	Hypothermia–rewarming
Cavernous hemangiomas (Kasabach-Merritt	Shock
syndrome)	Cocaine-induced rhabdomyolysis
Aneurysms	Use of Factor IX concentrates

Colman RW, et al: Disseminated intravascular coagulation. Ann Rev Med 30:359, 1979.

114. When disseminated intravascular coagulation (DIC) is present, what coagulation tests should be abnormal?

DIC occurs when there is inappropriate activation of thrombin and disseminated clotting, which in turn is associated with increased fibrinolysis. During this process multiple coagulation factors are consumed. By-products of thrombin and plasmin activity circulate as well. As endothelial cell damage occurs, there is consumption of platelets and in some instances fragmentation of RBCs, resulting in significant intravascular hemolysis. Although DIC is often a hemorrhagic condition, certain patients will present with thrombotic complications: digital ischemia, decreased mentation, migrating thrombophlebitis, and renal involvement. The typical profile of commonly used tests in DIC is shown below.

Laboratory Findings in DIC

Peripheral blood smear	Decreased platelets
	Red cell fragmentation
PT, PTT	Both prolonged
Fibrinogen	Decreased
Fibrin degradation products	Increased
Platelet count	Decreased

115. How does the bleeding diathesis associated with liver disease resemble DIC?

The liver may not be the seat of the soul, but it is definitely the site of production of all the clotting factors except for VIII:vWF. Severe liver disease compromises hemostasis in a number of ways. What is usually most readily detected is a decrease in the activity of the vitamin K-dependent Factors II, VII, IX, and X. Patients with severe liver disease will have a prolonged PT and PTT that does not improve after the administration of vitamin K. Low fibrinogen levels are seen. They also elaborate a poorly functioning fibrinogen. Dysfibrinogenemia produces prolongation of the PT, PTT, and the thrombin time. With the onset of cirrhosis and portal hypertension, splenomegaly and a reduced platelet count occur. The liver is also an important organ of clearance of plasminogen activators, so that increased fibrin degradation products may be measured. Thus the laboratory abnormalities in severe liver disease may mimic DIC.

116. Patients receiving certain antibiotics develop prolongation of the PT and PTT. What is the most likely cause and how may this be avoided?

It is now recognized that certain beta-lactam antibiotics reduce the prothrombin level. This characteristic is associated with a methylthiotetrazole substitution that appears to inhibit microsomal carboxylase activity. This results in decreased gamma carboxylation of the vitamin K-dependent factors. Antibiotics in general may reduce vitamin K levels by destroying the bacterial flora of the gut, which also provide vitamin K. Thus the combination of prolonged, reduced feeding and antibiotic administration is associated with vitamin K deficiency and a bleeding diathesis. When beta-lactam antibiotics with the methylthiotetrazole substitution are administered, the inhibition of the vitamin K-dependent carboxylase results in the more rapid onset of a bleeding diathesis.

Platelet function can be impaired by a number of antibiotics such as carbenicillin or ticarcillin. It appears that platelet function may also be affected by some of the newer beta-lactam antibiotics. Thus, moxalactam has been reported to prolong the bleeding time. Presumably, antibiotics interact with the platelet membrane to block receptor-mediated aggregation. Unfortunately, some patients who receive the beta-lactam antibiotics experience a "double whammy" of hypoprothrombinemia and platelet dysfunction. Bleeding may be avoided by concomitant administration of vitamin K and using the lowest antibiotic dose possible. The patient who develops bleeding while receiving this antibiotic may also benefit from platelet transfusions.

Sattler FR, et al: Potential for bleeding with the new beta-lactam antibiotics. Ann Intern Med 105:924, 1986.

117. What are the congenital disorders associated with increased incidence of deep venous thromboembolism (DVT)?

The occurrence of DVT in a young person, a family history of thrombosis, thrombosis at unusual sites (such as mesenteric vein), or recurrent thrombosis without precipitating factors should persuade the clinician that the patient has a hypercoagulable state. The most important hereditary conditions that predispose to venous thrombotic events are deficiencies of antithrombin III (ATIII) and protein C and S. Dysfibrinoginemia, factor XII deficiency, and certain disorders of the fibrinolytic system are also predisposing conditions. As mentioned before, the acquisition of a lupus anticoagulant may also result in a tendency to venous (and also arterial) thrombi. A relative ATIII deficiency may also occur in patients with liver disease or DIC. Proteins C and S are vitamin K-dependent anticoagulant proteins. When patients are placed on warfarin for treatment of DVT, the goal of therapy is to reduce the activity of procoagulant factors (VII included). This is monitored by following the PT, which detects early changes in the activity of factor VII. When coumarin therapy is initiated, particularly when started at high doses, or in patients with congenital deficiency, the levels of protein C may drop precipitously before the onset of anticoagulation due to decreased factor VII activity. A consequence of this is a serious disorder, coumarin skin necrosis. ATIII, protein C, and protein S deficiency states are heterozygous conditions. Neonates with homozygous protein C deficiency develop fatal thrombosis. Patients with these disorders need careful evaluation and family screening. Symptomatic individuals are cautiously managed with coumarin anticoagulation. The acquired or secondary causes of hypercoagulability are numerous and have been well reviewed by Schafer.

The Secondary Hypercoagulable States

Abnormalities of coagulation and fibrinolysis	Abnormalities of blood vessels and rheology
Malignancy	Conditions promoting venous stasis
Pregnancy	(immobilization, obesity, advanced
Use of oral contraceptives	age, postoperative state)
Infusion of prothrombin complex concentrates	Artificial surfaces
Nephrotic syndrome	Vasculitis and chronic occlusive arterial
Abnormalities of platelets	disease
Myeloproliferative disorders	Homocystinuria
Paroxysmal nocturnal hemoglobinuria	Hyperviscosity (polycythemia, leukemia,
Hyperlipidemia	sickle cell disease, leukoagglutination,
Diabetes mellitus	increased serum viscosity)
Heparin-induced thrombocytopenia	Thrombotic thrombocytopenic purpura

(From Schafer AI: The hyercoagulable states. Ann Intern Med 102:814, 1985, p 818, with permission.)

BIBLIOGRAPHY

1. Rappaport S: Introduction to Hematology, 2nd ed. Philadelphia, J.B. Lippincott, 1987.
2. Williams WJ, et al (eds): Hematology, 4th ed. New York, McGraw-Hill, 1990.
3. Wintrobe MM, et al: Clinical Hematology, 9th ed. Philadelphia, Lea & Febiger, 1989.

10. PULMONARY SECRETS

Sheila Goodnight White, M.D., and Anthony J. Zollo, Jr., M.D.

When man grows old . . . there is much gas within his thorax, resulting in panting and troubled breathing.

Huang Ti (The Yellow Emperor) (2697–2597 B.C.)
Nei Chung Su Wen, Bk. 6, Sect. 19 (tr. by Ilza Veith in: The Yellow Emperor's Classic of Internal Medicine)

DIAPHRAGM, n. A muscular partition separating disorders of the chest from disorders of the bowels.

Ambrose Bierce (1842–1914?)
The Devil's Dictionary

A PULMONOLOGIST'S VALENTINE

Roses are red
Violets are blue
Without your lungs
Your blood would be too.

David D. Ralph, M.D.
(Submitted by Susan Ott, M.D.,
Mrs. David Ralph)
From *The New England Journal of Medicine,* 304:739, 1981.

1. What are the principles of intensive care?
1. Air goes in and out.
2. Blood goes 'round and 'round.
3. Oxygen is good.
(From Matz R: Principles of medicine. NY State J Med 77:1984–1985, 1977, with permission.)

DIAGNOSTIC TECHNIQUES

2. What are the five basic mechanisms of hypoxemia?
Hypoxemia is defined as deficient oxygenation of the blood. There are five basic pathophysiologic mechanisms that can cause hypoxemia, and they are listed below:

1. **Decreased P_IO_2:** Any condition that leads to a decrease in the oxygen content of the inspired gas can lead to hypoxemia. This can be expressed as a decrease in the F_IO_2 (the fraction of the inspired gas made up of oxygen) or the P_IO_2 (the partial pressure of oxygen in the inspired gas). Situations leading to this problem include high altitudes, flying in a non-pressurized airplane cabin, or rebreathing expired gases (as in a paper bag or closed space).

2. **Hypoventilation:** Any condition that interferes with the normal movement of gas in and out of the alveoli will lead to hypoxemia. Examples include choking, COPD, asthma, and respiratory muscle paralysis.

3. **Diffusion abnormality:** Any condition that interferes with the normal diffusion of oxygen from the alveolar space into the capillaries can lead to hypoxemia. Examples include diffuse interstitial fibrosis, berylliosis, and collagen-vascular diseases.

4. **Ventilation-perfusion (V/Q) abnormalities:** Any condition that leads to a mismatching of ventilation and perfusion can cause hypoxemia. Most pulmonary disorders are associated with some degree of V/Q mismatching.

5. **Shunt:** Any condition that leads to perfusion of nonventilated tissue can lead to hypoxemia. A shunt is an absolute mismatching of ventilation and perfusion in which there is perfusion of alveoli with absolutely no ventilation. Examples include pulmonary arteriovenous fistulae, intracardiac shunts, and conditions in which there is perfusion of alveoli that are filled with pus, fluid, or other substances (pneumonia, pulmonary edema, intrapulmonary hemorrhage, etc.).

3. How can the five basic mechanisms of hypoxemia be differentiated?

The values of P_aCO_2, alveolar-arterial oxygen (A-aO_2) gradient, and the response to breathing 100% oxygen can be used to separate the basic causes of hypoxemia:

Differentiation of the Causes of Hypoxemia*

MECHANISM	P_aO_2	P_aCO_2	A-aO_2 GRADIENT	RESPONSE TO 100% O_2
↓ P_IO_2	↓	→ or ↓	→	N/A
Hypoventilation	↓	↑	→	N/A
Diffusion abnormality	↓	→ or ↓	↑	Yes
V/Q mismatch	↓	→ or ↓	↑	Yes
Shunt	↓	→ or ↓	↑	No

*↓ = decreased, → = normal, ↑ = increased, N/A = not applicable.

4. What is the alveolar-arterial oxygen gradient ($P_{A-a}O_2$)?

The $P_{A-a}O_2$ is the difference in the partial pressure of oxygen between the alveolar air (P_AO_2) and the arterial blood (P_aO_2). This can be stated as follows:

$$P_{A-a}O_2 = P_AO_2 - P_aO_2$$

A normal $P_{A-a}O_2$ is 10–15 mmHg in a patient breathing room air. In conditions that interfere with oxygen exchange between the alveoli and pulmonary capillaries, the $P_{A-a}O_2$ will increase.

5. Does the $P_{A-a}O_2$ increase with age?

Yes. A normal $P_{A-a}O_2$ can be estimated by multiplying the patient's age by 0.04. Thus, a healthy 70-year-old would be expected to have a $P_{A-a}O_2$ of approximately 28 mmHg. Of course, this is only an approximation and there is a great deal of individual variation.

6. How do you calculate a patient's A-aO_2 gradient ($P_{A-a}O_2$)?

The $P_{A-a}O_2$ can be calculated by estimating the alveolar PO_2 (P_AO_2) using a simplified form of the alveolar air equation, and then subtracting from that estimate the measured value of the arterial blood PO_2 (P_aO_2). The P_AO_2 is calculated as follows:

$$P_AO_2 = P_IO_2 - (P_aCO_2 / RQ)$$

The P_IO_2 is the partial pressure of oxygen in the inspired gas and is calculated as follows:

$$P_IO_2 = F_IO_2 (P_{atm} - P_{H_2O})$$

The RQ is the respiratory quotient (usually 0.8), the F_IO_2 is the fraction of the inspired gas that is oxygen (21% in room air), the P_{atm} is the atmospheric pressure (760 mmHg at sea level), and the P_{H_2O} is the vapor pressure of water (assumed to be 47 mmHg). Therefore, in a patient breathing room air with P_aO_2 of 94 mmHg and a $PaCO_2$ of 40 mmHg, the P_AO_2 would be:

$$P_{A\text{-}a}O_2 = 0.21 (760\text{–}47) - 40/0.8 = 150 - 50 = 100 \text{ mmHg}$$

Therefore, his $P_{A\text{-}a}O_2$ would be:

$$P_{A\text{-}a}O_2 = P_AO_2 - P_aO_2 = 100 - 94 = 6 \text{ mmHg (within normal limits)}$$

7. What is the respiratory quotient (RQ) used in the alveolar air equation and what factors affect its value?

The RQ is the ratio of CO_2 produced per unit of oxygen consumed at the cellular level. It ranges from 0.7 when fatty acids are the substrate to 1.0 when carbohydrates are the substrate. Usually, a value of 0.8 can be used, to reflect the normal mixture of substrates. The RQ will increase towards 1.0 with increasing exercise due to the greater contribution of the high RQ of actively contracting muscles.

8. What is the oxyhemoglobin equilibrium curve and what does it demonstrate?

The oxyhemoglobin equilibrium curve (or dissociation curve) is a plot of the hemoglobin percent saturation (S_aO_2) against the P_aO_2. It demonstrates the binding reaction of hemoglobin and oxygen. This sigmoid shaped curve is shown below:

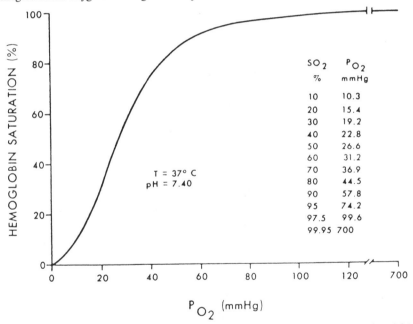

The normal oxyhemoglobin dissociation curve for humans. Values for hemoglobin saturation (SO_2) at different PO_2 values, under standard conditions of temperature and pH, are indicated. (From Murray JF: The Normal Lung, 2nd ed. Philadelphia, W.B. Saunders, 1986, p 174, with permission.)

The curve shows that the binding (or releasing) of oxygen and hemoglobin is not a linear relationship (as is the case with dissolved oxygen). Oxygen is readily released at the lower range of P_aO_2 values but very tightly held at the upper range of P_aO_2 values. In other words, the affinity of hemoglobin for oxygen increases as more and more oxygen molecules bind to it. This enables the oxygen content of blood to remain high at high P_aO_2 levels, but still allows hemoglobin to release oxygen readily as the P_aO_2 drops below 60 mmHg (the "steep" part of the curve).

9. How do you calculate the oxygen content of blood?

The oxygen content of blood (C_aO_2) includes the oxygen bound to hemoglobin, represented by the hemoglobin (Hgb) and the percent saturation (S_aO_2), and the oxygen dissolved in solution in the plasma, represented by the P_aO_2. It can be calculated as follows:

$$C_aO_2 = \text{oxygen bound to Hgb} + \text{oxygen dissolved in plasma}$$
$$= (1.34 \times Hgb \times S_aO_2) + (P_aO_2 \times 0.003)$$

The normal value is 16–20 ml per 100 ml of blood.

The vast majority (over 99%) of the oxygen content of blood is represented by that which is bound to hemoglobin. Only a very minor part of the total is represented by dissolved oxygen (that which is measured by P_aO_2). The clinical importance of this fact should be evident. Any therapy that raises the P_aO_2 while allowing a patient to remain anemic will not be affecting the maximal increase in the oxygen-carrying capacity of the blood.

10. What is meant by the P_{50}?

The P_{50} is the P_aO_2 that corresponds to a hemoglobin saturation (S_aO_2) of 50% under conditions of standard temperature (37°C) and pH (7.40). Normally it is 26.6 mmHg. It is a measure of the affinity of hemoglobin for oxygen. A higher P_{50} represents less hemoglobin affinity for oxygen and vice versa. The P_{50} varies with conditions that shift the oxyhemoglobin equilibrium curve.

11. Clinicians refer to a shift of the oxyhemoglobin equilibrium curve to the left or the right. What does this mean?

Since the curve represents the affinity of hemoglobin for oxygen over the range of P_aO_2, a shift in the curve in either direction represents a change in that affinity. A shift of the curve to the left represents an increase in the affinity of hemoglobin for oxygen, meaning that oxygen is taken up more readily and released less readily for any given P_aO_2. Conversely, a shift in the curve to the right represents a decrease in the affinity, meaning that oxygen is taken up less readily and released more readily.

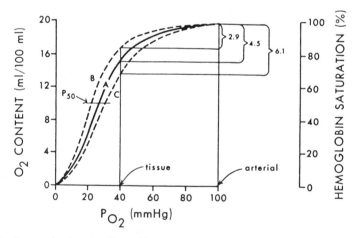

Schematic diagram showing the effects of increases and decreases in O_2 affinity on the amount of O_2 available at the PO_2 values prevailing in arterial blood and at the tissues. $P_{50} = PO_2$ at which hemoglobin saturation is 50 per cent. Hemoglobin concentration is assumed for convenience to be 14.9 gm/100 ml; therefore, O_2 content at 100 per cent saturation is 20 ml/100 ml. Curve A = normal blood; curve B = blood with increased affinity (decreased P_{50}); curve C = blood with decreased affinity (increased P_{50}). (From Murray JF: The Normal Lung, 2nd ed. Philadelphia, W.B. Saunders, 1986, p 175, with permission.)

12. What factors shift the oxyhemoglobin equilibrium curve?

Factors Influencing the Oxyhemoglobin Equilibrium Curve

SHIFT TO THE LEFT ($\uparrow$ Hgb/O_2 Affinity)	SHIFT TO THE RIGHT ($\downarrow$ Hgb/O_2 Affinity)
Hyperthermia/fever	Hypothermia
Alkalosis	Acidosis
Hypocapnia	Hypercapnia
$\downarrow$ 2,3 DPG	$\uparrow$ 2,3 DPG
$\uparrow$ Carboxyhemoglobin	$\downarrow$ Carboxyhemoglobin
Hemoglobin F, Chesapeake, Yakima, Ranier	Hemoglobin E, Seattle, Kansas

13. If the dissolved oxygen content of blood, measured by the P_aO_2, is so small compared to the oxygen bound to hemoglobin, why do we measure the P_aO_2 and follow it as we treat patients?

The oxyhemoglobin equilibrium curve answers this question. The P_aO_2, although directly measuring only a tiny fraction of the total oxygen content of blood, is related to the total oxygen content through the curve described above. As can be seen, as the P_aO_2 drops below 60 mmHg, the curve is very steep, whereas at a P_aO_2 over 60 mmHg, the curve is flat. A drop of P_aO_2 from 100 mmHg to 60 mmHg (a drop of 40 mmHg) represents a drop of hemoglobin saturation (S_aO_2) from 99% to 90% (a loss of only 9% of the blood's total oxygen content). However, a further drop of 40 mmHg, from a P_aO_2 of 60 mmHg to 20 mmHg, would represent a drop in S_aO_2 from 90% to about 30% (a loss of 60% of the blood's total oxygen content). Therapeutic guidelines call for maintaining the P_aO_2 above a level of 60 mmHg. Below this level, small decreases in P_aO_2 are accompanied by very large drops in the S_aO_2, and therefore very large drops in the total oxygen content of blood.

14. When is oxygen toxic?

Oxygen toxicity is an iatrogenic disease caused by prolonged administration of high concentrations of supplemental oxygen (in spite of the third law of intensive care—see Q. #1). Initially it is manifested by an acute exudative phase consisting of a decrease in vital capacity (within 6 hours), interstitial and alveolar edema, decreased lung compliance, decreased diffusion capacity, and an increased A–aO_2 gradient. The chronic proliferative phase has also been seen in humans and animals on prolonged oxygen therapy.

15. What is the good of oxygen therapy?

Because of oxygen toxicity, use of high concentrations of therapeutic oxygen (>60%) should be limited to a short duration (<24 hours) if possible. The goal of oxygen therapy should be to use the minimum oxygen concentration needed to maintain the P_aO_2 just over 60 mmHg. Attempts to further increase the P_aO_2 will not result in significant increases in the oxygen content of blood, but will increase the risk of oxygen toxicity.

16. What are the indications for bronchoscopy?

Flexible fiberoptic bronchoscopy (FOB) is a valuable diagnostic and therapeutic tool.
Diagnostic uses include:
- Evaluation of indeterminate lung lesions.
- Assessment of airway patency, including problems associated with endotracheal tubes.
- Investigation of unexplained symptoms (cough, hemoptysis, stridor, etc.) or unexplained findings (recurrent laryngeal nerve paralysis or recent diaphragmatic paralysis).
- Evaluation of suspicious or malignant sputum cytology.
- Preoperative staging of cancer.

- Specimen collection for selective cultures.
- Determination of the extent of injury secondary to burns, inhalation, etc.

Therapeutic uses include:
- Removal of mucous plugs/secretions, foreign bodies.
- Assist in difficult endotracheal intubations.

ATS Position Paper: Guidelines for fiberoptic bronchoscopy. ATS News, No. 4, Winter 1983.

17. What are the contraindications and complications of fiberoptic bronchoscopy?

Although there are no *absolute* contraindications to bronchoscopy, sound clinical judgment should guide any decision concerning an invasive procedure with potential risk for morbidity and mortality. In a large series of over 24,000 cases, mortality was 0.01% and complications 0.08%. Complications resulting from fiberoptic bronchoscopy include: reaction to topical anesthetic, trauma, laryngospasm, bronchospasm, hypoventilation, pneumothorax, hemorrhage, cardiac arrhythmia, myocardial infarction (MI), hypoxemia, ruptured lung abscess with flooding of airways, and postbronchoscopy fever/infection.

Credle WF, et al: Complications of fiberoptic bronchoscopy. Am Rev Respir Dis 109:67, 1974.

18. Which patients are at increased risk during bronchoscopy?

High-risk patients include patients with a bleeding diathesis, inability to cooperate with the examination, hypoxia, cardiac arrhythmias, unstable asthma, recent MI, acute hypercapnia, partial tracheal obstruction, hepatitis, uremia, lung abscess, immunosuppression, superior vena cava syndrome, and respiratory failure requiring mechanical ventilation.

19. State the most common clinical use of pulmonary function tests (PFTs).

By far the most common use of PFTs is the evaluation of obstructive airway disease. Causes of an obstructive ventilatory defect include: emphysema, bronchitis, asthma, bronchiolitis, and upper airway obstruction (by tumors, foreign bodies, stenosis, and edema.)

20. What are the lung volumes and capacities measured with PFTs?

Glossary for Static Lung Volumes

VOLUME/CAPACITY	SYMBOL	DEFINITION
Residual volume	RV	That volume of air remaining in the lungs after maximum expiration
Expiratory reserve volume	ERV	The maximum volume of air expired from the resting end-expiratory level
Tidal volume	TV*	That volume of air inspired or expired with each breath during quiet breathing
Inspiratory reserve volume	IRV	The maximum volume of air inspired from the resting end-inspiratory level
Inspiratory capacity	IC	The sum of IRV and TV
Vital capacity	VC	The maximum volume of air expired from the point of maximum inspiration
Inspiratory vital capacity	IVC	The maximum volume of air inspired from the point of maximum expiration
Functional residual capacity	FRC	The sum of RV and ERV (the volume of air remaining in the lungs at the end-expiratory position)
Total lung capacity	TLC	The sum of all volume compartments or the volume of air in the lungs after maximum inspiration

*The symbol TV is traditionally used for tidal volume to indicate a subdivision of static lung volume. The symbol V_T is used in gas-exchange formulas.
(From Fishman AP: Pulmonary Disease and Disorders. New York, McGraw-Hill, 1980, p 1752, with permission.)

The subdivisions of the lung volume. The term *capacity* is applied to a subdivision composed of two or more *volumes*. The definitions of these subdivisions are found in the table above. (From Fishman AP: Pulmonary Disease and Disorders. New York, McGraw-Hill, 1980, p 1752, with permission.)

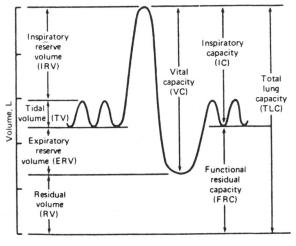

21. What are common causes of a restrictive ventilatory defect?

Common causes of restriction include:

- Interstitial lung disease (fibrosis, pneumoconiosis, edema)
- Chest wall disease (kyphoscoliosis, neuromuscular disease)
- Space-occupying lesions (tumors)
- Pleural disease (effusion)
- Extrathoracic conditions (obesity, ascites, pregnancy)

22. What are the PFT findings suggestive of a restrictive ventilatory defect?

A restrictive ventilatory defect is suggested by a decreased vital capacity, normal expiratory flow rates, and normal maximum voluntary ventilation. Supporting data confirming a restrictive defect are a decreased total lung capacity (TLC), decreased lung compliance, and decreased diffusion of carbon monoxide (DL_{co}).

23. Which test can help differentiate the etiology of an obstructive ventilatory defect secondary to emphysema versus chronic bronchitis?

The findings of an obstructive pattern associated with a normal single breath diffusing capacity (DL_{co}) argues against emphysema, whereas an obstructive defect with a decreased diffusion capacity suggests the presence of anatomic emphysema.

Gelb AF, et al: Physiologic diagnosis of subclinical emphysema. Am Rev Respir Dis 107:50–63, 1973.

PLEURAL EFFUSION

24. What are the two basic types of pleural effusions?

A pleural effusion represents an increase in fluid in the pleural space. The two basic categories are transudative and exudative effusions. A **transudative effusion** is classically associated with volume overload states, such as congestive heart failure, nephrotic syndrome, and cirrhosis. An **exudative effusion** is a protein-rich effusion secondary to inflammation or failure of lymphatic protein removal. Exudates occur in neoplasms, infection, and the various collagen vascular diseases.

25. What findings on physical examination are suggestive of a pleural effusion?

Small effusions (less than 500 cc) frequently have minimal findings. Larger effusions demonstrate dullness to percussion, diminished breath sounds, and reduced tactile and vocal fremitus over the involved hemithorax. Large effusions (greater than 1500 cc), with concomitant atelectasis, demonstrate bronchial breath sounds, egophony (a sound on auscultation like the bleating of a goat), and inspiratory lag.

26. Which diagnostic tests are used to distinguish transudative from exudative pleural effusions?

Thoracentesis (percutaneous removal of pleural fluid) is employed to obtain pleural fluid for analysis. The fluid is analyzed to help determine the etiology of the pleural effusion. An exudative pleural effusion meets one or more of the following criteria, whereas a transudative meets none:

    a. Pleural fluid protein/serum protein ratio of greater than 0.5.

    b. Pleural fluid LDH/serum LDH of greater than 0.6.

    c. Pleural fluid LDH greater than two-thirds the upper normal limit for serum.

Other tests that may be helpful include pleural fluid glucose, pH, cell count, and white blood cell (WBC) differential, amylase, Gram stain, special stains as indicated, and culture. Pleural glucose less than 60% of serum suggests infection, rheumatoid arthritis, or neoplasm. A pH less than 7.30 suggests empyema/infection. An elevated amylase in a left-sided pleural effusion may be secondary to pancreatitis. Pleural fluid WBC counts and differentials are usually of limited value. Transudative effusions usually have less than 1000 WBC/mm^3 and results are very variable in exudative effusions. Cytologic examination is indicated if a neoplasm is suspected.

Light RW, et al: Pleural effusion: The diagnostic separation of transudates and exudates. Ann Intern Med 77:507, 1972.

27. Which radiologic test should be performed in a patient with suspected pleural effusion?

A small amount of pleural fluid can be detected as the obliteration of the posterior part of the diaphragm on lateral chest x-ray. When a larger amount of fluid is present, the lateral costophrenic angle on the posteroanterior (PA) radiograph is blunted. When pleural fluid is suspected, lateral decubitus films should be obtained to detect free fluid gravitating to the dependent side and accumulating between the chest wall and lung (see accompanying figure). The amount of fluid present can be roughly quantitated by measuring the distance between the inner border of the chest wall and the outer border of the lung. When this distance is less than 10 mm, the amount of fluid present is small and usually a diagnostic thoracentesis should not be performed.

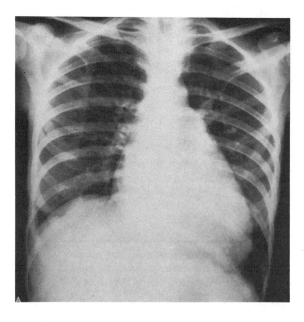

Value of lateral decubitus roentgenography in the assessment of pleural effusion. A posteroanterior roentgenogram in the erect position *(A)* reveals what appears to be marked elevation of the right hemidiaphragm, although slight thickening of the axillary pleura in the region of the costophrenic sulcus suggests the possibility of infrapulmonary effusion. *(Continued on next page.)*

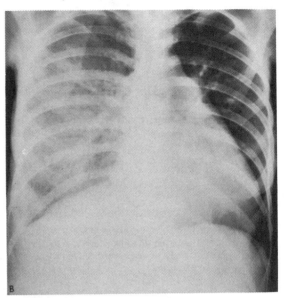

Roentgenography in the supine position *(B)* reveals a marked increase in the opacity of the right hemithorax, owing to the presence of fluid in the posterior pleural space; the right hemidiaphragm is now viewed in proper perspective, whereas in *A* it was obscured by subpulmonic effusion.

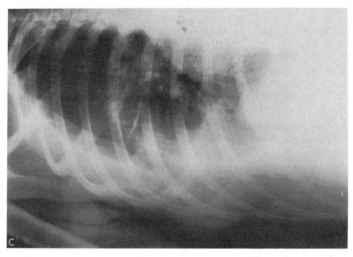

A lateral decubitus roentgenogram *(C)* shows the fluid to much better advantage along the costal margin and reveals how much fluid can be accommodated in the subpulmonic space. (From Pare JAP, Fraser RG: Synopsis of Diseases of the Chest. Philadelphia, W.B. Saunders, 1983, p 104, with permission.)

28. What is an empyema?

Empyema describes the presence of infected liquid or frank pus in the pleural space. It may result from infection of a contiguous structure, instrumentation of the pleural space, or hematogenous spread of infection. The diagnosis is made by examination of the pleural fluid obtained from thoracentesis. An empyema should be suspected when the pleural fluid has a high WBC count (>5000 cells/mm^3, with predominantly polymorphonuclear leukocytes [PMNs]), high protein (>3 g/dl), low glucose (<40 mg/dl), high LDH (>600 mg/dl) and low pH (<7.2). A Gram stain and culture of the pleural fluid may reveal the causative organism.

29. What other procedures are available if routine diagnostic pleural fluid analysis fails to diagnose an exudative effusion?

It is important to note that in approximately 20% of all exudative pleural effusions, no diagnosis will be made. In patients with a suspected neoplasm or tuberculous pleural effusion, a closed needle biopsy of the parietal pleura may establish the diagnosis. Although the overall yield from pleural fluid cytology is slightly higher, needle biopsy of the pleura will be positive in 40% of patients with malignant pleural disease.[1] When tuberculous pleuritis is suspected, a portion of the biopsy should be sent for culture. The initial biopsy is positive for granuloma in 50% to 80% of the patients.[2] Other procedures to be considered are:

- Bronchoscopy if the patient has a parenchymal abnormality on chest x-ray or CT scan.
- Pleuroscopy which allows direct visualization of the pleural surface and guided biopsy.
- Open pleural biopsy.

1. Prakash UBS, et al: Comparison of needle biopsy with cytologic analysis for the evaluation of pleural effusion: Analysis of 414 cases. Mayo Clin Proc 60:158–164, 1985.

2. Levine H, et al: Diagnosis of tuberculous pleurisy by culture of pleural biopsy specimen. Arch Intern Med 126:269–271, 1970.

HEMOPTYSIS

30. What is hemoptysis and what is its differential diagnosis?

Hemoptysis can be defined as blood in the sputum and includes the full range of bloody sputum from blood streaks to frank blood. In addition to history and physical examination, all patients should have a chest x-ray. Further diagnostic procedures should be guided by the findings of these studies.

Differential Diagnosis of Hemoptysis

Pulmonary Vasculature	Pulmonary Parenchyma
Vasculitis	Trauma
Wegener's granulomatosis	Foreign body
Goodpasture's syndrome	Bronchitis
Arteriovenous malformation	Neoplasm
Bleeding diathesis	Tuberculosis
Pulmonary embolus with infarction	Pneumonia
Pulmonary hypertension	Abscess
Oropharynx	Bronchiectasis
Trauma	**Cardiac**
Gum bleeding	Mitral stenosis
Palate bleeding	Left ventricular failure
Other	Trauma
Factitious	

Adelman M, et al: Cryptogenic hemoptysis: Clinical features, bronchoscopy findings and natural history in 67 patients. Ann Intern Med 102:829–834, 1985.

31. What is massive hemoptysis?

The term massive hemoptysis implies copious bleeding and has been defined as the expectoration of greater than 600 cc of blood in a 24-hour period. This potentially lethal and alarming clinical situation requires expeditious evaluation, close observation, and possible surgical intervention.

PNEUMOTHORAX

32. Which population of patients is most likely to experience a primary spontaneous pneumothorax? In which patients is a secondary spontaneous pneumothorax most often seen?

Primary spontaneous pneumothorax, occurring in patients with no history of pulmonary disease, is believed to result from spontaneous rupture of a subpleural emphysematous bleb. Primary spontaneous pneumothorax has a peak incidence at 20–30 years of age, is more common in smokers and ex-smokers, has a 4:1 male to female ratio, and is most often seen in tall, thin individuals.[1] **Secondary spontaneous pneumothorax,** occurring in patients with underlying pulmonary disease, is most often seen with COPD.[2]

    1. Gobbel WG Jr, et al: Spontaneous pneumothorax. J Thorac Cardiovasc Surg 46:331–345, 1963.
    2. Dines DE, et al: Spontaneous pneumothorax in emphysema. Mayo Clin Proc 45:481–487, 1970.

33. What is the likelihood that spontaneous pneumothorax will reoccur?

Recurrence rates for both primary and secondary spontaneous pneumothorax are similar. Recurrence rates for a second spontaneous pneumothorax range from 10–50%, and approximately 60% of those patients will have a third recurrence. After three episodes, the recurrence rate exceeds 85%. Therefore, repeated spontaneous pneumothorax should be treated by pleurodesis or surgical intervention, including parietal pleurectomy.

34. What are the causes of pneumothorax?

Spontaneous pneumothorax, although not common, should be considered in any patient with a history of underlying lung disease and unexplained clinical decompensation. Causes of pneumothorax secondary to underlying lung disease include COPD, asthma, lung abscess, adult respiratory distress syndrome (ARDS), neoplasm, and eosinophilic granuloma. Pneumothorax may be iatrogenic (following thoracentesis, transbronchial biopsy, or secondary to barotrauma, etc.) or traumatic. Catamenial pneumothorax is rare and occurs in females at the time of the menstrual period.

35. Which symptoms are associated with pneumothorax?

Chest pain and dyspnea are the two most common complaints. The acute pleuritic pain, which is localized to the side of the pneumothorax, may become more of a dull ache with time. Symptoms are more pronounced in patients with underlying pulmonary disease.

36. What is a tension pneumothorax?

Tension pneumothorax is due to continued pumping of air into the pleural space from which it cannot escape. Tension pneumothorax develops when intrapleural pressure exceeds atmospheric pressure during expiration, causing collapse of the involved lung and shift of the mediastinum.

37. When should the diagnosis of tension pneumothorax be suspected?

Tension pneumothorax is a medical emergency and requires prompt relief of the positive pleural pressure. It is usually heralded by sudden deterioration in cardiopulmonary status. It should be suspected (1) in any patient with a history of pneumothorax, (2) after a procedure known to cause pneumothorax, (3) in patients receiving mechanical ventilation, and (4) during cardiopulmonary resuscitation, if it is difficult to ventilate the patient or if there is electromechanical dissociation.

    On physical exam, tension pneumothorax should be suspected if the patient has signs of a significant pneumothorax (no tactile fremitus, markedly decreased or absent breath sounds, and hyperresonance on percussion), cardiopulmonary compromise (rapid pulse, hypotension, cyanosis, electromechanical dissociation), and possibly a shift of the trachea.

38. What is Hamman's sign?

Mediastinal emphysema or pneumomediastinum can be detected on auscultation by the presence of a mediastinal "crunch" (Hamman's sign) coinciding with cardiac systole and diastole. Named after the American physician, Louis Hamman, 1877–1946.

INFECTIONS

39. What is the most common cause of community-acquired pneumonia?

The commonest cause of community-acquired pneumonia is the **pneumococcus**. It accounts for about 60% of cases severe enough to be hospitalized. Other causes include *Mycoplasma, Legionella,* and viral pneumonia. However, the incidence of occurrence varies depending on the community and the patient population. Staphylococci and gram-negative rods are uncommon causes of community-acquired pneumonia.

40. Which community-acquired pneumonias are seen more commonly in the alcoholic patient?

As in the nonalcoholic patient, pneumococcal pneumonia is the most frequent community-acquired pneumonia. Although they are still at risk for the usual community-acquired pneumonias, alcoholics have higher incidence of gram-negative organisms (including *Klebsiella pneumonia* and *Hemophilus influenzae*), anaerobic pneumonia secondary to aspiration, and *Staphylococcus aureus.*

41. Which risk factors predispose for the development of nosocomial (hospital-acquired) pneumonia?

Risk factors for the development of nosocomial pneumonia include:
- Severity of the underlying illness
- Previous hospitalization
- Indwelling urethral catheters
- Presence of intravascular catheters
- Intubation (especially prolonged intubation)
- Recent thoracic or upper abdominal surgery
- Use of broad-spectrum antibiotics (increased risk of superinfection).

42. Which organisms most commonly cause nosocomial pneumonia?

Nosocomial pneumonia is most commonly caused by **gram-negative organisms**, including *Pseudomonas aeruginosa, Klebsiella pneumonia, Escherichia coli,* and *Enterobacter* species. Mortality from gram-negative nosocomial pneumonia remains high (30–75%), despite antimicrobial therapy.

  Steven RM, et al: Pneumonia in an intensive care unit: A 30-month experience. Arch Intern Med 134:106, 1974.

43. What are the predisposing risk factors for developing pneumococcal pneumonia?

Patients with severe underlying illness such as multiple myeloma, lymphoma and leukemia, cirrhosis and renal failure, poorly controlled diabetes mellitus, sickle cell anemia, patients who have undergone splenectomy, and the elderly are more likely to develop pneumococcal pneumonia.

44. What factors determine the prognosis of pneumococcal pneumonia?

The mortality associated with pneumococcal pneumonia ranges from 6% to 19% in hospitalized patients without complications. Prognosis is worsened by the presence of the following:

Underlying illnesses that include:

Alcoholism	Bronchiectasis
Chronic obstructive pulmonary disease	Hemoglobin SS and SC disease
Congestive heart failure	Bronchogenic carcinoma
Diabetes mellitus	Multiple myeloma

Other factors include:

Hypogammaglobulinemia	Bacteremia
Age over 60 years	Delay in onset of therapy
Multilobar involvement	Pneumococcal serotype 3
Leukopenia	Extrapulmonary involvement

Mufson MA: Pneumococcal infections. JAMA 246:1942, 1981.

45. What are the most common risk factors for the development of anaerobic pneumonia?

Approximately 25% of patients with anaerobic pneumonia report a history of transient loss of consciousness, especially seizures or alcohol-related loss of consciousness. Other predisposing factors include poor oral hygiene, dysphagia, and endobronchial obstruction.

46. What three radiographic patterns of pulmonary infiltrates are observed in immuno-compromised patients?

Patterns of Pulmonary Infiltrates in Immunocompromised Patients

PATTERN	COMMON CAUSES	LESS COMMON CAUSES
Diffuse	*Pneumocystis* Cytomegalovirus (CMV) Pulmonary edema NIP* Drug-induced Lymphangitic carcinomatosis	*Cryptococcus* *Aspergillus* *Candida* Hemorrhage Leukemic involvement Varicella-zoster virus Leukoagglutinin reaction
Nodular or cavitary	*Cryptococcus* *Nocardia* Bacterial lung abscess Neoplasm *Aspergillus*	*Legionella* Septic emboli *Pneumocystis*
Segmental/lobar	Bacteria, including *Nocardia* *Cryptococcus* Mucormycosis NIP* Pulmonary emboli	Tuberculosis Viral *Legionella* Radiation pneumonitis *Pneumocystis* Mixed infection

*NIP = nonspecific interstitial pneumonitis
(From Young LS: The lung and immunosuppressive disease. In Murray JF, Nadel JA (eds): Textbook of Respiratory Medicine. Philadelphia, W.B. Saunders, 1988, p 1935, with permission.)

47. Which bronchopulmonary segments are most commonly involved in lung abscesses and why?

The **posterior segment of the right upper lobe** and **superior segment of the right lower lobe** are the most commonly involved, followed by the posterior segment of the left upper lobe and the superior segment of the left lower lobes. Individuals usually aspirate while in the supine position. In this position, these are the dependent segments. The right lung is more frequently involved than the left, because the right main stem bronchus comes off at a less acute angle than the left.

Radiographic Distribution of 326 Cases of Anaerobic Lung Abscesses

LOBE	SEGMENT	RIGHT (%)	LEFT (%)
Upper	Posterior	30	10
	Apical	4	
	Anterior	7	3
Middle	(Lingula)	6	3
Lower	Superior	14	11
	Basal	8	3
	TOTAL	69%	31%

Bartlett JG, et al: Anaerobic infections of the lung and pleural space. Am Rev Respir Dis 110:56, 1974.
Pierce A: Pneumonia due to anaerobic bacteria: Medical Grand Rounds, Parkland Memorial Hospital,
Dallas, Texas, January 23, 1986.

TUBERCULOSIS

48. What symptoms are associated with tuberculosis (TB)?
The symptoms associated with TB are often nonspecific. Common complaints include
productive cough, weight loss, weakness, anorexia, night sweats, and generalized malaise.
These nonspecific symptoms are most often subacute or chronic (greater than 8 weeks) in
duration. Both fever, present in one-third to one-half of the patients, and hemoptysis
correlate with cavitary disease and positive sputum smears.

Holmes P, et al: Presentation of pulmonary tuberculosis. Aust NZ J Med 11:651, 1981.

**49. What is the most common anatomic distribution of roentgenographic changes in post-
primary (reactivation) TB?**
In post-primary TB, roentgenographic abnormalities are predominantly located in the
apical and posterior segments of the upper lobes (85%). Although the anterior segment of
the upper lobes may be affected, a lesion found *only* in the anterior segment suggests a
diagnosis other than TB (i.e., malignancy). The superior segments of the lower lobe account
for approximately 10% and the remainder of the lower lobe less than 7%. The right lung is
more often affected than the left.

50. What specific clinical entities are associated with increased risk for developing active TB?
- Silicosis
- Chronic renal failure
- Alcoholism
- Diabetes mellitus
- Postgastrectomy
- HIV infection

51. How is active *Mycobacterium tuberculosis* infection diagnosed?
Because many months of medical therapy are required to adequately treat TB, a definitive
diagnosis **by culture** is recommended. A negative tuberculin skin test (PPD) in a patient who
does not have an underlying disease (a patient who is not anergic) or overwhelming TB infection
makes the diagnosis of TB unlikely. A positive PPD without chest x-ray changes also makes
the diagnosis of *active pulmonary* TB unlikely and reflects previous exposure. A positive tuberculin test and typical chest x-ray findings or response to antituberculosis medications may
provide a presumptive diagnosis of TB, which should be verified by culture if at all possible.

52. What are the clinical problems associated with the treatment of TB?
1. **Drug resistance**, which may be further divided into primary drug resistance and
acquired drug resistance, is one clinical problem. Acquired drug resistance represents drug
resistance in patients previously treated with antituberculous medication. Primary drug
resistance (resistant organisms present in a patient not previously treated for TB) occurs in
approximately 7% of patients. Resistance to both isoniazid and rifampin has been reported.

Primary drug resistance can vary with location and ethnic background and is higher in Asian and Hispanic patients.

2. **Compliance** with therapy is another problem associated with TB treatment. Multiple drug regimens over an extended period of time (6 months or more) can be complicated, and this may lead to failure to successfully complete therapy.

3. **Side-effects** of medication also represent a clinical problem associated with therapy. The most important side-effect of antituberculous treatment is hepatitis. Hepatotoxicity, indicated by a rise in serum transaminases, is seen in 2–5% of patients treated. It occurs most frequently with INH (isoniazid) therapy, less frequently with rifampin, and rarely with PZA (pyrazinamide). Other side-effects include retrobulbar optic neuritis, hyperuricemia, thrombocytopenia (ethambutol), hyperglycemia (rifampin), and peripheral neuropathy (INH).

Carpenter JL, et al: Antituberculosis drug resistance in South Texas. Am Rev Respir Dis 128: 1055, 1983.

Dutt AK, et al: Undesirable side effects of isoniazid and rifampin in largely twice weekly short-course chemotherapy for tuberculosis. Am Rev Respir Dis 128:419, 1983.

53. What is the basis for multiple drug therapy in the treatment of TB?

Work done by Canetti over 25 years ago established the large numbers of organisms found in tuberculous cavities. Spontaneous resistance develops in one in 100,000 or 1,000,000 organisms. Therefore, single drug therapy may lead to the selection of resistant organisms and treatment failure.

Canetti G: Present aspects of bacterial resistance in tuberculosis. Am Rev Respir Dis 92:687, 1965.

54. Which groups of individuals are candidates for isoniazid (INH) chemoprophylaxis to prevent TB (prophylaxis vs. treatment)?

Chemoprophylaxis is a misleading term. INH or any other antimycobacterial agent has little effect on an infection in which microbial multiplication is minimal or absent. What is actually taking place is treatment of a subclinical but active infection. The following is a list of candidates for treatment ("prophylaxis") with INH:

Indications for INH Prophylaxis (300 mg per day for 1 year)

1. Persons of any age should receive INH if they:
   a. Are positive for antibody to the human immunodeficiency virus (HIV) or are suspected to be HIV positive and have a tuberculin skin test (TST) of 5 mm or more of induration.
   b. Are close contacts of newly diagnosed TB cases and have a TST of 5 mm or more of induration.
   c. Have an abnormal chest x-ray (CXR) with fibrotic lesions suggesting old TB and have a TST of 5 mm or more of induration.
   d. Are IV drug abusers, negative for HIV, and have a TST of 10 mm or more of induration.
   e. Have a medical condition that increases their risk of TB (including silicosis, gastrectomy, jejunoileal bypass, weight loss of 10% or more of ideal body weight, chronic renal failure, diabetes mellitus, high dose corticosteroid use, immunosuppression, leukemia, lymphoma, or malignancy), and have a TST of 10 mm or more of induration.

2. Persons less than 35 years of age should receive INH if they have a TST of 10 mm or more of induration and they:
   a. Are born in a high-prevalence country.
   b. Are in a medically underserved population (especially blacks, Hispanics and native Americans).

3. Recent converters (within the past 2 years):
   a. With a TST of 10 mm or more of induration and age less than 35 years.
   b. With a TST of 15 mm or more of induration and age greater than 35 years.

4. All persons less than 35 years of age who are likely to have a low incidence of TB but have a TST of 15 mm or more of induration.

Centers for Disease Control: Screening for tuberculosis and tuberculosis infections in high-risk populations, and the use of preventive therapy for tuberculosis infection in the United States: Recommendations of the Advisory Council for the Elimination of Tuberculosis. MMWR 39(No. RR-8):1–12, 1990.

55. Which infectious agents can mimic TB?

Fungal infections, especially histoplasmosis and coccidioidomycosis, can mimic pulmonary TB. Histoplasmosis has similar presenting symptoms and chest x-ray findings and should be considered in any differential where TB is considered. Lymph node involvement is more common with histoplasmosis than TB. Complications secondary to lymph node and mediastinal involvement include fibrosing mediastinitis (rare), pericarditis (rare), esophageal encroachment, superior vena cava syndrome, and tracheal/airway encroachment. *Nocardia*, a gram-positive, aerobic, partially acid-fast organism can mimic pulmonary TB. Symptoms include fever, night sweats, and productive cough. Chest x-ray findings with cavitation are frequent. Previously nocardiosis was viewed as infection by a primary pulmonary pathogen. It is now more frequently recognized as an opportunistic infection in patients with underlying disease, such as pulmonary alveolar proteinosis. Most strains are susceptible to sulfonamides.

56. What are the mechanisms of hemorrhage from the site of previous pulmonary TB?

- Reactivation of TB
- Bronchiectasis
- "Scar carcinoma" (adenocarcinoma)
- Erosion of a vessel by a broncholith (calcified lymph node)
- Fungal infection (usually aspergillosis) in the site of the cavity
- Rasmussen's aneurysm (terminal pulmonary artery)

NEOPLASTIC DISEASE

57. Which roentgenographic and clinical criteria can help distinguish between a benign and a malignant pulmonary nodule?

A pulmonary nodule can be described as a rounded lesion on a chest x-ray measuring less than 3 cm at maximum diameter. Although no single or group of characteristics can definitely predict the nature of a solitary pulmonary nodule, the following chart can be useful:

Differentiation of Benign and Malignant Solitary Pulmonary Nodules

FACTORS	BENIGN	MALIGNANT
Clinical		
Age	<40 years (except with hamartoma)	>45 years
Sex	Female	Male
Symptoms	Absent	Present
Past History	Lives in area of high granuloma incidence, exposure to TB, mineral oil medication	Diagnosis of primary lesion elsewhere
Skin tests	Positive, usually with specific infectious organisms	Negative or positive
Roentgenographic		
Size	Small (<2 cm in diameter)	Large (>2 cm in diameter)
Location	No predilection (except for TB [upper lobes])	Predominantly upper lobes (except for lung metastases)
Definition & contour	Margins well defined and smooth	Margins ill defined, lobulated, umbilicated
Calcification	Almost pathognomonic of a benign lesion, particularly if of a laminated, multiple punctate, or "popcorn" variety	Very rare, may be eccentric (scar carcinoma)
Satellite lesions	More common	Less common
Serial studies with no change over 2 years	Almost diagnostic of a benign lesion	Most unlikely
Doubling time	<30 or >490 days	Between 30 and 490 days

(From Frazer RG, et al: Diagnosis of Diseases of the Chest, 3rd ed. Philadelphia, W.B. Saunders, 1989, p 1390, with permission.)

58. What is the appropriate evaluation following an abnormal chest x-ray?

Evaluation needs to be directed by the symptoms of the patient. If there is evidence of infection, this needs to be treated before further evaluation. If the chest x-ray is still abnormal after treatment or reveals an obvious mass, then tissue diagnosis is imperative. This may be obtained by expectorated sputum cytology, bronchoscopy with biopsy, or percutaneous fine needle aspiration and cytology. Once the tissue diagnosis is established, treatment plans can be made.

If the abnormality is a solitary pulmonary nodule, the accompanying algorithm may be used:

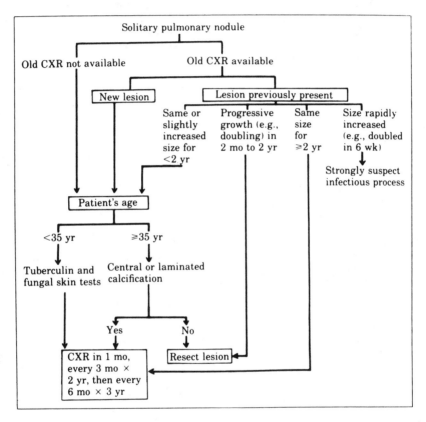

Guidelines for approaching the solitary pulmonary nodule. CXR = chest roentgenogram; mo = months; yr = years. (From Casciato DA, Lowitz BB: Manual of Clinical Oncology, 2nd ed. Boston, Little, Brown, 1988, p 120, with permission.)

59. What are the relative incidence and roentgenographic manifestations of the four most common lung cancers based on cell type?

The most common carcinomas of the lung are **squamous cell carcinoma** (35%), **adenocarcinoma** (25%), **small cell carcinoma** (25%), and **large cell undifferentiated carcinoma** (14%). Lung cancer is slightly more frequent in the right lung, in the upper lobes, and in the anterior segment. Both squamous cell and small cell carcinomas occur more commonly in a central location, whereas adenocarcinoma usually develops more peripherally.

The differences in presentation between the pathologic types of lung cancer are summarized below:

Type	Symptoms	Chest X-ray
Squamous cell	Local ± hypercalcemia	Central lesion, cavitation
Adenocarcinoma	Local or metastatic	Peripheral lesions
Small cell	Metastatic, paraneoplastic	Central lesions

Auerbach O, et al: Histologic type of lung cancer in relation to smoking habits, year of diagnosis, and site of metastasis. Chest 67:382, 1975.

60. What are the symptoms and location of a Pancoast tumor?

First described by Henry Khunrath Pancoast, a Philadelphia radiologist, in 1932, the term is used to described a tumor located in the extreme apex of the upper lobe of the lung. This type of tumor represents approximately 4% of all lung cancers. Although the tumor may be of various cell types, the most common is squamous cell carcinoma. Pancoast's original criteria included the following characteristics: arm/shoulder pain, Horner's syndrome, destruction of bone, and atrophy of the hand muscles.

Pancoast HK: Superior pulmonary sulcus tumor; tumor characterized by pain, Horner's syndrome, destruction of bone, and atrophy of hand muscles. JAMA 99:1391, 1932.

61. Name the most common *pulmonary* complications of lung cancer.

Pulmonary complications of lung cancer include atelectasis, postobstructive pneumonia secondary to endobronchial obstruction, hemoptysis, pleural effusion, and respiratory failure.

62. What is Eaton-Lambert syndrome?

Eaton-Lambert syndrome is a paraneoplastic myopathy. This means that it is associated with a malignancy but not secondary to the direct effects of the tumor or its metastases. This syndrome is most often seen with small cell carcinoma. Clinically, it resembles myasthenia gravis, but it can be distinguished by careful neurological examination and electromyography (EMG). Unlike myasthenia gravis, Eaton-Lambert syndrome involves proximal muscle groups, includes muscular strength *increases* with repetitive stimulation, has little response to neostigmine challenge, and EMG tracings demonstrate increased muscular response to repetitive stimulation.

63. What are the other paraneoplastic syndromes associated with pulmonary malignancy?

Overall, paraneoplastic syndromes are more often associated with small cell carcinoma. The spectrum of paraneoplastic syndromes, however, is quite broad and includes the following:

- Systemic symptoms (anorexia, cachexia, weight loss, and fever)
- Clubbing
- Hypertrophic pulmonary osteoarthropathy (HPO)
- Cushing's syndrome (secondary to ectopic ACTH production)
- Hypercalcemia
- Eaton-Lambert syndrome
- Hyponatremia (secondary to syndrome of inappropriate secretion of anti-diuretic hormone [SIADH])
- Migratory thrombophlebitis (Trousseau's syndrome)
- Myopathy
- Peripheral neuropathy
- Other less common paraneoplastic syndromes.

64. What are the symptoms and x-ray changes associated with hypertrophic pulmonary osteoarthropathy (HPO)?

HPO is one of the many varied paraneoplastic syndromes. It is more often associated with squamous cell carcinoma. The patient complains of a deep burning pain, usually in the distal extremity. There is usually clubbing of the fingers and/or toes, periostitis of the long bones, and occasionally polyarthritis. The most commonly involved bones are the tibia, fibula, humerus, radius, and ulna. The x-ray of the extremity reveals subperiosteal new bone formation. The etiology is unknown, and the abnormalities resolve with treatment of the primary tumor.

Rassam JW, et al: Incidence of paramalignant disorders in bronchogenic carcinoma. Thorax 30:86, 1975.

65. What are the causes of hypercalcemia secondary to pulmonary malignancy?

The most common pulmonary carcinoma associated with hypercalcemia is squamous cell. Causes of hypercalcemia include osseous metastasis, a tumor-produced parathyroid hormone-like substance, prostaglandin E2, and osteoclast-activating factor. Symptoms of hypercalcemia include drowsiness or altered mental status, hypotonia, abdominal pain, constipation, polyuria, and polydipsia.

66. Which tumors commonly metastasize to the lung?

The most common primary sites that metastasize to the lung include:

- Lung cancer itself
- Colorectal carcinoma
- Thyroid cancer
- Ovarian cancer
- Renal cell carcinoma
- Breast cancer
- Testicular cancer
- Prostatic carcinoma.

Endobronchial metastases occur most commonly in renal cell carcinoma, melanoma, and breast carcinoma.

PULMONARY THROMBOEMBOLISM

67. What predisposing factors increase the risk for pulmonary emboli (PE)?

Predisposing factors for the development of PE include:

- Injury or surgery of the pelvis and lower extremities
- Previous history of deep venous thrombosis (DVT)
- Prolonged general anesthesia
- Burns
- Pregnancy and the postpartum period
- Right ventricular failure
- Immobility
- Age
- Obesity
- Cancer
- Estrogen-containing medications
- Coagulation disorders (including deficiency of protein C, anti-thrombin III, or protein S).

68. What is the mortality rate for PE?

PE are responsible for approximately 50,000 deaths per year. The mortality rate is 10% and fewer than 30% are diagnosed antemortem.

69. Where is the usual origin of the thrombus that leads to PE?

The likelihood of a PE depends heavily upon the location of the thrombus. It is very rare for PE to result from a thrombus originating in the right ventricle or upper extremity unless there is overt right ventricular failure or the presence of an indwelling catheter. A thrombus below the knee rarely results in PE. However, the risk of embolism is quite high in thrombi located above the knee.

70. What chest x-ray findings are associated with PE?

The most common interpretation of the chest roentgenogram of a patient with acute PE is that of a normal roentgenogram. Chest x-ray changes associated with acute PE are subtle, if present at all. They include differences in diameters of vessels that should be similar in size, abrupt cutoff of a vessel when followed distally, and increased radiolucency in some

71. What are the findings associated with pulmonary infarction?
Approximately one in ten PE result in pulmonary infarction. Pleuritic chest pain, hemoptysis, and low-grade fever are present when infarction has occurred. Pulmonary infarction is classically described as a wedge-shaped infiltrate that abuts the pleura. Pulmonary infarction is often associated with a small pleural effusion that is usually exudative in character and may be hemorrhagic.

72. How is the diagnosis of PE established?
It is impossible to diagnose PE on clinical grounds alone. Therefore, one must proceed to further testing to establish the diagnosis. The ventilation-perfusion (V/Q scan) lung scan, although highly sensitive, is nonspecific. Interpretation is difficult in the patient with underlying pulmonary disease. Pulmonary angiography is the only established means that can demonstrate the embolus itself, but the procedure is not without risk. Therefore, the tests used to establish the diagnosis depends on the clinical situation and information obtained in less invasive testing.

73. What are two types of nonthrombotic PE?
The pulmonary vasculature filters the venous circulation and is exposed to nonthrombotic emboli. The two most common of these are **fat emboli** and **amniotic fluid emboli.** Fat embolism usually follows bone trauma or fracture and its symptoms begin 12–36 hours following the event. Clinical manifestations include altered mental status, respiratory decompensation, anemia, thrombocytopenia, and petechiae. Amniotic fluid embolism is secondary to entrance of amniotic fluid into the venous circulation, with resulting shock and disseminated intravascular coagulation (DIC).

OBSTRUCTIVE AIRWAY DISEASE

74. What are the causes of chronic obstructive pulmonary disease (COPD)?
Although cigarette smoking is generally acknowledged as having a primary role in most cases of COPD, the disease does not have a single cause. There is a normal loss of pulmonary function with increasing age. COPD occurs in patients who experience a rate of loss that significantly exceeds the norm. Contributing factors in the etiology include:

Associated Factors in COPD

---

1. **Cigarette smoking:** Cigarette and other forms of tobacco smoking are firmly established as the primary cause of COPD. There is a dose-related risk (usually expressed in pack-years) of cigarette consumption and COPD, although there is great individual variation. All smokers do not develop COPD, even among those with a high dose history.

2. **Air pollution:** Although difficult to measure, there is an association between air pollution and COPD. Sulfur dioxide and particulate matter are the components most highly correlated with COPD.

3. **Mucosal hypersecretion and bronchial infection:** Both have been associated with COPD but the causal relation is uncertain.

4. **Sex and race:** The data suggest that the higher prevalence of COPD in men is associated with sex-related differences in cigarette smoking. Some studies have suggested that white males may be more susceptible than black males.

5. **Allergic factors:** Patients with a history of allergic disorders may be at higher risk, but the role is probably minor.

6. **Hereditary factors:** Certainly the hereditary deficiency of alpha$_1$-antiprotease is associated with diffuse emphysema. There may be other genetic factors that contribute to the risk of COPD.

Table continued on next page.

Associated Factors in COPD (Continued)

7. **Sociological factors:** The increased association of COPD and lower socioeconomic groups is probably due to differences in cigarette smoking, occupational factors, and exposure to air pollution.

8. **Occupation factors:** Several occupations and occupational exposures may be associated with an increased risk of developing COPD, but none has equaled that of cigarette smoking. Occupations that are at increased risk include coal miners, fire fighters, grain handlers, and copper smelter workers (sulfur dioxide exposure). Occupational exposures that cause increased risk include poison gas (mustard gas and lewisite), granite dust, carbon black, cotton (byssinosis), hemp, and toluene diisocyanate.

Niewoehner DE: Clinical aspects of chronic airflow obstruction. In Baum GL, Wolinsky E (eds): Textbook of Pulmonary Diseases, 4th ed. Boston, Little, Brown, 1989.

75. How is chronic bronchitis defined?
Chronic bronchitis is defined by symptoms. Chronic bronchitis is a condition associated with a productive cough on most mornings for 3 or more consecutive months for 2 or more consecutive years.

Meneely GR, et al: Chronic bronchitis, asthma, and pulmonary emphysema: A statement by the committee on diagnostic standards for non-tuberculosis respiratory disease. Am Rev Respir Dis 85:762–768, 1962.

76. What is the definition of emphysema?
Unlike chronic bronchitis, which is described in terms of symptoms, emphysema is an anatomical/structural term. Emphysema is an abnormal enlargement of air-containing space distal to the terminal bronchioles accompanied by destruction of alveolar tissue.

Meneely GR, et al: Chronic bronchitis, asthma, and pulmonary emphysema: A statement by the committee on diagnostic standards for non-tuberculosis respiratory disease. Am Rev Respir Dis 85:762–768, 1962.

77. What are the physical examination findings in COPD?
The physical examination of a patient with COPD may be normal in the early stages. With advancing disease, the patient will manifest signs of lung hyperinflation (hyperresonance to percussion, increased anterior-posterior [AP] diameter, barrel-shaped chest, decreased vocal fremitus), diffusely diminished breath sounds, prolonged expiratory time, diffuse wheezes on forced expiration, and use of the accessory muscles of ventilation. Patients with chronic bronchitis will have signs of increased secretions (such as rhonchi). In more severe airway obstruction, the increased forces required for inspiration and expiration may result in large changes in intrathoracic pressure, which can lead to a drop in systolic blood pressure of as much as 15–20 mmHg on inspiration, and engorgement of the neck veins with expiration.

78. What radiographic changes are associated with COPD?
The associated findings on chest x-ray are secondary to overdistension of the lungs. These findings include a low, flat diaphragm, increased retrosternal airspace (on lateral x-ray), and an elongated, narrow heart shadow. Bullae, which appear as rounded radiolucent areas greater than 1 cm in diameter, are occasionally seen and reflect emphysematous changes.

79. What are the pulmonary function test (PFT) findings in patients with COPD?
The early signs, symptoms, and radiographic changes of COPD are variable and nonspecific. Therefore, PFTs are important in the diagnosis of COPD. Patients with COPD will show evidence of airway obstruction, such as decreased vital capacity (VC) and expiratory flow rates (i.e., forced expiratory volume in the first second of expiration [FEV_1] or a forced expiratory flow rate between 25% and 75% of the expiration [$FEF_{25-75\%}$]). There

will also be evidence of lung hyperinflation and air trapping, manifested by increases in residual volume (RV), functional residual capacity (FRC), and total lung capacity (TLC). There is generally a response to bronchodilators which, although variable, is usually only about 15–20% of the prebronchodilator values.

80. What is meant by a "pink puffer" or a "blue bloater"?
The patterns of gas exchange abnormalities differ among patients with advanced COPD. Two distinct clinical patterns have been described and labelled the "pink puffers" and "blue bloaters." The following table illustrates the differences between these two groups:

Differentiating Features in Advanced Chronic Airflow Obstruction

FEATURES	TYPE A (PINK PUFFER)	TYPE B (BLUE BLOATER)
Symptoms	Dyspnea (first and predominant symptom); patients are usually thin, weight loss is common; minimal or no cough; hyperinflated lung fields; no signs of cor pulmonale	Cough and sputum production with frequent chest infections; stocky build; recurrent or persistent signs of right heart failure
Routine Laboratory Studies		
Chest x-ray	Hyperinflation; decreased vascular markings	Normal or increased markings at lung bases (so-called dirty-chest appearance)
Arterial blood gases	Mildly reduced P_aO_2; normal or decreased P_aCO_2	Marked reduction in P_aO_2; increased P_aCO_2
Total lung capacity	Increased	Normal or slightly increased
DL_{CO}	Decreased	Normal
Hematocrit	Normal	Increased
Specialized Laboratory Studies		
Inspiratory resistance	Normal	Increased
Pulmonary compliance	Increased	Normal
Ventilation-perfusion distribution	Increased V_D/V_T	Increased regions of low $\dot{V}_A/\dot{Q}$
Hemodynamics	Normal or decreased cardiac output Mild pulmonary hypertension	Normal cardiac output Marked pulmonary hypertension
Ventilatory Performance and Gas Exchange during Exercise	Increased ventilatory equivalent ($\dot{V}_E/\dot{V}O_2$) DL_{CO} fails to increase normally Decreased P_aO_2; small rise in P_aCO_2	Decreased $\dot{V}_E/\dot{V}O_2$ DL_{CO} increases normally P_aO_2 may increase; moderate rise in P_aCO_2
Gas Exchange during Sleep	Moderate degree of oxygen desaturation	Frequent periods of profound oxygen desaturation

The "pink puffers" tend to be thin and dyspneic but maintain relatively normal P_aO_2 and P_aCO_2 levels. They breathe with hyperinflated lungs and fast, shallow respirations. They remain relatively free of cor pulmonale. The pathophysiology seems to be that of severe emphysema and their symptoms are largely the result of the loss of lung elastic recoil, with relatively little intrinsic airways disease.

The "blue bloaters," on the other hand, tend to be overweight, with minimal dyspnea but significant coughing and sputum production. They suffer from cor pulmonale, respiratory infections, and chronic CO_2 retention. Although they usually have some degree of emphysema, the pathophysiology is that of significant small and large airway inflammation and the symptoms are largely due to the intrinsic airway disease.

Both patterns are usually a result of long-term cigarette smoking. The reason for the two different presentations is not clearly defined.

(From Rubenstein E, Federman D (eds): Scientific American Medicine. New York, Scientific American Medicine, Inc., 1988, Chapter 14 (Respiratory Medicine), Part III, Table 1, page 11, with permission.)

81. What are the complications associated with COPD?

COPD is a chronic pulmonary illness characterized by frequent exacerbations and decompensation. The exacerbations can be induced by upper respiratory tract infections, pneumonia, medical noncompliance, and environmental changes (temperature, allergens, irritants, etc.). Complications associated with COPD include sleep disturbances due to nocturnal desaturation, acute and chronic respiratory failure, chronic cor pulmonale, spontaneous pneumothorax, and impairment of pulmonary function secondary to large bullae.

82. What is cor pulmonale?

Cor pulmonale, or pulmonary heart disease, is right-sided congestive heart failure (CHF) that is caused by an increase in pulmonary vascular resistance (pulmonary hypertension) due to intrinsic lung disease. It can be caused by pulmonary parenchymal diseases such as COPD, sarcoidosis, pneumoconiosis, and restrictive lung disease. It can also be caused by pulmonary vascular diseases such as primary pulmonary hypertension, recurrent pulmonary embolism, or scleroderma. It is a major cause of morbidity and mortality in COPD.

83. What is the prognosis of severe COPD?

The mortality rate of a patient with an FEV_1 less than 0.75 liters is 30% at one year and 95% at 10 years.

84. What is the treatment of COPD?

The components of therapy for COPD include:

1. **Removal of risk factors:** The most important component is the cessation of smoking and the removal of any other risk factors (i.e., environmental and occupational).

2. **Bronchodilators:** Although the airway obstruction is largely fixed, with only a small reversible component, most patients will experience a small improvement in their symptoms with the use of bronchodilator therapy.

3. **Corticosteroids:** Studies have given mixed conclusions on the efficacy of steroids in COPD. Patients who are most likely to respond include those with recurrent attacks of wheezing and a relatively significant response to inhaled bronchodilators (FEV_1 increase >20%). Due to the risk of side-effects, the lowest possible dose should be used, preferably on an alternate day regimen.

4. **Diuretics:** Indicated for the symptomatic relief of the symptoms of cor pulmonale.

5. **Vasodilators:** Studies have shown that long-term vasodilator therapy can decrease the pulmonary hypertension in patients with COPD, but it is not certain that this improves morbidity or mortality.

6. **Antibiotic therapy:** If indicated, broad-spectrum agents should be used (preferably the least expensive agent or an agent that the patient has tolerated well in the past).

7. **Continuous oxygen therapy:** In patients for whom it is indicated, long-term oxygen therapy has been shown to decrease the morbidity and mortality of COPD.

8. **Phlebotomy:** In the past, this procedure was commonly performed in patients with COPD and a secondary erythrocytosis. At present, with the advent of long-term oxygen therapy, phlebotomy is rarely necessary.

85. Which classes of bronchodilator drugs are available for the therapy of the obstructive airway diseases?

There are several classes of bronchodilators available for the treatment of obstructive airway diseases (both acute and chronic). These are:

1. **The methylxanthines:** These agents, available for oral or parenteral use, include aminophylline, theophylline, and related compounds. It was previously taught that the bronchodilation produced by this class of drugs was due solely to their inhibition of phosphodiesterase, an enzyme involved in the conversion of cyclic AMP (cAMP) to non-cyclic 5' AMP. This inhibition of the breakdown of cAMP increased levels of cAMP, which in turn led to bronchial smooth muscle relaxation and bronchodilation. In fact, it has been shown that at pharmacologic doses less than 10% of phosphodiesterase activity is inhibited. Therefore, there are probably other mechanisms responsible for the bronchodilation.

To achieve maximal benefit from theophylline, and to minimize toxic effects, the serum level must be maintained within the therapeutic range of 10–20 g/ml.

2. **Beta-adrenergic agonists:** These agents, available for oral, parenteral or inhalational use, produce bronchodilation by directly stimulating the beta$_2$ receptors on the bronchial smooth muscle cell. Epinephrine was the first available agent, but newer agents have been developed that offer increased duration of action and increased beta$_2$ selectivity. The beta-agonists offer an additive bronchodilator effect when combined with a methylxanthine.

3. **Anticholinergic agents:** These agents, which can be given via parenteral or inhalational use, compete with acetylcholine at its receptors. The currently available congener, ipratropium bromide (Atrovent), is available for inhalational use and causes far fewer systemic side-effects than atropine. It also has an extended duration of action over that of atropine.

86. What are the possible beneficial actions of theophylline in patients with COPD?

Theophylline is classified as a bronchodilator. However, since patients with COPD may have a very small reversible component to their obstruction, the significance of its bronchodilatory effects in COPD have been questioned. However, a variety of beneficial actions other than bronchodilation have been attributed to theophylline. These include:

- Increased mucociliary clearance
- Increased respiratory drive
- Improved cardiovascular function
- Increased diaphragmatic contractility
- Decreased dyspnea
- Improved exercise capacity.

Hill NS: The use of theophylline in "irreversible" chronic obstructive pulmonary disease. Arch Intern Med 148:2579–2584, 1988.

87. Are there toxic effects of theophylline therapy?

The toxic effects of theophylline occur with increasing frequency as the serum level exceeds 20 g/ml, although they can be seen even within the therapeutic range of 10–20 g/ml. Whereas the serious toxicities (especially seizures and cardiac arrhythmias) are usually not seen until the serum levels rise above 30 g/ml, they can be seen at lower serum levels and are often not preceded by any less severe sign of toxicity. The common toxic effects are:

1. **GI:** Nausea, vomiting, diarrhea and abdominal pain.
2. **Cardiac:** Various arrhythmias (including sinus tachycardia, multifocal atrial tachycardia, extrasystoles).
3. **Neurologic:** Headache, nervousness, insomnia, tremor, seizures.

88. What factors affect the clearance of theophylline?

The clearance of theophylline occurs mainly through the hepatic oxidation and demethylation. Hepatic metabolites and unmetabolized theophylline are excreted in the urine. The clearance rate is affected by many factors. Any increase or decrease in theophylline clearance will necessitate increasing or decreasing the maintenance dose to maintain therapeutic serum levels.

Factors Affecting Theophylline Clearance

1. **Clearance increased** (increased maintenance dose)
   Cigarette & marijuana smoking
   Therapy with phenytoin, phenobarbital, rifampin, carbamazepine
   Ingestion of charcoal-broiled and barbecued meats
   Childern (>*1 year old*)

2. **Clearance decreased** (decreased maintenance dose)
   Congestive heart failure
   Hepatic dysfunction
   Elderly patients and infants (<1 year of age)
   Viral or bacterial infections with fever
   Therapy with cimetidine, oral contraceptives, erythromycin, cipro-
   floxacin (and all quinolone antibiotics), allopurinol, propranolol.

---

89. What criteria suggest a course of antibiotics be given to a patient presenting with an acute exacerbation of COPD?

Increasing dyspnea
Increased sputum production
Purulent sputum

Anthonisen NR, et al: Antibiotic therapy in exacerbations of COPD. Ann Intern Med 106:196–204, 1987.

90. What are the criteria for continuous low-flow oxygen therapy?

The role of continuous low-flow oxygen therapy was largely established by the Nocturnal Oxygen Therapy trial in the U.S. and the Medical Research Council trial in Great Britain. This therapy is indicated for any one of the following conditions:

1. A patient at rest and on an optimal medical regimen, whose P_aO_2 is <55 mmHg.
2. A patient at rest and on an optimal medical regimen, whose P_aO_2 is >55 mmHg, if there is evidence of hypoxic end-organ dysfunction manifested by one or more of the following:

   - Cor pulmonale
   - Secondary pulmonary hypertension
   - Secondary erythrocytosis
   - Impaired mentation

3. A patient whose P_aO_2 drops below 55 mmHg on exercise, and who has evidence of significant improvement in one or more of the following with oxygen therapy:

   - Exercise duration
   - Exercise performance or capacity

4. A patient whose P_aO_2 drops below 55 mmHg during sleep and has evidence of one or more of the following:

   - Hypoxic organ dysfunction
   - Disturbed sleep pattern
   - Significant cardiac dysrhythmia

Nocturnal Oxygen Therapy Trial Group: Continuous or nocturnal oxygen therapy in hypoxemic chronic obstructive lung disease. Ann Intern Med 93:391–398, 1980.

Medical Research Council Working Party: Long term domiciliary oxygen therapy in hypoxemic cor pulmonale complicating chronic bronchitis and emphysema. Lancet i:681–686, 1981.

91. Does the cessation of smoking have an effect on patients with COPD?

Yes. The morbidity and mortality associated with COPD are favorably affected by the cessation of smoking. Studies have shown a small but significant improvement in objective tests of pulmonary function and subjective symptom severity following cessation. COPD patients who stop smoking have been shown to revert to the normal, age-related loss of pulmonary function seen in nonsmokers. These benefits appear to be more dramatic in patients with mild COPD than in those with more advanced disease.

92. What are the poor prognostic signs in an acute exacerbation of asthma?
The poor prognostic signs are:

- Pulse rate $> 100/$minute
- Pulsus parodoxus > 10 mmHg
- PEFR $< 16\%$ of predicted
- $PaCO_2 > 45$ mmHg
- Retraction of sternocleidomastoid muscles
- $FEV_1 < 600$ cc before treatment
- $FEV_1 < 1600$ cc after treatment

93. What is bronchiectasis?
Bronchiectasis is defined as a fixed dilatation of bronchi due to destructive changes in the elastic and muscular layers of the bronchial wall. It was a more common disease prior to the advent of appropriate antibiotic therapy for pulmonary infection. Currently it is seen in patients with a history of gram-negative pulmonary infection or chronic pulmonary inflammatory condition, immunodeficiency state, cystic fibrosis, and occasionally asthma. Patients usually present with a chronic cough productive of large quantities of foul, often blood-tinged sputum. The diagnosis is made with contrast bronchoscopy or CT scan.

INTERSTITIAL LUNG DISEASE

94. What is Hamman-Rich syndrome?
In 1944, Hamman and Rich first described rapidly progressive and fatal pulmonary fibrosis for which no etiology could be identified. Today the term idiopathic pulmonary fibrosis (IPF) is used to describe this entity except in rapidly progressive cases.

Hamman L, Rich AR: Acute diffuse interstitial fibrosis of the lungs. Bull Johns Hopkins Hosp 74:177–212, 1944.

95. Which connective tissue disease can be associated with chronic interstitial lung disease?
Rheumatoid arthritis is associated with interstitial pulmonary changes. The condition is more common in men, rarely precedes joint disease, and may be associated with cutaneous nodules. The most common pulmonary complication of rheumatoid arthritis is pleural effusion. Other connective tissue diseases associated with interstitial changes include systemic lupus erythematosus, systemic sclerosis, polymyositis, dermatomyositis, and Sjögren's syndrome.

96. What is Goodpasture's syndrome?
Goodpasture's syndrome usually refers to a combination of glomerulonephritis and diffuse pulmonary hemorrhage associated with the development of antiglomerular basement membrane (anti-GBM) antibodies and less frequently antipulmonary basement membrane antibodies. Some use the eponym more broadly to refer to all diseases characterized by glomerulonephritis and pulmonary hemorrhage.

97. What diagnostic tests can help differentiate Goodpasture's syndrome from other pulmonary-renal syndromes?
Anti-GBM antibodies can be demonstrated in serum, renal tissue, and less frequently in pulmonary tissue. Immunofluorescent staining of tissue reveals a *linear* pattern of deposition of IgG.

Goodpasture's syndrome is predominantly a disease of young adults (mean age 21 years) and is more common in males. The most common initial presentation is hemoptysis, but rarely renal involvement will present first. The differential diagnosis should include other pulmonary-renal syndromes including vasculitis, Wegener's granulomatosis, polyarteritis nodosa, uremia with pulmonary edema, and immune complex disease (systemic lupus erythematosus).

98. What is pulmonary alveolar proteinosis?

Pulmonary alveolar proteinosis is a rare pulmonary disorder in which proteinaceous material is deposited into the alveoli and bronchioles. The chest x-ray reveals bilateral peripheral infiltrates similar to pulmonary edema. The etiology is not known. Diagnosis can be made with bronchoalveolar lavage or bronchoscopic biopsy revealing strongly PAS positive material. Complications include superinfection, pulmonary fibrosis, cor pulmonale, and spontaneous pneumothorax. Nocardiosis is a common superinfection.

ADULT RESPIRATORY DISTRESS SYNDROME (ARDS)

99. What are the hallmarks of the adult respiratory distress syndrome (ARDS)?

The term ARDS is applied to diverse etiologies of lung injury in which there is an initial noxious event followed by an interval of normal lung function and then progressive and rapid hypoxemia and diffuse pulmonary infiltrates.

100. What is the "lesion" in ARDS?

ARDS is a type of pulmonary edema. Pulmonary edema is of two types: (1) cardiogenic, in which alteration of Starling forces is responsible for increases in water content of the interstitium and alveoli, and (2) noncardiogenic, in which the Starling forces are not deranged, but interstitial and alveolar water accumulates because of an increase in capillary permeability. The "lesion" in ARDS is an injured pulmonary capillary epithelium. (The Starling forces are the hydrostatic pressure inside the capillary, the hydrostatic forces in the interstitium, the oncotic pressure inside the capillary, and the oncotic pressure in the interstitium.)

101. Can cardiogenic pulmonary edema be distinguished from noncardiogenic pulmonary edema based on clinical and radiographic findings?

It is impossible to distinguish cardiogenic pulmonary edema from noncardiogenic pulmonary edema (ARDS) on the basis of the clinical presentation and radiographic findings. The two conditions can be differentiated by measurement of the pulmonary wedge pressure. The pulmonary capillary wedge pressure (PCWP), which reflects left ventricular (LV) filling pressures, is normally 6–12 mmHg. The PCWP is elevated in cardiogenic pulmonary edema, reflecting the elevated LV filling pressures. It is normal in ARDS, because LV filling pressures are normal—the defect is at the alveolocapillary membrane.

102. Name some of the known causes of ARDS.

The etiologies of ARDS are diverse and include:

- Shock (hemodynamic, septic, hypovolemic)
- Diffuse pulmonary infection
- Exposure to drugs or toxins
- Pancreatitis
- Immunologic disorders
- Hematologic disorders (DIC, transfusion, cardiopulmonary bypass)
- Trauma
- CNS disease
- Uremia
- Aspiration

103. What are the complications of ARDS?

Complications of ARDS include left ventricular failure, secondary bacterial infection, disseminated intravascular coagulation, pulmonary oxygen toxicity, barotrauma secondary to mechanical ventilation (pneumothorax, pneumomediastinum), and multisystem organ failure.

104. What is the prognosis of ARDS? How is the syndrome managed?

Despite the increased understanding of the pathophysiology of ARDS, the mortality rate remains high (greater than 50%). Management of the ARDS patient involves ruling out treatable causes, maintaining arterial PO_2 above 55 mmHg, supporting hemodynamics and nutritional status, and avoiding complications.

SARCOIDOSIS

105. What is the prevalence of sarcoidosis?

Sarcoidosis is a multisystem disorder with an unknown etiology. The prevalence of sarcoidosis is approximately 20 cases per 100,000. Although it may occur at any age, patients are usually between 20–40 years of age. Many organs may be involved, but the lung is the organ most frequently involved (greater than 90%), hence sarcoidosis appears in this chapter. Females have a slightly higher prevalence. In the U.S., sarcoidosis is more common in blacks than whites, with a 10:1 ratio.

Fanburg BL (ed): Sarcoidosis and Other Granulomatous Diseases of the Lung. New York, Marcel Dekker, 1983.

106. What chest x-ray abnormalities are observed in sarcoidosis?

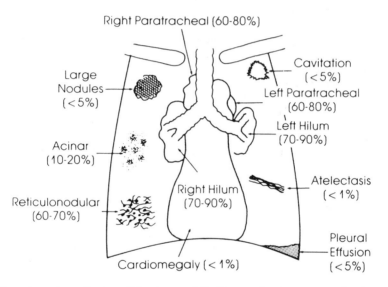

The figure is a schematic view of the abnormal findings on the chest x-rays of patients with sarcoidosis. Shown are changes observed and the average frequency of occurrence.

(From Crystal RG: Sarcoidosis. In Wilson JD, et al: Harrison's Principles of Internal Medicine, 12th ed. New York, McGraw-Hill, 1991, p 1466, with permission.)

107. How is sarcoidosis staged by chest x-ray?

About 90% of patients have an abnormality on chest x-ray sometime during the course of the disease.

Stage	Chest X-ray Findings
0	Clear chest roentgenogram (less than 10%)
I	Bilateral hilar adenopathy (25% to 40%)
II	Bilateral hilar adenopathy with pulmonary infiltrate (25% to 50%)
III	Pulmonary infiltrate without adenopathy (less than 15%)

These categories represent chest x-ray patterns and are not "stages" of the disease, as is usually understood. However, patients with stage I disease are more likely to have acute, reversible sarcoidosis.

108. What are the clinical and laboratory abnormalities associated with sarcoidosis?

Because sarcoidosis is a multisystem disease, clinical manifestations can be nonspecific, and approximately 20% of patients will be asymptomatic. When symptomatic, patients may complain of malaise, fever, weight loss, or symptoms referable to the specific organ involved.

Laboratory abnormalities are also nonspecific and include: increased erythrocyte sedimentation rate (ESR), hyperglobulinemia, increased angiotensin converting enzyme (ACE) activity, and occasionally hypercalcemia and/or hypercalciuria.

109. How is the diagnosis of sarcoidosis established?

The diagnosis of sarcoidosis rests upon the combination of history and radiographic and histological findings. The typical pathologic finding is the noncaseating granuloma. This pathological finding, in conjunction with the appropriate clinical picture and lack of infectious etiology (TB, fungal, etc.), establishes the diagnosis. Although any involved organ may be biopsied for pathologic changes, transbronchial lung biopsy is positive in approximately 90% of the cases.

110. What organs, other than the lung, are most frequently involved in sarcoidosis?

The most frequently involved organs other than the lung include the lymph nodes (greater than 75%), skin (25%), eyes (25%), and musculoskeletal system (arthralgias). Although the bone marrow, spleen, and liver are frequently involved, this finding is usually not clinically significant. Skin manifestations include erythema nodosum and plaques. Ocular manifestations include both anterior and posterior uveitis and can lead to blindness. Central nervous system and cardiac involvement are present in approximately 5%.

111. Which patients with sarcoidosis should be treated?

Sarcoidosis is usually a self-limited disease, with 30–50% of cases spontaneously remitting, 20–30% remaining stable, and 30% demonstrating progression.[1] Because therapeutic intervention is not without side-effects, close observation of patients who are asymptomatic and without organ dysfunction is warranted. Therapy should be initiated in patients with systemic organ impairment (lung, eyes, heart, CNS, or extensive skin lesions), or evidence of hypercalcemia or hypercalciuria. Steroids are considered the first line of therapy for sarcoidosis.[2]

1. Sones M, et al: Course and prognosis of sarcoidosis. Am J Med 29:84–93, 1960.
2. MacGregor RR, et al: Alternate day prednisone therapy. Evaluation of delayed hypersensitivity response, control of disease and steroid side effects. N Engl J Med 280:1427–1431, 1969.

ENVIRONMENTAL LUNG DISEASE

112. To what does the term pneumoconiosis refer?

The term is derived from Greek (pneumo = lung; konis = dust). It currently refers to an accumulation of inorganic dust in the lungs and the consequences of the tissue's response secondary to the presence of the dust. The most common pneumoconioses are silicosis, asbestosis, and coal worker's pneumoconiosis.

113. What are the radiographic abnormalities and clinical complications associated with silicosis?

Silicosis refers to pulmonary disease secondary to the inhalation of quartz dust or silica. The disease is characterized by focal pulmonary fibrosis that has a tendency to occur first in the upper lobes. Enlargement of the hilar lymph nodes and eggshell calcifications are suggestive of silicosis. Complications associated with silicosis include spontaneous pneumothorax, cor pulmonale, and infection with mycobacteria (tuberculosis and atypical mycobacteria) and fungi.

Ziskind M, et al: Silicosis. Am Rev Respir Dis 113:643, 1976.

114. What is Caplan's syndrome?
Caplan's syndrome or rheumatoid pneumoconiosis refers to the association of rheumatoid arthritis and nodules on chest x-ray in patients with coal worker's pneumoconiosis (CWP).

115. What are the clinical problems associated with asbestos exposure?
Asbestosis, pleural plaques, pleural effusions, and malignancies are associated with a history of asbestos exposure. Asbestosis is a fibrotic disease of the lung and visceral pleura. The chest x-ray shows interstitial fibrosis beginning usually at the bases and progressing upwards. There is usually no hilar adenopathy. Asbestos exposure increases the risk of malignancy, including lung cancer, gastrointestinal cancer, and mesothelioma.

116. Which diagnostic tests are useful in diagnosing mesothelioma?
Because generous biopsy specimens are needed to diagnose mesothelioma, diagnosis is usually made following open thoracotomy. Periodic acid-Schiff (PAS) stain, immunoperoxidase staining for carcinoembryonic antigen (CEA) and keratin, and electron microscopy are useful in differentiating mesothelioma from adenocarcinoma. Mesothelioma lacks PAS-positive vacuoles and has weak staining with CEA antigen.

   Antman KH, et al: Benign and malignant mesothelioma. In Light RW (ed): Clin Chest Med 6:141–152, 1985.

MEDIASTINUM

117. Name the three major compartments of the mediastinum viewed on lateral chest x-ray.
The three are the anterior, middle, and posterior compartments, as shown in the accompanying figure and described in the table.

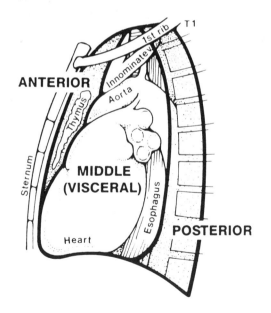

By convention the mediastinum is divided into anterior, middle, and posterior compartments, according to its appearance on lateral chest roentgenograph. Although other, more complex subdivisions exist, this one is most helpful to the clinician. (From Shields TW: Chest wall, pleura, mediastinum and diaphragm. In James EC, Corry RJ, Perry JF (eds): Basic Surgical Practice. Philadelphia, Hanley & Belfus, 1987, p 179.)

Normal Mediastinal Contents

Anterior mediastinum: Consists of everything forward of and superior to the heart shadow, which includes:

Thymus gland	Innominate veins
Aortic arch and major branches	Lymphatic vessels and lymph nodes
Substernal extension of the thyroid or parathyroid glands	

Middle mediastinum: Extends from the anterior heart border to the anterior vertebral border. This includes:

Heart and pericardium	Lymph nodes
Trachea and mainstem bronchi	Phrenic and vagus nerves
Pulmonary hila	

Posterior mediastinum: Occupies the space within the margins of the vertebrae on lateral film. This includes:

Esophagus	Thoracic duct and lymph nodes
Descending aorta	Vagus nerves and sympathetic chains
Azygous and hemiazygous veins	Areolar connective tissue

(From Pierson, DJ: Disorders of the mediastinum. In Murray JF, Nadel JA (eds): Textbook of Respiratory Medicine. Philadelphia, W.B. Saunders, 1988, Table 80-1, p 1782, with permission.

118. Name the various masses that can be commonly found in the anterior mediastinum of the adult patient.

The most common masses of the anterior mediastinum of the adult include thymoma, teratoma, lymphoma, thyroid and parathyroid tissue, germ cell tumor, and metastatic malignancy.

119. What is the most common type of mediastinal tumor in adults and in which compartment is it located?

The most common tumors arising in the mediastinum are **neurogenic tumors** (approximately 20% of adult cases) that arise in the posterior compartment.

120. What are the manifestations and causes of superior vena cava (SVC) syndrome?

The SVC, because of its location and thin walled structure, is vulnerable to compression and/or obstruction. Radiographically, there is usually a pulmonary mass (more often on the right) and a widened mediastinum in SVC syndrome. Symptoms are due to increased venous pressure secondary to obstructed drainage of the upper thorax and head. The patient complains of headache, changes in vision, or disturbed level of consciousness. Of note are the dilated collateral veins on the upper thorax and neck, and edema and plethora of face, neck, and conjunctiva.

Bronchogenic carcinoma accounts for 75% of the cases of SVC syndrome, and only 2–3% are due to nonmalignant etiologies.

Lokich JJ, et al: Superior vena cava syndrome: Clinical management. JAMA 231:58–61, 1975.

121. What are the presenting signs and symptoms of SVC obstruction?

Headache, and fullness in the chest, head, and neck are reported. Chest pain, cough (sometimes associated with syncope or headache), lacrimation, and periorbital edema are also seen. Symptoms are present in most patients for 2–4 weeks prior to hospitalization. Physical findings include neck vein distention; edema, plethora, and cyanosis of the face; tachypnea; edema of the upper extremities; paralysis of the vocal cords; and distention of retinal veins or veins beneath the tongue. Veins of the upper extremities do not empty when lifted above the level of the heart.

122. Which clinical entities are associated with thymoma?
Thymomas, located in the anterior mediastinum, account for approximately 10% of the primary mediastinal masses and are malignant in approximately 25% of the cases. Agammaglobulinemia, Cushing's syndrome, and pure red cell aplasia have been associated with thymomas. Myasthenia gravis occurs in almost 50% of patients with thymoma, but the majority of patients with myasthenia gravis do not have thymomas.

THE DIAPHRAGM

123. Name the three major diaphragmatic hernias.
Herniation of abdominal contents into the chest can occur through a region of congenital defect or weakness. **Hiatal hernias** (via the esophageal hiatus), with displacement of the stomach into the posterior mediastinum, are the most common. **Herniation via the retrosternal foramen of Morgagni** is often asymptomatic and appears as an abnormal shadow frequently on the right heart border. **Herniation via the posterolateral foramen of Bochdalek** is more common in infancy.

124. What are the causes of elevation of a hemidiaphragm on chest x-ray?
Normally, the right hemidiaphragm is several centimeters higher than the left because of displacement of the liver. Elevation of a hemidiaphragm may be secondary to:
- Unilateral diaphragmatic paralysis
- Displacement secondary to intraabdominal masses or ascites
- Loss of lung volume on the affected side
- Eventration of the diaphragm (a rare, congenital disorder)
- Subpulmonic effusion.

125. What are the most common causes of unilateral diaphragmatic paralysis?
Each diaphragm is innervated by a phrenic nerve originating from the third, fourth, and fifth cervical roots. Paralysis results from disruption of this nerve. The most common causes include invasion by bronchogenic carcinoma, thoracic trauma, surgical resection or disruption, and possibly postviral neuropathy. Slightly more than one-half of the cases remain unexplained. Occasionally recovery occurs. Unilateral diaphragmatic paralysis is usually asymptomatic.

126. How is the "sniff" test useful in evaluating unilateral diaphragmatic paralysis?
The diagnosis of unilateral diaphragmatic paralysis is suggested by elevation of one hemidiaphragm on chest x-ray. Under fluoroscopy this diagnosis can be confirmed by asking the patient to "sniff," which rapidly increases intraabdominal pressure, lowers intrathoracic pressure, and causes an upward (paradoxical) movement of the affected diaphragm.

VENTILATORY SUPPORT

127. What are the indications for initiation of mechanical ventilation?

General Guidelines for Mechanical Ventilation

Absolute indications:	Arterial blood gas values plus clinical evaluation:
Apnea	Hypoxemia not corrected by other means
Administration of paralyzing agents	Progressive hypercarbia with acidosis
Clinical examination alone:	
Ineffectual respiratory efforts	
Inspiratory muscle fatigue	

(From Johanson WG Jr, Peters JI: Critical care. In Murray JF, Nadel JA (eds): Textbook of Respiratory Medicine. Philadelphia, W.B. Saunders, 1988, p 1994, with permission.)

128. What physiologic guidelines should be used to evaluate the need for ventilatory support in respiratory failure?

Guidelines for Ventilatory Support in Respiratory Failure

PARAMETER	READING	PARAMETER	READING
Respiratory rate	> 35/minute	$PaCO_2$	> 55 mmHg
Vital capacity	< 15 ml/kg	A-aO_2 Gradient	> 450 mmHg
FEV_1	< 10 ml/kg	PaO_2	< 70 mmHg with oxygen
Inspiratory force	< 25 cm H_2O	V_D/V_T	> 0.60

(From Johanson WG Jr, Peters JI: Critical care. In Murray JF, Nadel JA (eds): Textbook of Respiratory Medicine. Philadelphia, W.B. Saunders, 1988, p 1994, with permission.)

129. What are the complications of endotracheal intubation?

Complications of Endotracheal Intubation

Immediate	Delayed	Late
Difficult intubation	Self-extubation	Tracheomalacia
Local trauma	Infections (tracheobronchitis,	Tracheal perforation
Malposition of the	pneumonia)	Laryngeal dysfunction
endotracheal tube	Mucosal edema, denudation	Subglottic/tracheal stenosis

(From Johanson WG Jr, Peters JI: Critical care. In Murray JF, Nadel JA (eds): Textbook of Respiratory Medicine. Philadelphia, W.B. Saunders, 1988, p 1979, with permission.)

APNEA SYNDROMES

130. What are the differentiating characteristics of central apnea and obstructive sleep apnea?

Apnea refers to a pause in respiration of greater than 10 seconds. Both central apnea and obstructive sleep apnea (OSA) result in cessation of respirations (apnea), but are differentiated by a lack of respiratory effort in central apnea, versus continued but *ineffective* respiratory effort in OSA. The figure below demonstrates the different airflow and respiratory effort tracings in the two conditions.

Apnea Type

Central   Obstructive

AIRFLOW

10 sec

RESPIRATORY EFFORT

Strain Gauge or Esophageal Balloon

The relationship between airflow and respiratory effort in both central and obstructive apnea is demonstrated. During a central apnea there is cessation of airflow for at least 10 seconds with no associated ventilatory effort. An obstructive apnea is defined as a similar cessation of airflow, but with continued respiratory effort. (From White DP: Central sleep apnea. Med Clin North Am 69:1206, 1985, with permission.)

131. What clinical characteristics help to differentiate central and obstructive sleep apnea?

Clinical Characteristics of Patients with Sleep Apnea

CENTRAL	OBSTRUCTIVE	
Normal body habitus	Commonly obese	Sexual dysfunction
Insomnia; hypersomnia rare	Daytime hypersomnia	Morning headache
Awaken during sleep	Rarely awaken during sleep	Nocturnal enuresis
Snoring mild and intermittent	Loud snoring	
Depression	Intellectual deterioration	
Minimal sexual dysfunction		

(From White DP: Central sleep apnea. Med Clin North Am 69:1208, 1985, with permission.)

132. What underlying mechanisms explain the events occurring during obstructive sleep apnea?

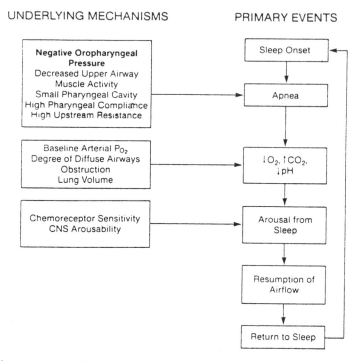

The primary sequence of events in patients with obstructive sleep apnea, and the pathogenetic mechanisms that contribute to these events. (From Bradley TD, Phillipson EA: Pathogenesis and pathophysiology of obstructive sleep apnea syndrome. Med Clin North Am 69:1170, 1985, with permission.)

CASE STUDIES

133. A 43-year-old male with a history of brittle diabetes complicated by several recent admissions for diabetic ketoacidosis (DKA) is admitted with fever (to 102°F), cough productive of scant clear sputum, left-sided chest pain, and a dense left upper lobe infiltrate on chest x-ray (see figure). His physical examination revealed only scattered rhonchi. Laboratory evaluation was significant for leukocytosis with absolute neutrophilia, moderate hypoxemia, and sputum studies revealing numerous neutrophils, a paucity of bacteria, and

negative potassium hydroxide (KOH) and Ziehl-Nielson stains. The patient was not improved after 24 hours of penicillin therapy. What diagnosis should be suspected?

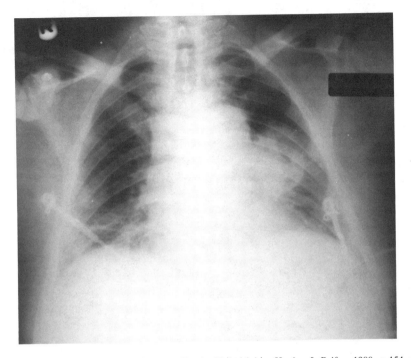

(From Sahn SA, Heffner JE: Pulmonary Pearls. Philadelphia, Hanley & Belfus, 1988, p 154, with permission.)

Community-acquired pneumonia is usually caused by a limited spectrum of pathogens. However, patients with comorbid disorders or an underlying immunodeficiency can present with unusual opportunistic pathogens. This patient had pulmonary mucormycosis. Brittle diabetics, especially those with a recent history of DKA, are predisposed to infection with this ubiquitous fungus. Rhinocerebral, cutaneous, gastrointestinal, and disseminated mucormycosis are also associated with brittle diabetes.

The diagnosis of pulmonary mucormycosis usually depends on detection of the organism in lung biopsy specimens or pulmonary secretions, since the organism does not grow well in culture. Therapy must include reversal of the underlying immunosuppression whenever possible. Amphotericin B has resulted in complete cure in some cases, but surgical resection of the infected lobes may be indicated in failures of medical treatment.

(Adapted from Sahn SA, Heffner JE: Pulmonary Pearls. Philadelphia, Hanley & Belfus, 1988, pp 154–156, with permission.)

134. A 50-year-old alcoholic male with a history of chronic pancreatitis is admitted with dyspnea on exertion (DOE). Physical examination shows a thin male in no acute distress, with dullness to percussion, decreased fremitus, and decreased breath sounds in the right chest. His blood counts are normal except for mild anemia, and his serum amylase is 581 IU/L. His chest x-ray is shown in the accompanying figure. A thoracentesis revealed serosanguinous fluid with 1500 nucleated cells (5% PMNs, 47% macrophages, and 29% lymphocytes), amylase 25,000 IU/L, protein 4.0 g/dl, LDH 221 IU/L, glucose 119 mg/dl, pH 7.35. The fluid reaccumulated in 3 days. What is your diagnosis?

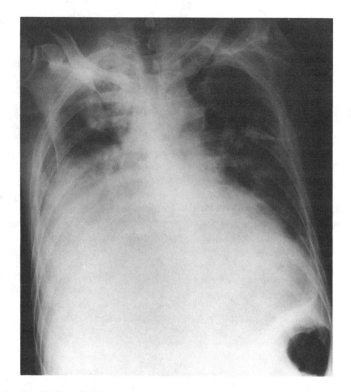

(From Sahn SA, Heffner JE: Pulmonary Pearls. Philadelphia, Hanley & Belfus, 1988, p 39, with permission.)

The patient had a pancreatic pleural effusion. Unlike patients with effusions from acute pancreatitis, patients with large pleural effusions from chronic pancreatitis usually present only with signs of dyspnea, chest pain, or cough. They do not usually have concurrent abdominal symptoms. In contrast to pleural effusions due to acute pancreatitis, the pleural fluid caused by chronic pancreatitis almost always has an elevated amylase, which may reach 100,000 IU/L.

(Adapted from Sahn SA, Heffner JE: Pulmonary Pearls. Philadelphia, Hanley & Belfus, 1988, pp 39–40, with permission).

135. A 32-year-old female was resuscitated from near-drowning. Her physical examination was significant for tachycardia (pulse 120/minute), tachypnea (respiratory rate 22), lethargy, diffuse rhonchi, and the presence of an endotracheal tube. CBC and serum electrolytes are normal. ABGs on 60% O_2: pH 7.53, P_aCO_2 29 mmHg, and P_aO_2 68 mmHg. The chest x-ray is normal except for the presence of an adequately positioned endotracheal tube. What is her expected course and how would you manage this patient?
The course of near-drowning victims varies based on the duration of submersion, the degree of aspiration, and the severity of the resultant hypoxemia. The traditional wisdom that serum electrolyte abnormalities are dependent on the salinity of the aspirated fluid has not been supported by recent studies. The amount aspirated is usually less than 10 ml/kg and should therefore have negligible effects on serum electrolyte balance.

The hypoxemia in these patients does vary with the type and amount of aspirated fluid. Up to 12% of these patients develop laryngospasm, which prevents significant aspiration and leads to hypoxemia on the basis of hypoventilation. The remaining 80–85%

of patients have hypoxemia on the basis of aspiration. Sea water causes alveolar filling due to exudative flooding from irritated mucosa. Fresh water removes alveolar surfactant, leading to collapse. Both fluids can lead to noncardiogenic pulmonary edema, progressing to the adult respiratory distress syndrome (ARDS).

The degree of change in mental status varies with the degree and duration of cerebral anoxia. The prognosis for recovery varies with the temperature of the submersion, age of the patient, and the presence of comorbid medical conditions.

Management of these patients is primarily supportive. Respiratory failure may require mechanical ventilation with positive end-expiratory pressure (PEEP). Prophylactic corticosteroids or antibiotics are of no benefit.

(Adapted from Sahn SA, Heffner JE: Pulmonary Pearls. Philadelphia, Hanley & Belfus, 1988, pp 69–70, with permission.)

136. A 34-year-old woman with a history of pulmonary tuberculosis (TB) treated 1 year ago with isoniazid (INH) and rifampin now complains of a chronic cough and poor exercise tolerance. Physical examination, CBC, electrolytes, and sputum smear for acid-fast bacilli (AFB) and fungi are all negative. Her chest x-ray (see figure) shows several calcified granulomas and a poorly visualized left mainstem bronchus, which appears narrowed on a right anterior oblique view. Tomograms demonstrate left bronchostenosis. What is the diagnosis and how common is it?

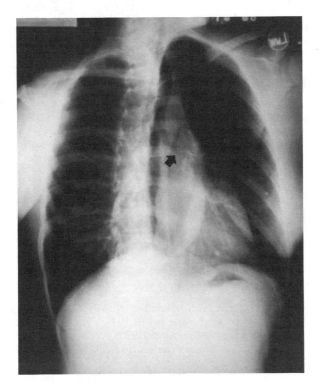

(From Sahn SA, Heffner JE: Pulmonary Pearls. Philadelphia, Hanley & Belfus, 1988, p 77, with permission.)

The diagnosis is bronchial stenosis as a complication of healed endobronchial TB. Endobronchial involvement in pulmonary TB is a common occurrence. Ten to 37% of patients with active pulmonary TB have evidence of endobronchial infection on bronchoscopy. The major sequelae of endobronchial TB is bronchostenosis. Over 90% of patients with endobronchial TB will have some degree of stenosis. Symptoms may be delayed as long as 20 years after treatment of the TB. The diagnosis can be made on tomography or CT scanning of the airway.

(Adapted from Sahn SA, Heffner JE: Pulmonary Pearls. Philadelphia, Hanley & Belfus, 1988, pp 77–78, with permission.)

137. A 57-year-old man presents with a 5-day history of progressive dyspnea, orthopnea, and pedal edema. His history is significant for TB treated in childhood, an 80 pack-year smoking history, a 20-pound loss of weight over the past 4 months, low grade fevers, and occasional night sweats. His physical examination reveals a pulse of 140, blood pressure 100/90 with a 40 mmHg paradoxic pulse, distant heart sounds, nonpalpable cardiac impulse, slight dullness at both lung bases, and bilateral pedal edema. His chest x-ray is shown below (see figure). An echocardiogram confirmed a large pericardial effusion. What is the most likely etiology of this patient's pericardial effusion?

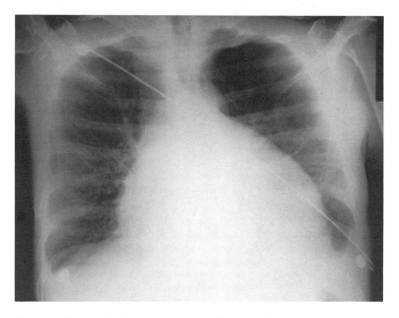

(From Sahn SA, Heffner JE: Pulmonary Pearls. Philadelphia, Hanley & Belfus, 1988, p 89, with permission.)

The most likely etiology is a malignant pericardial effusion. Cancer is the most frequent cause of pericardial tamponade, accounting for 16 to 41% of cases. This patient's smoking history, age, and history of weight loss are strong predictors of a malignant etiology. Lung and breast cancers are the most common cancers involving the pericardium, followed by leukemia, lymphoma, sarcoma, and melanoma.

Unlike this case, malignant pericardial effusions are usually asymptomatic. Symptoms, when present, are nonspecific and can be obscured by symptoms of the malignancy. Only 30% of the effusions are correctly diagnosed antemortem.

The diagnosis is most often suggested by enlarged cardiac silhouettes on chest x-ray and is confirmed by echocardiography. Pericardial biopsies in cases of malignant pericardial effusions are positive in only 55% of patients.

Treatment of symptomatic malignant pericardial effusions is aimed at prevention of long-term fluid reaccumulation and can include subxyphoid pericardiotomy, placement of an intrapericardial catheter with sclerotherapy by the instillation of tetracycline, or a pericardial window.

(Adapted from Sahn SA, Heffner JE: Pulmonary Pearls. Philadelphia, Hanley & Belfus, 1988, pp 89–90, with permission.)

138. A 54-year-old male farmer presents with a 1-month history of increasing dyspnea on exertion (DOE), nonproductive cough, and occasional fevers and chills. He occasionally works in silos and has had symptoms of coughing following entrance into the silo. His last silo exposure was 2 months prior to admission. His physical examination is normal except for minimal basilar rales. CBC and electrolytes are normal and ABGs reveal pH 7.43, P_aCO_2 39 mmHg, and P_aO_2 75 mmHg. His chest x-ray (see figure) shows diffuse nodular opacities. What is the diagnosis and what agent is responsible for the disease?

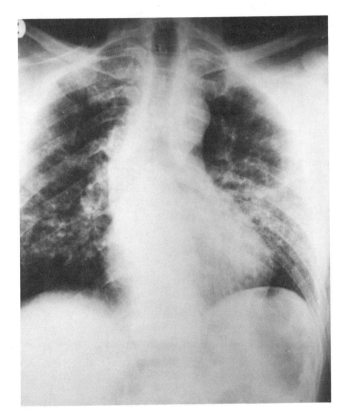

(From Sahn SA, Heffner JE: Pulmonary Pearls. Philadelphia, Hanley & Belfus, 1988, p 91, with permission.)

The diagnosis is silo-filler's disease. The agent responsible is nitrogen dioxide (NO_2). It has been known for almost 200 years that NO_2 can cause an acute, fatal lung injury, but it was not until 1949 that it was found that high concentrations of NO_2 are present in silo gas. The NO_2 is formed from the fermentation of plant nitrates during silo storage. There are three clinical phases of NO_2 inhalational disease:

1. **Superacute stage:** a rare condition with severe hypoxemia rapidly leading to death.

2. **Acute phase:** occurs within a few hours of exposure and is characterized by cough, dyspnea, bronchospasm, headache, and chest pain. Pulmonary edema may develop. If the patient survives, this is followed by a relatively asymptomatic period that lasts 2–5 weeks.

3. **Subacute and chronic phase:** Develops after the asymptomatic period and is characterized by fever, cough, and progressive dyspnea. The chest x-ray will show multiple nodular densities. Severe cases will result in bronchiolitis obliterans, which is probably related to the long-term sequelae of this syndrome. Corticosteroids can be helpful in treating this condition, if treatment is begun early enough.

(Adapted from Sahn SA, Heffner JE: Pulmonary Pearls. Philadelphia, Hanley & Belfus, 1988, pp 91–92, with permission.)

BIBLIOGRAPHY

1. Andreoli TE, et al (eds): Cecil Essentials of Medicine, 2nd ed. Philadelphia, W.B. Saunders, 1990.
2. Baum GL, Wolinsky E (eds): Textbook of Pulmonary Diseases, 4th ed. Boston, Little, Brown, 1989.
3. Fishman AP: Pulmonary Diseases and Disorders, 2nd ed. New York, McGraw-Hill, 1988.
4. Guenter CA, Welch MH (eds): Pulmonary Medicine. Philadelphia, J.B. Lippincott, 1977.
5. Murray JF, Nadel JA (eds): Textbook of Respiratory Medicine. Philadelphia, W.B. Saunders, 1988.
6. Wilson JD, et al (eds): Harrison's Principles of Internal Medicine, 12th ed. New York, McGraw-Hill, 1991.
7. Wyngaarden JB, Smith LH (eds): Cecil Textbook of Medicine, 18th ed. Philadelphia, W.B. Saunders, 1988.

11. RHEUMATOLOGY SECRETS

Richard A. Rubin, M.D.

*The rheumatism is a common name for many aches and pains,
which have yet got no peculiar appellation, though owing to
very different causes.*

William Heberden (1710–1801)
*Commentaries on the History and Cure
of Diseases, Ch. 79.*

*I cannot conceive why we who are composed of over 90 per cent
water should suffer from rheumatism with a slight rise in the
humidity of the atmosphere.*

John W. Strutt, Baron Rayleigh (1842–1919)
(Letter)

GENERAL

1. State an operational definition for rheumatic diseases.
Rheumatic diseases are syndromes of pain or inflammation or both in articular or
periarticular tissues.

2. What is a "joint mouse"?
Osteocartilaginous bodies within a joint are often termed "joint mice" or "loose bodies"
and occur commonly in osteoarthritis. They are thought to arise when bits of articular
cartilage and subchondral bone break off the surface and are released into the joint. There
may be proliferation and deposition of new bone on these fragments.

Resnick D, Niwayama G: Degenerative disease of extraspinal locations. In Diagnosis of Bone
and Joint Disorders, 2nd ed. Philadelphia, W.B. Saunders, 1988, pp 1364–1479.

3. What is chondromalacia patella?
Chondromalacia is a softening and degeneration of articular cartilage. In the patella, it is
often associated with disease of the menisci, knee laxity, or recurrent trauma. Typically,
pain is associated with activity, most commonly descending stairs.

4. What is a bunion?
A bunion is a deviation of the proximal phalanx of the great toe ("big toe") toward
the fibular (or lateral) side of the foot. It is called more formally in Latin a **hallux
valgus,** hallux meaning "big toe" and valgus meaning "bending outward." (See the figure
with Q. 6.)

5. How does a bunion occur?
It can be caused by biomechanical factors, such as tight and pointed-toe shoes that push the
proximal phalanx laterally (**B** panel in figure); inflammatory disease, for example, gout or
rheumatoid arthritis; or abnormal alignment at the first metatarsal-cuneiform joint. If the
cuneiform is abnormal (panel **A** in figure), the first metatarsal may deviate excessively
toward the midline (a primary varus, or bending inward, deformity), which will lead to a
valgus deformity (lateral deviation) of the proximal phalanx when the abnormal foot is
placed into standard shoes.

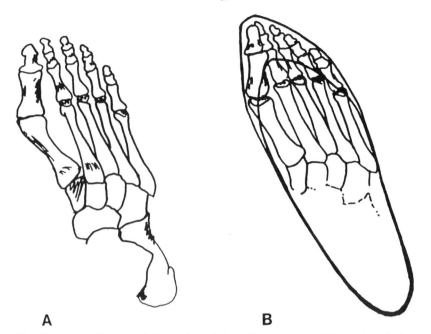

A, A bunion showing deviation of the proximal phalanx of the great toe. B, Formation of a bunion by pointed-toe shoes.
Forrester DM, Brown JC: The foot. In The Radiology of Joint Disease, 3rd ed. Philadelphia, W.B. Saunders, 1987, pp 139–198.

6. List some conditions associated with avascular necrosis of bone.

Some conditions associated with avascular necrosis (also called osteonecrosis or aspetic necrosis) of bone include:

- Trauma (femoral head fractures)
- Sickle cell disease and other hemoglobinopathies
- Hyperphysiologic concentrations of exogenous or endogenous glucocorticoids
- Alcoholism
- Diabetes mellitus
- Gaucher's disease
- Pregnancy
- Systemic lupus erythematosus
- Polyarteritis
- Kidney transplantation
- Lymphoproliferative diseases
- Caisson disease (decompression sickness, or the "bends")
- Heroin abuse
- Idiopathic
    Legg-Calve-Perthes (femoral head)
    Kohler's disease (tarsal navicular)
    Freiberg's disease (metatarsal head)
    Osgood-Schlatter disease (tibial tubercle)

7. What are cryoglobulins and how do they cause disease?

Cryoglobulins are immunoglobulin molecules that have the unusual property of reversibly precipitating at low temperatures. The development of these abnormal immunoglobulins can lead to symptoms. They can be classified into three groups:

Type I cryoglobulinemia involves monoclonal immunoglobulins (as in multiple myeloma and Waldenstrom's macroglobulinemia). These are often asymptomatic but can also cause vascular occlusive disease (Raynaud's phenomenon, cutaneous ulcers, and gangrene).

Type II cryoglobulinemia involves both mono- and polyclonal immunoglobulins. It usually presents as a systemic vasculopathy with arthralgias, neuropathy, leukocytoclastic skin lesions, and perhaps renal involvement.

Type III cryoglobulinemia involves only polyclonal immunoglobulins, and the clinical presentation is the same as in type II disease.

8. Which rheumatologic syndromes are associated with complement deficiencies?

Protein	Disease
C1q	Glomerulonephritis, poikiloderma congenita
C1r	Glomerulonephritis, lupus-like syndrome
C1s	Lupus-like syndrome
C1INH	Discoid lupus, lupus-like syndrome
C4	Systemic lupus, Sjögren's syndrome
C2	Systemic lupus, discoid lupus, polymyositis, Henoch-Schonlein purpura, Hodgkin's disease, vasculitis, glomerulonephritis
C3	Glomerulonephritis, vasculitis, lupus-like syndrome
C5	Systemic lupus, *Neisseria* infection
C6	*Neisseria* infection
C7	Systemic lupus, rheumatoid arthritis, Raynaud's sclerodactyly, vasculitis, *Neisseria* infection
C8	Systemic lupus, *Neisseria* infection
C9	*Neisseria* infection

(From Ruddy S: Complement deficiencies and the rheumatic diseases. In Kelley WN, et al (eds): Textbook of Rheumatology, 3rd ed. Philadelphia, W.B. Saunders, 1989, p 1389, with permission.)

DIAGNOSIS

9. What volume of synovial fluid is present in the normal knee?
The knee normally has up to 4 ml of fluid. Detection of a joint effusion is important in the evaluation of patients with articular symptoms.

Gatter RA: Gross synovial analysis at the bedside. In A Practical Handbook of Joint Fluid Analysis. Philadelphia, Lea & Febiger, 1984, pp 15–20.

10. Which studies should generally be performed on synovial fluid after arthrocentesis?
Important information can be gained by evaluating joint fluid using selected tests. Gram stain and bacterial culture may confirm the presence of an infective agent. In the right clinical setting, similar procedures for mycobacteria or fungi may cinch the diagnosis. A WBC count with differential count is one of the best indicators of the degree of inflammation. Evaluation of the fluid using polarized light is the simplest way to establish the diagnosis of a crystalline arthropathy. Although a good deal has been written about various other tests (glucose, complement, rheumatoid factor [RF], antinuclear antibody [ANA], LDH, protein), they add little diagnostic information.

McCarty DJ: Synovial fluid. In McCarty DJ (ed): Arthritis and Allied Conditions, 11th ed. Philadelphia, Lea & Febiger, 1989, pp 69–90.

11. What are the "string" and "mucin clot" tests?
The primary component of joint fluid is hyaluronic acid. It is quite viscous and will normally make a "string" when expressed from a syringe as a single drop. Likewise, dilute acetic acid added to normal joint fluid causes hyaluronic acid and protein to clump and fall to the bottom of a test tube, producing the notable "mucin clot." Inflammatory mediators cause fragmentation of the hyaluronic acid-protein complex, leaving the fluid less viscous (more watery) and therefore unable to form a good mucin clot. Both viscosity and mucin clot are indirect measures of inflammation. Evaluation of the wet prep and total WBC count are probably better indicators.

Gatter RA: Chemistry, serology, and immunology. In A Practical Handbook of Joint Fluid Analysis. Philadelphia, Lea & Febiger, 1984, pp 55–62.

12. What findings of synovial fluid analysis are considered normal?

Normal findings and those of various rheumatic disease states are shown in the following table:

Synovial Fluid Analysis

DIAGNOSIS	APPEARANCE	TOTAL WBC COUNT (Per Cubic mm)	PMN %	MUCIN CLOT TEST	FLUID/BLOOD GLUCOSE DIFF. (mm/dl)	MISCELLANEOUS (CRYSTALS/ ORGANISMS)
Normal	Clear, pale	0–200 (200)	<10%	Good	NS	—
Group I (noninflammatory; degenerative joint disease, traumatic arthritis)	Clear to slightly turbid	50–4000 (600)	<30%	Good	NS	—
Group II (noninfectious, mildly inflammatory; SLE, scleroderma)	Clear to slightly turbid	0–9000 (3000)	<20%	Good (occ. fair)	NS	Occ. LE cell, decreased complement
Group III (noninfectious, severely inflammatory)						
Gout	Turbid	100–160,000 (21,000)	70%	Poor	10	Uric acid crystals
Pseudogout	Turbid	50–75,000 (14,000)	70%	Fair– poor	Insuff. data	Calcium pyro- phosphate
Rheumatoid arthritis	Turbid	250–80,000	70%	Poor	30	Decreased
Group IV (infectious, inflammatory)						
Acute bacterial	Very turbid	150–250,000 (80,000)	90%	Poor	90	Positive cul- ture for bac- teria
Tuberculosis	Turbid	2,500–100,000 (20,000)	60%	Poor	70	Positive cul- ture for M. tuberculosis

(From Wyngaarden JB, Smith LH (eds): Cecil Textbook of Medicine, 18th ed. Philadelphia, W.B. Saunders, 1988, p 1994, with permission.)

13. Straight leg raising is a useful diagnostic maneuver in which common condition?

The straight leg raising test is designed to reproduce back pain secondary to nerve root compression. The leg is lifted by the calcaneus with the knee remaining straight.

Hoppenfeld S: Physical Examination of the Spine and Extremities. Norwalk, CT, Appleton-Century-Crofts, 1976, pp 237–264.

14. How does one distinguish neurogenic from arterial claudication?

Progressive leg or back pain with walking (claudication) can occur because of either arterial insufficiency or nerve compression. Distinguishing between these entities can be difficult. Absence of pedal pulses suggests arterial disease, although one study reported this sign in 9% of patients with spinal stenosis. Patients with arterial insufficiency can often get relief of pain simply by pausing, or slowing their pace. Patients with nerve compression rarely get relief unless they sit or lie down. Neurologic signs such as weakness, abnormal reflexes, and abnormal electromyograms and nerve conduction velocities (EMG/NCV) are present in spinal stenosis, but absent in patients with arterial disease.

Hall S, et al: Lumbar spinal stenosis: Clinical features, diagnostic procedures and results of surgical treatment in 68 patients. Ann Intern Med 103:271–275, 1985.

15. What is onychodystrophy and with which diseases is it associated?

Separation of the nail plate beginning at the free margin and progressing proximally is called onychodystrophy. Both systemic and local processes are associated with this physical examination finding. Some of these include hypo- and hyperthyroidism; pregnancy; syphilis; trauma (particularly clawing); mycotic, pyogenic, or viral infections; psoriasis; systemic lupus erythematosus; Reiter's syndrome; atopic dermatitis; eczema; and use of solvents (including nail hardeners).

Domonkos AN, et al: Diseases of the skin appendages. In Andrews' Diseases of the Skin: Clinical Dermatology, 7th ed. Philadelphia, W.B. Saunders, 1982, pp 930–984.

16. Which rheumatic syndromes have been reported to be associated with uveitis?

A partial list of rheumatic conditions associated with uveitis includes:

- Ankylosing spondylitis
- Reiter's syndrome
- Psoriasis
- Inflammatory bowel disease
- Kawasaki disease
- Juvenile rheumatoid arthritis
- Sjögren's syndrome
- Sarcoidosis
- Behcet's disease
- Relapsing polychondritis

17. Where is chondrocalcinosis commonly demonstrated roentgenographically?

- Menisci of the knee
- Radiocarpal joints
- Annulus fibrosus of the intervertebral discs
- Symphysis pubis

18. How does the polarizing microscope work and how is it useful in the diagnosis of rheumatic diseases?

Identification of crystals in synovial fluid by polarizing microscopy is often essential in establishing a diagnosis in a patient with articular inflammation. Because crystals rotate light (they are birefringent), polarized light passing through a crystal will no longer be parallel to light not passing through the crystal. If a second polarizer is then added so that its axis is rotated 90 degrees to the light as it emerged from the first polarizer (extinction), the only light reaching the observer's eye will be the light that the crystal has rotated. This allows for the identification of the type of crystal present.

Dieppe P, Calvert P: Crystals and Joint Disease. London, Chapman & Hall, 1983.

19. Which diseases are associated with soft tissue calcification?

Soft tissue calcification detected by plain roentgenograms can be an important adjunct to the diagnosis of rheumatic conditions. A partial list of associated conditions includes:

- Parathyroid disease
- Sarcoidosis
- Diabetes mellitus
- Neoplasms
- Neuropathic arthropathy
- Calcific tendinitis
- Renal osteodystrophy
- Scleroderma
- Trauma
- Ehlers-Danlos syndrome
- Chondrocalcinosis
- Dermatomyositis (especially in children)

20. What conditions commonly mimic systemic necrotizing vasculitis?

Bacterial endocarditis, atrial myxoma, and multiple cholesterol embolization syndrome have many of the same presenting signs and symptoms as systemic vasculitis.

21. What are Gottron's papules?

Patches of erythematous scaly plaques on the knuckles in patients with dermatomyositis are sometimes referred to as Gottron's papules.

RHEUMATOID ARTHRITIS

22. State an operational definition for rheumatoid arthritis (RA).

RA is a *systemic* disease characterized clinically and pathologically by inflammation of diarthrodial joints (movable joints lined with synovial membrane). Although often accompanied by a variety of extra-articular manifestations, *arthritis* represents the major expression of the disorder.

23. What is the approximate frequency of rheumatoid arthritis?

About 1% of the adult population.

24. What are rheumatoid factors, and what conditions are associated with their presence in the circulation?

Rheumatoid factors are antibodies (usually IgM, IgA, or IgG) directed at the F_c portion of the IgG molecule. The presence of circulating rheumatoid factor is not specific for RA. Patients with other rheumatic conditions, including SLE, scleroderma, and Sjögren's syndrome, may have circulating rheumatoid factor. Viral, parasitic, and other infectious diseases, including mononucleosis, hepatitis, malaria, tuberculosis, and bacterial endocarditis, may be associated with these antibodies.

25. In what percentage of RA patients is no circulating rheumatoid factor detectable?

Up to 25% of patients with clinical RA have no circulating rheumatoid factors.

26. What are the approximate frequencies of joint involvement in rheumatoid arthritis?

Joint	Frequency	Joint	Frequency
MCP/PIP*	90%	Hip	50%
MTP*	90%	Acromioclavicular	50%
Wrist	80%	Cervical spine	40%
Ankle/subtalar	80%	Sternoclavicular	30%
Knee	80%	Temporomandibular	30%
Shoulder	60%	Cricoarytenoid	10%
Elbow	50%		

*MCP = metacarpophalangeal joint; PIP = proximal interphalangeal joint; MTP = metatarsophalangeal joint.

27. The classic swan-neck and boutonnière deformities occur by which mechanisms?

The **swan-neck deformity** describes flexion at the metacarpophalangeal (MCP) and distal interphalangeal (DIP) joints, with extension at the proximal interphalangeal (PIP) joints (see figure). This results from inflammation and subsequent contraction of interosseus and flexor muscles and tendons. Also contributing are the synovitis and destruction leading to MCP subluxation. There is flexion at the MCP, leading to exaggerated pull on the extensor tendon of the PIP. Flexion at the DIP is caused because the pull of the flexor tendon overcomes the pull of the extensor tendon.

The **boutonnière deformity** is caused by flexion contracture at the PIP with extension of the DIP (see figure). The pathogenesis of this deformity is thought to relate to an injury of the extensor tendon. If it becomes lengthened or torn, the flexor tendons are unopposed. The altered mechanics and location of the joint lead to functional shortening of the lateral tendons and hyperextension of the DIP joint.

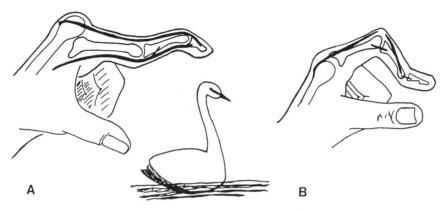

A, Swan-neck deformity; B, boutonnière deformity.

28. What are rheumatoid nodules and where are they found?

The classic rheumatoid nodule has a central area of necrosis enclosed by a rim of palisading fibroblasts surrounded by a collagenous capsule with perivascular collections of chronic inflammatory cells. They occur in 20–35% of rheumatoid arthritis patients and can be found at the elbow and wrist, and on the soles, Achilles tendon, head, and sacrum. Rheumatoid factor is usually present in patients with rheumatoid nodules.

29. When does "gelling" occur?

Gelling describes the achiness and stiffness that occur in the joints of patients with rheumatoid arthritis after a period of inactivity.

30. What is pannus?

The synovium is a primary target for the inflammatory process in rheumatoid arthritis. In established disease, an infiltrate of mononuclear cells, primarily T-lymphocytes, is seen. In addition, activated macrophages and, later, plasma cells are present. The synovial cells become hyperplastic, and the synovium becomes grossly boggy and edematous, with villous projections. This congested, proliferative synovium is called **pannus**. Destruction of the joint occurs not only from the direct effect of this invading granulation tissue (pannus) but also from degradation by enzymes of the synovial fluid.

31. Which five types of lung disease occur in rheumatoid arthritis?

1. **Pleural disease:** Although common at post mortem examination, it is relatively uncommon clinically.
2. **Pneumonitis and interstitial fibrosis.**
3. **Nodules:** Singly or in clusters, they may cavitate and occasionally precede articular involvement.
4. **Arteritis:** From pulmonary hypertension.
5. **Airway disease:** Obstructive lung disease, including bronchiolitis obliterans.

32. How does pregnancy affect rheumatoid arthritis?

Signs and symptoms of rheumatoid arthritis lessen in approximately 70% of women during pregnancy. Post partum flares of disease occur in approximately 90% of women who experience improvement.

Klipple GL, Cecere FA: Rheumatoid arthritis and pregnancy. Rheum Dis Clin North Am 15:213–239, 1989.

33. Describe the classic clinical setting for the development of vasculitis associated with rheumatoid arthritis.

The development of vasculitis in patients with rheumatoid arthritis classically occurs after longstanding disease, with evidence of joint destruction, high circulating titers of rheumatoid factor, and nodules. There is generally associated fever.

34. What are the cocked-up toes of rheumatoid arthritis?

Inflammation of the metatarsophalangeal joints in rheumatoid arthritis can often result in subluxation of the metatarsal heads, leading to collapse of the arch of the foot. A claw-like or cocking-up appearance of the toes follows.

35. Is there increased mortality in rheumatoid arthritis?

Multiple studies reveal patients with RA have decreased survival compared to the general population.

Pincus T: Is mortality increased in rheumatoid arthritis? J Musculoskel Med 5:27–46, 1988.

36. In which diseases are subcutaneous nodules found?

Subcutaneous nodules are found in rheumatoid arthritis, rheumatic fever, and systemic lupus erythematosus. Additionally, gouty tophi, synovial cysts, and xanthomas can sometimes appear as subcutaneous nodules.

37. Which ocular abnormalities occur in rheumatoid arthritis?

Both episcleritis and scleritis are ocular manifestations of rheumatoid arthritis. If scleral inflammation progresses, scleral thinning or scleromalacia may be noted.

Bacon PA: Extra-articular rheumatoid arthritis. In McCarthy DJ (ed): Arthritis and Allied Conditions, 11th ed. Philadelphia, Lea & Febiger, 1989, pp 1967–1998.

38. What percentage of patients with rheumatoid arthritis have a positive antinuclear antibody (ANA) assay?

Up to 25% of patients with established rheumatoid arthritis have circulating ANA. Patients with rheumatoid arthritis and Sjögren's syndrome often have anti-Ro antibodies. Patients with positive ANA are often considered to have a poorer prognosis.

39. Is there an HLA association with rheumatoid arthritis?

There is an established relationship between HLA DR4 and DR1 and rheumatoid arthritis. Approximately 93% of rheumatoid arthritis patients have one or the other of these antigens. Exactly how these molecules confer increased susceptibility to the disease is unclear, but is an area of active research.

McDermott M, McDevitt H: Immunogenetics of rheumatic diseases. Bulletin on Rheum Dis 38(1):1–10, 1989.

40. How do you classify the functional capacity of patients with rheumatoid arthritis?

Class I: No restrictions; able to perform normal activities.
Class II: Moderate restriction, but able to perform normal activities.
Class III: Marked restriction; inability to perform most duties of the patient's usual occupation or self care.
Class IV: Incapacitation or confinement to a wheelchair.

41. What are the extra-articular manifestations of rheumatoid arthritis?

- Nodules
- Leukocytoclastic vasculitis
- Pericardial disease
- Pulmonary involvement
- Eye involvement
- Felty's syndrome

42. What is the mechanism for low pleural glucose in pleural effusions of rheumatoid arthritis?

The mechanism for low pleural glucose in pleural effusions of patients with RA appears to be a defect of the transport of glucose into the fluid.

43. Describe the stages of progression of rheumatoid arthritis.

Stage I: Early
- No destructive changes on roentgenologic examination.
- Roentgenologic osteoporosis acceptable.

Stage II: Moderate
- Roentgenologic evidence of osteoporosis with or without slight cartilage destruction.
- Adjacent muscle atrophy.
- Extra-articular soft tissue lesions such as nodules or tenosynovitis may be present.

Stage III: Severe
- Roentgenologic evidence of cartilage and bone destruction in addition to osteoporosis.
- Joint deformity, such as subluxation, ulnar deviation, or hyperextension without fibrosis or bony ankylosis.
- Extra-articular soft tissue lesions such as nodules or tenosynovitis may be present.

Stage IV: Terminal
- Bony or fibrous ankylosis.
- Criteria of Stage III.

44. An aggressive disease course in rheumatoid arthritis is suggested by what factors?
a. High titer rheumatoid factor (RF)
b. Positive ANA
c. Nodules

45. Do patients with rheumatoid arthritis develop gout with increased, decreased, or the same frequency as the general population?

There is a negative association between RA and gout.

46. Does Still's disease occur in the adult? How is it diagnosed?

Still's disease (from Sir George Frederick Still, 1868–1941) is the eponym assigned to systemic onset juvenile arthritis. It has been reported in adults as a seronegative polyarthropathy associated with sudden onset high fever and chills, with evanescent rash on the trunk and extremities. Bony erosions are uncommon, although fusion of the carpal bones may occur.

47. Describe Felty's syndrome.

Felty's syndrome describes the syndrome of circulating neutropenia and splenomegaly in patients with established RA. It is also associated with recurrent infections.

48. How does the effect of aspirin (ASA) on platelets differ from that of other nonsteroidal anti-inflammatory drugs (NSAIDs)?

NSAIDs, including ASA, decrease platelet aggregation that is induced by adenosine diphosphate (ADP), collagen, or epinephrine by inhibiting the enzyme cyclo-oxygenase. ASA, an acetylated salicylate, irreversibly destroys this enzyme, whereas other NSAIDs (including nonacetylated salicylates) leave the enzyme able to function again once the drug level has dropped. Thus, patients taking ASA should discontinue the drug 10 days to 2 weeks before a surgical procedure, whereas a much shorter period is possible with the other NSAIDs.

SJÖGREN'S SYNDROME

49. What is Sjögren's syndrome and how is it classified?

Sjögren's syndrome is an inflammatory disease of exocrine glands manifested primarily by dryness of the eyes and mouth. It can occur as an isolated entity (primary Sjögren's syndrome) or in association with another rheumatic disease, commonly rheumatoid arthritis or SLE (secondary Sjögren's syndrome).

50. Which glands are most commonly involved in Sjögren's syndrome?

Major and minor salivary glands as well as lacrimal glands are commonly involved in Sjögren's syndrome. These include parotids and submandibular glands.

51. What is keratoconjunctivitis sicca (KCS) and how is it documented?

KCS (or sicca complex) is the loss of integrity of the corneal epithelium due to desiccation from inadequate tear production. It is most commonly associated with Sjögren's syndrome and is characterized by hyperemia of the conjunctiva, lacrimal deficiency, thickening of the corneal epithelium, itching and burning of the eye (often described as a "gritty" or foreign-body sensation), and frequently reduced visual acuity.

52. Is Sjögren's syndrome rare?

Many believe that Sjögren's syndrome is underdiagnosed, because the signs and symptoms are subtle and easy to misinterpret. In both its primary and secondary forms, it may be the second most common rheumatic disease in the U.S.

Lane HC, Fauci AS: Sjögren's syndrome. In Wilson JD (ed): Harrison's Principles of Internal Medicine, 12th ed. New York, McGraw-Hill, 1991.

53. How is Sjögren's syndrome diagnosed?

The first step is to ask the appropriate historical questions to document sicca complex and other symptoms. Inquiries about eye grittiness or the ability to eat crackers without drinking water have been suggested as nonleading ways to ask about dryness. The Schirmer's test (the measurement of tear production using filter paper) can document diminished output of the lacrimal glands that cause the sicca complex. Likewise, biopsy of the salivary glands (usually in the lower lip) showing the presence of infiltrating lympho-cytes establishes the diagnosis (along with the presence of keratoconjunctivitis sicca and xerostomia).

54. What percent of patients with primary Sjögren's syndrome subsequently develop a connective tissue syndrome?

If symptoms of an underlying connective tissue disease do not appear within 12 months of the keratoconjunctivitis sicca, then the chances are approximately 10% that it will appear later in life.

55. Which neoplasms are associated with Sjögren's syndrome?

There is an increased incidence of non-Hodgkin's lymphoma in patients with Sjögren's syndrome. The lymphomas are usually B-cell derived, and some patients may also have serum protein spikes. The diagnosis of tumor may be difficult, given that the nonmalignant lymphoid infiltration of lymphocytes can often simulate neoplasm (pseudolymphoma).

THE SPINE

56. What is spinal stenosis?

Progressive narrowing (or stenosing) of the spinal canal leads to spinal stenosis. This is most commonly caused by osteoarthritis of the lumbar or cervical spine. With cervical disease, patients often present with pain and limitation of motion. Hyperrreflexia is common. Other signs present may include muscle weakness, spastic gait, and Babinski's sign. In the lumbar region, the clinical manifestations are mostly those of compression of the cauda equina, especially claudication.

57. What is cauda equina syndrome?

A central midline herniation of a disc can bring on a surgical emergency termed cauda equina syndrome. Sacral nerve roots are paralyzed and there is loss of bowel and bladder function (often with limited return). The patient may not be able to walk. The herniated disc must be removed surgically.

Lipson SJ: Low back pain. In Kelley WN, et al (eds): Textbook of Rheumatology, 2nd ed. Philadelphia, W.B. Saunders, 1985, p 461.

58. What is the difference between spondylolysis and spondylolisthesis?

Spondylolysis refers to an interruption of the pars interarticularis of the vertebra. The pars interarticularis is the portion of the vertebral arch on each side between the superior and inferior articular processes. The term spondylolisthesis refers to displacement of one vertebra on another. The most common etiology of spondylolisthesis is bilateral spondylolysis. Severe osteoarthritis of the apophyseal joints can produce spondylolisthesis without spondylolysis.

59. What is the vacuum sign?

The vacuum sign is a radiographic sign of intervertebral osteochondrosis. These radiolucencies represent gas (nitrogen) appearing at the site of negative pressure produced by abnormal spaces or clefts. Clefts are produced by degeneration of the intervertebral disc, especially the nucleus pulposus.

60. What is meant by the term spondyloarthropathy, and which diseases are usually included in this classification?

The term spondyloarthropathy describes a group of diseases of uncertain etiology that have a predilection for inflammatory lesions of the spine and sacroiliac joints. In addition, they are characterized by the absence of rheumatoid factors or other autoantibodies. Other unifying features include peripheral oligoarthropathy, enthesopathy (disease of the muscular or tendinous attachment to bone), extra-articular foci of inflammation, and an association with HLA B27 antigen. Diseases classified under this rubric include ankylosing spondylitis, Reiter's syndrome, the arthropathy of psoriasis, and the arthropathy associated with inflammatory bowel disease. Some authorities also include the arthropathy associated with Whipple's and Behcet's disease.

Arnett FC: Seronegative spondyloarthropathies. Bulletin on Rheum Dis 37(1):1–12, 1987.

61. How do syndesmophytes and osteophytes differ?

Syndesmophytes are thin, vertical outgrowths and represent calcifications of the annulus fibrosis. As syndesmophytes enlarge, ossification can involve adjacent anterior longitudinal and paravertebral connective tissue. Syndesmophytes predominate on the anterior and lateral aspects of the spine, particularly near the thoracolumbar junction, eventually bridging the disc space and connecting one vertebral body with its neighbor. Osteophytes are triangular and arise several millimeters from the discovertebral junction.

62. What are the extra-articular features of ankylosing spondylitis?

- Anterior uveitis
- Aortitis
- Pulmonary fibrosis

63. How is inflammation of the sacroiliac (SI) joint graded radiographically?

Grade I	Normal
Grade II	Sclerosis of bone adjacent to the SI joints
Grade III	Erosion at the SI joints
Grade IV	Bony fusion across the SI joints

Arnett FC: Seronegative spondyloarthropathies. Bulletin on Rheum Dis 37(1):1–12, 1987.

64. Where is an enthesis located?

An enthesis is the junction of muscle or ligament and bone. It is the site of inflammation in the spondyloarthropathies, termed enthesopathy. In response to this inflammation, reactive new bone is formed. This process accounts for the formation of syndesmophytes in ankylosing spondylitis.

65. DISH is an acronym for which syndrome?

Diffuse idiopathic skeletal hyperostosis is a syndrome characterized by extensive ossification of tendinous and ligamentous attachments to bone. Involvement of the spine with flowing calcification over the anterior longitudinal ligament is the most common finding. Extraspinal manifestations have also been reported. Clinical symptoms are often mild. When present they consist of morning stiffness and deep aching of the affected portion.

66. Are there specific radiographic findings for DISH?

Radiographic criteria have been stated and are designed to help distinguish between DISH and ankylosing spondylitis, degenerative spine disease, and spondylosis deformans:

   1. The presence of flowing calcification and ossification along the anterolateral aspect of at least four contiguous vertebral bodies, with or without associated localized pointed excrescences at the intervening vertebral body intervertebral disc junctions.

   2. The presence and relative preservation of intervertebral disc height in the involved vertebral segment and the absence of extensive radiographic changes of "degenerative" disc disease, including vacuum phenomena and vertebral body marginal sclerosis.

   3. The absence of apophyseal joint bony ankylosis and sacroiliac joint erosion, sclerosis, and intra-articular osseous fusion.

   Resnick D, et al: Diffuse idiopathic skeletal hyperostosis (DISH): Ankylosing hyperostosis of Forestier and Rotes-Querol. In Resnick D, Niwayama G (eds): Diagnosis of Bone and Joint Disorders, 2nd ed. Philadelphia, W.B. Saunders, 1988, pp 1548–1602.

SYSTEMIC LUPUS ERYTHEMATOSUS (SLE)

67. What are the most common clinical features of SLE?

Feature	Frequency	Feature	Frequency	Feature	Frequency
Arthritis/arthralgia	91%	Adenopathy	58%	Nephritis	46%
Fever	83%	Anemia (<11 g)	56%	Pleurisy	45%
Skin involvement	71%	Myalgia	48%	CNS symptoms	25%

Dubois EL, Wallace DJ: Clinical and laboratory manifestations of systemic lupus erythematosus. In Wallace DJ, Dubois EL (eds): Dubois' Lupus Erythematosus, 3rd ed. Philadelphia, Lea & Febiger, 1987, pp 317–349.

68. What is the LE cell and how does it relate to the antinuclear antibody (ANA)?

The LE or lupus erythematosus cell was first described by Malcolm Hargraves. It is a polymorphonuclear leukocyte (PMN) that has ingested the nucleus of a damaged cell. The damage occurred secondary to an autoantibody directed towards nuclear components. Thus the LE cell is really a manifestation of circulating ANA.

   Hargraves MM, Richmond H, Morton R: Presentation of two bone marrow elements: the "tart" cell and the "L.E." cell. Proc May Clin 23:25–28, 1948.

69. What conditions are associated with a positive ANA?

A brief list of diseases in which circulating ANA has been detected includes:

   a. Systemic lupus (SLE)   e. CREST syndrome   i. Chronic hepatitis
   b. Drug-induced lupus   f. Polymyositis   j. Infectious mononucleosis
   c. Rheumatoid arthritis   g. Dermatomyositis
   d. Systemic sclerosis   h. Mixed connective tissue disease

70. Is the ANA one antibody?

No. The detection of the LE cell initiated the study of autoantibodies. With the development of immunofluorescent techniques, different staining patterns were discovered, and it became clear that many different nuclear antigens could elicit an antibody response. Detecting the specific antibody reaction requires more refined techniques.

Antigen	Antibody
Deoxyribose phosphate backbone of DNA	Anti-DNA (double-stranded or native)
Purine and pyrimidine bases	Anti-single-stranded DNA
H1, H2A, H2B, H3, H2A/H2B, and H3/H4 complexes	Anti-histones
DNA topoisomerase I	Anti-SCL-70
Histidyl t-RNA transferase	Anti-Jo-1
Kinetochore	Anti-centromere
RNA polymerase I	Anti-nucleolar
Y^1-Y^5 RNA and protein	Anti-Ro
U1-6 RNA and protein	Anti-RNP (includes anti-Sm)

Hardin JA: The molecular biology of autoantibodies. In Schumacher HR Jr (ed): Primer on the Rheumatic Diseases, 9th ed. Atlanta, Arthritis Foundation, 1988, pp 32–35.

71. Do ANA staining patterns detect specific ANA present? What is their clinical significance?

The immunofluorescence technique for detecting ANA is performed by incubating human epithelial cells with the patient's serum. If antinuclear antibodies are present, they will bind to the nuclear component of the substrate. Next, fluorescent anti-immunoglobulin is added. This antibody is designed to bind to antibodies in the test serum. With the fluorescent tag, the ANA can be directly visualized under fluorescent light. Different patterns of staining occur, and although they can provide some diagnostic information, they do not identify the specific antibody present. For example, the rim pattern usually associated with the presence of circulating antibody to native DNA may be obscured if another autoantibody (staining a homogeneous pattern) is present.

72. Why is it helpful to know the specific ANA present in a patient?

Although no laboratory test is 100% diagnostic for any rheumatic disease, the presence of certain autoantibodies in the appropriate clinical setting can be helpful. Some common disease associations include:

ANA	Disease
Ro/SSA	SLE, neonatal lupus, subacute lupus, Sjögren's syndrome, rheumatoid arthritis
Double-stranded DNA	SLE
Sm	SLE
JO-1	Polymyositis
Centromere	CREST syndrome
SCL-70	Systemic sclerosis

Reichlin M: Antinuclear antibodies. In Kelley WN, et al (eds): Textbook of Rheumatology, 2nd ed. Philadelphia, W.B. Saunders, 1985, pp 690–707.

73. What drugs are commonly associated with the development of a positive ANA?

Historically, a clinical syndrome of arthritis, fever, rash, and positive ANA was seen after initiating antihypertensive therapy with the drug hydralazine. The development of circulating ANA (primarily to histones) has been subsequently demonstrated with many drugs, including procainamide, isoniazid (INH), chlorpromazine, D-penicillamine, sulfasalazine, methyldopa, and quinidine.

74. What are the common skin manifestations of SLE?
The skin is a frequent target organ in SLE. The classic lesion of acute lupus is the malar (butterfly) rash. This is often exacerbated by UV light (either artificial or sunlight). Symmetric, superficial, non-scarring, annular lesions of the shoulders, upper arms, and back are the classic lesions of subacute cutaneous lupus. Non-scarring alopecia often occurs concurrently. These patients may or may not have circulating anti-Ro antibodies. These lesions are very photosensitive. The skin lesions of discoid lupus most commonly occur over the face and neck. Alopecia can be particularly troublesome. These lesions eventually become hypopigmented and atrophic.

75. What is subacute cutaneous lupus (SCLE)?
Some consider this cutaneous eruption to lie between chronic discoid lupus and acute cutaneous lupus. The lesions generally occur in the shoulders, upper chest, and neck. They are symmetric and non-scarring. They can be annular or resemble psoriasis. Between 25–50% of patients will have constitutional symptoms. The patients may have circulating antibodies to Ro antigen, and there is an association with HLA DRw3.

76. Is there a relationship between discoid lupus and systemic lupus?
This is an area of some controversy. Approximately 25% of patients with classic discoid lesions may have constitutional symptoms but do not meet the American College of Rheumatology's criteria for systemic lupus. Approximately 10% of discoid lupus patients go on to develop systemic lupus.

Dubois EL, et al: Relationship between discoid lupus and systemic lupus erythematosus. In Wallace DJ, Dubois EL (eds): Dubois' Lupus Erythematosus, 3rd ed. Philadelphia, Lea & Febiger, 1987, pp 302–313.

77. Does SLE recur in a transplanted kidney?
Disease activity in SLE often quiets with the onset of uremia and dialysis. Several studies note the ability to discontinue glucocorticoid therapy without a return of the extra-renal manifestations of the disease once dialysis has been initiated. Although there are reports of subsequent disease exacerbations, kidney transplantation can usually be accomplished without a return of disease activity.

78. What percentage of SLE patients have a positive rheumatoid factor?
Approximately one-third of patients with SLE have circulating rheumatoid factor present. It is often present in a low titer.

79. What are the common GI manifestations of SLE?
There are many GI manifestations in SLE, and they may be present in up to 50% of SLE patients. Anorexia, nausea, and vomiting are among the most common. Oral ulceration (most commonly buccal erosions) were identified in 40% of one group studied. Esophageal involvement, either as esophagitis, esophageal ulceration, or esophageal dysmotility, have all be reported. The latter seems to correlate with the presence of Raynaud's phenomenon. Intestinal involvement results in abdominal pain, diarrhea, and occasionally hemorrhage. Intestinal ischemia may be present and may progress to infarction and perforation. Pneumatosis intestinalis in SLE is usually benign and transient but may represent an irreversible necrotizing enterocolitis. Pancreatitis, elevated liver function tests, and abdominal serositis are also well recognized. A vasculitic process has been implicated in the pathogenesis of these GI manifestations.

Hoffman BI, et al: The gastrointestinal manifestations of systemic lupus erythematosus: A review of the literature. Semin Arthritis Rheum 9:237–247, 1980.

80. What are the most characteristic histologic manifestations of SLE?
Hematoxylin bodies are the tissue correlates of the LE cell. Although only present in approximately 15% of SLE patients, the onion-skin lesions of the arterioles of the spleen are characteristic of lupus. The concentric arteriolar fibrosis may be a manifestation of earlier active arteritis. The Libman-Sacks verrucous endocarditis lesions, most commonly found on the mitral valve, also represent characteristic pathologic changes in SLE.

81. What is the most common pathologic abnormality found in patients with lupus CNS disease?
Commonly used designations like "lupus cerebritis" suggest that CNS lesions in lupus patients are usually inflammatory. However, small infarcts and hemorrhages are more frequently encountered than vasculitis.

82. How do pregnancy and systemic lupus interact?
There has been considerable evolution of thought regarding pregnancy in patients with systemic lupus; however, a number of points are clear. First, fertility is unaffected by the disease (i.e., lupus patients get pregnant just as readily as controls). Second, there is increased risk of miscarriage, abortion, and prematurity in patients with lupus compared to controls. Antibodies to phospholipids may contribute to this risk. Third, it has been established that the Ro antibody crosses the placenta and is responsible for most of the neonatal lupus syndromes, including the skin manifestations and congenital heart block. There are recent data suggesting that pregnant lupus patients do not have disease flares more frequently than nonpregnant lupus patients.

Mintz G, et al: Pregnancy in patients with rheumatic diseases: Systemic lupus erythematosus. Rheum Dis Clin North Am 15:255–274, 1989.

Lochshin MD: Pregnancy does not cause systemic lupus erythematosus to worsen. Arthritis Rheum 32:665–670, 1989.

83. What is the incidence of renal involvement in SLE?
This depends on criteria used to define renal disease. If abnormal urinary sediment or proteinuria is used as a criterion, 35–90% of patients with SLE have renal disease. If light microscopic examination of renal biopsy or autopsy material is used, nearly 90% have renal disease. Almost 100% of patients with SLE have abnormalities if tissue is examined with electron microscopy or immunofluorescence regardless of clinical disease activity.

84. What is the role of cytotoxic therapy in the treatment of nephritis in lupus patients?
Cytotoxic agents such as azathioprine and cyclophosphamide are useful in the management of many rheumatic diseases. Because of toxicity, they should be used only where careful clinical trials point to specific advantages. One such condition is lupus nephritis. Patients with inflammatory renal lesions had slower progression to end-stage renal disease and diminished mortality when their regimens included cyclophosphamide.

Austin HA III, et al: Therapy of lupus nephritis: Controlled trial of prednisone and cytotoxic drugs. N Engl J Med 314:614–619, 1986.

GOUT

85. Which crystals are currently associated with joint inflammation, and how are they differentiated?
The three principal crystalline deposits associated with joint disease are:

1. **Uric acid** (monosodium urate) crystals are seen in gouty arthritis. These crystals are needle-shaped and vary in length (2 to 10 μm). They may be seen either extracellularly or within polymorphonuclear leukocytes. They exhibit strong negative birefringence under a polarizing microscope. This means that they appear yellow when the long axes of the

crystals are aligned parallel to the rays of the first-order red-plate compensator (and blue when aligned in a perpendicular fashion). This can possibly be remembered as "Yellow = parallel = gout."

2. **Calcium pyrophosphate** crystals are seen in pseudogout. They appear as broad-, rod- or rhomboid-shaped crystals. They exhibit positive birefringence and therefore appear blue when aligned parallel with the red-plate compensator (and yellow when aligned in a perpendicular fashion).

3. **Hydroxyapatite** crystals are also associated with joint inflammation but are very difficult to visualize with light microscopy.

86. Describe the most common pathogenic mechanism for the development of hyperuricemia in gout.

Hyperuricemia can develop secondary to overproduction or underexcretion of urate. Of gout patients 5–15% are found to be urate overproducers. The remaining patients have decreased renal clearance of urate, accounting for their hyperuricemia. Although nonrenal mechanisms for the removal of urate are known (the GI tract for example), diminished clearance by these routes does not lead to hyperuricemia.

87. What are the four stages of gout?

Stage 1 consists of **asymptomatic hyperuricemia**. There is elevated serum urate without articular disease or nephrolithiasis. Not all patients with asymptomatic hyperuricemia will go on to develop gout, but the higher the serum level, the greater the likelihood of developing articular disease. In most cases, 20–30 years of sustained hyperuricemia will occur before an attack of nephrolithiasis or arthropathy.

Stage 2 is reached with **the first attack of articular disease.** It is exquisitely painful and usually occurs in a single joint. There may be associated fever, swelling, erythema, and skin sloughing. Of initial attacks 50% occur as podagra (inflammation and pain at the metatarsophalangeal joint of the great toe). If left untreated, 90% of patients with gout will have podagra at some stage of the disease.

Stage 3 is the **period between attacks described as intercritical gout.** Generally patients are completely asymptomatic. Classic studies by Gutman and Yu reveal that 62% of patients had a second attack of articular disease within 1 year of the first attack. An additional 16% of patients had their second attack 1–2 years after their first, and 11% of patients had their second attack 2–5 years after their first. Likewise, an additional 4% did not have a second attack until 5–10 years after their first. Only 7% of patients had no second attack after 10 years of follow-up.

Stage 4 is termed **chronic tophaceous gout** and occurs with the development of chronic arthritis, with tissue deposition of urate. The principle determinant of the rate of urate deposition is the serum urate concentration.

Gutman AB: The past four decades of progress in the knowledge of gout with an assessment of present status. Arthritis Rheum 16:431, 1973.

88. What is the mechanism for the development of hyperuricemia after organ transplantation?

Hyperuricemia and acute gout are common complications in patients undergoing organ transplantation. One study of renal transplant patients found that hyperuricemia was significantly more common in those receiving cyclosporin A (CSA) as opposed to those who were receiving azathioprine. Another study of patients receiving heart or heart-lung transplants also found CSA to be a major risk factor for hyperuricemia and acute gout. These authors felt that the course of the disease is more aggressive and treatment more difficult. The hypothesized mechanism for the development of the disease is a CSA-induced decrease in renal urate clearance.

Lin HY, et al: Cyclosporin-induced hyperuricemia and gout. N Engl J Med 321:287–292, 1989.

OSTEOARTHRITIS

89. Compare the biochemical changes of the aged joint with the osteoarthritic joint.
Although age is the single most significant epidemiologic association with osteoarthritis, there are biochemical differences between an old joint and an osteoarthritic one. The major components of the joint are bone and cartilage. The major components of the cartilage include the chondrocytes and the matrix (which in turn is composed of collagen, water, and proteoglycans).

	Aging	*Osteoarthritis*
Bone	Osteoporosis	Thickened cortices, osteophytes, subchondral cysts, remodeling
Chondrocyte activity	Normal	Increased
Matrix		
Collagen	Increased fibril cross-linking	Irregular weave, smaller fibrils
Water	Slight decrease	Significant increase
Proteoglycans	Normal total content	Decreased total content
	Decreased chondroitins	Increased chondroitins
	Increased keratin	Decreased keratin
	Normal aggregation	Decreased aggregation

Brandt KD, et al: Aging in relation to the pathogenesis of osteoarthritis. Clin Rheum Dis 12:117–130, 1986.
Hough AJ Jr, et al: Pathology of osteoarthritis. In McCarthy DJ (ed): Arthritis and Allied Conditions, 11th ed. Philadelphia, Lea & Febiger, 1989, pp 1571–1594.

90. Name the classic radiographic findings of osteoarthritis.
- Subchondrial cyst formation
- New bone formation (osteophytes)
- Sclerosis of bone
- Joint space narrowing
- Lack of subchondral osteoporosis

91. What is the prevalence of osteoarthritis in the population?
The prevalence of osteoarthritis increases with age. It also depends on which criteria are used to make the diagnosis. The prevalence of osteoarthritis by autopsy is nearly 100% in patients over 65 years old. Roentgenographic studies reveal a prevalence of osteoarthritis ranging from approximately 4% in patients between 18–24 years old to over 85% in patients older than 75.

INFECTIOUS DISEASE

92. What is pyoderma gangrenosum?
Pyoderma gangrenosum is the term applied to skin lesions that begin as pustules or erythematous nodules and break down to form spreading ulcers with necrotic undermined edges. It is associated with inflammatory bowel disease, but also occurs in chronic active hepatitis, seropositive rheumatoid arthritis (without evidence of vasculopathy), leukemia, and polycythemia vera. Differential diagnosis of the lesions includes necrotizing vasculitis, bacterial infection, and spider bites.

Braverman IM: Diseases of the gastrointestinal tract. In Skin Signs of Systemic Disease, 2nd ed. Philadelphia, W.B. Saunders, 1981, pp 566–618.

93. Do the manifestations of acute rheumatic fever differ when presenting in the child compared to the adult?

The classic signs of rheumatic fever include arthritis, rash, chorea, nodules, and carditis. The frequency of the clinical features exhibited varies with age, as indicated in the following table:

	Children	*Adults*
Fever	Present	Present
Arthritis	Less common than in adults	May be the only manifestation in 80–85% of adults
Carditis	Present in 75–90% of childhood cases	Present in 15% of adult cases
E. marginatum	Present in 10–20%	Rare
Nodules	Present in 2–22%	Absent
Chorea	Present in <5%	Absent

Pope RM: Acute rheumatic fever and Jaccoud's arthropathy. In Schumacher HR Jr (ed): Primer on the Rheumatic Diseases, 9th ed. Atlanta, Arthritis Foundation, 1988, pp 156–160.

94. What is the mechanism for acute rheumatic fever?

Rheumatic fever occurs after group A streptococcal pharyngitis (although the infection may not be symptomatic). Data indicate that the immune response initiated against the bacteria plays an important role. The antibodies produced are known to cross-react with human antigens, leading to a persistent autoimmune reaction and tissue destruction (molecular mimicry). Development of immune complexes has also been documented.

95. Which common viral illnesses are associated with arthropathy?

The development of arthralgia or frank arthritis is common with a variety of viral infections. Common viruses that often have an associated arthropathy include: hepatitis B, parvovirus, rubella, and human immunodeficiency virus (HIV or AIDS virus). Some uncommonly encountered viral infections strongly associated with arthropathy include the group A arboviruses (Ross River virus, chikungunya, O'nyong-nyong fever, Sindbis, Mayaro). Commonly occurring viral infections that occasionally produce arthropathy include: mumps, smallpox (including vaccinia), Epstein-Barr virus, cytomegalovirus, and enteroviruses (echo viruses and coxsackieviruses).

96. What are the most common bacterial pathogens responsible for septic arthritis?

Septic arthritis is usually classified as gonococcal or nongonococcal. Of the nongonococcal bacteria causing joint infections, *Staphylococcus* remains most common. Species of streptococcus are the next most frequent when grouped together. Finally, gram-negative bacilli may cause 20–30% of septic joints.

97. What is the mechanism by which septic arthritis develops?

Septic arthritis generally develops by hematogenous spread of bacteria. Less commonly, direct inoculation may occur either by trauma, adjacent osteomyelitis (a more common mechanism in children), or placement of an infected prosthesis. Bacteria then multiply and inflammation occurs, leading to cartilage destruction. Predisposing factors include an immunocompromised state, an underlying systemic disease (including diabetes mellitus, chronic liver disease, and sickle cell anemia), or previous joint damage (rheumatoid arthritis or previous trauma).

98. What are the common clinical manifestations of gonococcal (GC) arthritis?

GC arthritis occurs in approximately 0.1–0.5% of patients with gonorrhea. The arthropathy is commonly migratory and is often accompanied by tenosynovitis. Skin lesions are often present, usually as a small macule or papule on a distal extremity. Clinical manifestations of GC arthritis may differ from other bacterial arthropathies. Even under optimal conditions, joint fluids are culture-positive in less than 50% of cases.

99. What is reactive arthritis?

Reactive arthritis is an inflammatory arthropathy of at least one month's duration occurring after a bout of urethritis or dysentery. The mechanism for the development of the arthropathy is unclear.

OTHER SYNDROMES AND ENTITIES

100. What is reflex sympathetic dystrophy (RSD)?

RSD (also called Sudeck's atrophy, causalgia, post-traumatic osteoporosis, and shoulder-hand syndrome) is a syndrome characterized by pain and swelling of distal extremities, trophic skin changes, and signs and symptoms of vasomotor instability. The latter may vary from frank Raynaud's phenomenon to hyperemia. Additionally, hyperhidrosis may be observed. Roentgenographic changes include localized osteopenia, which may occur rapidly and be quite severe, but there usually is preservation of the joint space. The syndrome may be idiopathic, although there is a long list of reported associations, including Colles' fracture, myocardial infarction, stroke, neoplasm, and others. Radionuclide blood flow studies show increased blood flow to the affected side. Although the actual data are limited, most authors suggest some abnormality of the sympathetic nervous system as an explanation for the syndrome.

101. What are the muscles in the musculotendinous structure of the rotator cuff?

The muscles of the rotator cuff include the supraspinatus, infraspinatus, teres minor, and subscapularis.

102. Which syndrome is associated with malfunction of the muscles of the rotator cuff?

Disorders of the rotator cuff are a common cause of shoulder pain. **Impingement syndrome** occurs when the supraspinatus tendon gets caught between the head of the humerus and the acromion, resulting in pain (see figure). The motion most likely to bring these structures into proximity (and thereby cause pain) is repetitive overhead movement and internal rotation of the arm, as might be found in manual laborers or athletes. Night pain is characteristic. If the tendon ruptures (rotator cuff tear), significant weakness of these muscles may be found. Impingement syndrome usually results from injury to the supraspinatus. Rotator cuff tendonitis is often an acute problem and may be associated with calcification.

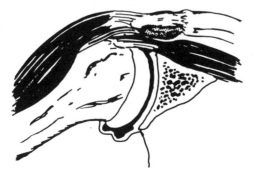

Illustration of the rotator cuff.

103. Why does a neuropathic joint cause problems?
Without sensation and proprioception as regulators of joint function, there is a gradual relaxation of supporting structure, abnormal mechanics, and ultimately joint destruction.

104. What are the most common causes of the neuropathic joint in the upper extremity?
Many diseases, including congenital pain insensitivity, amyloidosis, diabetes mellitus, alcoholism, and tabes dorsalis, can lead to neuroarthropathy. In the upper extremities, particularly the elbow, syringomyelia is a common cause of sensory abnormalities leading to arthropathy.
    Forrester DM, Brown JC: The elbow. In The Radiology of Joint Disease, 3rd ed. Philadelphia, W.B. Saunders, 1987, pp 318–358.

105. What are the rheumatic manifestations of sarcoidosis?
Sarcoidosis is a systemic disease characterized by a noncaseating granulomatous reaction of unknown origin. Besides the lungs, involvement of the eyes, skin, and joints is not uncommon. Skin involvement, including erythema nodosum, occurs in approximately 30% of patients. Asymptomatic sarcoid granulomas have been found in muscle biopsy. Sarcoid granulomas may occur in bones, appearing radiographically as cysts, and osteolysis has also been described. Articular symptoms are present in most patients presenting with acute sarcoidosis (hilar adenopathy, fever, erythema nodosum). Ankles and knees are the most common joints involved. This articular syndrome is usually self-limited, lasting up to 4 weeks. When the disease is less acute in onset, articular involvement is less common. It can, however, be recurring and protracted. Joint destruction is infrequent. The articular involvement may predate the pulmonary involvement, or occur after 10 years of disease.

106. What patterns of arthritis are associated with psoriasis?
The five clinical subgroups of arthritis associated with psoriasis include:
    1. distal interphalangeal joints of the hands and/or feet
    2. peripheral asymmetric oligoarthropathy
    3. symmetric polyarthritis resembling rheumatoid arthritis
    4. arthritis mutalans ("opera glass hands")
    5. sacroiliitis with or without higher levels of spinal involvement.
    Arnett FC: Seronegative spondyloarthropathies. Bulletin on Rheum Dis 37(1):1–12, 1987.

107. Reiter's syndrome has which mucocutaneous manifestations?
Skin and mucus membranes are commonly involved in Reiter's syndrome. Small, painless areas of **desquamation of the tongue** may not even be noticed. Conversely, **circinate balanitis** is rarely missed by the patient. It primarily affects the glans penis and can range from small erythematous macules to larger areas of dry flaking skin. **Keratoderma blennorrhagicum** is a thickening and keratinization of the skin found in patients with Reiter's syndrome. It generally involves the feet, hands, and nails. The lesions resemble psoriasis.

108. What are the common radiographic manifestations of Reiter's syndrome?
Periostitis at areas of tendinous insertions, frank articular erosions, and syndesmophyte formation have all been documented in Reiter's syndrome.

109. What patterns of arthritis are associated with inflammatory bowel disease (IBD)?
Both a peripheral and axial arthropathy have been associated with IBD. The arthropathy occasionally precedes the bowel symptoms. Approximately 20% of patients with IBD have a peripheral arthropathy. This arthropathy is often accompanied by fever, oral ulcers, eye

or skin lesions (erythema nodosum or pyoderma gangrenosum). The activity of this arthropathy usually parallels the gut disease. There is no increased frequency of HLA B27 phenotype among patients with IBD and peripheral arthritis. Sacroiliitis and spondylitis occurs in approximately 10% of IBD patients. This arthropathy is independent of bowel disease. Treatment of bowel disease does not influence outcome of spondylitis. There is an association of HLA B27 with sacroiliitis and spondylitis.

110. What possible mechanisms exist to explain the association of HLA B27 with arthropathy?
The mechanism by which HLA B27 predisposes to the development of arthritis after urogenital or intestinal infection is unknown. Hypotheses to explain the interaction include:
  1. B27 is directly involved in disease predisposition:
    • B27 could act as a receptor for a microorganism.
    • B27 might be modified by a microorganism eliciting an immune reaction against the new antigen.
    • B27 might resemble microbial epitopes; antibodies directed against the microorganism might cross-react with host antigens (molecular mimicry).
  2. An independent gene closely linked with, but not identical to, B27 is involved in disease susceptibility.
  3. Disease susceptibility conferred by a particular configuration of the T cell receptor.

  Schiffenbauer J, et al: The major histocompatibility complex and reactive arthritis. In Espinoza L (ed): Infections in the Rheumatic Diseases. New York, Grune & Stratton, 1988, pp 303–310.

111. What is Raynaud's phenomenon and with which rheumatic conditions is it characteristically associated?
Raynaud's phenomenon is the eponym given to the occurrence of color change (usually red, white, and then blue) in the hands (or any distal part of the body) on exposure to cold. When making inquires about Raynaud's, it is sometimes difficult not to suggest a positive answer. Thus, one might ask "When you are in a grocery store, do you notice any problems in the frozen food section?" Many conditions have Raynaud's phenomenon as a part of their clinical presentation. Some of these include:
  • Systemic lupus erythematosus (SLE)
  • CREST (calcinosis, Raynaud's, esophageal dysmotility, sclerodactyly, and telangiectasias) syndrome
  • Systemic sclerosis
  • Idiopathic Raynaud's phenomenon
  • Polymyositis and dermatomyositis
  • Sjögren's syndrome
  • Drug-induced Raynaud's phenomenon
  • Cold agglutinins
  • Reflex sympathetic dystrophy

112. What is the difference between Raynaud's disease and Raynaud's phenomenon?
When the syndrome of pallor and cyanosis of the digits is the primary disorder, it is called Raynaud's disease. When it is secondary to another disease or ascertainable cause, it is Raynaud's phenomenon. The disease is the most common cause of the phenomenon.

113. What is the CREST syndrome and what does the acronym represent?
The CREST syndrome is one of a number of sclerosing skin conditions. It is associated with the anti-centromere antibody and has the following manifestations:
  Calcinosis
  Raynaud's phenomenon
  Esophageal dysmotility
  Sclerodactyly
  Telangiectasias

114. What factors may predict the development of systemic sclerosis in a patient presenting with Raynaud's phenomenon?

Patients presenting with Raynaud's phenomenon are at increased risk of developing a rheumatic disease. Positive serology, abnormal nail-bed capillaries, or abnormal pulmonary function studies suggest increased risk of development of disease.

   Fitzgerald O, et al: Systemic sclerosis. Am J Med 84:718–726, 1988.

115. What are the noncutaneous features of scleroderma?

Noncutaneous features of systemic sclerosis (scleroderma) include arthritis, inflammatory muscle disease, GI dysmotility with resulting malabsorption, pulmonary interstitial fibrosis with resulting pulmonary hypertension, and scleroderma renal crisis.

116. What is Jaccoud's deformity?

Arthropathy of the hands, usually the metacarpophalangeal joints, that occurs secondary to chronic inflammation of the joint capsule, ligaments, and tendons is called Jaccoud's deformity. The changes may mimic those of rheumatoid arthritis (ulnar deviation of the fingers, metacarpophalangeal joint subluxation); however erosions are generally not present. Patients can correct these changes voluntarily. Although originally described as a rare condition in rheumatic fever, this eponym has been extended to include arthropathy occurring in other conditions, most commonly SLE.

117. What is Dupuytren's contracture and with which conditions is it associated?

Fibrosis and thickening of the palmar fascia can lead to the flexion contracture first described by Dupuytren in 1831. Disease associations include diabetes mellitus, chronic liver disease, epilepsy, plantar fasciitis, carpal tunnel syndrome, rheumatoid arthritis, trauma to the hand, pulmonary TB, and alcoholism, to name a few.

118. What are the characteristic features of Churg-Strauss vasculitis?

The Churg-Strauss syndrome, described in 1951, is one of the systemic necrotizing vasculopathies. It is associated with eosinophilia (circulating or tissue infiltration), and the onset, later in life, of atopic disease (asthma or allergic rhinitis). This disease has been hypothesized to represent an overlap between the hypereosinophilic syndromes and the vasculitides.

119. Which conditions are associated with mononeuritis multiplex?

Mononeuritis multiplex is a peripheral neuropathy involving one or more nerves. It is sometimes difficult to distinguish from other mononeuropathies caused by local factors such as trauma, compression (acoustic neuroma or peroneal palsy), and entrapment syndromes (carpal tunnel syndrome). Reported associations with mononeuritis multiplex include diabetes mellitus, polyarteritis, SLE, rheumatoid arthritis, Lyme disease, Sjögren's syndrome, cryoglobulinemia, giant cell arteritis, scleroderma, leukemia, leprosy, AIDS, carcinoma, and lymphoma. One recent study found that even after extensive workup almost half of all nondiabetic patients with electromyographic evidence of mononeuritis multiplex did not have an established diagnosis.

   Hellmann CB, et al: Mononeuritis multiplex: The yield of evaluations for occult rheumatic disease. Medicine 67:145–153, 1988.

120. What is leukocytoclastic vasculitis?

Leukocytoclastic vasculitis is a necrotizing lesion of venules and postcapillary venules of the skin. It can occur independently or as a part of another systemic vasculitis. Exudation and hemorrhage account for the clinical manifestation of palpable purpura. When small vessels deeper in the dermis are involved, livedo reticularis can be seen.

   Braverman I: The angiitides. In Skin Signs in Systemic Disease, 2nd ed. Philadelphia, W.B. Saunders, 1981, pp 378–454.

121. Identify the most devastating complication of temporal arteritis.

Temporal arteritis is a granulomatous inflammatory condition of the temporal arteries. It is a disease of the elderly and of women (female to male ratio is 2:1). The clinical manifestations include nonspecific achiness, primarily of the neck, shoulder, and pelvic girdles. Headaches and jaw claudication are noted by patients. Involvement of the posterior ciliary or ophthalmic arteries may lead to sudden loss of vision, which is usually permanent.

122. What is erythema nodosum?

Erythema nodosum is one of the panniculitides. In other words it is associated with inflammation of veins in the fibrous septa of fat. The etiology and pathogenesis remain unclear, although many conditions have been found in association. Infections associated with erythema nodosum include streptococci, TB, most pulmonary fungi, leprosy, and cat scratch disease. Sarcoidosis, Behcet's syndrome, SLE, rheumatic fever, drugs, and inflammatory bowel disease are also associated. Erythema nodosum can also occur without recognizable associations.

123. What systemic vasculopathy is associated with hepatitis B antigenemia?

The presence of circulating hepatitis B antigen has been reported in 10–50% of patients with polyarteritis nodosa (PAN). The disease and its treatment progress similarly in patients with or without circulating hepatitis B antigens.

124. Which autoantibodies are associated with polymyositis (PM)?

Polymyositis patients may have circulating autoantibodies. A positive ANA is not uncommon. Specifically, anti-Jo-1 is found in PM patients, particularly in those who have concomitant pulmonary fibrosis. The antigen has been found to be histidyl-tRNA synthetase.

125. What is the antiphospholipid syndrome?

Antiphospholipid syndrome refers to the clinical syndrome made up of one or more of the following: multiple miscarriages, arterial and venous thromboses, and thrombocytopenia in association with a laboratory finding of antibodies to phospholipids. The common laboratory tests that indicate the presence of antibodies to phospholipids include prolonged PTT, falsely positive VDRL, or positive anticardiolipin antibodies. Another clotting time that may indicate the presence of an antiphospholipid antibody is the Russell viper venom time. Antiphospholipid syndrome can occur by itself (primary antiphospholipid syndrome) or in association with another underlying connective tissue syndrome, primarily lupus (secondary antiphospholipid syndrome).

126. What is the approximate frequency of antibody to phospholipid in established SLE?

A biological false-positive test for syphilis is reported to occur in 10% of cases. The lupus anticoagulant is reportedly present in 6–10% and antibodies to cardiolipin in 15–40% of patients.

127. What common arthritic conditions are associated with Ehlers-Danlos syndrome?

Ehlers-Danlos syndrome is a familial disorder of connective tissue. Because it is associated with several inheritance patterns and variable penetrance, there is marked clinical heterogeneity. There are three basic clinical criteria: (1) fragile skin, (2) bleeding diathesis, and (3) hyperplastic joints. The hypermobility of joints can lead to frequent dislocations (patients may be able to spontaneously dislocate and reduce their joints), kyphoscoliosis, pes planus (flat feet), and premature degenerative joint disease. Additionally, multiple subcutaneous dense lesions that may calcify are noted radiographically. There is a tendency toward muscle calcification (myositis ossificans), particularly adjacent to the hips (from the iliac spines to the inferior trochanter). Joint effusions, hemarthrosis (particularly the knee) secondary to ligamentous laxity, and repetitive trauma are described. Olecranon and prepatellar bursitis are likewise common. There is an association with Raynaud's phenomenon and acro-osteolysis.

BIBLIOGRAPHY

1. Kelley WN, et al (eds): Textbook of Rheumatology, 3rd ed. Philadelphia, W.B. Saunders, 1989.
2. McCarthy DJ (ed): Arthritis and Allied Conditions, 11th ed. Philadelphia, Lea & Febiger, 1989.
3. Resnick D, Niwayama G (eds): Diagnosis of Bone and Joint Disorders, 2nd ed. Philadelphia, W.B. Saunders, 1988.
4. Schumacher HR Jr (ed): Primer on the Rheumatic Diseases, 9th ed. Atlanta, Arthritis Foundation, 1988.
5. Sheon RP, et al (eds): Soft Tissue Rheumatic Pain: Recognition, Management, Prevention, 2nd ed. Philadelphia, Lea & Febiger, 1987.

12. ALLERGY AND IMMUNOLOGY SECRETS

Robert Bressler, M.D. and Anthony J. Zollo, Jr., M.D.

All that wheezes is not asthma.

Chevalier Jackson (1865–1958)
Boston Medical Quarterly 16:86, 1965.

1. Name the two major limbs of the immune system and the principal components of each.
The two major limbs of the immune system are **humoral immunity** and **cellular** or **cell-mediated immunity** (CMI). Although this division has some usefulness, there are many interactions and areas of overlap between the two limbs. The humoral immune response is primarily mediated by antibodies produced by terminally differentiated B cells (plasma cells), but the complement system also plays an important role. Humoral immunity serves as the principal host defense against bacterial infections and also functions in other important immune responses, such as antibody-dependent cellular cytotoxicity (ADCC).

The principal effector of CMI is the T cell, although macrophages and other cellular components are important participants. Intact CMI is critical for host defense against viral, fungal, and protozoal infections, and against development of malignancies, particularly of the lymphoreticular system. An important example of CMI is delayed-type hypersensitivity.

2. What is the major histocompatibility complex (MHC)?
The MHC is a cluster of genes (located on chromosome 6 in man) whose products play critical roles in regulation of immune recognition and responsiveness. In man, MHC genes code for class I (HLA-A,B,C), Class II (HLA DR,DQ,DP), and class III (complement components C2, C4, factor B) antigens, as well as a number of other molecules with important immunoregulatory properties, including tumor necrosis factor alpha and tumor necrosis factor beta (lymphotoxin).

3. What are B lymphocytes (B cells)?
B cells are derived from hematopoietic stem cells and are precursors of plasma cells, which are the antibody- or immunoglobulin-producing cells in the body. They are found primarily in the bone marrow, spleen, lymph nodes, and peripheral blood.

4. What is an antibody? What is its basic structure?
An antibody or immunoglobulin (Ig) molecule is a protein produced by B cells in response to antigen and has the ability to bind to the antigen that induced its formation. The basic Ig structure (see figure) consists of four polypeptide chains, two light and two heavy chains. The two heavy chains, and the light chains and heavy chains, are bound together by inter-chain disulfide bonds. The exception to this is IgA2, in which the light and heavy chains are not covalently linked to each other. There are two types of light chains, kappa (κ) and lambda (λ), but all light chains of any individual Ig molecule are either kappa or lambda. The carboxy-terminal half is the constant region of the light chain (C_L) and heavy chain (C_H), and the amino-terminal half is the variable region (V_L and V_H). The heavy chain constant region contains three domains in IgG, IgD, and IgA, and four domains in IgE and IgM. These constant regions are responsible for the functional aspects of the Ig molecules (i.e., complement binding to the C_H2 region), whereas the light and heavy chain variable regions together determine antibody specificity and binding to antigen. IgG, IgD, and IgE are monomeric in form. IgM is pentameric, and IgA is either monomeric or polymeric (some serum and all secretory IgA are dimers). Some of the major characteristics and biologic functions of the five isotypes of Ig are shown in the table on page 366.

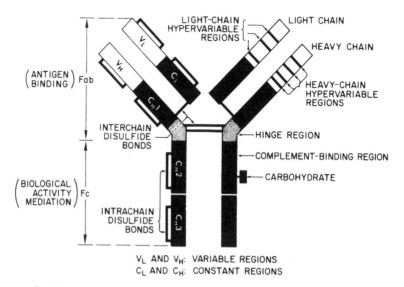

V_L AND V_H: VARIABLE REGIONS
C_L AND C_H: CONSTANT REGIONS

Structure of an Ig molecule. The figure is a schematic representation of an Ig molecule indicating the chain and domain structure of the molecule and the existence of hypervariable regions within variable regions of both H and L chains. Fab and Fc refer to fragments of the IgG molecule formed by papain cleavage. The former contains the V_H and C_{H1} H chain regions and an intact L chain; the latter consists of C_{H2} and C_{H3} region of two H chains, linked to one another by disulfide bonds. (From Wasserman RL, Capra JD: Immunoglobulins. In Horowitz MI, Pigman W (eds): The Glycoconjugates. New York, Academic Press, 1977, pp 323–348, with permission.)

5. What are the physical and biologic properties of the different classes of Ig?

Physical and Biologic Properties of Human Immunoglobulins

PROPERTY	IgG	IgA	IgM	IgD	IgE
Molecular form	Monomer	Monomer, polymer	Pentamer	Monomer	Monomer
Subclass	IgG 1,2,3,4	IgA 1,2	None		
Molecular weight	150,000 for IgG 1,2,4 180,000 for IgG3	160,000	950,000	175,000	190,000
Serum level (mg/cc)	9,3,1,0.5	2.1	1.5	4	0.03
Serum half-life (days)	IgG 1,2,4:23 IgG 3:7	6	10	3	2
Complement fixation	IgG 1,2,3+ but IgG4–	–	+	–	–
Placental transfer	+	–	–	–	–
Other properties	Secondary response	Mucous secretions	Primary response, rheumatoid factor	Class switching	Allergy

*The plus and minus signs indicate whether the pathway exists (+) or not (–).
(Modified from Samter M, et al (eds): Immunological Diseases, 4th ed. Boston, Little, Brown, 1988, p 44, with permission.)

6. What are the features of primary and secondary antibody responses?

A primary antibody response occurs following the first exposure to an antigen, while secondary antibody response occurs with the second and subsequent exposures. Major features of these two responses are illustrated below.

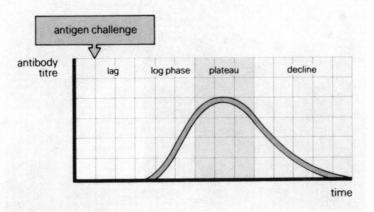

The four phases of a primary antibody response. Following antigen challenge the antibody response proceeds in four phases:

  1. a lag phase when no antibody is detected;
  2. a log phase when the antibody titer rises logarithmically;
  3. a plateau phase during which the antibody titer stabilizes; and
  4. a decline phase during which the antibody is cleared or catabolized.

(From Roitt IM, et al: Immunology. New York, Gower Medical, 1985, Fig. 8.1, p 8.1, with permission.)

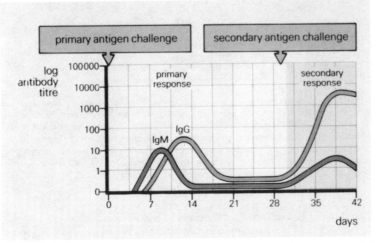

Primary and secondary antibody responses. In comparison with the antibody response following primary antigenic challenge, the antibody level following secondary antigenic challenge in a typical immune response:

  1. appears more quickly and persists for longer;
  2. attains a higher titer;
  3. consists predominantly of IgG. In the primary response the appearance
     of IgG is preceded by IgM.

(From Roitt IM, et al: Immunology. New York, Gower Medical, 1985, Fig. 8.2, p 8.1, with permission.)

7. Summarize the functions of the complement system.

The complement system functions as part of humoral immunity and also promotes inflammatory reactions. Specific functions of the complement system are summarized in the figure below.

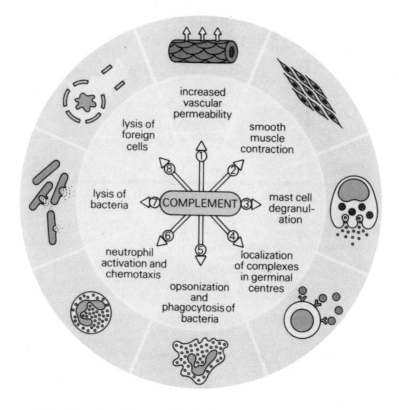

Summary of the actions of complement and its role in the acute inflammatory response. Note how the elements of the reactions are induced: increased vascular permeability (1) due to the action of C3a and C5a on smooth muscle (2) and mast cells (3) allows exudation of plasma protein. C3 facilitates both the localization of complexes in germinal centers (4) and the opsonization and phagocytosis of bacteria (5). Neutrophils, which are attracted to the area of inflammation by chemotaxis (6), phagocytose the opsonized microorganisms. The membrane attack complex, C5–9, is responsible for the lysis of bacteria (7) and other cells recognized as foreign (8). (From Roitt IM, et al: Immunology. New York, Gower Medical, 1989, Fig. 13-22, p 13.11, with permission.)

8. What factors cause activation of the classical complement pathway?

The classical pathway is principally activated by antibody-antigen (immune) complexes. A single IgM or two IgG molecules (IgG doublet) of IgG subclasses 1, 2, and 3, but not 4, bind C1, causing complement activation. Certain viruses, urate, and DNA also may activate the classical pathway.

9. What factors cause activation of the alternative complement pathway?

Substances that activate the alternative pathway include zymosan; cobra venom factor; bacterial lipopolysaccharide; aggregated IgG, M, A, and E; and cells that are free of sialic acid on their surface. Most bacteria, some parasites and virtually all plant cells lack sialic acid. Some of the pathogenicity of encapsulated bacteria that have sialic acid as part of their capsule may be due to their ability to evade destruction by the alternative pathway.

10. Compare the activation sequences of the classical and alternative complement pathways.
Classical complement pathway activation utilizes components C1–9. Activation of the alternative pathway also consumes C5–9 but not C1, 2, and 4. The classical and alternative pathways are diagrammed below.

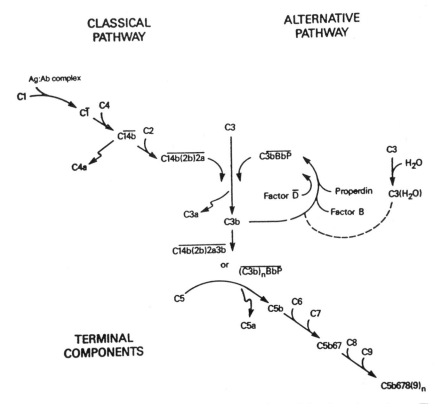

An overview of the complement cascade showing the classical and the alternative pathways. The central position of C3 in both pathways is indicated. (From Samter M (ed): Immunological Diseases, 4th ed. Boston, Little, Brown, 1988, p 205, with permission.)

11. What considerations limit the usefulness of serum complement levels in assessing the role of complement pathway activation in a disease process?
When interpreting serum complement levels (C3 and C4), one must realize that a normal level does not rule out either complement activation or complement-mediated tissue damage. In some diseases, complement synthesis is increased (i.e., acute inflammation), thereby potentially masking increased consumption. In addition, under certain conditions, complement may be extremely efficient at causing cell damage without lowering serum levels. Furthermore, serum complement levels do not necessarily reflect activity in other body compartments. For example, in rheumatoid arthritis complement levels may be normal in serum but decreased in joint fluid. Finally, low serum complement levels may occur in hepatic failure due to decreased synthesis of complement components.

12. What patterns of serum C3 and C4 levels are seen with activation of the classical and alternative complement pathways? Name at least one disease associated with each pattern.

Serum Complement Levels in Disease

PATHWAY	C4	C3	DISEASE
Classical	↓	↓	Systemic lupus erythematosus, serum sickness
Classical (Fluid phase)	↓	N	Hereditary angioedema
Alternative	N	↓	Endotoxemia (gram negative sepsis)
Alternative (Fluid phase)	N	↓	Type II membranoproliferative glomerulo-nephritis (C3 nephritic factor)

↓ = Decreased, ↑ = Increased, N = Normal

13. What are the two major pathways of arachidonic acid metabolism and what effects do aspirin, nonsteroidal anti-inflammatory drugs, eicosapentaenoic acid (fish oil), and cortico-steroids have on mediator production by these pathways?

Prostaglandins (PG) and thromboxanes are produced via the cyclo-oxygenase (CO) and leukotrienes (LT) by the lipoxygenase pathways of arachidonic acid metabolism. These eicosanoids exhibit an array of potent inflammatory and immunoregulatory properties. Aspirin and NSAIDs inhibit CO and, therefore, PG/thromboxane but not LT production. Eicosapentaenoic acid (fish oil) inhibits both PG/thromboxane and LT formation by preferential fatty acid substitution for arachidonic acid in the cell membranes of eicosanoid-producing cells. Corticosteroids also inhibit both PG/thromboxane and LT generation by stimulating production of the intracellular protein, lipocortin, which inhibits the activity of phospholipase A. Specific lipoxygenase inhibitors are currently undergoing clinical trials.

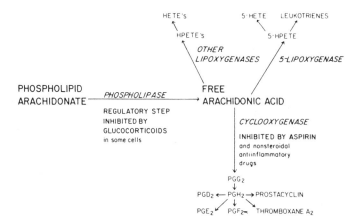

Sites of inhibition of arachidonic acid release and metabolism by pharmacologic agents. (From Wyngaarden JB, Smith LH: Cecil Textbook of Medicine, 17th ed. Philadelphia, W.B. Saunders, 1985, p 1240, with permission.)

14. What are alpha, beta and gamma interferons (IFNs)?

Since their discovery, interferons have been divided into three classes, IFN-α, IFN-β, and IFN-γ. IFN-α and IFN-β were previously classified as Type I and IFN-γ as Type II. IFN-α is comprised of 20 or more subtypes, all of which have a high degree of homology. IFN-β has at least two subtypes. IFN-β_1 has only about a 34% sequence homology with IFN-α, but their biologic effects are similar. IFN-β_2 has been found to be "B cell differentiation factor-2," now named interleukin-6 (IL-6). It has essentially no homology with IFN-α. IFN-γ is unrelated to the other IFNs in either structure or function.

15. Which cells produce interferons and what are their major function(s)?

IFN-α is produced by leukocytes, fibroblasts (to a lesser degree), and many other cells. IFN-β_1 is produced by fibroblasts, leukocytes (to a lesser degree), and many other cells. Both IFN-α and IFN-β_1 function in the immunomodulation of antibody production, graft rejection, and delayed-type hypersensitivity (DTH) reactions. They can induce autoimmune and inflammatory reactions, and they play a role in antiviral, antibacterial, antifungal, and antitumor responses.

IFN-β_2 (IL-6) is produced by fibroblasts, T cells, monocytes, and endothelial cells, and has poor antiviral activity. It has also been called "B cell differentiation factor," because it stimulates the differentiation of mature B cells to immunoglobulin-secreting plasma cells. It also plays a role in early hematopoiesis and may be an important autocrine growth factor for multiple myeloma and other malignancies.

IFN-γ is produced by activated T lymphocytes, natural killer (NK) cells, and lymphokine-activated killer (LAK) cells. Its biologic effects include enhancing cytotoxic T cell and NK cell activity; induction of class II antigen expression on B cells, multiple antigen presenting cells, dendritic cells, endothelial cells, and fibroblasts; induction of IL-2 receptor expression on T cells; down-regulation of collagen synthesis; and inhibition of IL-4-induced IgE synthesis.

16. What is the bursa of Fabricius and which lymphoid organ is its equivalent in humans?

The bursa of Fabricius is the site of B cell development in the chicken (*Gallus domesticus*). In humans, B cell maturation occurs primarily in the bone marrow.

17. Outline B cell ontogeny from stem cell to plasma cell.

Stem cell $\longrightarrow$ Pre-B cell $\longrightarrow$ Immature $\longrightarrow$ Mature $\longrightarrow$ Activated $\longrightarrow$ Secretory $\longrightarrow$ Plasma cell

18. What is the role of surface Ig on B cells?

Surface Ig serves as the antigen-binding site and as an activation receptor for B cells. Receptor function includes both signal transduction and participation in antigen processing and presentation for cognate interaction with T cells.

19. What are the major subtypes of T cells? Describe the principal function of each.

T cells function both as effectors and regulators of the immune response. They, like B cells, are derived from the embryonic hematopoietic stem cells.

The major types of T cells are:

1. CD4$^+$ T cells: These function primarily as helper/inducer T cells by providing soluble and cognate signals to B cells for stimulating antibody production. Antigen recognition is MHC class II restricted.

2. CD8$^+$ T cells: These cells function as cytotoxic and suppressor T cells. Cytotoxic T cell function includes recognition and destruction of cells bearing antigen recognized as foreign. Examples include tumor cells, virally infected cells, and allogeneic cells. An example of suppressor cell function is inhibition of antibody synthesis by B cells. CD8$^+$ T cell function is MHC class I restricted.

20. What is the CD nomenclature of phenotyping cells?

The CD (cluster designation) nomenclature is a system for universal identification of cell surface antigens that have been defined by monoclonal antibodies. Some of the major CD markers are listed below:

CD	Cell Expression of Antigens
2	T cells, approximately 50% of NK cells (E rosette receptor)
3	T-cell receptor complex for antigen recognition
4	Helper T cells (HLA Class II restricted)
5	T cells, mature thymocytes, B-cell subsets
7	T cells, NK cells
8	Suppressor/cytotoxic T cells (HLA Class I restricted), NK cells
10	Pre-B cells, common acute lymphoblastic leukemia cells (common acute lymphoblastic leukemia antigen, or CALLA)
14	Monocytes
19	Pan-B cell
20	B cells, dendritic cells
21	Complement receptor 2 and receptor for Epstein-Barr virus
23	Activated B cells, subset of T cells, monocytes, eosinophils, platelets (low affinity IgE receptor)
25	Activated T and B cells, monocyte subset (low affinity IL-2 receptor)
34	Lymphoid and myeloid precursors

21. Peripheral blood lymphocyte phenotyping has what use in the diagnosis of AIDS?

The normal $CD4^+$ (helper/inducer cells, formerly called T4 cells) to $CD8^+$ (cytotoxic/suppressor cell) ratio in peripheral blood ranges from approximately 1:1 to 3:1. An inverted ratio can be caused by a decrease in $CD4^+$ cells, an increase in $CD8^+$ cells, or alterations in both populations. With AIDS, the ratio is typically inverted. Early in the course of the disease, the inversion may be caused by a decrease in $CD4^+$ and/or an increase in $CD8^+$ cells. With advanced disease, the ratio becomes markedly inverted because of a severe loss of $CD4^+$ cells. However, other diseases, particularly other viral infections (such as cytomegalovirus, Epstein-Barr virus, and influenza A), can also cause an inverted CD4/CD8 ratio because of increases in the $CD8^+$ cell populations. These changes may persist for months before returning to normal.

22. What is the role of the thymus in T cell development and maturation?

The thymus is derived from the third and fourth pharyngeal pouches and is the principal site of T cell maturation. Stem cells migrate into the thymus where, under the influence of the microenvironment comprised of epithelial cells and of dendritic cells rich in MHC class II antigens, they are educated to differentiate between self and foreign antigens, and they acquire the surface phenotype of mature T cells. Most thymocytes leaving the thymus bear CD3, the α/β T cell receptor, and either CD4 (helper phenotype) or CD8 (cytotoxic-suppressor phenotype).

23. What are some of the T-cell-derived lymphokines?

T-cell–derived Lymphokines

LYMPHOKINE	OTHER NAMES	FUNCTIONS
Interleukin 2 (IL-2)	T cell growth factor	T cell growth regulation Regulation of Ig synthesis
Interleukin 4 (IL-4)	B cell stimulatory factor 1	Co-stimulation of B cell growth Ig class switching T cell growth regulation Macrophage activation Regulation of mast cell growth Co-stimulation of hematopoietic precursor cells

Table continued on next page.

T-cell–derived Lymphokines (Continued)

LYMPHOKINE	OTHER NAMES	FUNCTIONS
Interleukin 5 (IL-5)	B cell growth factor 2 T cell replacing factor Eosinophil differentiation factor	Stimulation of B cell growth and Ig synthesis Stimulation of eosinophil growth and differentiation
Interleukin 6 (IL-6)	B cell stimulatory factor 2 Interferon β2 Hybridoma/plasmacytoma growth factor Hepatocyte stimulatory factor	Control of Ig synthesis Stimulation of plasmacytoma and hybridoma growth Multiple other functions
Interferon γ (IFN-γ)		Macrophage activation Ig class switching Multiple other functions
Lymphotoxin (LT)	Tumor necrosis factor β (TNF β)	Inhibition of cell growth Differentiation of certain cell lines
Interleukin 3 (IL-3)	Multicolony stimulating factor	Stimulation of hematopoietic precursors of multiple lineages Mast cell growth factor
Granulocyte-macrophage colony stimulating factor (GM-CSF)		Stimulation of myeloid precursor cells

(From Paul WE (ed): Fundamental Immunology, 2nd ed. New York, Raven Press, 1989, p 13, with permission.)

24. What is anergy and what is its clinical significance?
Anergy is the lack of delayed-type hypersensitivity (DTH) reactivity to a battery of common antigens following intradermal challenge. The presence of anergy is a very sensitive reflection of depressed cell-mediated immunity (particularly T-cell function). Anergy may be temporary, such as in viral infections (measles), or prolonged, as in sarcoidosis, AIDS, and malignancies. The accurate assessment of anergy by DTH skin testing is dependent on a number of factors, including use of an appropriate battery of skin test reagents, proper reagent dilution and storage, injection technique (intradermal), and interpretation of results.

25. What are antigen-presenting cells (APCs) and what is their role in the immune response?
APCs are a heterogeneous population of cells that are capable of surface presentation of antigen to immune responder cells, resulting in immunostimulation. In most cases, it is obligatory that antigen be presented in close proximity to MHC molecules on the presenting cell. For example, CD4+ (helper) T cells will not recognize antigen on the surface of macrophages (an APC) unless it is presented in conjunction with MHC class II molecules. Viral and foreign tissue antigens are presented in association with class I MHC molecules and are recognized primarily by cytotoxic (CD8+) T cells. T cell antigen recognition requires intimate association between antigen and MHC molecules on the APC and the CD4 or CD8 and the CD3/T cell receptor complex on the T cell. This interaction leads to T cell activation and effector function with resultant immune responsiveness. APCs may have constitutive antigen-presenting capability or capability only after induction of MHC molecules on their surface, such as occurs with fibroblasts (Class I) and some types of macrophages (Class II). APCs include macrophages, Langerhans cells, dendritic cells, B cells, Kupffer cells, microglial cells, astrocytes, fibroblasts, and endothelial cells.

26. What are the principal chemotactic factors for neutrophils and eosinophils?

A number of factors have been shown to be chemoattractant for neutrophils or eosinophils, or both. C5a and leukotriene B4 (LTB_4) are very potent chemoattractants for neutrophils, and platelet-activating factor (PAF) is an extremely potent eosinophil chemoattractant. Since eosinophils produce large quantities of PAF, this mediator may play an important role in amplification of the eosinophilic response.

Chemotactic Factors for Eosinophils[1]

FACTOR	MAJOR SOURCE(S)
Platelet activating factor (PAF)	Monocytes/macrophages, neutrophils, eosinophils, platelets, other cells
Eosinophil chemotactic factor of anaphylaxis (ECF-A)	Mast cells
Interleukin 5	T cells
C5a, C567	Complement cascade
Leukotriene B4	Monocytes/macrophages, neutrophils

Chemotactic Factors for Neutrophils[1]

FACTOR	MAJOR SOURCE(S)
Leukotriene B4	Monocytes/macrophages, neutrophils
C5a, C5a des arg[2], C567	Complement cascade
fMet-Leu-Phe	Synthetic peptide (not naturally produced)
Neutrophil chemotactic factor	Mast cells
PAF	(see above PAF)

[1] Factors not necessarily listed in order of potency.
[2] Formed by cleavage of terminal arginine by carboxypeptidase, less potent than C5a.

27. What is major basic protein (MBP)?

MBP is the principal protein of the cytoplasmic granules of eosinophils and has been localized to the crystalline core. It is also present in much smaller amounts in basophils. Its biologic effects include:

1. Nonspecific toxicity to many parasites (including *Schistosoma mansoni, Trichinella spiralis,* and *Trypanosoma cruzi.*
2. Toxicity to a wide variety of mammalian cells (including human cells).
3. Stimulation of histamine release from basophils and mast cells.
4. Neutralization of heparin.

An example of the potential clinical significance of MBP is that MBP deposition by eosinophils may play an important role in the pathophysiology of asthma by causing desquamation of respiratory tract epithelium.

28. What are the four types of hypersensitivity reactions?

The four classic types of hypersensitivity reactions, also referred to as the Coombs and Gell classification of immunologically mediated inflammation, are summarized in the table below.

Types of Immunologically Mediated Inflammation

TYPE OF INFLAMMATION	RECOGNITION COMPONENT	SOLUBLE MEDIATOR	INFLAMMATORY RESPONSE	DISEASE EXAMPLE
I. Reagenic, allergic	IgE	Basophil and mast cell products	Immediate flare and wheal, smooth muscle constriction	Atopy, anaphylaxis

Table continued on next page.

Types of Immunologically Mediated Inflammation (Continued)

TYPE OF INFLAMMATION	RECOGNITION COMPONENT	SOLUBLE MEDIATOR	INFLAMMATORY RESPONSE	DISEASE EXAMPLE
II. Cytotoxic antibody	IgG, IgM	Complement	Lysis or phagocytosis of circulating antigens, acute inflammation in tissues	Autoimmune hemolytic anemia, thrombocytopenia associated with systemic lupus erythematosus
III. Immune complex	IgG, IgM	Complement, lipid mediators	Accumulation of polymorphonuclear leukocytes and macrophages	Rheumatoid arthritis, lupus erythematosus
IV. Delayed hypersensitivity	T lymphocytes	Cytokines	Mononuclear cell infiltrate	Tuberculosis, sarcoidosis, polymyositis, granulomatosis, vasculitis

(From Wyngaarden JB, Smith LH: Cecil Textbook of Medicine, 18th ed. Philadelphia, W.B. Saunders, 1988, p 1989, with permission.)

29. Describe the mechanism of immediate hypersensitivity reactions and give some clinical examples.

Type I, or immediate hypersensitivity, reactions are classic allergic reactions initiated by the binding of an antigen to IgE attached to the surface of mast cells or basophils. This results in cross-linkage of high-affinity IgE receptors, cell activation, and noncytolytic degranulation, with release of potent mediators (including histamine, prostaglandins, and leukotrienes). The reaction becomes clinically manifested within seconds to minutes and is almost always apparent within 1 hour. Clinical examples include anaphylaxis, allergic rhinitis (hay fever), food allergy, extrinsic (allergic) asthma, immediate drug allergy (such as to penicillin), and acute urticaria (hives).

30. Describe the mechanism of cytotoxic reactions and give some clinical examples.

Type II, or cytotoxic, reactions occur when antibody binds to specific antigens on circulating cells or in tissue. Antibody binding can lead to cytotoxicity by complement activation or interaction with Fc receptors on effector cells, such as neutrophils, macrophages, eosinophils, and natural killer (NK) cells. Examples include hemolytic disease of the newborn, autoimmune hemolytic anemia, and Goodpasture's syndrome.

31. Describe the mechanism of immune complex reactions and give some clinical examples.

Type III, or immune complex, reactions are caused by the formation of immune complexes (antigen and antibody bound together) and their deposition in tissue. The immune complexes may cause complement activation that results in neutrophil accumulation and tissue damage. Examples include the Arthus reaction and serum sickness (glomerulonephritis, endocarditis).

32. Describe the mechanism of delayed type hypersensitivity (DTH) reactions. What are the four major types?

Type IV, or DTH, reactions are a reflection of cell-mediated immunity and are primarily mediated by T cells. Unlike reaction types I–III, DTH can be transferred by T cells, but not by serum. When antigen-sensitized T cells are re-exposed to that specific antigen by antigen-presenting cells, T cell activation occurs, resulting in secretion of gamma interferon and multiple other cytokines. Monocyte/macrophage influx and activation occur, leading to release of an array of inflammatory mediators and cytokines. Chronic presence of antigen leads to continued lymphocyte and macrophage activation. This results in the characteristic pathologic changes, including granuloma formation and tissue destruction.

Key Features of the Four Types of Delayed Hypersensitivity Reactions

TYPE	INDUCING ANTIGEN	REACTION TIME	EXTERNAL SIGNS	HISTOLOGICAL APPEARANCE
Tuberculin	Tuberculin, typhoidin, abortin, leishmanial antigens	48 h	Indurated, painful skin swelling	Dermal reaction, lymphocyte and monocyte infiltration
Jones–Mote	Innocuous proteins such as ovalbumin	24 h	Slight skin thickening	Dermal reaction, lymphocyte and basophil infiltration
Contact	Urushiol, varnish, resins, nickel	48 h	Eczema	Epidermal reaction, lymphocyte and monocyte infiltration
Granuloma-tous	Persistent Ag or Ag–Ab complexes, talcum powder	4 weeks	Skin induration	Epithelioid cell granuloma formation, giant cells, macrophages, fibrosis, necrosis

Ab, antibody; Ag, antigen; h, hour.
(From Klein J: Immunology. Oxford, Blackwell Scientific Publications, 1990, with permission.)

33. What is an Arthus reaction? When does it occur in a clinical setting?

Arthus reactions are caused by antigen-antibody complexes (immune complexes) and were first described by Nicolas-Maurice Arthus, a French physiologist, in 1903. The reaction is an acute, hemorrhagic, inflammatory skin lesion elicited in the dermis by injection of an antigen. It relies on high serum levels of complement-fixing antibodies, which lead to the formation of immune complexes in the blood vessel walls of the dermis and a localized vasculitis. It is dependent on both neutrophil and complement function.

In humans, Arthus reactions have been reported after tetanus and diphtheria immunization, and in some diabetics after insulin injection.

34. What is an allergen?

An allergen is an antigen (usually a protein) that induces IgE synthesis and sensitization with IgE. The IgE response to an allergen is dependent on multiple factors including cellular (i.e., T and B cell) function, soluble mediators, and genetic factors.

35. Are all mast cells alike?

No. Mast cell heterogeneity exists in both animals and man. This has been most extensively studied in the mouse, where there appear to be two major mast cell populations. These have been labelled mucosal mast cells (MMC) and connective tissue mast cells (CTMC). MMC are found principally at mucosal surfaces, whereas CTMC are found within connective tissue, lining blood vessels, and at serosal surfaces. They differ with respect to histamine content, degranulation to non-IgE stimuli, arachidonic acid metabolite production, and histochemical-staining characteristics caused by differences in proteoglycan content of their granules. MMC are dependent on the T cell cytokine interleukin-3 (IL-3). In contrast, expression of the CTMC phenotype is dependent on the presence of fibroblasts.

In man, there also appear to be two major mast cell populations. The two types of human mast cells are identified by differences in neutral protease content of their cytoplasmic granules. Both populations of human mast cells contain tryptase, but only one contains both tryptase and chymase. The **tryptase-only mast cells (MC^T)** are located primarily at mucosal surfaces, whereas the **tryptase and chymase-positive mast cells (MC^{TC})** are located primarily in connective tissue, lining blood vessels, and at serosal surfaces. Unlike the mouse, the factors responsible for human mast cell growth remain to be clearly defined. Although human IL-3 appears to have some mast cell growth-promoting activity, its effect in man is less well defined. Whether an additional factor(s) is needed for human mast cell growth and differentiation remains to be determined. However, it is of interest that MC^T mast cells, but not MC^{TC} mast cells, appear to be T-lymphocyte dependent. This is suggested by a marked decrease in MC^T but not MC^{TC} mast cell numbers in the tissues of patients with severe T cell immunodeficiency disorders.

36. Which special stains are useful for identifying human mast cells?

The following stains are particularly useful in the histochemical identification of human mast cells:

1. **Toluidine blue (TB):** This is the classic stain for mast cells. TB is a metachromatic dye that binds to highly acidic (negatively charged) proteoglycans (especially highly sulfated heparin) in the cytoplasmic granules. The reaction results in metachromasia (a change in color), with the positive-staining granules staining purple as opposed to the blue background. Basophils also stain positively with TB because of the proteoglycans (chondroitin sulfate) in their granules. However, mast cells and basophils can usually be differentiated by morphologic criteria.

2. **Chloroacetate esterase:** This enzyme is present in mast cells, neutrophils, and myeloid precursor cells. Mast cell granules stain bright red and basophils are negative. The mast cells can easily be differentiated from the other positively staining cells based on morphologic characteristics.

3. **Giemsa stain:** This stain has no specificity for mast cells, although the cytoplasmic granules will stain purple. It may be particularly useful in identifying mast cells in bone marrow biopsy specimens, where metachromatic dyes react poorly.

4. **Tryptase:** These stains utilize antibodies against human mast cell tryptase. Tryptase is also present in very small quantities in basophils but is not detected using the appropriate concentrations of antibodies to identify mast cells. It is therefore specific for mast cells.

37. What are the major differences between mast cells and basophils?

Comparison of Mast Cells and Basophils

PARAMETER	MAST CELL	BASOPHILS
Life span	? weeks to years	Days
Origin	Probably bone marrow	Bone marrow
Location	Tissues, noncirculating	Normally circulating, may egress into tissues under certain conditions
Size	8–20 μm	5–7 μm
Nucleus	Round to oval, may be indented	Multi-lobulated
Cytoplasmic granules	Smaller, more numerous, relatively homogeneous	Larger, fewer, variable in size
Ultrastructure	Scroll structure of granules, filopodia on cell surface	Scroll patterns absent, smooth cell surface
High affinity IgE receptor	Present	Present
Histamine release	+	+
Major arachidonic acid metabolites	PGD2, LTC4,* LTD4,* LTE4*	LTC4
Staining characteristics:		
Toluidine blue	+	+
Tryptase	+	–
Chloroacetate esterase	+	–

* = previously collectively referred to as slow-reacting substance of anaphylaxis (SRS-A).
PG = prostaglandin, LT = leukotriene.

38. Which single procedure or test is most useful in the diagnosis of systemic mastocytosis?
A bone marrow biopsy is the procedure of choice because of its high sensitivity and specificity. A positive skin biopsy does not indicate internal organ involvement. Plasma histamine levels may be normal or elevated (although very high levels are highly suggestive of systemic disease). Bone scan findings are nonspecific. Hepatomegaly and splenomegaly may or may not be seen and are not diagnostic.

The bone marrow is characterized by prominent aggregates of mast cells in association with spicules, lymph tissue, or blood vessels. Eosinophils are often prominent, and variable degrees of fibrosis are present. If the diagnosis of systemic mastocytosis is suspected, the pathologist should be notified, since the standard bone marrow preparation involves decalcification, which results in poor staining of mast cell granules by metachromatic dyes such as toluidine blue. A Giemsa stain may be useful in identifying mast cells in these samples. It is emphasized that bone marrow *aspiration* without biopsy is insufficient to rule in or rule out systemic mastocytosis.

39. Which biologic functions are mediated via H_1, H_2, or a combination of H_1 and H_2 histamine receptors?

Biologic Effects of H_1 and H_2 Histamine Receptor Stimulation

H_1 RECEPTORS	H_2 RECEPTORS	H_1 AND H_2 RECEPTORS
Smooth muscle contraction	Gastric acid secretion	Hypotension
↑ vascular permeability	↑ cyclic AMP	Tachycardia
Pruritus	Mucous secretion	Flushing
Stimulation of prostaglandin synthesis	Inhibits basophil, but not mast cell histamine release	Headache
Tachycardia	↑ suppressor cell function	
↑ cyclic GMP production	↓ lymphocyte cytotoxicity	

↑ = increased, ↓ = decreased.

40. What is the reticuloendothelial system (RES) and what are its principal functions?
The RES (mononuclear/phagocyte system) comprises a heterogeneous population of fixed-tissue phagocytic cells throughout the body which are critical in the removal of particulate and soluble substances from the circulation and tissues. Examples of substances removed by the RES are immune complexes, bacteria, toxins, and exogenous antigens. These molecules may be internalized by nonspecific endocytosis, nonimmune but receptor-mediated phagocytosis, or immunologic phagocytosis mediated by binding to Fc or complement receptors. Components of the RES include Kupffer cells of the liver, microglial cells of the brain, pulmonary alveolar macrophages, and macrophages in the bone marrow, lymph nodes, gut, and other tissues. Blockade of the RES is one postulated mechanism for prevention of platelet destruction by high-dose IV gamma globulin (IVGG) in idiopathic thrombocytopenic purpura (ITP). The binding of IgG-sensitized platelets to the IgG-Fc receptors on RES cells, particularly in the liver and spleen, leads to phagocytosis and platelet destruction in ITP. This IgG-Fc receptor mechanism may be "blocked" or overwhelmed by the infusion of high dose IVGG. IgG-Fc receptors are lost during phagocytosis and may take as long as several days to be re-expressed.

41. What maneuver elicits Darier's sign?
Darier's sign is the erythema and whealing that occurs following gentle stroking of the characteristic, reddish-brown skin lesions of urticaria pigmentosa. It is presumably caused by degranulation and mediator release from the large numbers of dermal mast cells in these patients.

42. What is the cold-agglutinin syndrome and how is it diagnosed?

The cold agglutinin syndrome is characterized by hemolytic anemia secondary to IgM antibodies, which cause increasing red blood cell (RBC) lysis with decreasing temperature. Agglutination of normal RBCs at $20°C$ occurs with serum from virtually all patients with the cold agglutinin syndrome. The direct Coombs' test is typically positive for complement and negative for immunoglobulin. The cold agglutinin syndrome is typically idiopathic, with the presentation of hemolytic anemia in the sixth or seventh decade of life. These patients have a high titer of monoclonal IgM kappa antibody, with anti-I specificity. Despite the monoclonal nature of the antibody response, these patients typically do not develop multiple myeloma or Waldenstrom's macroglobulinemia.

Cold agglutinin syndrome may also occur in association with the lymphoproliferative disorders (i.e., non-Hodgkin's lymphoma), infections (*Mycoplasma* pneumonia, infectious mononucleosis), and rarely in connective tissue disorders (systemic lupus erythematosus [SLE]). With the lymphoproliferative disorders, the IgM is often monoclonal. The cold agglutinin in these disorders is often anti-I, but other antibodies may be present, particularly in infectious mononucleosis when anti-i is often found. Determination of antibody specificity is not necessary for either diagnosis, or as a prerequisite for blood transfusion.

43. Name some of the clinical characteristics of antibody deficiency disorders.

Antibody deficiency disorders, whether acquired or congenital, have several general characteristics that are manifestations of the defect in humoral-mediated immunity. These include:

1. Recurrent infections with high-grade extracellular encapsulated pathogens.
2. Few problems with fungal or viral (except enteroviral) infections.
3. Chronic sinopulmonary disease.
4. Growth retardation is *not* a striking feature.
5. Low antibody levels measured in serum and secretions.
6. Patients may or may not lack B lymphocytes with surface immunoglobulins or complement receptors.
7. Absence of cortical follicles in lymph nodes and spleen in X-linked agammaglobulinemia.
8. Paucity of palpable lymphoid and nasopharyngeal tissue in X-linked agammaglobulinemia.
9. Compatible with survival to adulthood or for several years after onset except for those with persistent enterovirus infections, autoimmune disorders or malignancy.

(From Wyngaarden JB, Smith LH: Cecil Textbook of Medicine, 18th ed. Philadelphia, W.B. Saunders, 1988, p 1943, with permission.)

44. What is the most common immunoglobulin deficiency disorder?

Selective IgA deficiency has a frequency of approximately 1 in 500–700 in the population. Many patients are asymptomatic, but some have recurrent infections, particularly of the respiratory tract. IgG2 deficiency sometimes accompanies IgA deficiency and these patients are particularly prone to infectious complications with encapsulated bacteria (such as *Hemophilus influenzae*) because IgG2 is the principal IgG antibody response against bacterial polysaccharide. In selective IgA deficiency, the serum IgA level is less than 5 mg/dl (0.05 mg/cc). IgA in secretions is almost always depressed as well. IgG and IgM levels are normal. The patients have an increased incidence of autoimmune disorders (including SLE and rheumatoid arthritis). Treatment is supportive unless frequent infections and IgG2 deficiency are present. In that case, IV gamma globulin (IVGG) may be helpful, but severe anaphylactoid reactions may occur due to the presence of anti-IgA antibodies, which may occur in as many as 50% of IgA-deficient patients.

45. What are the clinical characteristics of disorders of cell-mediated immunity?

The manifestations of cellular immunodeficiency disorders, due to a partial or total defect in T cell function, include:

1. Recurrent infections with low-grade or opportunistic infectious agents, such as fungi, viruses, or protozoa (e.g., *Pneumocystis carinii*).
2. Delayed cutaneous anergy.
3. Accompanied by growth retardation, short life span, wasting, and diarrhea.
4. Susceptible to graft-versus-host disease (GVHD) if given fresh blood, plasma, or unmatched allogeneic bone marrow.
5. Fatal reactions from live virus (including BCG) vaccination.
6. High incidence of malignancy.

(From Wyngaarden JB, Smith LH: Cecil Textbook of Medicine, 18th ed. Philadelphia, W.B. Saunders, 1988, p 1945, with permission.)

46. What is the common variable immunodeficiency disease (CVID)?

CVID is a heterogeneous group of disorders characterized by hypogammaglobulinemia (total IgG < 250 mg/dl and usually total Ig < 350 mg/dl), decreased ability to produce antibody following antigenic challenge, and recurrent infections. It is apparent, however, that a significant number of patients who have a depressed serum IgG level, but which is greater than 250 mg/dl, may also have a similar clinical presentation. The most common serum Ig pattern is panhypogammaglobulinemia with a deficiency of IgG, IgM, and IgA.

The usual presentation of CVID is in late childhood or early adulthood, but it can present at any age. Recurrent bacterial infections of the upper and lower respiratory tract with encapsulated bacteria (*Streptococcus pneumoniae, Hemophilus influenzae*, etc.) are common pathogens and bronchiectasis may develop. Patients may also have defective cell-mediated immunity and may also have mycobacterial, fungal, and protozoal (i.e., *Giardia lamblia*) infections.

CVID patients have an increased frequency of a number of autoimmune disorders including pernicious anemia, Coombs' positive hemolytic anemia, autoimmune thrombocytopenia, and thyroiditis. GI disorders are common, including diarrhea, malabsorption, and nodular lymphoid hyperplasia of the small intestine. Finally, these patients have an increased incidence of malignancy, particularly of the lymphoreticular system and the gastrointestinal tract.

47. Identify the principal immunologic defects in CVID.

The immunologic abnormality that affects most patients appears to be a defect in B cell maturation, in which the B cells cannot terminally differentiate into antibody-producing plasma cells. These patients generally have normal numbers of circulating, surface Ig-positive, B cells. Up to 20% of patients may have increased suppressor-cell activity causing decreased antibody production. Other T cell immunoregulatory defects have also been described. Depressed cell-mediated immunity, as demonstrated by cutaneous anergy, may be present in up to 30% of patients.

48. Is there a specific treatment for CVID?

The principal therapy for CVID is IV gamma globulin (IVGG) replacement and aggressive management of infections with appropriate antibiotics. IVGG is given every 3 to 4 weeks. The usual dose is 200 mg/kg and the infusion is given slowly over several hours. Adverse reactions consisting of pruritus, headache, and nausea usually resolve with slowing or stopping of the infusion. IVGG often dramatically decreases the frequency and severity of infections and may also alleviate some of the symptoms, such as arthralgias, that sometimes accompany CVID.

49. What are some of the secondary causes of hypogammaglobulinemia?

Causes of Secondary Hypogammaglobulinemia

CAUSE	MECHANISM
Drugs	Drugs
a. Anticonvulsants (esp. phenytoin)	a. Increased suppressor cell activity (any or all isotypes affected)
b. Cytotoxic agents	b. Decreased Ig production
Multiple myeloma	Decreased Ig production
Chronic lymphocytic leukemia	Decreased Ig production
Myotonic dystrophy	Selective hypercatabolism of IgG
Nephrotic syndrome	Ig loss in urine (particularly IgG)
Intestinal lymphangiectasia	Ig loss through GI tract, increased catabolism
Radiation therapy	Decreased Ig production

50. How is the radioallergosorbent test (RAST) performed?

The RAST is used for measurement of specific IgE antibody in serum. The test is only semiquantitative. Purified allergen is coupled to a carrier (particles, paper discs, plastic wells) and incubated with the patient's serum. After washing, ^{125}I-labelled anti-IgE is added and radioactivity present on the immunoabsorbent material (carrier) is measured. The RAST is increasingly being converted to an ELISA system that uses enzymatic color change rather than radioactivity.

51. How does the RAST compare with skin testing in the diagnosis of allergy?

The RAST is less sensitive, and its correlation with some allergies is poorer than with skin testing. Furthermore, validity of the RAST is highly dependent on proper controls and interpretation of the results by the reporting laboratory. However, the RAST may be particularly useful in patients in whom skin testing performance or interpretation is compromised. This includes patients with extensive skin disease such as dermatographism, urticaria pigmentosa, and diffuse cutaneous mastocytosis. It may also be useful in patients receiving H_1 antihistamines and patients in whom skin testing is considered to carry a high risk of severe anaphylaxis. By itself, a positive RAST does not diagnose a specific allergy but should be used only in conjunction with the clinical history.

52. Describe the basic technique for performance of the enzyme-linked immunosorbent assay (ELISA).

The ELISA has, to a great extent, replaced the radioimmunoassay (RIA) in diagnostic testing. Compared to the RIA, the ELISA eliminates the radioactive hazards and has a sensitivity that is comparable or better (sensitivity of 1 ng or less, depending on the test substance and the various components used in the assay). The ELISA is typically performed in plastic, flat-bottomed, 96-well, microtiter plates. The basic ELISA procedure used to test for antibody against specific antigen is outlined below. The concentration of the substance to be measured is determined by comparing the optical density of the test samples against negative controls and a standard curve.

ELISA Test Procedure

1. Coat wells with antigen (by incubation of appropriate concentration of antigen in the wells) and then wash.	4. Add enzyme-linked anti-species immunoglobulin and incubate.
2. Add test sample and incubate.	5. Wash.
3. Wash.	6. Add developing substrate and measure optical density.

53. Which principal components of house dust have been implicated in causing allergic disease?

House dust is a frequent cause of allergic rhinitis and asthma. House dust is a mixture of variable amounts of antigens from dust mites, cockroaches, cats, dogs, pollens, molds and other environmental substances. Dust mites are often the most important source of offending allergen and are particularly prevalent in clothing, carpets, and mattresses. The principal mite in house dust is *Dematophagoides pteronyssimus* and the allergen is the mite feces. Dust mites thrive optimally at 25°C and 80% relative humidity. Human epidermal scales are a major substrate for dust mite growth. Efforts to minimize exposure to dust and to decrease favorable environments available for dust mite growth may be very beneficial for allergic patients. Treatment with antiallergic medications and, when necessary, immunotherapy (allergy shots) is an effective form of therapy.

54. What are the modes of therapy available for allergic rhinitis?
  1. Avoidance of the offending allergens
  2. Medical therapy
     a. H_1 antihistamines
     b. Sympathomimetics
     c. Cromolyn sodium
     d. Corticosteroids (nasal spray; systemic therapy only for severe acute exacerbations)
  3. Allergen specific immunotherapy

55. What immunologic changes occur in patients who undergo allergen-specific immunotherapy?

Allergen-specific immunotherapy involves the subcutaneous injection of extracts of the specific allergens responsible for a patient's symptoms. Immunologic changes that have been reported in response to allergen-specific immunotherapy include:
  1. Diminished seasonal increases of allergen-specific IgE.
  2. Increased allergen-specific IgG.
  3. Decreased basophil histamine release.
  4. Development of allergen-specific suppressor T cells.

Despite these observations, the specific cause(s) for the effectiveness of immunotherapy remains to be precisely determined.

Rubenstein E, Federman D (eds): Scientific American Medicine. New York, Scientific American, Inc., 1990.

56. What is the mechanism of action of cromolyn?

Cromolyn is available for use via inhalational, intranasal, and topical ophthalmic routes. It inhibits the degranulation of mast cells, thereby preventing the release of the mediators of immediate hypersensitivity. The mechanism by which this occurs is unknown, although inhibition of calcium influx is one of several proposed explanations. It has no intrinsic antihistamine, bronchodilator, or anti-inflammatory activity. Cromolyn sodium is used as a prophylactic agent in patients with sufficiently frequent symptoms to justify continuous therapy, because it is most effective when administered prior to exposure to an allergen (i.e., prior to mast cell degranulation). Cromolyn inhibits both immediate hypersensitivity and late-phase reactions.

57. How would 2 weeks of treatment with H_1 antihistamines, H_2 antihistamines, or corticosteroids (CS) be expected to affect the results of (A) allergy and (B) delayed type hypersensitivity (DTH) skin testing?

  A. Allergy skin testing is used to evaluate a patient for potential immediate hypersensitivity reactivity (a type I reaction) against a specific allergen. Thus, if a patient's mast cells have been sensitized with IgE antibody against the injected allergen, mast cell degranulation will occur, resulting in release of mediators such as histamine into the skin. The wheal and flare reaction of a positive skin test is primarily due to histamine stimulation of H_1 receptors. Thus, H_1 antihistamines would markedly inhibit positive skin test reactivity and must be discontinued for a period of time (depending on the antihistamine) prior to skin testing. H_2 antihistamines do not typically, but may occasionally, have significant effects on skin test reactivity. This emphasizes the importance of always using a histamine standard as a positive control when performing allergy skin testing. CS do not affect mast cell degranulation nor do they affect the biologic effects of histamine. Thus, CS do not alter allergy skin test results.

B. In contrast DTH skin testing is a type IV reaction and is a sensitive measurement of T-cell function. Histamine does not play a significant role in DTH, and antihistamines (both H_1 and H_2) do not affect DTH skin testing. However, corticosteroids may substantially depress cell-mediated responses, including T-cell function, so that DTH responsiveness may be profoundly depressed with CS treatment.

58. Which types of infections play a role in the exacerbation of asthma?

There is strong evidence implicating upper respiratory infections (URI) caused by viruses and *Mycoplasma pneumoniae* as important causes of exacerbations of asthma. The association is especially pronounced in the pediatric age group. Respiratory syncytial virus (RSV) is an especially important offending organism. Other implicated viruses include parainfluenza, influenza A, and adenovirus. The severity of the exacerbation depends on multiple factors, including age, severity of the underlying asthma, concurrent medical problems, the site and severity of the infection, and the specific infectious agent. Bacterial infections of the respiratory tract, with the exception of chronic sinusitis, have not been commonly associated with exacerbations of asthma.

59. A 22-year-old patient complains of symptoms of asthma after playing basketball. What is a likely explanation?

The patient probably has exercise-induced asthma (EIA). Bronchoconstriction typically begins following cessation of exercise and is usually maximal 3 to 12 minutes later. The severity of the asthma varies, but it is almost always short-lived. The diagnosis of EIA is confirmed by a decrease in the forced expiratory volume (FEV) following exercise or isocapnic hyperventilation, although the former is the preferred form of testing. The etiology of EIA is believed to be water loss from the bronchial mucosa, resulting in hyperosmolarity in the bronchial tissue. This has been demonstrated by prevention of EIA during exercise by means of air that is fully saturated with water vapor at body temperature. Water content of the inspired air is probably the single most important factor affecting bronchospasm, but level of ventilation achieved, temperature of the inspired air, and the interval since the previous episode of EIA are also contributing factors. The last factor is important because a refractory period usually occurs for as long as 2 hours following the previous episode. During this period a second challenge will invoke less than half of the initial airway response. The severity of EIA cannot be predicted by baseline pulmonary function tests (PFTs).

60. What treatment is available for prevention of exercise-induced asthma?

Inhaled beta agonists are the most effective pharmacologic treatment (90% or greater response rate). Approximately 60–70% of patients will respond to inhaled cromolyn alone. Some patients will require combination therapy and ipratropium bromide (an anticholinergic agent) may offer additional relief. Treatment should be administered by a hand-held nebulizer immediately before exercise. The protective effects of pharmacologic therapy may last for only 2 hours, even though in nonexercise related bronchospasm there may be continued benefits for an additional 2 to 4 hours. Inhaled corticosteroids, when taken over several weeks, may decrease both the severity of EIA and the doses of the other medications required for control. Finally, nasal breathing may attenuate EIA but it is not practical in strenuous exercise.

61. In a patient who complains of nocturnal worsening of asthma, what potential factors should be considered?

Considerable attention has been directed toward the role of circadian rhythms in nocturnal exacerbations of asthma (usually between 3 am and 7 am). Cortisol levels decrease, plasma histamine levels increase, and epinephrine levels decrease during the night. The decrease in plasma cortisol is not thought to be a major factor since administration of corticosteroids in the evening is ineffective in preventing nocturnal exacerbations. Plasma histamine levels do not correlate with changes in pulmonary function tests (PFTs). However, epinephrine levels do correlate, suggesting a possible important physiologic role.

Circadian changes in the airways themselves are also important. Both airway caliber and reactivity are affected, with an overall 5–10% decrease in flow rates in normal individuals, but up to a 50% decrease in asthmatics. Increased vagal tone, impaired muco-ciliary clearance, and airway cooling and drying have also been reported as contributing factors in nocturnal asthma. Gastroesophageal reflux (GER) may also exacerbate asthma at night by microaspiration or reflex bronchoconstriction caused by stimulation of nerve endings by acid in the lower esophagus. GER may be exacerbated by theophylline, which decreases lower esophageal sphincter tone.

The patient's pharmacologic regimen should be carefully examined and compliance assured. Theophylline absorption may be decreased at night, leading to lower serum levels. If necessary, the evening dose should be adjusted so that peak levels occur approximately 6 hours later. H_2 antihistamines may be helpful in some patients with GER. Evening corticosteroids should not generally be given because of marked suppression of the adrenal axis and lack of demonstration of a beneficial effect. Patients who have an allergic component to their asthma and who are on maximal pharmacologic therapy should be considered for immunotherapy.

Potential environmental and dietary agents should be considered as exacerbating factors. For example, dust mites may cause immediate hypersensitivity reactions during the night. Allergen or irritant exposure several hours before going to sleep can also be important. The late-phase response that may occur following such exposure typically peaks 6–12 hours later and may cause severe prolonged bronchospasm. Finally nonasthmatic causes of wheezing such as cardiac disease should be considered as potential contributing factors. Nocturnal asthma is not related to any particular stage of sleep. The contribution of sleep "per se" is unclear but does not appear to be of major significance.

62. Why is it critical that nocturnal asthma be aggressively treated?

The importance of the treatment of nocturnal asthma cannot be overemphasized, since the majority of fatalities due to asthma occur during the early morning hours.

63. What are Charcot-Leyden crystals, Creola bodies, and Curschmann's spirals?

Charcot-Leyden crystals are composed of lysophospholipase, and their presence in tissue or secretions has been considered as specific for eosinophil activity. However, lysophospholipase is also found in basophils.

Creola bodies are clumps of epithelial cells and suggest a desquamating disease process.

Curschmann's spirals are mucus plugs composed of mucus, proteinaceous material, and inflammatory cells in a swirling, spiraling pattern. They usually conform to the configuration of the involved airways.

These findings may be seen alone or together as part of the clinical presentation of asthma. They are characteristically seen in patients who have died from status asthmaticus.

64. What are the clinical manifestations of anaphylaxis?

Clinical Manifestations of Anaphylaxis

General:	Flushing, sense of foreboding
Skin:	Urticaria/angioedema, flushing, pruritus
Eyes:	Lacrimation, pruritus
Upper respiratory tract:	Sneezing, nasal pruritus, discharge, and congestion, hoarseness, laryngeal edema, stridor
Lower respiratory tract:	Bronchospasm, tachypnea, intercostal retractions, use of accessory muscles of respiration
Cardiovascular:	Hypotension, tachycardia, arrhythmia
GI:	Nausea, vomiting, abdominal pain, diarrhea
Neurologic:	Headache, syncope, seizure

65. A 20-year-old patient presents with hypotension, wheezing, and urticaria 30 minutes after a bee sting. What is the appropriate treatment?

This patient's presentation is that of systemic anaphylaxis. Anaphylaxis is an immediate hypersensitivity reaction caused by mast cell/basophil release of multiple potent mediators, including histamine, prostaglandins, and leukotrienes, into tissues and the circulation. Prompt treatment is critical, and therapy should be directed toward maintaining cardiovascular and pulmonary function. Initial treatment should be administration of epinephrine either by subcutaneous or intramuscular (IM) routes (0.3–0.5 cc of a 1:1000 dilution). In the face of cardiovascular collapse, intravenous (IV) epinephrine may be indicated. Other immediate steps include applying a tourniquet proximal to the site of allergen inoculation (for example, a bee sting or allergen injection in the forearm). If the anaphylaxis is due to oral intake of an allergen (such as food ingestion), a nasogastric (NG) tube may be inserted and residual gastric contents removed to prevent further antigen absorption. The patient's legs should be elevated, oxygen and airway support provided as needed, and IV fluids (such as normal saline) given for blood pressure support. Parenteral H_1 (diphenhydramine) and H_2 (ranitidine) antihistamines may also be administered. Inhaled beta-1 agonists can be given prophylactically or if bronchospasm is present. Repeat doses of medication such as epinephrine should be given as needed and vasopressor agents given when indicated. Although steroids will not alter the acute course of anaphylaxis, they may be given to attenuate a subsequent late phase response. The aggressiveness of the above outlined therapy depends on the severity of the anaphylaxis and the response to treatment.

66. What are the major distinguishing factors between Churg-Strauss syndrome (allergic angiitis and granulomatosis) and classic polyarteritis nodosa (PAN)?

Both of these diseases are systemic necrotizing vasculitides. It is important to recognize that some patients may have characteristics of both Churg-Strauss and PAN. These patients are classified as having polyangiitis overlap syndrome. Patients who fail corticosteroid therapy or who have fulminant disease should receive cytotoxic drug therapy.

Comparison of Churg-Strauss and PAN

	CHURG-STRAUSS	PAN
Pulmonary involvement	+	–
Histology	Necrotizing vasculitis with granulomas	Necrotizing vasculitis
Vessel involvement	Small-to-medium arteries	Medium muscular arteries; veins, venules with aneurysmal dilation

Table continued on next page.

Comparison of Churg-Strauss and PAN (Continued)

	CHURG-STRAUSS	PAN
Asthma/atopic disease	+*	–
Eosinophilia (blood and/or tissue)	+	–
Association with serum hepatitis B surface antigen	–	+

*Often present for years before onset of vasculitis.

67. What does palpable purpura indicate?
Palpable purpura indicates cutaneous vasculitis.

68. What is the classic triad of Wegener's granulomatosis (WG)?
WG is a systemic necrotizing vasculopathy of unknown etiology. The classic triad includes (1) necrotizing granulomatous vasculitis of the upper respiratory tract and (2) lungs, in addition to (3) glomerulonephritis. Vasculitis of many other organs, including the skin, ears, eyes, joints and central nervous system, may also be present. Vasculitis typically involves small arteries and veins. The glomerulonephritis is usually focal or crescentic without vasculitis or granulomas. Since the original description by Wegener in Germany in 1939, many more limited forms of the disease have been recognized. The clinical presentation may include fever, chronic sinusitis, otitis media, cough, chest pain, hemoptysis, and arthralgias. Upper airway infections are common, with *Staphylococcus aureus* the most common pathogen. Such infections may mimic exacerbation or recurrence of disease following remission. With the inflammatory process unchecked, nasal septal perforation may occur, leading to a saddle-nose deformity. Laboratory data are generally nonspecific, although recently an antibody to cytoplasmic components of the polymorphonuclear leukocyte (anti-neutrophil cytoplasmic antibody, or ANCA) has been associated with active disease. The erythrocyte sedimentation rate (ESR) is markedly elevated (often > 100 mm/hr) and is a sensitive indicator of disease activity. Mild anemia, leukocytosis, and an increase in serum IgG and IgA levels are commonly seen. Chest x-ray patterns of the disease include multiple nodules (which frequently cavitate), infiltrates, and solitary nodules. The mean age of onset is 40 years with a male predominance.

69. What is the treatment for Wegener's granulomatosis (WG)?
Prior to the use of cytotoxic drugs, specifically cyclophosphamide, WG was an almost uniformly fatal disease, with a mean survival of 5 months. Corticosteroid therapy did not significantly alter the disease's outcome. However, treatment with cyclophosphamide results in complete remission in over 90% of patients. Combination treatment with corticosteroids and cyclophosphamide should be given initially to gain benefits from the rapid anti-inflammatory effects of the steroid while the cytotoxic actions of the cyclophosphamide are taking effect. Prednisone may be started at 1 mg/kg daily, maintained for 1 month, tapered to alternate day therapy, and then gradually discontinued, depending on the patient's response to the taper. Cyclophosphamide should be started at 2 mg/kg orally and continued for at least a year. If, at the end of the year, clinical remission has been obtained, the cyclophosphamide may be tapered and discontinued. The patient's hematologic parameters should be closely monitored for cyclophosphamide toxicity. The patient's WBC count should be maintained above 3,000/mm³ with a neutrophil count above 1,000/mm³ to lessen the risk of infectious complications. Other cytotoxic drugs, such as azathioprine, are less effective than cyclophosphamide in the treatment of WG.

70. What are the principal toxicities of cyclophosphamide therapy for immunologic diseases?
Bone marrow toxicity is primarily manifested as leukopenia with relative sparing of red blood cells and platelets. However, any or all myeloid and erythroid precursors may be

affected. Nausea and/or vomiting is common, especially with intravenous administration. Alopecia frequently occurs, but hair growth usually resumes after discontinuation of the drug. The bladder is an important site of toxicity, and hemorrhagic cystitis, though not common, may be life-threatening. Its incidence may be lessened by maintaining a well-hydrated state and monitoring urine sediment during therapy. Bladder fibrosis and carcinoma of the bladder rarely occur. Development of other malignancy, especially of the lymphoproliferative type, has been reported. The degree of gonadal dysfunction and sterility caused by fibrosis of the reproductive organs is variable. Finally, because of adverse effects on sperm, egg, and fetus, neither male nor female patients should attempt conception while on cyclophosphamide therapy or for at least a year following therapy. Counseling should be obtained prior to family planning regarding the potential genetic risk following cessation of cyclophosphamide therapy.

71. What are the major differences between Wegener's granulomatosis and Goodpasture's syndrome?

Wegener's Granulomatosis Versus Goodpasture's Syndrome

	WEGENER'S	GOODPASTURE'S
Etiology	Unknown	Unknown, but hydrocarbon exposure increases risk
Patients	Male > female 5th decade	Male >> female Young adults
Histopathology	Necrotizing granulomatous vasculitis of upper/lower respiratory tract	Linear deposition of IgG along basement membrane of lung and kidney demonstrated by immunofluorescence, vasculitis absent
Target organs	Lung > kidney May also affect: CNS, eyes, ears, joints skin, heart, others	Kidney > lung
Primary symptoms	Chronic sinusitis/rhinitis, fever, weight loss, cough, chest pain, hemoptysis may occur.	Hemoptysis, dyspnea, easy fatigability
Typical chest x-ray finding	Pulmonary nodule(s) with or without cavitation	Diffuse bilateral infiltrates
Diagnosis	Clinical picture with biopsy showing necrotizing vasculitis with granulomas of small arteries and veins.	Demonstration of circulating or tissue-bound anti-basement membrane antibodies, pulmonary hemorrhage, glomerulonephritis
Treatment	Cyclophosphamide, corticosteroids	Plasmapheresis, corticosteroids, cyclophosphamide

72. What clinical and laboratory findings are most important in determining the cause of angioedema?

In a patient who presents with recurrent angioedema, a careful history is of the utmost importance. For example, allergic angioedema might be suggested by a temporal relationship to exposure to specific allergens (such as food). Cold urticaria/angioedema would be indicated by onset following exposure to cold temperatures. A number of findings might indicate hereditary angioedema (HAE), including a positive family history, low C4 during and between attacks, and low antigenic or functional activity of C1 esterase inhibitor. The majority of angioedema cases are idiopathic, and an extensive evaluation fails to reveal a specific cause or associated underlying disease. The list of diseases reported to be associated with angioedema is exhaustive, but some of the most widely recognized are connective tissue diseases, malignancies, thyroid disease, and liver disease (such as hepatitis B).

73. What is the cause of angioedema in the hereditary angioedema syndrome (HAE)?

HAE is caused by deficiency of C1 esterase inhibitor enzyme (C1INH). Eighty-five percent of HAE patients have depressed serum levels of C1INH (by antigenic assay), whereas the remaining 15% have normal enzyme levels but lack functional activity. The clinical presentation and inheritance patterns are similar for both groups. Decreased C1INH leads to unchecked activation of the classical complement pathway and decreased inhibition of Hageman factor-dependent activation of the kinin and plasmin pathways. This results in increased generation of C2 kinin, bradykinin, and other putative molecules.

74. What are some of the most important clinical characteristics of hereditary angioedema (HAE)?

HAE is transmitted in an autosomal dominant pattern, although sporadic cases do occur. The age of onset is variable and the diagnosis can be hindered by a predilection for nonlaryngeal sites, such as the abdominal viscera. Inciting causes are not usually identified, although trauma, even if minor, can lead to attacks. Most patients have a high propensity for life-threatening laryngeal edema that is not characteristic of angioedema due to other causes. Urticaria, although commonly seen in association with other causes of angioedema, is not part of the HAE syndrome. Pain, not pruritus, is typical of HAE lesions. Patients typically have depressed serum C4 levels even when they are asymptomatic between attacks. Attenuated androgen (i.e., stanazolol) therapy dramatically decreases the severity and frequency of attacks. Androgens should be tapered to the lowest dose that adequately controls disease activity in order to minimize potential adverse effects such as virilization and hepatic toxicity.

75. How would you evaluate a previously healthy 26-year-old patient who presents with an 8-week history of daily urticaria?

Urticaria persisting for longer than 6 weeks is deemed chronic. A careful history should be obtained to determine whether the urticaria is related to the ingestion of a specific food or liquid, environmental exposure, animal exposure, physical condition (heat, cold, water, sunlight, pressure, exercise, etc.), or stress. The history should also seek to rule out symptoms suggestive of an underlying systemic disease. A careful medication history should also be obtained for the ingestion of both prescription and over-the-counter medications (particularly aspirin and aspirin-containing compounds). A thorough physical examination should be performed to identify potential underlying illnesses, such as thyroid disease, malignancy, infection, and rheumatic diseases.

A chest x-ray usually should be obtained, particularly if the patient has not had one within 6 months. If the patient has poor dental health, or if there are findings suggestive of a dental abscess, dental x-rays may reveal the source of an occult infection. Screening laboratory tests should include a complete blood count (CBC) with white blood cell (WBC) count and differential, urinalysis, erythrocyte sedimentation rate (ESR), antinuclear antibody (ANA) screen, and liver function tests. In patients over the age of 40, a serum protein electrophoresis should be obtained. Other tests that may be helpful include C3, C4, rheumatoid factor, stool for ova and parasites, thyroid function studies, hepatitis B surface antigen (HB$_s$Ag), and cryoglobulins. Whether these and other tests for the evaluation for systemic diseases are obtained depends upon the degree of clinical suspicion based on the history, physical examination, and initial laboratory results. Tests for specific types of the physical urticarias can be performed as indicated and are eloquently reviewed in the provided reference.

Despite extensive evaluation, as many as 90% of the cases of chronic urticaria may be classified as idiopathic, since an etiology cannot be determined. Typical urticarial lesions do not usually require biopsy. However, in particularly severe, persistent cases, and especially when urticarial lesions are very painful (as opposed to pruritic), very erythematous, or persist longer than 24 hours, a biopsy may reveal urticarial vasculitis. Some of these cases are accompanied by hypocomplementemia and may require more aggressive medical therapy.

Kaplan A: Urticaria and angioedema. In Middleton E, et al (eds): Allergy: Principles and Practice, 3rd ed. St. Louis, C.V. Mosby, 1988.

76. What is the usefulness of rheumatoid factors (RFs) in the diagnosis of rheumatoid arthritis? (See also pp. 346–349.)

RFs are autoantibodies (most commonly IgM) that react with the Fc portion of IgG. The presence of RF is not diagnostic of rheumatoid arthritis. In fact, RF may *not* be detected in approximately 20% of patients with rheumatoid arthritis. When present, RF may be detected in blood, synovial fluid, and pleural fluid. The potential pathogenic significance of RF is indicated by the more aggressive joint and extra-articular disease (especially vasculitis) in patients with rheumatoid arthritis who have a high titer of RF.

It should be appreciated that RF is also found in a long list of other illnesses, including other systemic inflammatory diseases, malignancies, infectious diseases (such as tuberculosis, viral, subacute bacterial endocarditis), and sarcoidosis. Furthermore, RF can be detected in a small percentage of normal individuals, particularly in the elderly population.

77. What is the single best test for the diagnosis of Sjögren's syndrome? (See also pp. 349–350.)

Sjögren's disease is a chronic inflammatory disease of the exocrine glands characterized by keratoconjunctivitis sicca and xerostomia. The inflammatory infiltrate is comprised primarily of lymphocytes and plasma cells. Primary Sjögren's disease is exocrine gland disease alone, whereas secondary Sjögren's is the occurrence with another connective tissue disease, most commonly rheumatoid arthritis. Eye involvement may be confirmed by the Schirmer test (a measurement of tearing on filter paper with < 10 mm wetting in 5 minutes defining a positive test), rose bengal staining of the conjunctiva, or the finding of keratitis on slit lamp examination. Parotid salivary flow rates and salivary radionuclide scanning may be used to assess salivary gland function. Autoantibodies present include Ro(SS-A), La(SS-B), rheumatoid factor, and Epstein-Barr-related nuclear antigen (RANA). Although all of the above tests may be helpful in the evaluation of Sjögren's syndrome, biopsy of the labial minor salivary glands is the most specific diagnostic procedure available.

78. What is the Prausnitz-Kustner (P-K) reaction?

The P-K reaction was used in the past to demonstrate the passive transfer of reaginic (IgE) antibodies in humans. Serum was removed from an allergic individual and injected into the skin of a person known not to be allergic to the specific allergen being tested. Twenty-four hours later, the antigen (allergen) was injected intradermally into the sensitized skin and observed for a wheal and flare response. A positive response indicated passive transfer of IgE antibodies from the donor serum, which bound to the dermal mast cells in the recipient's skin, leading to an immediate hypersensitivity reaction.

79. What do the direct and indirect Coombs' tests measure and what is the diagnostic usefulness of each?

Once the presence of hemolytic anemia has been confirmed, additional testing should be performed to determine whether an immune mechanism is causing the hemolysis. The direct Coombs' test (direct anti-globulin test, or DAT) measures antibody or complement on the surface of the RBC. Titrations are performed to determine the degree of RBC sensitization.

Briefly, the test is performed by incubation of the patient's RBCs with anti-Ig or anti-C3 reagent. If surface-bound immunoglobulin or complement is present, then agglutination will occur with the appropriate antisera.

The indirect Coombs' test (indirect antiglobulin test, or IAT) measures the presence of antibody in the patient's serum. The patient's serum is added to normal RBCs, and after incubation and washing, anti-Ig reagent is added. If the antibody from the patient's serum has bound to the RBCs, agglutination will occur. The usefulness of the DAT and IAT in the diagnosis of autoimmune hemolytic anemia (AIHA) is outlined in the table.

Usefulness of the Coombs' Test in Autoimmune Hemolytic Anemias

TYPE OF ANEMIA	RESULT OF DIRECT COOMBS' TEST IgG, C3	RESULT OF INDIRECT COOMB'S TEST	ANTIBODY SPECIFICITY	COMMENT
Autoimmune				
Warm antibody (most common type)	+ + (67%) + – (20%) – + (13%)	Majority + (57%)	Most often within Rh system	With SLE, DAT usually positive for both C3 and IgG
Cold agglutinin syndrome	– +	High titer at 4°C	Usually anti-I, but also anti-i, especially with infectious mononucleosis	Agglutinating activity up to 30°C in albumin; high titer (usually >500) at 4°C
Paroxysmal cold hemoglobinuria	– +	Biphasic hemolysin	anti-P	Donath-Landsteiner antibody
Drug-induced				
Alpha-methyldopa (Aldomet)	+ –	Similar to warm anti-body AIHA	Usually within Rh system	IgG autoantibody directed against RBC surface antigen, DAT positivity is dose-dependent, occurs after 3–6 months of treatment, and may remain (+) for up to 2 years after stopping the drug. Hemolysis improves in 1–3 weeks after stopping.
Penicillin	+ – (mostly)	(–) unless testing with penicillin-coated RBCs	Reacts with penicillin-coated RBCs	Haptenic mechanism, penicillin binds to RBCs
Other drugs (such as quinidine)	– +	Negative unless drug, normal RBCs, and serum incubated together		Immune complex mechanism (innocent bystander), intra-vascular hemolysis with anti-drug anti-body (usually IgM).

(From McMillan R (ed): Immune cytopenias. In Methods in Hematology. New York, Churchill Livingstone, 1983, p 30, with permission.)

80. When does a food allergy occur, and what can mimic a food allergy?

True food allergy occurs when ingested food antigens bind to IgE on the surface of intestinal mast cells, causing an immediate hypersensitivity reaction. Basophils may also participate if food antigens appear in the circulation. The diagnosis of food allergy is complicated by a bewildering array of other factors that may cause adverse reactions to food and that mimic allergic reactions. These include reactions to food additives, preservatives, dyes, and toxins. Gastrointestinal disorders such as eosinophilic gastroenteritis, malabsorption syndromes, enzyme deficiencies, gluten-sensitive enteropathy, gallbladder disease, peptic ulcer disease, and scromboid poisoning are among a long list of important, nonimmunologic causes of adverse food reactions. Finally, the psychological aspect may be important, particularly in patients who are convinced that allergy is the cause of their GI symptoms. A partial list of some of the foods that most commonly cause true food allergies are: peanuts, true nuts, shellfish, eggs, and wheat. Cooking may destroy a food's allergenicity.

81. How is a food allergy diagnosed?

A careful history and physical examination should be performed to rule out other potential causes of adverse reactions to food. In an allergic reaction, symptoms should occur following each ingestion of the specific food. This and the resolution of symptoms with elimination of the food from the diet support a diagnosis of food allergy. The onset of symptoms may occur for up to 2 hours. The longer time until onset of symptoms with some GI reactions compared to typical ($<$1 hr) immediate hypersensitivity reactions may be due to the need for transport of the antigen into the GI tract, processing of antigen by digestion, and absorption into the intestinal mucosa. Symptoms of food allergy may be localized to the GI tract (including nausea, vomiting, diarrhea, bloating, and pain), or may be systemic (urticaria, angioedema, headache, wheezing, hypotension, and other symptoms of anaphylaxis).

Of the immunologic diagnostic procedures, skin testing is the most useful. By itself, a positive skin test is not diagnostic of food allergy and must be interpreted in the context of other clinical findings. A positive skin test in the presence of a positive clinical history is highly suggestive of specific food allergy, whereas a negative skin test suggests that allergy to that specific food is highly unlikely. The RAST may also be helpful, but its use should be limited to patients in whom skin testing cannot be properly performed and interpreted, or in those thought to be at particular risk of a severe anaphylactic reaction to skin testing.

A clinical diagnosis of food allergy can be confirmed by food challenge. If the challenge is negative, there is strong evidence against allergy to that specific food. Food challenge should be performed only in an appropriate medical setting, since life-threatening anaphylaxis may occur. The double-blinded, placebo-controlled food challenge is the ideal method for confirming food allergy. In some patients, such as those with a low probability of a positive reaction, an open challenge may be useful. If positive, then a double-blinded, placebo-controlled challenge may be necessary.

Bock SA: Double-blind, placebo-controlled food challenge (DBPCFC) as an office procedure: A manual. J Allergy Clin Immunol 82:986, 1988.

82. What is the treatment for food allergy?

The treatment for food allergy is avoidance. Treatment with antiallergic medications, such as antihistamines or oral cromolyn, cannot be expected to decrease the risk of life-threatening reactions. Anaphylaxis caused by food ingestion should be treated like any other anaphylactic reaction, except that nasogastric (NG) tube placement and lavage may be useful to remove residual food antigen. Immunotherapy has no place in the treatment of food allergy.

83. What is the difference between a drug allergy, drug intolerance, and an idiosyncratic drug reaction?

All three are types of adverse drug reactions. A true **drug allergy** is an **immunologically mediated** adverse reaction to a drug. It can occur with very small doses of the offending agent and accounts for only 5–6% of all adverse drug reactions. **Drug intolerance,** which also can occur with very small doses, is the result of an undesirable **pharmacologic effect** of the drug. An **idiosyncratic drug reaction** is based on an individual patient's **biochemical alterations** of a drug's metabolism.

84. What are the indications for skin testing for penicillin allergy?

Skin testing for penicillin allergy is indicated in patients with a possible or definite past history consistent with immediate hypersensitivity to penicillin and in whom penicillin therapy is indicated and effective alternative antibiotic therapy is not available. Penicillin sensitization occurs by the haptenation mechanism and may involve a number of structural components (or "determinants") of the penicillin molecule. The penicilloyl determinant is referred to as the major determinant, and the penicillin G, penicilloate, and penilloate determinants are referred to as the minor determinants. This "major" and "minor" nomenclature refers only to abundance of breakdown product and does not indicate relative clinical importance, as the minor determinants are responsible for the majority of life-threatening anaphylactic reactions.

85. What is the predictive value of skin testing for penicillin allergy?

Negative skin testing in patients with a positive prior history indicates that clinically significant amounts of IgE antibodies against penicillin are not present and the risk of anaphylaxis is extremely low. When an allergic reaction occurs in these patients it is usually not life-threatening.

A positive reaction with skin testing indicates that the patient is at significant risk for anaphylaxis to the administration of penicillin. In these patients, alternative antibiotic therapy should be given, if at all possible. If penicillin must be given, desensitization may be performed. Thereafter, penicillin must be given without significant interruption, or the risk of anaphylaxis will return.

86. What is the "innocent bystander" mechanism of drug-induced hemolysis?

Some drugs (such as sulfonamides, phenothiazines, quinidine, and quinine) can cause an immune hemolytic anemia even though they do not bind to RBCs. These drugs, bound to plasma proteins, stimulate the formation of complement-fixing antibodies that activate the classical complement pathway. Generated C3b binds to the RBC, which leads to intravascular hemolysis of these "innocent bystanders."

87. Which class of medications should be used with particular caution in patients prone to develop anaphylaxis?

Beta blockers should be avoided whenever possible, because they may accentuate the severity of anaphylaxis and prolong its cardiovascular and pulmonary manifestations. They may also markedly decrease the effectiveness of epinephrine in reversing the life-threatening manifestations of anaphylaxis.

88. What is C3 nephritic factor?

C3 nephritic factor (C3NF) is an IgG_3 antibody that binds to the C3 convertase (C3b,Bb) of the alternative pathway of complement. This results in stabilization of C3b,Bb, which prevents its inactivation and results in uncontrolled C3 cleavage and alternative pathway activation. C3NF is found in partial lipodystrophy, some patients with SLE, and in most patients with type II membranoproliferative glomerulonephritis. The pathologic significance of the antibody is unknown. The antibody level and degree of lowering of the serum C3 level do not correlate with the severity of tissue damage or with disease activity.

89. What is the mechanism of action of cyclosporine and what are its principal adverse effects?

Cyclosporine A inhibits the production of multiple cytokines, but its principal immunosuppressive effect appears to be mediated through inhibition of interleukin-2 (IL-2) production. The principal side-effects are listed in the table below.

Principal Side-effects of Cyclosporine

Renal dysfunction	Central nervous system toxicity:
Hypertension	Tremor
Hirsutism	Seizures
Hepatotoxicity	Hypomagnesemia
Gingival hyperplasia	

90. What are the serum half-lives and relative potencies of the following steroid preparations: prednisone, prednisolone, methylprednisolone, dexamethasone, hydrocortisone, and cortisone?

Relative Potencies and Effects of Common Glucocorticoids

PREPARATION	POTENCY RELATIVE TO HYDROCORTISONE	RELATIVE SODIUM-RETAINING POTENCY	APPROXIMATELY EQUIVALENT DOSE OF ACTION (mg)	DURATION
Hydrocortisone	1	1	20	Short
Cortisone	0.8	0.8	25	Short
Prednisolone	4	0.8	5	Intermediate
Prednisone	4	0.8	5	Intermediate
6α-Methyl-prednisolone	5	0.5	4	Intermediate
Triamcinolone	5	0	4	Intermediate
Dexamethasone	25	0	0.75	Long
Betamethasone	25	0	0.75	Long

(From Schleimer RP: Glucocorticosteroids. In Middleton E, et al (eds): Allergy: Principles and Practice, 3rd ed. St. Louis, C.V. Mosby, 1988, p 742, with permission.)

91. What are the effects of corticosteroids on circulating leukocytes?

Effects of Corticosteroids on Leukocytes

CELL TYPE	EFFECT ON NUMBERS	EFFECT ON FUNCTION	COMMENT
Neutrophil	Increase	Minimal effect on chemotaxis, phagocytosis, bactericidal activity	Decreased from circulation marginating pool, increased production and release from bone marrow, increased half-life in circulation
Lymphocytes	Decrease	Decreased profliferative response, inhibition of mediator production and release, altered helper and suppressor function	Greater effect on T cells than on B cells
Lymphocytes T cells	Decrease a. Helper/inducer (CD4)-decrease b. Cytotoxic/suppressor (CD8) —no change		
B cells	Minimal decrease or no change		

Table continued on next page.

Effects of Corticosteroids on Leukocytes (Continued)

CELL TYPE	EFFECT ON NUMBERS	EFFECT ON FUNCTION	COMMENT
Monocytes	Decrease	Depressed chemotaxis, suppression of cytotoxic activity	Possible sequestration
Eosinophils	Decrease	Inhibition of mediator production and release	Possible sequestration
Basophils	Decrease	Inhibition of degranulation	Possible sequestration
NK cells	No effect	No effect	
Null cells	No effect	Unknown	

92. What is the recommended treatment for Guillain-Barré syndrome (GBS)?

The cause of GBS remains obscure and the principal therapy is supportive, particularly with regard to decreased respiratory function. Plasmapheresis, particularly when instituted within 7 days of the onset of symptoms, has been shown to be beneficial in acute GBS. Typically 6–10 plasmapheresis procedures are performed. Each procedure consists of the exchange of total plasma volume (usually 2–3 liters in an adult) with an albumin/saline/electrolyte solution. The frequency of procedures varies with the overall medical condition of the patient and the availability of venous access.

93. What is the Chinese restaurant syndrome?

It is a reaction to glutamate ingested as MSG (monosodium glutamate), a flavoring agent commonly used in Chinese cooking. It occurs within 15–30 minutes of ingestion and consists of a sensation of warmth and tightness on the face and anterior chest. It is occasionally confused with angina pectoris, but is benign and requires no therapy except avoidance of foods cooked with MSG.

Kwok RHN: Chinese restaurant syndrome. N Engl J Med 278:1122, 1968.

94. What is the triad of Kartagener's syndrome?

Originally described by Kartagener in 1904, the syndrome consists of the triad of situs inversus, bronchiectasis, and chronic sinusitis. It is an autosomal recessive disorder resulting in a defect of the cilia, which lack dynein arms. Patients also suffer from chronic sinopulmonary infections and sterility may occur in males (due to immotile spermatozoa).

Eliasson R, et al: The immotile cilia syndrome. N Engl J Med 297:1–6, 1977.

95. Chronic or recurrent meningococcemia and gonococcemia have been particularly associated with which host immune defects?

Deficiencies of the late components of complement (C6, C7, and C8) are the predominant defects associated with these disorders. Several reports of C3, C5, properdin, IgG_2 subclass, and IgM deficiencies have also been reported with these syndromes.

Ross S, et al: Complement deficiency and infection: Epidemiology, pathogenesis and consequences of neisserial and other infections in an immune deficiency. Medicine 63:243–273, 1984.

96. A patient with a history of hypotension following an intravenous pyelogram (IVP) now requires a radiocontrast study. What procedure should be followed?

Systemic reactions to radiocontrast media administration occur in 1–2% of patients. The reaction may begin from just after the onset of the infusion to 30 minutes after its completion. Cardiovascular collapse results in death in approximately 1 in 50,000 test procedures. The cause is unknown, but it does not appear to be a true immediate hypersensitivity (IgE mediated) reaction. A method for detection of patients at risk is not available, and skin testing with contrast or iodine is of no value. A patient who experiences a reaction has approximately a 33% chance of having another reaction with repeated radiocontrast exposures.

Management of patients who *require* the radiocontrast procedure includes careful evaluation and documentation of the essential nature of the procedure and obtaining informed consent from the patient and the family (especially with regard to the potentially fatal outcome). The presence of necessary personnel and supplies for emergency treatment, adequate patient hydration, and preprocedure medical prophylaxis are also necessary. The usual prophylactic regimen consists of steroids (usually prednisone 50 mg orally at 13, 7 and 1 hour before the procedure) and H_1 antihistamines (diphenhydramine 50 mg parenterally or orally 1 hour before radiocontrast media administration). When not contraindicated, ephedrine, 25 mg orally, may offer additional benefit. The usefulness of H_2 antihistamines and/or ephedrine is controversial.

Reactions after prophylactic therapy are usually mild. However, it is important that the procedure be started at the scheduled time or the efficacy of the prophylaxis may be decreased. Newer, lower osmolality contrast media are much less likely to cause systemic reactions. However their high expense greatly limits their routine use. Furthermore, in patients with a history of radiocontrast media reactions, nonionic media do not seem to offer significant protective advantage over medical prophylaxis.

Patterson R, et al: Drug allergy & protocols for the management of drug allergies. New England & Regional Allergy Proceedings 7(4):325–342, 1989.

97. A patient with systemic lupus erythematosus (SLE) asks whether or not she should be vaccinated against measles. What would be your recommendation? (See also pp 352–355.)

The major live attenuated vaccines currently available are rubeola (measles), poliomyelitis, BCG (bacille Calmette-Guerin), mumps, and yellow fever. Vaccinia (small pox) is no longer given. Live vaccines should not be administered to immunologically compromised patients, particularly those with depressed cell-mediated immunity (CMI), including SLE. Conditions in which live vaccination of patients should be avoided include:

1. Patients treated with primary immunodeficiency disorders (especially those with defective CMI such as severe combined immunodeficiency syndrome [SCID]).

2. Patients given immunosuppressive therapy (including corticosteroids, cytotoxic drugs, and radiation therapy).

3. Patients with malignancies, including leukemia, lymphoma and Hodgkin's disease.

4. Patients with systemic immunoregulatory, inflammatory, or infectious diseases associated with defective CMI (such as SLE, diabetes mellitus, sarcoidosis, AIDS, and atopic dermatitis).

5. Children less than 1 year of age.

6. Patients with severe malnutrition or burns.

7. Live vaccines should not be given to pregnant women because of the potential harm to the fetus. The exception is yellow fever when the mother must travel to an endemic area. In this case, the risk of infection and detrimental effects without the vaccine are greater than that of receiving the immunization.

Also noteworthy, household contacts of immunocompromised patients should not receive oral live polio vaccine, since the live attenuated strain may revert back to the wild type in the GI tract and be spread by the fecal-oral route.

98. Do the major histocompatibility complex (MHC) genes affect susceptibility to and expression of SLE?

There are data showing that disease expression is affected by MHC-associated genes. Deficiencies in complement (particularly C2 and C4, which are both part of the MHC) have significant associations with SLE. HLA DR2 and HLA DR3 occur in increased frequency in white lupus patients (almost 75% of SLE patients express one of these antigens). Newer data suggest that alleles of the DQ locus may also influence disease. Some clinical subsets have been outlined. In patients with onset at a young age and nephritis, DR2 DQwl has been found in higher frequency. In SLE patients with onset at an older age, sicca symptoms, photosensitive skin rash, and circulating anti-Ro and anti-La antibodies, expression of DR3 and DQw2 has been noted.

99. What is the lupus band test?

It is a test that may be of value in questionable cases of SLE. It involves demonstration of granular deposition of C3 and IgG along the dermal-epidermal junction in a biopsy of normal skin. The test is most likely to be positive in hypocomplementemic patients. However, the test rarely correlates with renal involvement.

100. What is the lupus anticoagulant (LA)?

The LA was so named because of its initial discovery in association with systemic lupus erythematosus (SLE). The name is actually a misnomer, because these patients are prone to hypercoagulability with recurrent venous and, less commonly, arterial thrombosis. Patients do not exhibit increased bleeding tendency unless concomitant hematologic dysfunction such as thrombocytopenia (which may be seen in association with LA) or clotting factor deficiency is present. LA may be present in autoimmune disorders (SLE and others), malignancies, nephrotic syndrome, and AIDS (especially during opportunistic infections). LA has also been reported to be associated with recurrent spontaneous abortions. LA may be seen with drug therapy (especially chlorpromazine, procainamide, hydralazine, and phenytoin) and usually correlates positively with dosage and duration of therapy. The LA is initially identified in the laboratory by the finding of a prolonged partial thromboplastin time (PTT) that does not correct with the addition of normal plasma. The PTT can usually be corrected by substitution of platelets for the addition of phospholipid in performance of the PTT. The LA is an antibody (most commonly IgG, but also IgM and rarely IgA), is usually polyclonal and is directed against determinants on anionic phospholipids. This antiphospholipid binding is responsible for the in vitro prolongation of the PTT. Some of these antibodies will cross-react with cardiolipin (thus explaining the false-positive VDRL test that may occur in these patients) and with DNA.

101. What percent of patients with systemic lupus erythematosus (SLE) have a negative antinuclear antibody test (ANA)?

Five percent or less of patients with SLE have been reported to be ANA negative. However, these patients have probably been tested using mouse kidney as the test substrate. This substrate will not readily detect antibody against Ro/SSA, ssDNA, Jo, and centromere. Antibodies against Ro and ssDNA are found in SLE.

The HEp-2 cell line, which is now widely used as the substrate for ANA testing, *will* detect these antibodies. Virtually all SLE patients probably are ANA positive using this testing protocol.

102. What are the most common clinical manifestations of drug-induced lupus? Which organs are characteristically spared in this syndrome when compared to idiopathic SLE?

Hydralazine and procainamide are the most common causes of drug-induced lupus. Up to 50% of patients receiving these drugs may have a positive antinuclear antibody test (ANA), although fewer will actually develop symptoms. Slow acetylators of these drugs are particularly susceptible for developing clinical disease. Hydralazine-induced lupus is most commonly encountered when the total daily dose administered exceeds 400 mg, with 10–20% of these patients developing a lupus-like syndrome. Other causes include D-penicillamine, isoniazid, and phenytoin. The ANA pattern in drug-induced lupus is usually homogeneous or speckled and is caused by anti-histone antibodies. Antibodies to double-stranded DNA, often seen in SLE, are not found in drug-induced lupus.

Drug-induced lupus manifests many of the same symptoms as idiopathic SLE, although they are generally milder. However, lupus nephritis and cerebritis rarely, if ever, complicate the syndrome. Drug-induced lupus is more frequent in women than men and in those with HLA DR4 phenotype. Symptoms resolve shortly after discontinuation of the drug, although laboratory abnormalities may persist for months or years.

Clinical and Serologic Features of Drug-induced Lupus and Systemic Lupus Erythematosus

	DRUG-INDUCED LUPUS	IDIO-PATHIC SLE		DRUG-INDUCED LUPUS	IDIO-PATHIC SLE
Polyserositis	+	+	Nephritis	–	+
Arthritis	+	+	Cerebritis	–	+
Fever	+	+	Positive ANA	+	+
Rash	+	+	Positive anti-dsDNA	–	+
Photosensitivity	+	+	Reversible*	+	–
Hemolytic anemia	+	+			

* Within several months of drug discontinuation.
Cush JJ, et al: Drug-induced lupus: Clinical spectrum and pathogenesis. Am J Med Sci 290:36, 1985.

103. What is the Donath-Landsteiner antibody, and in which disease is it found?

The Donath-Landsteiner antibody is an IgG cold-reacting antibody. It was described in patients with syphilis who developed paroxysmal cold hemoglobinuria (Donath-Landsteiner hemolytic anemia) on exposure to cold temperatures. The clinical syndrome consists of paroxysmal chills, fever, headache, and diffuse pain in the abdomen, back, and legs, in addition to the hemoglobinuria.

104. What is erythema multiforme (EM)?

EM is an immunologic reaction of the skin and mucous membranes to a variety of antigenic stimuli, but no such stimulus can be identified in up to 50% of cases. The lesions may be localized or widespread, and consist of bullae, erythematous plaques, and epidermal cell necrosis. The lesions are usually bilaterally and symmetrically distributed on the extensor surfaces of the limbs, on the dorsal and volar aspects of the hands and feet, and on the trunk. The lesions, which resemble "targets" or "bull's eyes," are diagnostic. They appear as a central vesicle or dark purple papule, surrounded by a round, pale zone that is in turn surrounded by a round area of erythema.

105. What are the precipitating factors in EM?

Precipitating Factors in Erythema Multiforme

1. **Viral diseases:** Herpes simplex, hepatitis, influenza A, vaccinia, mumps.
2. **Fungal diseases:** Dermatophytoses, histoplasmosis, coccidioidomycosis.
3. **Bacterial diseases:** Hemolytic streptococcal infections, tuberculosis, leprosy, typhoid.
4. **Collagen vascular disease:** Rheumatoid arthritis, SLE, dermatomyositis, allergic vasculitis, polyarteritis nodosa.
5. **Malignant tumors:** Carcinoma, lymphoma after radiation therapy.
6. **Hormonal changes:** Pregnancy, menstruation.
7. **Drugs:** Penicillins, sulfonamides, barbiturates, salicylates, halogens, phenolphthalein.
8. **Miscellaneous:** Rhus dermatitis, dental extractions, mycoplasma pneumonia infection.

(From Rubenstein E, Federman D (eds): Scientific American Medicine. New York, Scientific American Medicine, Inc., 1990. Section 2 (Dermatology), Subsection IX, with permission.)

106. What is Stevens-Johnson syndrome?
Stevens-Johnson syndrome is a severe form of erythema multiforme associated with fulminant, disseminated, multi-system involvement. The patients appear toxic, with fever, chills, malaise, tachycardia, tachypnea, and prostration. Diffuse vesicular, bullous, and ulcerative lesions of the skin and mucous membranes develop and desquamate, leading to secondary infections, which in turn may lead to sepsis and even death. It is associated with all the causes of erythema multiforme.

107. What is the role of immune complexes in bacterial infections?
Immune complex deposition can result in glomerulonephritis and vasculitis as a complication of many chronic bacterial infections. It is seen after pneumococcal, staphylococcal, and beta-hemolytic streptococcal infections. It is also seen in association with subacute bacterial endocarditis (SBE), infected arteriovenous shunts, disseminated gonorrheal infections, syphilis, and leprosy.

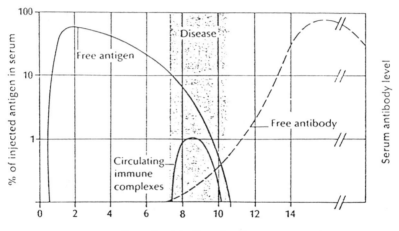

Relationships between antigen, antibodies, immune complexes, and serum sickness. (From Klein J: Immunology. Oxford, Blackwell Scientific Publications, 1990, with permission.)

108. Why is the Kviem test no longer performed?
The Kviem test was performed by intradermal injection of sarcoid spleen suspension into patients suspected of having sarcoidosis. The development of a skin reaction revealing noncaseating granulomas on biopsy was considered positive. However, the test lacked specificity and availability of the reagent was poor. Because of these problems and the risk of transmission of infectious diseases, the test is no longer performed.

109. How do you make the diagnosis of sarcoidosis? (See also pp 328–329.)
The diagnosis is one of exclusion in the presence of compatible clinical findings and noncaseating granulomas on biopsy.

110. What is the significance of erythema nodosum (EN) in sarcoidosis?
EN is a favorable prognostic sign, indicating a low propensity for development of chronic disease.

111. Hepatitis B surface antigenemia is associated with which of the vasculitides?
Polyarteritis nodosa. It is seen in 40% of HB_sAg-positive patients. The severity of the vasculitis and hepatitis is not correlated.

112. What is the differential diagnosis of a positive blood test for rheumatoid factor?

Differential Diagnosis of a Positive Rheumatoid Factor

Rheumatological diseases:	Pulmonary diseases:
Rheumatoid arthritis	Bronchitis or asthma
Juvenile rheumatoid arthritis	Coal miner's disease
SLE	Asbestosis
Mixed connective tissue disease	Idiopathic pulmonary fibrosis
Behçet's syndrome	Sarcoidosis
Sjögren's syndrome	
	Other diseases:
Infectious diseases:	Cirrhosis
Syphilis	Myocardial infarction
Viral hepatitis	Neoplasms
Parasitic infections	Essential mixed cryoglobulinemia
Granulomatous disease	
Mononucleosis	**Healthy persons—increases with age**

(From Coffey R, et al: Immunologic tests of value in diagnosis. 1. Acute phase reactants and autoantibodies. Postgrad Med 70:164, 1981, with permission.)

113. An 18-year-old male presents with abdominal pain, bloody diarrhea, peripheral neuropathy, and demonstration of IgA deposition on biopsy of the GI tract. What is the most likely diagnosis?
The clinical presentation is characteristic of Henoch-Schönlein purpura (HSP), although the age of onset is typically younger. The disease is almost always limited to males. This type of hypersensitivity vasculitis principally involves the skin, joints, intestine, and kidney. The disease is usually self-limited, although chronic renal failure may rarely occur. A history of recent infection, usually of the upper respiratory tract, is often reported. Circulating IgA immune complexes are common. Serum IgA levels may be elevated and IgA deposition can be demonstrated in the affected tissues.

114. Is skin testing useful for the diagnosis of histoplasmosis?
Skin testing is rarely useful in the diagnosis of histoplasmosis and should be principally limited to epidemiologic surveys. A positive skin test indicates prior exposure and not necessarily active infection. Furthermore, the histoplasmin reagent often causes a significant rise in antibody titers, thereby complicating interpretation of subsequent serologic studies. A negative skin test is highly suggestive of the absence of disease (even during dissemination stages), unless the patient is anergic.

115. How do anticentromere antibodies help differentiate between the CREST syndrome and scleroderma?
The anticentromere antibody, which is found by antinuclear antibody (ANA) testing, is characteristic of CREST patients but is usually absent in patients with diffuse scleroderma.

116. Which other laboratory and clinical findings distinguish the CREST syndrome from diffuse scleroderma (progressive systemic sclerosis)?
Skin involvement is principally limited to the extremities, and internal organ involvement generally develops more slowly and is less severe than in diffuse scleroderma. Particularly noteworthy of the CREST syndrome (but not in diffuse scleroderma) is the development of pulmonary arterial hypertension in the absence of pulmonary fibrosis. Intimal proliferation of the small and medium-sized pulmonary arteries is prominent. Pulmonary hypertension may be progressive and is almost uniformly fatal. Biliary cirrhosis also may occur in the CREST syndrome but is uncommon in diffuse scleroderma.

117. In a patient who complains of fatigue with hair-combing and stair-climbing, what are the most likely diagnoses?

Diseases characterized by proximal muscle weakness, such as myasthenia gravis, Eaton-Lambert syndrome (myasthenic syndrome), polymyositis, dermatomyositis, and polymyalgia rheumatica.

118. Explain the importance of HLA and ABO typing in solid organ and bone marrow transplantation (BMT).

HLA compatibility of donor and recipient affects graft outcome in both solid organ transplantation (such as kidney, heart, lung, and liver) and BMT. HLA compatibility is not a major graft survival factor for first-time, nonvascularized corneal transplants. HLA incompatibility may lead to graft rejection and destruction in solid organ transplantation and to graft-versus-host disease in BMT. In graft rejection, the graft is attacked by the recipient's immune system. In contrast, with graft-versus-host disease, the immunocompetent cells from the donor attack the recipient. ABO blood typing is critical in solid organ transplants, because ABO antigens are expressed on tissue cells of the transplanted organ. Thus, transplantation of a donor kidney from a type A donor into a type O recipient could lead to hyperacute rejection and graft death.

119. What are the four types of graft rejection and their immunologic mechanisms?

Types of Graft Rejection

TYPE	ONSET	MAJOR EFFECTOR MECHANISMS
Hyperacute	Minutes to hours	Humoral: preformed cytotoxic antibody in the recipient against donor graft antigen(s) a. ABO system b. Anti-HLA class I
Accelerated	2–5 days	Cell-mediated: due to prior T cell sensitization against donor antigen(s)
Acute	7–28 days	a. Principally cell-mediated immunity: allogeneic reactivity by recipient T cells against donor antigen(s) b. Humoral immunity
Chronic	>3 months	a. Principally cell-mediated immunity allogeneic reactivity by recipient T cells against donor antigen(s) b. Humoral immunity

120. What are the principal immunologic defects associated with recurrent bacterial infections?

The principal defects are antibody deficiency, complement deficiency, and defective neutrophil function. Infections in patients with antibody deficiencies are most commonly due to encapsulated organisms (i.e., *Hemophilus influenzae, Pneumococcus*). Screening for antibody deficiency first includes determination of serum immunoglobulin levels (IgG, IgM, and IgA) and IgG subclass levels if subclass deficiency is suspected. Further evaluation may include serum isohemagglutinin titers (these are IgM antibodies) and measuring serum IgG antibody levels against protein (tetanus toxoid) and carbohydrate (*Pneumococcus* and/or *Hemophilus influenzae*) antigens before and after immunization in order to determine antibody response capability following specific antigen challenge.

Isolated C3 deficiency is associated with severe, recurrent pyogenic (particularly gram negative) infections. Particularly noteworthy is the association of recurrent, disseminated *Neisseria* infections with terminal complement component deficiencies (except C9). Properidin deficiency may also be accompanied by recurrent pyogenic and *Neisseria* infections. Complement defiiciency can be evaluated by obtaining a CH50 (or CH100) and by measuring levels of specific complement components when indicated.

Most defects of neutrophil function associated with recurrent infections occur in the pediatric age group. However, it is now recognized that some adults may have a variant of chronic granulomatous disease of childhood (CGD) in which the defect in respiratory burst is qualitatively less than in typical CGD. A nitroblue tetrazolium test can be performed to assess neutrophil respiratory burst in patients with a clinical history suggestive of CGD. These patients are particularly susceptible to catalase-positive organisms. Bacteria infections are typically caused by *Staphyloccocus aureus, Escherichia coli* and *Serratia marcescens* and fungal infections by *Candida albicans, Aspergillus,* and *Nocardia.*

121. A 70-year-old female patient complains of fever, headache, and jaw claudication, and has an erythrocyte sedimentation rate (ESR) of 90 mm/hour. What is the most probable diagnosis?

This presentation is highly suggestive of temporal arteritis (TA). It usually occurs in patients over the age of 50 and is more common in females. Constitutional symptoms may be the only presenting manifestations, or headaches, visual symptoms (blurring, diplopia), and claudication (such as with mastication) may occur. On physical examination, the temporal arteries may be normal, tender, or nodular, and have normal or decreased pulsations. Mild anemia and a high ESR are characteristic but not obligatory laboratory findings. The definitive diagnosis is made by temporal artery biopsy. A 1-inch segment of one or both temporal arteries should be obtained. A positive biopsy will reveal granulomatous inflammation and giant cells. However, because of the "skipped" nature of the lesions, a patient with TA may have a negative biopsy even when multiple cuts are examined. This vasculitic syndrome has a predisposition for branches of the carotid artery. The aorta and other medium to large arteries may also be involved.

A dreaded complication of TA is sudden irreversible blindness. It is usually preventable by the daily administration of corticosteroids. Therefore, if a diagnosis of TA is suspected, one should not withhold steroid therapy while awaiting a biopsy. The pathologic findings will not be altered by steroid therapy for at least 24, and probably 48 hours. Symptoms typically show dramatic improvement over several days, after which the steroid dose may be tapered to the lowest dose that will maintain clinical remission. Steroid therapy should be continued for a minimum of one, and perhaps even two years after remission is induced.

122. What causes rhinitis medicamentosa (RM) and how is it treated?

RM is caused by rebound vasodilation due to long-term use of topical vasoconstrictors (decongestants, cocaine). The nasal mucosa typically is reddened in appearance. Treatment consists of discontinuation of the offending drug and beginning therapy with topical intranasal or, for severe cases, oral corticosteroids.

123. What are the differentiating clinical and immunologic features of primary biliary cirrhosis and idiopathic sclerosing cholangitis?

Comparison of Primary Biliary Cirrhosis and Idiopathic Sclerosing Cholangitis

PARAMETER	BILIARY CIRRHOSIS	SCLEROSING CHOLANGITIS
Etiology	Unknown	Unknown
Sex	Middle-aged women	Men
HLA association	None	B8
Histology	Destructive, nonsuppurative cholangitis, cirrhosis	Fibrosis with obliteration of intra- and extrahepatic bile ducts

Table continued on next page.

Comparison of Primary Biliary Cirrhosis and Idiopathic Sclerosing Cholangitis (Cont.)

PARAMETER	BILIARY CIRRHOSIS	SCLEROSING CHOLANGITIS
Cholangiography	Normal early, cirrhosis late	Narrowing and dilatation of intra- and extrahepatic bile ducts causing "beaded appearance"
Associated diseases	CREST form of scleroderma, hypothyroidism, keratoconjunctivitis sicca	Ulcerative colitis, biliary cholangiocarcinoma
Autoantibodies	Antimitochondrial	None
Immunologic	Polyclonal hypergamma-globulinemia, particularly ↑ IgM (may be monomeric) and also ↑ IgA, anergy, ↓ NK, and T cell function	No major defects known
Treatment	Supportive, liver transplantation for end-stage disease	Supportive, liver transplantation for end-stage disease
Prognosis	Variable	Variable

↑ = increased, ↓ = decreased.

124. Name some diseases associated with elevation of the total serum IgE level.

Diseases Associated with Increased Total Serum IgE

Atopic (allergic) diseases:	**Infections:**	
Allergic rhinitis	Parasitic infections	
Allergic asthma	Viral infections (infectious mononucleosis,	
Allergic bronchopulmonary	others)	
aspergillosis	Fungal infections (candidiasis, others)	
Primary immunodeficiency disorders:	**Malignancies:**	**Acute graft-versus-host**
Hyper IgE syndrome	Hodgkin's disease	**disease**
Wiskott-Aldrich syndrome	Bronchial carcinoma	**Dermatologic disorders:**
Nezelhof's syndrome (cellular	IgE myeloma	Atopic dermatitis
immunodeficiency with Ig's)		Bullous pemphigoid
Selective IgA deficiency (with		Others
concomitant atopic disease)		

In many of these diseases, IgE levels may be normal, mildly elevated, or markedly elevated. The clinical usefulness of measurement of total serum IgE is usually limited to diagnosis and monitoring of exacerbations, remissions, and/or treatment of allergic bronchopulmonary aspergillosis, parasitic infections, and immunodeficiency disorders.

BIBLIOGRAPHY

1. Klein J: Immunology. Oxford, Blackwell Scientific Publications, 1990.
2. Middleton E, et al (eds): Allergy: Principles and Practice, 3rd ed. St. Louis, C.V. Mosby, 1988.
3. Paul WE (ed): Fundamental Immunology, 2nd ed. New York, Raven Press, 1989.
4. Roitt IM, et al: Immunology, 2nd ed. Philadelphia, J.B. Lippincott, 1990.
5. Rubenstein E, Federman D (eds): Scientific American Medicine. New York, Scientific American, Inc. 1990.
6. Samter M, et al (eds): Immunological Diseases, 4th ed. Boston, Little, Brown, 1988.
7. Wyngaarden JB, Smith LH (eds): Cecil Textbook of Medicine, 18th ed. Philadelphia, W.B. Saunders, 1988.

13. AIDS AND HIV SECRETS

Christopher J. Lahart, M.D.

Dr. Rieux resolved to compile this chronicle . . . to state quite
simply what we learn in a time of pestilence: that there are more
things to admire in men than to despise.
                                                        Albert Camus
                              The Plague, Pt. V, tr. by Stuart Gilbert

***Virus**, L (akin to Sanskrit* visha *poison and Greek* ios *poison,*
esp. of serpents), a slimy or poisonous liquid, poison, venom.
                    Churchill's Illustrated Medical Dictionary, 1989.

GENERAL

1. In which family of viruses is the human immunodeficiency virus (HIV)?

The HIV is a retrovirus in the Retroviridae family. A retrovirus is an RNA virus that contains an enzyme, reverse transcriptase, which is capable of transcribing DNA from the viral RNA. This is the reverse of normal DNA to RNA transcription, hence the name.

2. My patient is HIV positive. Does he have AIDS?

Probably not. There is no simple test for AIDS (the acquired immune deficiency syndrome). A positive HIV test indicates infection with the HIV virus, but HIV infection is a wide spectrum of illness, and the vast majority of HIV-positive patients are asymptomatic. AIDS is a syndrome of explicitly defined conditions that represent severe immuno-suppression and is the final band in this spectrum of illness. A diagnosis of AIDS is usually made when a person with evidence of HIV infection develops a malignancy, opportunistic infection, or other symptomatic illness that meets the diagnostic criteria for AIDS.

To prematurely inform a patient that he or she has AIDS is to inappropriately set in motion a wide range of psychological, social, and medical processes, some of which may result in relatively adverse complications. When your patient has tested positive for infection by HIV, a comprehensive history and physical examination need to be performed in an attempt to iden-tify symptoms and signs of immunosuppression and any co-morbid conditions. In addition, laboratory examination can help place your patient in a relative position in the spectrum.

3. Why are HIV-ELISA tests confirmed by Western blot?

For a variety of reasons there can be a significant number of false-positive tests for the presence of antibodies to HIV using the ELISA (enzyme-linked immunosorbent assay). Due to the obvious need for proper diagnosis, most laboratories will repeat a positive ELISA. A repe-titively positive result should then be confirmed by Western blot to verify that the positive ELISA result is based upon true HIV antibodies and not some cross-reacting proteins. In *low-risk* populations, as many as 29 of every 30 positive ELISAs will be false positives. There-fore, across-the-board screening of such low-risk populations is not indicated at this time.

Meyer KB, Pauker SG: Screening for HIV: Can we afford the false positive rate? N Engl J Med 317(4):238–241, 1987.

4. Who should be tested for HIV?

A clinician should recommend HIV testing for any patient with a high index of suspicion for HIV infection. Early epidemiologic investigations and further refinements suggest that the following groups should be tested:

Gay or bisexual males	Patients in tuberculosis (TB) clinics
Intravenous (IV) drug users	Persons who received blood products from 1978 to 1985
Prostitutes	Anyone having sex with a member of a high-risk group.
Patients in STD clinics	

5. What is the follow-up for an "indeterminate" Western blot?

Assuming that your patient had an initial ELISA test repeatedly positive prior to the indeterminate Western blot, the Western blot should be repeated. If indeterminate again, both the ELISA and Western blot should be repeated in 3 months.

6. What are the diagnostic criteria for AIDS?

The diagnosis of AIDS depends on the status of the patient's laboratory evidence for or against HIV infection:

  1. **For patients with laboratory evidence for HIV infection**, a diagnosis of AIDS can be made if the patient has a presumptive or definitive diagnosis of one or more of a list of "indicator diseases."

  2. **For patients without laboratory evidence for HIV infection**, a diagnosis of AIDS can be made if there is no other cause for an underlying immunodeficiency state and the patient has a definitive diagnosis of one or more of a list of "indicator diseases."

  3. **For patients with laboratory evidence against HIV infection**, a diagnosis of AIDS can still be made if the patient has had a definitive diagnosis of *Pneumocystis carinii* pneumonia (PCP) or has a definitive diagnosis of one or more of a list of "indicator diseases" with a helper T-lymphocyte count of <400 cells/mm^3.

  (NOTE: The list of "indicator diseases" is different for each group. See reference for complete details.)

  CDC: Revision of the CDC Surveillance Criteria for AIDS. MMWR 36(Suppl):1987.

7. How much time elapses between infection with HIV and the diagnosis of AIDS?

This period is not easily defined. Studies of large patient cohorts indicate that 50% of HIV-positive patients will progress to AIDS in approximately 10 years. The 90% mark may be 13 years, but this is not currently confirmed. The rate of disease progression is not stable over this period, since few develop disease early on.

  Litson AR, et al: The natural history of human immunodeficiency virus infection. J Infect Dis 158:1360–1367, 1988.

8. What is ARC?

ARC is an eponym for AIDS-related complex. This is a term used to describe patients symptomatic with HIV infection (e.g., with oral candidiasis) but not yet diagnosed with an AIDS-defining condition. There is no clear-cut or generally accepted definition for this term, and it is no longer in common use.

9. What is a T4-lymphocyte count and why is it obtained?

A T4-lymphocyte count is a laboratory measurement of the number of T4, or CD4$^+$, or helper-inducer lymphocytes present in peripheral blood. Since very early in the HIV epidemic, it has been known that one of the most problematic effects of HIV infection is the depletion of these T4-lymphocytes. By measuring these cells, a clinician can attempt to place a patient in a general position on the spectrum of HIV-related illness. The T4 lymphocyte count is also used to determine the timing of various interventions, such as zidovudine therapy or prophylaxis against *Pneumocystis carinii* pneumonia. Thus it is of prognostic and therapeutic value.

10. Are any other laboratory tests of prognostic value?

The T4 lymphocyte count appears to be the best single indicator of prognosis. However, there may be some benefit obtained by also examining the serum level of beta-2 microglobulin or neopterin. Beta-2 microglobulin is a marker of generalized lymphoid activity, and high levels reflect a poorer prognosis. Neopterin is produced by T-cell-stimulated macrophages, and elevated levels are associated with disease progression.

However, there is no widely accepted serologic staging system, and experience with many of these tests is extremely limited.

11. What is the prognosis of HIV-1 infected patients?

In a review of 32 follow-up studies, Cooper and Jeffers reported the following:
- From the time of seroconversion, 10 to 20% of HIV-infected individuals will progress to AIDS after 3 to 6 years of follow-up.
- Once the patient has constitutional symptoms (such as fevers, night sweats, weight loss), herpes zoster, thrush, or lowered T4 (CD4$^+$) cell counts, there is more than a 40% chance of progressing to AIDS after 3 years of follow-up and more than a 50% chance after 5 years.

These data are from *untreated* patients. Recent studies show that the patient's prognosis can be modified by anti-retroviral therapy and general medical support.

Cooper GS, Jeffers DJ: The clinical prognosis of HIV-1 infection: A review of 32 follow-up studies. J Gen Intern Med 3:525–532, 1988.

12. Is AIDS invariably fatal?

Presently there is no final answer to this question. Certainly a large majority of patients with AIDS die, but it is not yet clear whether all will die from this disease. Figures obtained through nationwide reporting to the Centers for Disease Control reveal approximately 30% mortality 1 year after a diagnosis of AIDS, over 50% at 2 years, and over 75% at 3 years.

13. What is thrush?

Thrush is oropharyngeal pseudomembranous candidiasis that often presages AIDS. It most often presents as white plaques ("pseudomembranes") seen on any oral mucosal surface. There may be scattered small plaques or larger sheets of candidiasis. Significant oral pain may be present along with altered taste. The diagnosis can be made clinically, with potassium hydroxide smear examination, or by culture.

14. How is oral thrush treated?

Treatment can take any number of different courses depending on the extent of involvement and the patient's clinical condition.

Treatment of Oral Thrush

Limited involvement:	Extensive involvement:
Improved oral hygiene with peroxide rinses	Ketoconazole
Nystatin oral suspension	200 mg p.o. QD
Nystatin vaginal tablets—used orally	Fluconazole*
Clotrimazole tablets	50–100 mg p.o. QD

* FDA approved its use in early 1990.

It should be noted that thrush often indicates significant immune suppression and evaluation should begin for other HIV-related medical interventions, such as prophylaxis for PCP.

15. What are some common dermatologic conditions in HIV infection?

Besides Kaposi's sarcoma (KS), there is a multitude of skin findings including seborrheic dermatitis, psoriasis, and ichthyosis. Fungal infections such as candidiasis and tinea are common. Rarely, cryptococcus and histoplasma are seen. Viral infections with herpes simplex type 2, varicella zoster, molluscum contagiosum, and condylomata acuminata are common. Rashes due to syphilis must also be considered in these high-risk patients.

16. What are the recognized rheumatic conditions known to occur in HIV-positive patients?
As further advances are made in the treatment of HIV disease, the history of infection likewise changes. More and more frequently rheumatic manifestations of disease are becoming apparent. Patients are found to have inflammatory myopathy, Reiter's syndrome, and psoriasis. Additionally, cases of Sjögren's syndrome and vasculitis have been described, and patients with HIV infection sometimes develop an oligoarticular arthritis of severe proportions and variable duration. NSAIDs do not seem helpful. Also described are painful arthralgias of short duration that often require narcotics for relief. In addition to a variety of clinical syndromes, lab evaluations often reveal low titers of rheumatoid factors, antinuclear antibodies, and anticardiolipin antibodies. Generalized hypergammaglobulinemia is reported.

Calabrese LH: The rheumatic manifestation of infection with the human immunodeficiency virus. Sem Arthritis Rheum 18(4):225–239, 1989.

17. Do HIV-infected patients respond to the influenza vaccine?
Administration of the influenza vaccine is recommended for all persons infected with the HIV. Although the vaccine is safe in these patients, the antibody response to the vaccine has been shown to be lower than in non-HIV-infected controls. It has been shown that a two-dose regimen is not superior in efficacy to the traditional single-dose regimen.

Miotti PG, et al: The influence of HIV infection on antibody responses to a two-dose regimen of influenza vaccine. JAMA 262:779–783, 1989.

18. Do HIV-infected patients respond to the pneumococcal polysaccharide vaccine?
HIV-infected patients who are asymptomatic or have persistent generalized lymphadenopathy have been shown to respond to the vaccine. Patients with AIDS have been shown to have an impaired response to the vaccine. However, it is recommended that all HIV-infected individuals, regardless of the stage of their disease, receive the vaccine.

ACIP: Pneumococcal polysaccharide vaccine. MMWR 38(5):64–76, 1989.

19. Are heterosexuals at risk for HIV infection?
Most certainly. Although heterosexual contact does not appear to be an efficient transmitter of infection, it clearly does occur. In many developing countries the *equal* incidence of AIDS in both males and females provides evidence for this. As of September 1990, in the U.S., 2% of AIDS cases in males (2993 cases) and 32% of female cases (4425) were attributed to heterosexual contact. About 50% of the cases of heterosexually acquired AIDS resulted from sexual contact with an intravenous drug user.

20. How long is someone with HIV infectious?
It is thought that a person is infectious for life. There may be periods of increased infectiousness, but there is never a period of absolute noninfectiousness. This highlights the importance of changing high-risk behavior patterns. Such change must be consistent and permanent.

21. What is AIDS dementia complex?
Patients with AIDS may develop cognitive, behavioral, and motor dysfunction in the course of their illness. Although multiple opportunistic infections need to be ruled out (cryptococcus, toxoplasma, TB, etc.), direct CNS infection by HIV causes this complex of signs and symptoms. Early in its development, neuropsychologic testing may be needed to support a clinical suspicion. However, the dementia may progress to a vegetative state. Patients may first complain of concentration difficulties, and family and friends may note personality changes. A thorough neurologic evaluation and investigation into other causes are needed. There is some evidence that zidovudine is helpful in treatment of this dementia.

Navia BA, et al: The AIDS dementia complex: I. Clinical features. Ann Neurol 19:517–524, 1986.

22. Do neurologic conditions in AIDS only appear late in the course of the disease?

Not necessarily. Neurologic signs and symptoms may be the earliest manifestations of HIV infection in some patients. The most frequent cause of neurologic abnormality is subacute encephalitis.

Harter DH, Petersdorf RG: Viral diseases of the nervous system: Aseptic meningitis and encephalitis. In Wilson JD, et al: Harrison's Principles of Internal Medicine. New York, McGraw-Hill, 1991, p 2036.

23. What is HIV wasting syndrome?

This is an AIDS-defining diagnosis that includes profound weight loss of greater than 10% of body weight, with either chronic diarrhea or weakness and fever present for over 30 days. These clinical events should be evaluated for other HIV-related illnesses and, in the absence of other etiologies, a diagnosis of wasting can be made.

24. What is the risk of HIV transmission via a needle stick?

The average risk of transmission in a large group of health care workers having percutaneous exposure was one in 250 exposures, or 0.4%. However, each exposure needs to be evaluated individually. There is tremendous variation in the degree of exposure, and the likelihood of seroconversion will depend on the significance of the exposure.

Mosus R, et al: Surveillance of health-care workers exposed to blood from patients infected with the human immunodeficiency virus. N Engl J Med 319:1118–1123, 1988.

25. What variables may increase the risk of occupational exposure?

Exposure to a large volume of infectious material (or material with a high viral load), prolonged contact with the infectious material, and the body area (or portal of entry) are all important factors. Mucosal splashes and exposure on intact skin are rare routes of transmission (no transmission in over 12,500 exposures followed prospectively). Associated with increased risk are intramuscular (IM) injection, exposures via hollow needles (as opposed to suture needles, pins, etc.), and exposure to material from a viremic HIV-positive patient.

26. Does postexposure zidovudine therapy prevent transmission?

This is currently unknown. However, due to the overriding concern for the protection of exposed health care workers, this therapy is coming into general use. Drug therapy must be part of a well thought out program that includes immediate availability of counseling as well as medication. Close follow-up needs to be provided and confidentiality guaranteed.

Pneumocystis carinii INFECTION

27. What is "PCP"?

PCP stands for *Pneumocystis carinii* pneumomia. Prior to routine prophylactic treatments, this infection was the presenting diagnosis in 60% of patients with AIDS and eventually was seen in over 80% of patients with AIDS at some time during their illness. During discussions of AIDS-related conditions, you may hear someone mention extrapulmonary or disseminated pneumocystis infection and use a phrase similar to ". . . and PCP was identified in the bone marrow." This clearly is a misnomer, because it is difficult to have pneumonia in the marrow. The comment refers to *Pneumocystis carinii* infection elsewhere in the body and not pneumonia.

Glatt AE, Chirgwin K: *Pneumocystis carinii* pneumonia in human immunodeficiency virus-infected patients. Arch Intern Med 150:271–279, 1990.

28. How does PCP present?

Cough, fever, and dyspnea are the most common presenting symptoms. The cough is usually nonproductive or productive of only scant whitish sputum. Patients may also relate a sensation of chest tightness or an inability to take a full, deep inspiration. Other less common complaints include nonspecific weight loss, night sweats, and malaise. Findings on physical examination include fever, tachypnea, persistent cough, and dry rales. Rarely a patient may endure symptoms at home long enough to present with cyanosis. Laboratory findings include hypoxemia with an elevated alveolar-arterial oxygen gradient (A-a gradient). An elevated serum lactate dehydrogenase (LDH) can also be a finding.

29. What are the chest x-ray findings in PCP?

Typically seen is a diffuse, bilateral interstitial infiltrate, often more pronounced in the hilar region (butterfly distribution). Areas of local consolidation are less common, as are cystic and cavitary changes. Normal chest x-rays are also seen, especially in those patients presenting early in the illness. Pleural effusion is a rare finding and, if present, should raise the suspicion of another diagnosis.

30. How is PCP diagnosed?

Diagnosis of PCP requires pathologic demonstration of the organism. Since the lung is the most commonly involved organ, it is from here the specimens must be obtained. Several centers have reported success with examination of induced sputum. Although the expertise required may limit the technique to experienced centers, this is an inexpensive, noninvasive way to attempt to make the diagnosis. Most centers rely upon bronchoscopic examination with bronchoalveolar lavage (BAL). Lavage alone has a sensitivity around 95%; thus most bronchoscopists do not perform transbronchial biopsy during the initial procedure, withholding biopsy for those cases not diagnosed by BAL. Open lung biopsy is rarely needed. A diagnostic algorithm follows:

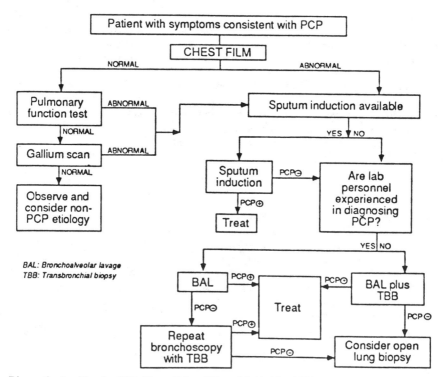

Diagnostic algorithm for PCP. (From Cohen PT, et al (eds): The AIDS Knowledge Base. Waltham, MA, The Medical Publishing Group, 1990, Fig. 6.5.3.a, with permission.)

31. How is PCP treated?

Conventional treatment comes down to a choice between two agents: trimethoprim-sulfamethoxazole (TMP-SMX) or pentamidine isethionate. These agents seem to be equally effective but differ in the routes of administration. Both are available for intravenous use, TMP-SMX three-to-four times daily and pentamidine once daily. TMP-SMX can also be administered orally, making outpatient therapy much more convenient. Much work is being done to evaluate the role of inhaled pentamidine in the acute treatment of PCP. The usual daily dose of TMP-SMX is 20 mg/kg of trimethoprim and 100 mg/kg of sulfamethoxazole in divided doses. It appears that a lower dose (15 mg/kg and 75 mg/kg) may be equally effective with fewer side-effects. Pentamidine is usually given at a dose of 4 mg/kg once a day. There is also evidence that a dose of 3 mg/kg once a day is effective in mild pneumonias.

Duration of therapy is usually 21 days, but some practitioners are moving to a 14-day acute treatment with immediate institution of prophylaxis.

32. What are the expected side-effects of treatment of PCP?

Side-effects in patients with AIDS treated with TMP-SMX greatly increase in incidence over non-AIDS patients. While the drug is very well tolerated in non-AIDS patients, side-effects occur in a range of 65–100% of patients with AIDS. Most commonly reported are rash, hepatitis, GI upset, anemia, and neutropenia. Severe rash and neutropenia often cause termination of therapy and both are reversible with drug cessation.

Pentamidine was formerly administered via IM injection; however, the incidence of sterile abscess is frequent enough to relegate this to unfavored status. Progressive renal insufficiency and pancreatitis with dysglycemias are the most serious side-effects of pentamidine infusion. Toxicity to pancreatic islet cells can occur, and acute hypoglycemia or chronic hyperglycemia can result. Thus, a finger-stick glucose level, followed with 50% dextrose in water (D50W) administration should be considered in disoriented PCP patients receiving pentamidine. Altered mental status may not always be due to hypoxemia.

33. Who should receive prophylaxis for PCP?

Prophylaxis is recommended for any patient who has already had an episode of PCP (secondary prophylaxis) or for any HIV-seropositive patient with CD4 lymphocyte count less than 200/mm^3 or CD4 lymphocytes less than 20% of total lymphocytes, regardless of previous PCP history (primary prophylaxis). In patients with thrush or fever, prophylaxis may be considered with a CD4 count above 200.

    1. Centers for Disease Control. MMWR 38(Suppl 5):1, 1989.

    2. Phair J, et al: The risk of *Pneumocystis carinii* pneumonia among men with human immunodeficiency virus type I. N Engl J Med 322:161–165, 1990.

34. What is the proper prophylaxis for PCP?

Although multiple agents are being investigated for use in PCP prophylaxis, the same two drugs used for treatment, TMP-SMX and pentamidine, remain the standards for prophylactic regimens. The dose of TMP-SMX most commonly employed to date has been TMP 160 mg/SMX 800 mg twice daily (one double-strength tablet bid). Side-effects are similar in nature to those seen in PCP treatment but are less common. Many clinicians are decreasing the dose by 50% (one double-strength tablet qd) in an attempt to decrease the incidence of side-effects while preserving efficacy. Early reports are favorable.

For prophylaxis, pentamidine can be administered as inhalation therapy. Given once a month, 300 mg of pentamidine via a nebulizer is effective. Side-effects are limited to transient taste alterations and coughing or wheezing. The coughing and wheezing, not seen in most patients, can be minimized by pretreatment with inhaled bronchodilators. Patients must be evaluated for active TB prior to starting this therapy.

While TMP-SMX appear virtually 100% effective in those who can tolerate the side-effects, pentamidine has a 5–10% failure rate per year. However, failure means episodes of PCP that may be mild and may appear atypical, with mostly peripheral or apical involvement.

35. Has aerosolized pentamidine changed the presentation of PCP?

Yes. Since this type of prophylaxis is not 100% effective, there are new episodes of PCP occurring during therapy. These episodes may present with an atypical radiographic appearance, weighted more toward upper-lobe infiltrates as opposed to the traditional diffuse interstitial infiltrates. In addition, the yield of bronchoscopy and BAL for pathologic diagnosis is decreased. However, the severity of the disease appears unchanged.

Jules-Elysee KM, et al: Aerosolized pentamidine: Effect on diagnosis and presentation of *Pneumocystis carinii* pneumonia. Ann Intern Med 112:750–757, 1990.

36. Should PCP patients be intubated?

The answer to this question is obviously individualized according to a patient's previously expressed desires and the clinical setting of respiratory failure. One group of patients who may benefit from mechanical ventilation has been identified. These patients have a shorter duration of symptoms of PCP, a precipitous decline of respiratory status postbronchoscopy, and better arterial oxygenation on admission ($PO_2 \geq 60$).

El-Sadr W, Simberkoff MS: Survival and prognostic factors in severe *Pneumocystis carinii* pneumonia requiring mechanical ventilation. Am Rev Respir Dis 137:1264–1267, 1988.

37. Should steroids be used as therapy for PCP?

In November 1990 the recommendations of a consensus conference convened by the National Institute of Allergy and Infectious Diseases and the University of California were published in conjunction with two major clinical trials addressing this question.[1] Prior to this, such treatment had been strongly debated due to potential adverse outcomes. The recommendations suggest that, in addition to specific anti-pneumocystis therapy, adjunctive corticosteroid therapy should be administered to patients with known or suspected HIV-related PCP if on room air there is moderate or severe pulmonary impairment as evidenced by an arterial PO_2 less than 70 mmHg or an alveolar-arterial oxygen gradient ($A-aO_2$ gradient) greater than 35 mmHg. Such adjunctive therapy should be initiated at the same time as specific anti-PCP therapy, since a delay seems to diminish its benefit.

The regimen recommended is that which was used in the largest study group with the most important endpoints.[2] On days 1 through 5, oral prednisone is given at a dose of 40 mg twice a day. This is followed by prednisone, 40 mg once a day on days 6 through 10, and 20 mg once a day on days 11 through 21. This regimen is but one of several that have been studied. The optimal steroidal agent, route of administration, dose, and frequency have not been determined.

Due to potential complications of steroid therapy when used in patients in whom pneumocystis is not the sole pulmonary pathogen, diagnostic testing for the presence of other agents (*Mycobacterium tuberculosis, Cryptococcus neoformans, Histoplasma capsulatum* and others) or other processes (Kaposi's sarcoma) should be performed.

1. Consensus Statement on the Use of Corticosteroids as Adjunctive Therapy for Pneumocystis Pneumonia in the Acquired Immunodeficiency Syndrome. N Engl J Med 323:1500–1504, 1990.

2. Bozzette SA, et al: A controlled trial of early adjunctive treatment with corticosteroids for *Pneumocystis carinii* pneumonia in the acquired immunodeficiency syndrome. New Engl J Med 323:1451–1456, 1990.

38. What is extrapulmonary pneumocystosis?

Multiple reports of extrapulmonary pneumocystosis have been published covering anatomical sites literally from head (otitis) to foot (vasculitis). The underlying theme appears to be the use of nonsystemic (i.e., inhaled) pentamidine therapy for prophylaxis for PCP. As more cases are reported, this could become a larger cause for concern.

Telzak EE, et al: Extrapulmonary *Pneumocystis carinii* infections. Rev Infect Dis 12:380–386, 1990.

39. Is the incidence of pneumothorax increased in pentamidine inhalation?

This question arose when patients enrolled in community trials of inhaled pentamidine had several episodes of pneumothorax. It appears that these episodes were related to recurrent episodes of PCP and not to the use of inhalation therapy.

TREATMENT OF HIV INFECTION

40. What drugs are currently available to treat HIV infection?

To date only one antiviral agent is available for general use. This is zidovudine (Retrovir, formerly known as azidothymidine, or AZT). This drug first became available for general use in 1986, following early termination of its phase-II placebo-controlled trial.

In late 1989 a second agent, didanosine (Videx, DDI), became available through the FDA's new parallel track program. By registering with its manufacturer, a physician may obtain DDI on a compassionate use basis for patients not able to take zidovudine. Also recently available through the manufacturer (effective mid-1990) is a third drug, dideoxy-cytidine (DDC).

Fischl MA, et al: The efficacy of azidothymidine in the treatment of patients with AIDS and AIDS-related complex. N Engl J Med 317:185–191, 1987.

41. How does zidovudine work?

Zidovudine acts as an inhibitor of viral reverse transcriptase. Zidovudine is a thymidine analog that becomes phosphorylated to a triphosphate form and interferes with viral replication, causing DNA chain termination.

42. What is the proper dose of zidovudine?

The optimal does has not been established at this time, and current dosing recommendations have arisen from several sources. For symptomatic HIV infection with an initial T4-lymphocyte count less than 200, 200 mg every 4 hours (1200 mg per day) is given for the initial month, followed by 100 mg every 4 hours (600 mg per day). In asymptomatic infection with a T4-lymphocyte count less than 500, the dose is 100 mg every 4 hours while awake (500 mg per day). Thus, at any one time a practitioner may have patients on three different dosing regimens of zidovudine.

In practice, most clinicians would now begin therapy at the 500 mg per day dose while awaiting completion of other dosing studies.

43. What are the side-effects seen in zidovudine treatment?

Subjective symptoms on higher dose zidovudine (1200 mg per day or more) include nausea, myalgia, and insomnia. Although headache, diarrhea, fever, and abdominal pain are also often noted, in a placebo-controlled study these were not seen more frequently in the zidovudine group. At the lower-dose zidovudine regimens (500–600 mg per day), only nausea was seen more frequently in zidovudine-treated patients when compared to placebo-treated patients.

Marked hematologic toxicity is seen in symptomatic HIV-infected patients treated with high-dose zidovudine. Anemia and/or granulocytopenia is seen in approximately half the patients. Lower-dose therapy in less-ill patients greatly minimized this toxicity, with only 1% of patients experiencing anemia with hemoglobin levels less than 8 g/dl and less than 2% developing granulocytopenia. No other clinical or chemical toxicity is frequently seen, although a zidovudine-related myositis can occur in rare instances.

Rickman DD, et al: The toxicity of azidothymidine in the treatment of patients with AIDS and AIDS-related complex. N Engl J Med 317:192–197, 1987.

Volberding PA, et al: Zidovudine in asymptomatic human immunodeficiency virus infection. N Engl J Med 322:941–949, 1990.

44. Does viral resistance to zidovudine develop?

There is early evidence that the HIV can develop decreased sensitivity to zidovudine. Clinical correlation with these laboratory findings is, as of yet, not known.

Larder BA, et al: HIV with reduced sensitivity to zidovudine isolated during prolonged therapy. Science 243:1731–1734, 1989.

45. How long does zidovudine work?

The answer to this question is unknown. In more advanced HIV infection, higher-dose zidovudine has been shown to continue to convey a survival advantage to those taking it over a 21-month period.

Creagh-Kirk T, et al: Survival experience among patients with AIDS receiving zidovudine. JAMA 260:3009–3015, 1988.

Fischl MA, et al: Prolonged zidovudine therapy in patients with AIDS and advanced AIDS-related complex. JAMA 262:2405–2410, 1989.

46. For whom is zidovudine recommended?

The most recent guidelines for prescribing zidovudine suggest use of this drug for HIV-infected individuals with a T4-lymphocyte count less than 500. This is an expansion of its previous indication, which was for use in symptomatic HIV infection with a T4-lymphocyte count less than 200 or a previous history of PCP. In those patients with a T4 count less than 200 or prior PCP, zidovudine has been shown to prolong life. In less ill patients with T4 counts between 200 and 500 zidovudine has been shown to delay the onset of HIV-related symptoms and AIDS-defining diagnoses. No improvement in survival has been demonstrated in this patient group. Study populations for these clinical trials have been predominantly comprised of white homosexual males. The generalization of these findings across race, risk group, or sex has not been verified. In fact, a study recently completed (but not yet published at the time of this writing) by the Veterans Affairs Cooperative Studies Program showed little or no benefit to zidovudine therapy in African-American or Hispanic-American males.

National Institute of Allergy and Infectious Diseases: Recommendations for zidovudine: Early infection. JAMA 263:1606–1609, 1990.

Volberding PA, et al: Zidovudine in asymptomatic human immunodeficiency viral infection. N Engl J Med 322:941–949, 1990.

47. What alternatives exist if a patient can't take zidovudine?

Patients who are intolerant of zidovudine or who have progression of their HIV disease while taking zidovudine are eligible to receive didanosine (Videx) therapy on a compassionate basis. A physician must register with the drug's manufacturer and request the drug on a case-by-case basis. Dideoxycytidine (DDC) is also available through a similar compassionate-use protocol.

48. Does a patient need PCP prophylaxis even though he is on zidovudine?

Yes. In patients with advanced HIV infection on zidovudine, but not on PCP prophylaxis, approximately half of the opportunistic infections observed were PCP. Therefore, it is recommended that patients on zidovudine also be given PCP prophylaxis if they meet the criteria discussed above.

49. What about taking acetaminophen with zidovudine?

With high-dose zidovudine therapy, the risk of granulocytopenia is increased in those taking acetaminophen and this risk increases with duration of therapy. There has been no further evidence of combined toxicity, and moderate acetaminophen use with lower dose zidovudine need not be avoided.

CRYPTOCOCCAL INFECTION

50. How often does cryptococcus cause infection in AIDS?

Depending upon which series is examined, cryptococcus may cause 5–10% of the AIDS-defining opportunistic infections. Additional patients will develop cryptococcal infections following a previous AIDS diagnosis, so an overall estimate is between 8 and 15%.

51. How does cryptococcal infection present?

Meningitis is the most common presentation of cryptococcal infection in AIDS. Extraneural disease is frequently seen with meningitis but is much less common in the absence of meningitis. Meningismus is present in only 25–30% of patients with meningitis, but fever and headache are seen in 80–90%. Focal neurologic symptoms or signs are seen in a small minority.

Features of Meningeal Cryptococcosis in 89 Patients

FEATURE			NO. (%)
*P. carinii**			12 (13%)
Cryptococcosis as initial manifestation of AIDS			40 (45%)
Symptoms			
Fever	58 (65%)	Altered mentation	25 (28%)
Malaise	68 (76%)	Focal deficits	5 (6%)
Headaches	65 (73%)	Seizures	4 (4%)
Stiff neck	20 (22%)	Cough or dyspnea	28 (31%)
Nausea or vomiting	37 (42%)	Diarrhea	19 (21%)
Photophobia	16 (18%)		
Signs			
Temperature	50 (56%)	Altered mentation	15 (17%)
Meningeal signs	24 (27%)	Focal deficits	13 (15%)

*Concurrent pneumonia due to *P. carinii.*
(From Chuck SL, Sanda MA: Infections with *Cryptococcus neoformans* in AIDS. N Engl J Med 321:795, 1989, with permission.)

52. Which patients with cryptococcosis need a lumbar puncture (LP)?

Any and all patients with a culture positive for cryptococcus or a serum antigen titer positive need an LP performed. This is irrespective of which site originally yielded the positive specimen. In any HIV-infected patient with an undiagnosed fever and/or headache, an LP should be considered to examine specifically the possibility of cryptococcal disease.

53. How often should an LP be done?

An LP is performed at the time of diagnosis of cryptococcal infection. If indicative of meningitis and the patient is clinically responding to therapy, an LP should be performed approximately 1 week into therapy to help evaluate microbial response. Subsequent LP examinations should be performed as clinically indicated or until adequate microbial response is documented. If response is poor, weekly LPs may be needed to guide therapy.

54. What cerebrospinal fluid (CSF) findings are seen in cryptococcal meningitis?

From three large series describing cryptococcosis in AIDS, the following table can be constructed for the patients with a diagnosis of meningitis:

CSF Findings in AIDS-related Cryptococcal Meningitis

	NO. WITH FINDING/NO. TESTED	%		NO. WITH FINDING/NO. TESTED	%
WBC <20 cells/L	96/128	75	Positive India ink	92/125	74
Glucose >40 mg/dl	87/127	68	Positive CSF	116/126	92
Protein <45 mg/dl	53/127	42	antigen		

As you can see from the data, the CSF can appear remarkably normal. However, you should always perform an India ink test, since this is usually positive and can yield an immediate diagnosis without waiting for other laboratory results.

Kovacs JA, et al: Cryptococcosis in the acquired immunodeficiency syndrome. Ann Intern Med 103:533–538, 1985.

Zugar A, et al: Cryptococcal disease in patients with the acquired immunodeficiency syndrome. Ann Intern Med 104:234–240, 1986.

Chuck SL, Sande MA: Infections with *Cryptococcus neoformans* in the acquired immunodeficiency syndrome. N Engl J Med 321:794–799, 1989.

55. What is proper treatment for cryptococcosis in AIDS?

No one therapeutic regimen has been evaluated specifically for patients with AIDS. Much of what has been published is based on case series reporting experience using standard regimens from the pre-AIDS era adapted for cryptococcosis in AIDS. Until recently there were few options. The only therapeutic question was whether to add flucytosine to amphotericin B therapy. In early 1990, the FDA approved the use of fluconazole, an oral triazole derivative for use in AIDS-related cryptococcosis. The National Institute of Allergy and Infectious Diseases (AIDS Clinical Trial Units) and the Mycoses Study Group have an ongoing trial comparing amphotericin B to fluconazole in patients with AIDS. For the time being, most practitioners would advise a short induction course of amphotericin B (0.4–0.6 mg/kg/day) over 14 days followed by oral fluconazole therapy if response has been judged adequate.

Larsen RA, et al: Fluconazole compared with amphotericin B plus flucytosine for cryptococcal meningitis in AIDS. Ann Intern Med 113:183–187, 1990.

56. Is maintenance anticryptococcal therapy needed?

The reports of cryptococcal infection in AIDS suggest a high relapse rate following primary therapy and a high mortality rate during relapse. Because of this combination of observations, the standard of care has been to give chronic maintenance, or suppressive therapy. This has been accomplished in a variety of ways. Intermittent infusions of amphotericin B as well as oral ketoconazole or fluconazole have been used. Should the early promise of fluconazole be borne out, this will be the agent of choice. For now all patients with AIDS and cryptococcal infection should be continued on maintenance therapy. Since no therapy has been shown completely successful, the use of the least toxic, least invasive agent should be considered.

Zugar A, et al: Maintenance amphotericin B for cryptococcal meningitis in the acquired immunodeficiency syndrome. Ann Intern Med 109:592–593, 1988.

Sugar AM, Saunders C: Oral fluconazole as suppressive therapy of disseminated cryptococcosis in patients with acquired immunodeficiency syndrome. Am J Med 85:481–489, 1988.

57. Are serum cryptococcal antigen levels good indicators of response to therapy?

No. Although the serum antigen test can be very helpful in the diagnosis of cryptococcal infection, it can't be used to judge therapeutic response. In most cases of meningitis, the CSF antigen titer should be determined by repeat lumbar puncture.

Eng RK, et al: Cryptococcal infections in patients with acquired immune deficiency syndrome. Am J Med 81:19–23, 1986.

58. How is a relapse of cryptococcal infection treated?

Depending upon the patient's previous therapeutic course and compliance with maintenance therapy, relapse should be treated with a re-induction regimen of amphotericin B.

59. What are the prognostic indicators in AIDS-related cryptococcosis?

In 1974, Diamond and Bennett described multiple prognostic factors in non-AIDS cryptococcal meningitis. Several of the reports of AIDS-related cryptococcosis have attempted to define similar factors in that illness but for the most part have been unsuccessful. The following table compares some of these findings:

Prognostic Factors Indicating Poor Response in Cryptococcosis

STUDY	PATIENTS	POOR PROGNOSTIC INDICATORS
Diamond (1974)	111	India ink +; high opening pressure; low CSF glucose; CSF WBC < 20; extra-CSF site of infection.
Kovacs (1985)	27	No reliable factor identified.
Zugar (1986)	34	India ink +; pre-treatment CSF antigen ≥ 1:10,000; posttreatment antigen ≥ 1:8.
Chuck (1989)	89	Hyponatremia, extra CSF site of infection.

It is difficult to directly compare these reports due to their differing study populations and intentions. However, it can be appreciated that cryptococcal disease, in patients with AIDS, is a less predictable illness than in non-AIDS patients. In AIDS patients, adequate response to anticryptococcal therapy is frequently disturbed by the development of new adverse clinical events related to the underlying HIV infection.

Diamond RD, Bennett JE: Prognostic factors in cryptococcal meningitis. A study of 111 cases. Ann Intern Med 80:176–181, 1974.

KAPOSI'S SARCOMA (KS)

60. What does Kaposi's sarcoma (KS) look like?
KS in HIV-infected patients is most often seen as cutaneous or oropharyngeal nodules. The nodules usually range in size from 0.5 to 2.0 cm in diameter, although multiple nodules may coalesce and form a large plaque. These nodules are most often raised and readily palpable, painless and nonpruritic, and have no evidence of inflammation or exudate. Rarely, lesions may become friable or verrucous-like (warty) and weep or bleed with trauma. The lesions are usually blue or violet-to-purple in color and in darker-skinned patients they often appear black. These nodules are usually multiple when first diagnosed, reflecting the rather aggressive nature of this malignancy in HIV infection. Any area of the body may be involved, although the palms of the hands are rarely affected despite more common involvement of the soles of the feet.

61. Does a lesion suspicious for KS need to be biopsied?
In general, yes. If a patient with HIV infection has no previous diagnosis of KS or any opportunistic infection, these suspicious lesions should be uniformly biopsied to establish such a diagnosis. In the instance of a patient who has had previously diagnosed opportunistic infections and is under your regular supervision and care, there may be some debate about the necessity for confirming a clinical diagnosis by biopsy. However, there are other etiologies for pigmented cutaneous lesions in HIV infection, and the decision to biopsy should be made individually. A patient with previously diagnosed KS does not need new lesions biopsied unless he had been in remission following therapy.

62. Is KS an AIDS diagnosis?
Yes. Since the Centers for Disease Control first established the surveillance definition of AIDS, KS has been on the list of indicator conditions.

63. What treatment is recommended for KS?
There is no single therapeutic approach to KS in patients with AIDS. The KS patient will often have concurrent conditions that should receive priority because, with the exception of pulmonary KS, the disease is rarely threatening to the patient's immediate health. The dichotomy stems from the realization that although AIDS-associated KS is a more aggressive variant of KS, it is relatively benign compared to other AIDS-related processes. In addition, response rates of KS to systemic therapy have not been high enough to recommend such

therapy across the board. Patients are often receiving other life-preserving antimicrobial or antiviral therapies that would need to be compromised for the use of myelosuppressive chemotherapy.

A general approach to AIDS-associated KS should start with an assessment of the possible course of KS disease and its effect upon the patient's overall condition. The table below can help you distinguish between patients with possible indolent disease or disease that may take a more aggressive course.

Prognostic Variables in Kaposi's Sarcoma

PREDICTS INDOLENT COURSE	PREDICTS AGGRESSIVE COURSE
Few lesions (< 25)	Many KS lesions (≥ 25)
Low rate of growth	Rapid appearance of new lesions
No visceral KS identified	Intraoral or visceral lesions
No fevers, drenching night sweats, weight loss	One or more constitutional symptoms
No prior opportunistic infection	One prior or concurrent opportunistic infection
Absolute CD4+ count $> 400/mm^3$	CD4+ cell count $< 200/mm^3$
Normal ESR	ESR > 40 mm/hr
HIV p24 antigen not detectable	HIV p24 detectable
Normal β_2-microglobulin	β_2-microglobulin > 5
Normal blood counts	Leukopenia or anemia present

(From Chaisson RE, Volberding PA: Clinical manifestations of human immunodeficiency. In Mandell GL, et al (eds): Principles & Practice of Infectious Diseases, 3rd ed. New York, Churchill Livingstone, 1990, p 1081, with permission.)

64. What is the life expectancy for a patient with AIDS and KS?

There are no firm numbers with which to answer this question. Since survival statistics were first calculated for patients with AIDS, an AIDS-defining diagnosis of KS, as opposed to another malignancy or an opportunistic infection, has carried the best prognosis. This is due to the frequent appearance of KS at a less advanced point in the progressive immuno-suppression. The exceptions are patients with pulmonary KS. This is a quickly progressive condition resulting in respiratory failure often within 3 to 6 months.

Rothenberg R, et al: Survival with the acquired immunodeficiency syndrome. Experience with 5833 cases in New York City. N Engl J Med 317:1297–1302, 1987.

65. Is KS always cutaneous?

No! Visceral involvement is relatively common and most often involves the gastrointestinal (GI) tract, the lungs, and lymph nodes. After the oropharynx, the most common GI sites are the stomach and duodenum.

Sites of Disease and Systemic Signs at Presentation in 49 Patients with Epidemic Kaposi's Sarcoma

MANIFESTATION	NO. (%)	MANIFESTATION	NO. (%)
Skin Lesions:		**Lymph node involvement:**	
None	4 (8%)	None	19 (39%)
Generalized	13 (27%)	Generalized	30 (61%)
Locally aggressive	1 (2%)	Splenomegaly	5 (10%)
Visceral involvement:		**Systemic signs:***	
Bone	1 (2%)	Fever and weight loss	9 (18%)
Hepatomegaly	5 (10%)	Fever only	4 (8%)
Lung	5 (10%)	Weight loss only	1 (2%)
GI Tract	22 (45%)	Total with symptoms	14 (29%)

* Unexplained fever $> 100°$F (orally) and 10% or greater weight loss.
(From DeVita, et al (eds): AIDS: Etiology, Diagnosis, Treatment and Prevention, 2nd ed. Philadelphia, J.B. Lippincott, 1988, p 252, with permission.)

66. Does zidovudine treat KS?

Zidovudine does not appear to provide any therapeutic response in KS. However, patients with AIDS-related KS should receive zidovudine therapy for its other antiviral actions. This therapy could complicate any myelosuppressive chemotherapy the patient may receive for KS, and care should be taken to recognize the priority of each individual patient's clinical needs.

CYTOMEGALOVIRUS INFECTION

67. What is the cause of blindness experienced by some patients with AIDS?

Chorioretinitis caused by cytomegalovirus (CMV) is a sight-threatening infection experienced by 5–10% of patients with AIDS during the course of their illness. It is an AIDS-defining diagnosis if it occurs as the initial opportunistic infection. Usually, however, this infection appears later in the disease process, after a patient has already been diagnosed with AIDS.

68. How is CMV retinitis diagnosed?

Often a patient will present with nonspecific complaints of blurred vision, decreased visual acuity, or increasing "floaters," but occasionally CMV retinitis may present with a clear visual field cut. Ophthalmologic examination is essential and will typically show large white granular areas with hemorrhage. Diagnosis is based upon this characteristic fundoscopic appearance because no tissue is obtained for pathologic examination.

69. How is CMV retinitis treated?

Ganciclovir (DPHG, Cytovene) has received FDA approval for this indication. It is given intravenously at a dose of 5 mg/kg every 12 hours, and the response can be rather rapid. This therapy is clearly indicated for those patients with involvement close to the optic disk or the macula. It is not clear whether treatment should be administered to those with more peripheral lesions, and studies are ongoing.

Depending upon clinical response as judged by repeated ophthalmologic exam, initial treatment is given for 14–21 days. If therapy is discontinued, relapse invariably occurs. Maintenance therapy should be administered 5–7 days per week at dose of 5 mg/kg once a day.

70. What are the major toxicities of ganciclovir?

By far the most common toxicity is bone marrow suppression, usually seen as neutropenia and/or thrombocytopenia. Almost 40% of patients treated with ganciclovir will develop neutrophil counts below 1000 cells/mm³, and this can become a dose-limiting toxicity. Also seen is CNS toxicity manifested as confusion, headaches, or, rarely, seizures. Nausea, vomiting, and hepatitis can also be seen.

71. Should all HIV-infected patients have eye exams?

As noted above, CMV retinitis usually presents later in HIV infection, so most patients do not need an immediate referral to an ophthalmologist. There should be a baseline examination performed with subsequent examinations as clinical symptoms and signs dictate.

72. How else can CMV infection manifest in HIV infection?

Besides chorioretinitis, CMV can cause an interstitial pneumonia, colitis, esophagitis, adrenal insufficiency, and encephalitis. The pneumonia, colitis, and esophagitis can be diagnosed via endoscopically obtained pathologic specimens. The diagnoses of encephalitis or adrenal involvement are most often made post mortem.

73. Can ganciclovir and zidovudine be used in combination?

Due to the overlapping bone marrow toxicity, as well as the usual poor status of the patients involved, this becomes a very problematic therapeutic combination. In a more stable patient tolerating therapy with ganciclovir, there is no overwhelming reason not to attempt zidovudine therapy. Extremely close hematologic monitoring must be used. There is no other real toxicity overlap. However, there is also no evidence for therapeutic synergy.

Hochster H, et al: Toxicity of combined ganciclovir and zidovudine for cytomegalovirus disease associated with AIDS. Ann Intern Med 113:111–117, 1990.

TUBERCULOSIS, OTHER MYCOBACTERIA, AND AIDS

74. What is the relationship between AIDS and tuberculosis (TB)?

Throughout this century there had been a steady, rapid decline in the morbidity and mortality attributed to TB. However, in the mid-1980s this decline halted, and in 1986 there occurred the first increase in new TB cases since nationwide reporting was initiated in 1953. Several investigators cross-matched statewide public health registers for TB and AIDS cases and found a remarkably high number of patients on both lists.

This occurrence is predictable from knowledge of the pathogenesis of each of these separate infections. Control of TB is dependent upon cell-mediated immunity, precisely the most profound deficit seen in HIV infection. The incidence of TB in an HIV-infected population can be expected to mirror that population's previous exposure to *Mycobacterium tuberculosis*. Thus, immigrants, inner-city minorities, and IV drug users, with a high prevalence of both HIV infection and previous TB infection, will develop a high number of active TB cases unless prophylaxis is used.

75. Is TB different in presentation in HIV-infected patients?

TB in HIV-infected patients remains primarily a pulmonary disease; however, the incidence of extrapulmonary disease is much higher in the HIV-positive population compared to that seen in the general population. Miliary and disseminated TB are often seen, and "typical" apical or cavitary disease is much less common. Although the symptoms of chronic productive cough and hemoptysis are less common, TB in HIV infection remains a progressive, febrile, wasting disease.

The more "typical" TB cases will appear in those HIV-infected patients with a more preserved immune status, whereas the more "atypical" cases will be in those further along in their HIV-related illness. There appears to be a temporal clustering of TB cases around the time of an AIDS diagnosis.

The evaluation of any pulmonary process must include examination of specimens for acid-fast bacilli (AFB), as should the evaluation of other biopsy specimens.

76. Is TB more contagious in patients with AIDS?

Mycobacterium tuberculosis, which is a pathogen in individuals with normal immunity, represents the rare organism that may be transmitted from an HIV-infected individual to a noninfected individual. Due to decreased episodes of cavitary disease, it may be that patients with AIDS will be less contagious than non-AIDS patients. The bottom line, however, is that any patient capable of aerosolizing respiratory droplets containing *Mycobacterium tuberculosis* is contagious.

From the other perspective, patients with AIDS are much more susceptible to TB infection, and care should be taken to minimize any new exposures.

77. What is the treatment of TB in HIV infection?

Thus far TB appears to be a curable infection in this patient population. The recommended treatment is isoniazid, 300 mg/day, rifampin, 600 mg/day, and pyrazinamide, 20–30 mg/kg/

day, for the first 2 months of therapy. Continuation of therapy should then include at least isoniazid and rifampin for a minimum of 9 months treatment or at least 6 months after culture conversion. Ethambutol, 25 mg/kg/day, should be added initially for those with central nervous system involvement, dissemination, or suspected isoniazid resistance.

Centers for Disease Control: MMWR 38:236–238, 243–250, 1989.

78. Is a PPD of any use in HIV-infected patients?

The benefits derived from PPD skin testing are dependent upon the prevalence of underlying TB infection in the population being screened and the degree of immunosuppression already present. The ability to detect underlying TB infection is another argument for early HIV testing, with prompt skin testing of all HIV-positive persons. It is currently recommended that all HIV-positive individuals have a PPD placed shortly after the diagnosis of HIV infection. Those persons with a reaction of 5 mm or greater are recommended to receive isoniazid prophylaxis for 12 months, regardless of their age at the time of diagnosis.

Centers for Disease Control: MMWR 38:236–238, 243–250, 1989.

79. What about TB reporting and contact tracing?

TB remains a reportable disease in all states, and cases should be reported as locally regulated. This reporting is wholly independent from reporting HIV infection or cases of AIDS.

80. Should TB patients be screened for HIV infection?

Since a larger number of TB cases are now related to HIV infection, and early diagnosis of HIV infection has many benefits, all TB patients should be asked to consent to HIV testing.

81. What other mycobacterial infections are seen in HIV-infected patients?

Very early in the HIV epidemic it was noted that a large number of patients with AIDS have disseminated *Mycobacterium avium-intracellulare* (MAI) infection. Autopsy series have demonstrated up to 50% prevalence of this infection at the time of death from AIDS. Multiple other mycobacteria have been found to cause infection in patients with AIDS, but the only additional one seen in any significant number is *M. kansasii.*

82. How does MAI infection present?

The answer to this question is less straightforward than it would appear. MAI infection is usually associated with advanced HIV disease, and the patient usually has multiple concurrent conditions. The contribution to the overall condition of the patient by the MAI infection can be difficult to ascertain.

Usually seen are systemic symptoms such as fever, night sweats, weight loss, fatigue, and malaise. Laboratory examination may reveal increasing anemia or mild hepatitis. Chronic diarrhea with abdominal pain and/or malabsorption is also seen. The frequency of GI symptoms and pathologic changes has led some to believe this is the portal of entry.

Diagnosis of MAI infection can be made by culture of biopsy specimens or blood culture. Although the yield from blood culture is excellent, there is often a delay while awaiting results. Specimens from biopsies will quickly reveal AFB organisms on stains, thus facilitating the diagnosis.

83. Is there a standard therapy for MAI in patients with AIDS?

To date, therapy for MAI in patients with AIDS has been very disappointing. MAI is resistant to most anti-mycobacterial agents. Often a clinician may institute therapy only in the hope of suppressing infection. Multiple drug regimens have been evaluated, with a few showing promise. Some regimens have included up to 5 or 6 drugs. Prolonged parenteral administration of amikacin, combined with rifampin, ethambutol, and ciprofloxacin or clofazimine, has resulted in a number of culture conversions on a short-term basis that coincided with clinical improvement.

SYPHILIS AND AIDS

84. In which HIV-infected patients should a serological test for syphilis serology be obtained?

Every HIV-infected patient needs a serological test for syphilis, as well as a detailed history for all sexually transmitted diseases and past treatments. There is a growing body of literature that raises the possibility of an accelerated course for syphilitic infection in patients also infected with HIV. There may also be an unusual progression of syphilis in these patients. With this in mind, and the fact that the route of transmission for HIV and syphilis is similar, all patients with positive serology for one of these infections should be tested for the other.

Hook EW: Syphilis and HIV infection. J Infect Dis 160:530–534, 1989.

85. What if serology is positive but the patient gives no history of syphilis?

Due to the concern over altered progression of syphilis in HIV infection, the discrimination between early syphilis, early latent syphilis, and late latent syphilis may be less important, because most practitioners may now more aggressively treat early infection. A question does arise over the use of lumbar puncture (LP) to evaluate neurosyphilis. This is not currently recommended in early syphilis but is recommended in late latent (over 1 year duration) syphilis. With no patient history to steer you, it may be best to err on the side of caution and proceed with LP in HIV-infected patients, especially those with any neurologic signs or symptoms or a serum antibody titer $\geq 1{:}32$.

An inquiry to your local public health office may provide additional history that the patient has not recalled.

Centers for Disease Control: Recommendations for diagnosing and treating syphilis in HIV-infected patients. MMWR 37:600–608, 1988.

86. Which HIV-infected patients with syphilis need a lumbar puncture (LP)?

Although a few authorities would recommend an LP in all of these patients, most would agree that patients with a clear episode of primary or secondary syphilis do not need an LP. Examination of the CSF should be done for all HIV-infected patients with syphilis of more than 1 year's duration or any clinical signs or symptoms of nervous system involvement. Patients with early syphilis whose serologic titers increase or fail to decrease appropriately (fourfold within 6 months) should also undergo an LP to evaluate CNS involvement prior to re-treatment.

87. What is the treatment for neurosyphilis in HIV-infected patients?

The treatment for neurosyphilis is the same whether or not a patient has simultaneous HIV infection: aqueous crystalline penicillin G, 2–4 million units IV every 4 hours (12–24 million units per day) for 10–14 days. No nonpenicillin-based therapy is considered wholly satisfactory. Patients with remote histories of unclear penicillin allergy may need skin testing.

88. If a chancre is present, is initial therapy changed?

Although the recommended regimen remains one dose of benzathine penicillin G, 2.4 million units IM, many authorities would more aggressively treat primary syphilis in patients co-infected with HIV and recommend a total of 7.2 million units given as 2.4 million units weekly for 3 consecutive weeks.

Musher DM: How much penicillin cures early syphilis? Ann Intern Med 109:849–851, 1988.

89. How should you follow patients with HIV infection and primary syphilis?
These patients should have repeat serologic testing at 1, 2, 3, 6, 9, and 12 months. If at any time there is a fourfold increase in titer, an LP should be done. If by 3 months there has not been a fourfold decrease in titer, CSF should be examined.

90. Is HIV-related syphilis reported to local health authorities?
By all means. The presence of concomitant HIV infection does not change the reporting requirement for syphilis.

91. Should all syphilis patients be tested for HIV?
Yes. Again, HIV infection may alter the course of syphilis or the response to treatment. Thus, for each syphilis patient you treat, it would behoove you to know their HIV status. Also, there are common risk factors for both infections.

TOXOPLASMOSIS AND AIDS

92. What are the most common causes of CNS mass lesions in AIDS?
The two most prevalent AIDS-related mass lesions are cerebral toxoplasmosis and primary CNS lymphoma. Other causes include progressive multifocal leukoencephalopathy (PML), cryptococcoma, tuberculoma, bacterial and fungal abscesses, and metastatic neoplastic disease.

93. How can the differential diagnosis between CNS toxoplasmosis and lymphoma be made?
Most clinicians would recommend empirical treatment for toxoplasmosis (pyrimethamine 100 mg loading dose, then 25 mg per day, and short-acting sulfonamide 4–6 grams daily in divided doses) and judge clinical response as well as response seen on CT scanning. This response should be rapid (3–5 days) and if not seen should raise the suspicion of an etiology other than toxoplasmosis.

94. Are there characteristic CT scan findings in CNS toxoplasmosis?
The following table may help differentiate between CNS toxoplasmosis and lymphoma. However, the high degree of overlap should be kept in mind.

CT Scan Findings in CNS Toxoplasmosis and Lymphoma

FINDING	TOXOPLASMOSIS	LYMPHOMA
Area involved	Deep gray matter and basal ganglia	White matter, periventricular areas
Mass effect	Yes	Yes
Enhancement	Ring-enhancement	Weakly, not ring shaped
Number of lesions	Multiple	1–2

95. How long should patients with AIDS be treated for toxoplasmosis?
This is another AIDS-related infection that appears to require life-long suppressive therapy, much like pneumocystis and cryptococcus.

AIDS-RELATED HEMATOLOGY

96. How often does HIV infection result in anemia or thrombocytopenia?
Patients with full-blown AIDS are frequently pancytopenic, with anemia occurring in up to 80%, neutropenia in 85%, and thrombocytopenia in 65% of cases. Seropositive, but asymptomatic, individuals are much less frequently cytopenic. Clinically significant thrombocytopenia indistinguishable from that seen in idiopathic thrombocytopenic purpura (ITP)

may be a presentation of HIV infection. Typically there is a normal bone marrow with adequate numbers of megakaryocytes present and behavior much like classic ITP in that patients respond to steroids and splenectomy. With the appearance of HIV infection in heterosexual contacts of IV drug users and bisexual men or other infected persons, it seems reasonable to obtain HIV serology in the majority of patients presenting with ITP. Recently, small numbers of thrombocytopenic patients have improved on zidovudine therapy. Of interest also is the recent recognition of thrombotic thrombocytopenic purpura (TTP) in association with HIV infection.

Walsh C, et al: Thrombocytopenia in homosexual patients. Ann Intern Med 103:542, 1985.

97. What are the characteristic bone marrow aspirate and biopsy findings in AIDS?

Most bone marrows examined from patients with AIDS have decreased cellularity, although a markedly hypocellular marrow is rare. In some instances a dyserythropoiesis has been observed. Increased numbers of lymphocytes and plasma cells are commonplace findings. Histiocytic hyperplasia with phagocytosis of red cells, platelets, and white cells has also been observed in the bone marrow of patients with AIDS. This finding has been associated with numerous infections, including herpes virus infections, typhoid fever, TB, and brucellosis. Perhaps the HIV virus itself, atypical mycobacterial infections, or toxoplasmosis causes this marrow picture in AIDS. Granulomas and marrow fibrosis are also common findings, as is serous fat atrophy. A form of pure red cell aplasia associated with giant pronormoblasts in the marrow in connection with parvovirus B_{19} infection has also been recently recognized. Patients receiving zidovudine often have ineffective hematopoiesis with megaloblastic maturation.

Namiki TS, et al: A comparison of bone marrow findings in patients with acquired immunodeficiency syndrome (AIDS) and AIDS-related conditions. Hematological Oncology 5:99, 1987.

98. What lymphomas are associated with AIDS? How often do they present with extra lymphatic presentations?

AIDS is associated with high-grade B-cell lymphomas that arise most often in extralymphatic sites. The histologic types that are most frequently seen are small noncleaved cell (resembling Burkitt's), large cell, and immunoblastic lymphoma. In one series nearly one-third of the patients presented with extranodal disease alone. The most frequent extranodal sites are: bone marrow, liver, meninges, lung, soft tissue, primary CNS, rectum, and Waldeyer's ring. Patients without prior histories of AIDS-related infections, such as pneumocystis pneumonia, and in good physical condition may respond to standard chemotherapy followed by institution of zidovudine therapy. Patients who develop lymphoma after other manifestations of AIDS typically do not fare well with chemotherapy. Supportive care only is a reasonable course in these patients.

Kaplan LD: AIDS-associated non-Hodgkin's lymphoma in San Francisco. JAMA 261:719, 1989.

BIBLIOGRAPHY

1. Cohen PT, Sande MA, Volberding PA: The AIDS Knowledge Base. Waltham, MA, Medical Publishing Group, Massachusetts Medical Society, 1990.
2. Harawi SJ, O'Hara CJ: Pathology and Pathophysiology of AIDS and HIV-related Diseases. St. Louis, C.V. Mosby, 1989.
3. Holmes KK, Mardh P-A, Sparling PF, Wiesner PJ (eds): Sexually Transmitted Diseases, 2nd ed. New York, McGraw-Hill, 1990.
4. Makadon HJ, et al: HIV Disease in Primary Care. J Gen Intern Med 6(Suppl 1):S1–S62, 1991.
5. Mandell GL, Douglas RG, Bennett JE: Principles and Practice of Infectious Diseases, 3rd ed. New York, Churchill Livingstone, 1990.
6. Sande MA, Volberding PA: The Medical Management of AIDS, 2nd ed. Philadelphia, W.B. Saunders, 1990.

14. NEUROLOGY SECRETS

Loren A. Rolak, M.D.

From the brain and from the brain only arise our pleasures, joys, laughter and jests, as well as our sorrows, pains, griefs and tears . . . It is the same thing which makes us mad or delirious, inspires us with dread, or fear, whether by night or by day, brings sleeplessness, inopportune mistakes, aimless anxieties, absent-mindedness, and acts that are contrary to habit. These things that we suffer all come from the brain, when it is not healthy, but becomes abnormally hot, cold, moist, or dry.

Hippocrates (460?–377? B.C.)
The Sacred Disease, Sect. XVII
(tr. by W. H. S. Jones)

APPROACH TO THE PATIENT

1. What is the best way to evaluate patients complaining of neurologic symptoms?

The first step is to localize the lesion, to determine specifically which part of the nervous system is affected. Only then should an etiology be sought, since defining the anatomy usually implies certain causes.

The brain is extraordinary among organs for its great degree of specialization. Because each individual part of the brain, spinal cord, and peripheral nerves has such specialized functions, lesions in these defined areas produce specific clinical deficits. Therefore, symptoms can often be localized, sometimes to the millimeter, to discrete parts of the nervous system. This property of the nervous system has been referred to as "eloquence"— the brain "speaks to" the clinician directly.

2. How can neuroanatomy be applied clinically, given the great complexity of the nervous system?

For clinical purposes, the most important neuroanatomy consists of only a few large regions. Finer detail can be left to the neurologic specialists. The regions where lesions should be localized are (proceeding from distal to proximal):

1. Muscle
2. Neuromuscular junction
3. Peripheral nerve
4. Root
5. Spinal cord
6. Brainstem
7. Cerebellum
8. Subcortical brain
9. Cortical brain

3. How are symptoms localized to these neuroanatomic regions?

As in all aspects of medicine, the history guides the diagnosis. By asking the proper questions during the history, most neurologic lesions can be localized accurately.

When approaching a patient with neurologic disease, a useful system for diagnosis is to begin distally (with the muscle) and ask questions about each part of the anatomy of the nervous system, working backward through the neuromuscular junction, peripheral nerve, root, spinal cord, cerebellum, brainstem, subcortex, and ending with the cortex of the brain. By sequentially asking about each of these areas of the nervous system, the neurologic patient can be "examined" thoroughly. Only after the lesion is localized by means of history-taking should the physical examination begin. If you do not know where the lesion is after you have finished the history, do not begin the neurologic examination—take a better history!

4. Which clinical features of muscle disease can be elicited by the history?

Muscle disease (myopathy) causes proximal symmetric weakness without sensory loss. Therefore, questions that elicit these symptoms should be asked. For example:

1. Can the patient arise from a chair, get out of a car seat, get off of the toilet, or go up stairs without using his hands? (This checks proximal leg weakness.) Can the patient lift or carry objects, such as briefcases, school books, children, grocery bags, or garbage bags? (This checks proximal arm weakness.)

2. Is the weakness relatively symmetric? (Minor differences are allowed because most generalized processes are slightly asymmetric, but weakness essentially confined to one limb or one side of the body is unlikely to be a myopathy.)

3. Is there numbness or other sensory loss? (Pain, cramping, and other sensations may occur with some myopathies, but there should not be sensory loss with disease that is confined to the muscle.)

5. After a history of muscle disease is elicited, what findings can be expected on physical examination?

The examination should show proximal symmetric weakness without sensory loss. Tone is usually normal or mildly decreased, reflexes are usually normal or mildly decreased, and there is seldom significant atrophy unless the process is very advanced.

6. Which clinical features of neuromuscular junction disease can be elicited by history?

Neuromuscular junction diseases closely resemble myopathies, causing proximal symmetric weakness without sensory loss. However, the hallmark of disease of the neuromuscular junction is fatigability; the weakness worsens with use and recovers with rest. Since strength improves with rest, this fatigability does not usually present as a steady progressive decline throughout the day. Instead, it presents as variability or fluctuation in weakness as the muscle first fatigues, then recovers, then fatigues again, then recovers, etc. (Almost every medical symptom can be worse at the end of the day. Look for variability or fluctuation as the characteristic of neuromuscular junction fatigability.)

Another feature of neuromuscular junction diseases is that they are usually extremely proximal. They often involve muscles of the face resulting in drooping of the eyelids (ptosis), double vision, difficulty chewing and swallowing, slurred speech, and facial weakness.

7. After a history of neuromuscular junction problems is elicited, what findings can be expected on physical examination?

The examination should show proximal symmetric weakness without sensory loss that results in fatigue. With repetitive testing of the muscles, they will weaken, but with a minute or so of rest they will regain their strength. Similarly, sustained muscular activity (such as upward gaze) will lead to fatigability and progressive weakness (such as ptosis). Tone, reflexes, and muscle bulk will all be normal.

8. Which clinical features of peripheral neuropathies can be elicited by history?

Peripheral neuropathies cause distal, often asymmetric, weakness with sensory changes. Atrophy and fasciculations may also appear. Questions to elicit these symptoms would include:

1. Does the patient wear out the toes of his shoes or catch his toes and trip, as would be expected with a foot-drop? (Checking distal weakness in the legs.) Does the patient have trouble with his grip, or frequently drop things? (Checking distal strength in the hands.)

2. Is the process asymmetric? (Some neuropathies are distal, symmetric, stocking-and-glove neuropathies, but most are asymmetric, such as carpal tunnel syndrome, radial nerve palsy, etc.)

3. Has the patient noticed a shrinkage or wasting of the muscle (atrophy) or quivering, twitching muscles (fasciculations)?

4. Is there numbness, tingling, or paresthesias?

9. After a history of peripheral neuropathy is elicited, what findings can be expected on physical examination?

The examination should show distal, often asymmetric weakness, with atrophy and fasciculations, and sensory loss such as decreased pinprick, vibration, and occasionally position sense. Tone is normal or decreased and reflexes are diminished. Sometimes there are also trophic changes, such as loss of hair and nails, and smooth, shiny skin.

10. Which clinical features of root diseases (radiculopathies) can be elicited by history?

The hallmark of root disease is pain. In addition, radiculopathies usually have similar features to peripheral neuropathies: denervation (weakness, atrophy, and fasciculations) with sensory loss. The weakness may be proximal (the most common radiculopathies in the arms involve C5/6 muscles, which are proximal), or distal (the most common radiculopathies in the legs involve L5/S1 muscles, which are distal). The history is therefore the same as for peripheral neuropathies, but with the added element of pain. This pain is usually severe, often described as sharp, hot, or electric, and commonly radiates down an arm or leg.

11. After a history of radiculopathy is elicited, what findings can be expected on physical examination?

The neurologic examination will show weakness in one myotomal group of muscles, such as C5/6 in the arm or L5/S1 in the leg, sometimes with atrophy and fasciculations. Tone will be normal or decreased, and the reflex in those muscles will be diminished or absent. There will be sensory loss in a dermatomal distribution. Sometimes maneuvers that stretch the root will elicit the pain, such as straight leg raising. (See figure on following page.)

12. Which clinical features of spinal cord disease can be elicited by history?

Spinal cord lesions cause a triad of symptoms:

1. **A sensory level.** This level, which may occur as a band of sensory change around the thorax or abdomen, or a sharp level below which sensation is lost, is the hallmark of spinal cord disease.

2. **Distal, usually symmetric weakness.**

3. **Bowel and bladder changes.**

Questions about spinal cord disease will therefore focus on eliciting these symptoms. For example:

1. Does the patient drag his toe or trip because of the distal leg weakness? (Lesions in the pyramidal tract, also called the corticospinal tract or upper motor neuron, cause weakness that is usually greatest distally, and thus can mimic a peripheral neuropathy.)

2. Are the patient's legs stiff? (Since pyramidal tract weakness causes spasticity, many patients report their legs are stiff, and their knees will not bend when they walk.)

3. Is a sensory level present? Sometimes patients describe this as a belt or band or "tight swimming trunks" around their waist or thorax.

4. Is there either retention or incontinence of bowel and bladder? (The bladder is usually much more sensitive to spinal cord injury than the bowel.)

13. After a history of spinal cord disease is elicited, what findings can be expected on physical examination?

The physical examination in a person with spinal cord disease will show distal weakness, usually worse in the legs than the arms, and usually worse in the extensors (dorsiflexors of

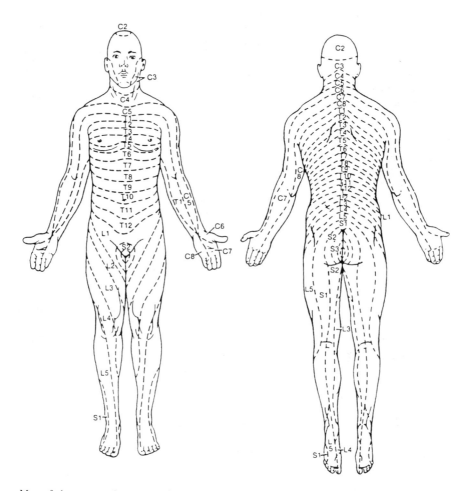

Map of the sensory dermatomes in the anterior and posterior aspects. (From DeJong RN: The Neurologic Examination. Hagerstown, Harper & Row, 1979, with permission.)

the feet and extensors of the wrists and fingers) than flexors. The tone will be increased, the reflexes will be brisk, and there are usually extensor plantar reflexes (positive Babinski signs). Superficial reflexes are commonly lost, such as anal wink, sphincter tone, cremasteric reflex, and abdominal reflexes. A sensory level can often be found, below which all sensory modalities are diminished.

14. Which clinical features of brainstem disease can be elicited by history?
The brainstem is essentially a spinal cord with cranial nerves stuck in it. Cranial nerve abnormalities are the hallmark of brainstem disease. Symptoms of brainstem disease will usually consist of a combination of long-tract findings (such as weakness from the pyramidal tract, numbness from the spinothalamic tract, etc.) plus cranial nerve findings. Because the long tracts have now crossed (decussated), the weakness and numbness will not be in the distribution of a level, but rather in a hemiparesis or a hemianesthesia. Because of the crossing of these long tracts, damage to one side of the brainstem, affecting the cranial nerves on that side, usually results in long tract symptoms that affect the opposite

side of the body. These crossed symptoms are another hallmark of brainstem disease—weakness of one side of the face and the opposite side of the body, for example.

Cranial nerve (CN) lesions commonly cause the big "Ds": **diplopia** (CN III, IV, or VI), **decreased** sensation in the face (CN V), **decreased** strength in the face (CN VII), **dizziness** and **deafness** (CN VIII), and **dysarthria** and **dysphagia** (CN IX, X, and XII). The history should therefore focus on eliciting these symptoms:

1. Is there diplopia, facial weakness or numbness, dizziness, deafness, dysarthria, or dysphagia?
2. Are there long-tract findings, such as hemiparesis or hemisensory loss?
3. Are the findings crossed or bilateral?

15. After a history of brainstem disease is elicited, what findings can be expected on physical examination?

The physical examination will show a combination of cranial nerve and long-tract abnormalities. Checking the cranial nerves may reveal ptosis, abnormalities of extraocular movements, diplopia, nystagmus, decreased corneal reflexes, facial weakness or numbness, decreased hearing, dysarthria, paralysis of the palate, decreased gag reflex, or tongue deviation. There are usually long-tract abnormalities resulting in hemiparesis, with a pyramidal pattern of distal weakness with increased reflexes, increased tone, and a positive Babinski sign. Hemisensory loss may include decreased sensation to all modalities.

16. Which clinical features of cerebellar disease can be elicited by history?

Cerebellar disease causes clumsiness and lack of coordination. The cerebellum is responsible for smoothing out voluntary movements, and impairments produce abnormalities in the rate and rhythm of movements. Questions should therefore focus on incoordination in the legs and the arms:

1. Does the patient have a staggering, drunken walk? Most laymen understand what is meant by a "drunken" walk and will use this term to describe cerebellar disease. (This is probably because drinking alcohol does in fact impair the cerebellum, and the characteristic wide-based, ataxic, staggering gait of the person intoxicated by alcohol is caused by cerebellar dysfunction.)
2. Does the patient have difficulty putting a key in a lock, lighting a cigarette, or other target-directed movements? The cerebellar tremor is worse with voluntary, intentional movements, especially as the hand approaches the target object. Fine coordinated movements, such as extending a key and inserting it into the narrow slot of a lock, are perfect examples of difficult tasks for people with cerebellar lesions.

17. After a history of cerebellar disease is elicited, what findings can be expected on physical examination?

Patients with cerebellar disease usually have a staggering gait, and difficulty with tandem walking. When sliding a heel down a shin, it will waver unsteadily. In the arms, there will be a tremor and wavering when touching the examiner's finger, the patient's own nose, or other targets. Similarly, rapid alternating movements in the limbs will be irregular in rate and rhythm.

18. Which clinical features of subcortical and cortical brain disease can be elicited by history and neurologic examination?

Clinically, disease of the brain itself can affect either subcortical or cortical regions. The main features differentiating these are:

1. The presence of specific cortical deficits (such as aphasia).
2. The pattern of motor and sensory loss.
3. The type of sensory change.
4. Visual field deficits.
5. Involuntary movements.
6. Seizures.

Questions to elicit these features would include:

1. Does the patient have aphasia (left hemisphere cortex) or visual-spatial deficits (right hemisphere cortex)?

2. Is the leg weak or numb? Motor and sensory neurons are arranged in the cortex in a manner that has been described as a homunculus. This "little man" is draped upside-down over the cortex, with a large face and lips, small neck, a large hand and thumb, and a small trunk. The leg is not over the outside cortex. Instead, it hangs down in the interhemispheric fissure, in the cortex lying deep between the two hemispheres of the brain. Most cortical processes, such as a stroke, affect the face and arm but cannot "get to" the leg fibers between the hemispheres. Deeper in the brain, in subcortical regions, fibers from the face, arm, and leg lie close together, in the pyramidal tract or spinothalamic tract. Even a small lesion in these tracts can affect the face, arm, and leg. So if the face and arm are involved, the lesion is cortical; if the face, arm, and leg are involved, it is subcortical.

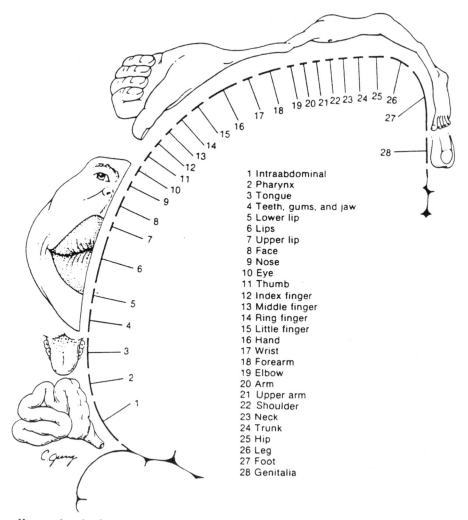

1 Intraabdominal
2 Pharynx
3 Tongue
4 Teeth, gums, and jaw
5 Lower lip
6 Lips
7 Upper lip
8 Face
9 Nose
10 Eye
11 Thumb
12 Index finger
13 Middle finger
14 Ring finger
15 Little finger
16 Hand
17 Wrist
18 Forearm
19 Elbow
20 Arm
21 Upper arm
22 Shoulder
23 Neck
24 Trunk
25 Hip
26 Leg
27 Foot
28 Genitalia

Homunculus showing sensory and motor representation over the cortex. (From Penfield W, Rasmussen T: The Cerebral Cortex. New York, Macmillan, 1950, with permission.)

3. Is the patient "numb"? Primary sensations, such as pain, temperature, touch, position, and vibration, are registered in the thalamus (subcortex) and are not much affected by cortical lesions. Destroying the cortex alone causes very little numbness or sensory loss. What are seen with cortical damage are secondary sensory changes, such as astereognosis, agraphesthesia, loss of two-point discrimination, etc. (these are difficult to elicit by history).

4. Does the patient have a visual field defect? Because visual fibers run subcortically (in the optic tract, lateral geniculate, and optic radiations), cortical lesions will not cause field cuts. (Damage to the occipital cortex causes field cuts, but since there are no motor or sensory fibers there, it will not cause any other focal deficits.)

5. Does the patient have a movement disorder? Most movement disorders are thought to arise from subcortical structures, such as the basal ganglia. A history of parkinsonism, chorea, dystonia, hemiballismus, etc. would thus suggest a subcortical lesion.

6. Does the patient have seizures? Seizures arise from the paroxysmal discharge of neurons, almost exclusively in the cortex. Subcortical lesions seldom cause seizures.

MAJOR DISEASES AFFECTING NEUROANATOMICAL REGIONS

MYOPATHIES

19. Which of the myopathies are most common on the medical ward?

Polymyositis is the most common myopathy seen on the medical ward. It is an inflammatory, probably autoimmune, disease of muscles. It has a variable course, generally characterized by the subacute onset of proximal weakness of the arms and legs, often with dysphagia. One-third of patients have muscle pain and cramps. About 15% have an accompanying skin rash, a condition known as **dermatomyositis**. Polymyositis may accompany connective tissue disease (such as systemic lupus erythematosus) or vasculitis, or it may occur as a remote effect of cancer in patients with underlying neoplasms, but usually it appears in isolation, as a discrete clinical entity. It runs a variable course but can be severe or even fatal, and is generally treated with steroids or more powerful immunosuppressants if those fail.

Other common myopathies include those secondary to systemic medical conditions, especially hypothyroidism, and those secondary to drugs, especially clofibrate and steroid myopathy. Rarer conditions would include metabolic abnormalities such as mitochondrial myopathies and infectious diseases such as trichinoses. Adult inherited muscular dystrophies are uncommon but include myotonic dystrophy, fascioscapulohumeral dystrophy, and limb-girdle dystrophy.

Bohan A, Peter JB: Polymyositis and dermatomyositis. N Engl J Med 292:344–347, 403–407, 1975.

20. Which tests and procedures are used in the diagnostic evaluation of a patient with a myopathy?

The diagnostic evaluation of a myopathy generally entails a triad of tests: (1) serum creatine phosphokinase (CPK), (2) electromyography (EMG), and (3) muscle biopsy. Muscle destruction usually liberates CPK. Elevation of this enzyme is a good screening test for muscle disease. (The MM isoenzyme of CPK is the most common.) An EMG is done by inserting a fine needle electrode into the muscle to record its contractions. Myopathies cause low-voltage, short-duration muscle contractions, and this test can thus confirm the presence of myopathy. Finally, a muscle biopsy is often needed to define the cause, since most myopathies clinically resemble one another. The tissue could show inflammation (polymyositis), mitochondrial abnormalities, or other specific diseases.

OF NOTE: Treatment depends upon the specific diagnosis, but attention should always be paid to breathing. Pulmonary arrest from respiratory muscle weakness is the most serious complication of most myopathies.

NEUROMUSCULAR JUNCTION

21. Which neuromuscular junction disease is most common on the medical ward?
Myasthenia gravis (MG), which is rare, has a prevalence of 1 case per 50,000 population. MG has a bimodal age distribution, occurring in young women in their teens and twenties, and old men aged 60 and above. It presents with proximal weakness, especially ptosis and diplopia, that fatigues with use and recovers with rest. Because it can involve the respiratory muscles, pulmonary failure is the most feared complication.

MG is an autoimmune disease. Acetylcholine is the neurotransmitter that makes muscles contract, and patients with MG produce antibodies that destroy the acetylcholine receptors on the muscle.

Although no definitive cure is yet available, advances in treatment now allow patients with MG to lead near normal lives.

Treatment consists of anticholinesterase inhibitors, which block the cholinesterase enzymes that break down acetylcholine, thus allowing for greater concentrations of acetylcholine at the receptor. Pyridostigmine is the drug of choice. However, immunosuppressive drugs, such as steroids are often necessary to attack the underlying autoimmune process.

22. Are some drugs contraindicated for use in patients with neuromuscular junction diseases?
Some drugs can worsen neuromuscular junction diseases. These include:

Drugs That Worsen Neuromuscular Junction Diseases

1. "Mycin" antibiotics (i.e., clindamycin)	6. Quinidine
2. Tetracycline antibiotics	7. Lidocaine
3. Corticosteroids (acutely)	8. Propranolol
4. Thyroid hormone	9. Lithium
5. Phenothiazines (i.e., chlorpromazine)	10. Dilantin

23. What is the second most common disease causing neuromuscular junction problems?
The most common condition after myasthenia gravis (MG) is the Lambert-Eaton myasthenic syndrome (LEMS). This is probably also an autoimmune condition, although the target is the mechanism that releases acetylcholine, not the receptor. It is commonly seen in association with occult carcinoma, especially small cell carcinoma of the lung. LEMS clinically resembles MG because of fluctuating proximal weakness. It is generally treated by therapy of the underlying neoplasm, sometimes accompanied by plasmapheresis and other immune suppressors, especially in those cases where no occult cancer can be discovered. Guanidine may provide symptomatic relief.

Other rare causes of neuromuscular junction problems are botulism and black widow spider bites.

Seybold ME: Myasthenia gravis: A clinical and basic science review. JAMA 250:2516–2521, 1983.
Rowland LP: Controversies about the treatment of myasthenia gravis. J Neurol Neurosurg Psychiatry 43:659–694, 1980.

24. How can we differentiate myasthenia gravis (MG) from the Lambert-Eaton myasthenic syndrome (LEMS)?
Although MG and LEMS strongly resemble each other clinically, LEMS does not involve extraocular muscles, so ptosis and diplopia, which are very common with MG, do not

occur. Also, by EMG testing, repetitive stimulation of the nerve in MG shows a progressive decline in each muscle contraction, documenting the fatigability with repetitive stimulation. With LEMS, there is actually a paradoxical increase, rather than decrease, in successive muscle contractions when the nerve is repetitively stimulated. This is due to a progressive increase in the amount of acetylcholine released presynaptically by the stimulated nerve.

25. What is the triad of tests in the diagnostic evaluation for patients with neuromuscular junction problems?
The triad of tests includes (1) a Tensilon test, (2) antibody levels in the serum, and (3) repetitive stimulation on EMG. The Tensilon test is performed by administering a small dose of intravenous Tensilon (edrophonium), which is a powerful but transient acetylcholinesterase inhibitor. This will cause a reversal of weakness within 30 seconds to 2 minutes, which will last approximately 10 minutes before returning back to baseline. For example, ptosis of the eyes may transiently resolve after a Tensilon test.

Antibodies against the acetylcholine receptor can be assayed directly in the serum, providing a useful diagnostic test for MG. Repetitive stimulation of the muscle on EMG testing can detect defects in acetylcholine transmission that are not apparent clinically.

PERIPHERAL NEUROPATHIES

26. Which peripheral neuropathies are most common on the medical ward?
Peripheral neuropathies are probably the most frequent neurologic problems seen on a medical ward, unlike myopathies and neuromuscular junction disease, which are rare. The most common peripheral neuropathies can be remembered by the mnemonic DANG THE RAPIST, as follows:

Mnemonic for the Most Common Causes of Peripheral Neuropathies

D = Diabetes
A = Alcohol
N = Nutritional (vitamin deficiencies, etc.)
G = Guillain-Barré

T = Trauma (carpal tunnel, etc.)
H = Hereditary
E = Environmental (toxins, drugs, etc.)

R = Remote effects of cancer
A = Amyloid
P = Porphyria
I = Inflammation (collagen vascular disease, etc.)
S = Syphilis
T = Tumors

27. The evaluation of a patient with a peripheral neuropathy usually begins with which study?
The evaluation of a patient with peripheral neuropathy usually begins with an **electromyogram and nerve conduction velocity** study (EMG/NCV). This test applies electrical current directly over the nerves and records with an electrode the speed with which the nerves conduct the current. It can thus document the extent and the degree of slowing and impairment of nerve conduction. The EMG also uses a needle electrode within the muscles to record muscle contractions and thus show denervation of the muscles.

Once a neuropathy has been confirmed, workup for the etiology will focus on the above mnemonic, requiring evaluation for diabetes, alcoholism, B_{12} deficiency, metabolic abnormalities such as thyroid disease or uremia, familial illnesses, toxic exposure, collagen vascular disease, etc. A spinal tap is often needed to detect inflammatory neuropathies. Only rarely is a nerve biopsy required. Therapy of peripheral neuropathies usually consists of treating the underlying cause.

Nakano KK: The entrapment neuropathies. Muscle Nerve 1:264–279, 1978.
Harati Y: Diabetic peripheral neuropathies. Ann Intern Med 107:546–559, 1987.

28. What is the Guillain-Barré syndrome?

The Guillain-Barré syndrome is an acute inflammatory polyradiculopathy, in which there is inflammation of the nerve roots and peripheral nerves. It is presumably autoimmune and often follows viral infections, surgery, pregnancies, and other immune-altering events. It runs a monophasic course, with weakness progressing for several days to weeks, reaching a plateau, and then recovering over a period of several weeks to months. The entire course may take up to 6 months. Clinically, the diagnosis is confirmed by weakness, often but not always in an ascending pattern (from legs up the trunk to the arms and face). The weakness is hyporeflexive but there is no significant sensory loss. **Rapidly progressive weakness with absent reflexes and no sensory change is almost always Guillain-Barré syndrome.**

29. What is the abnormality of Guillain-Barré syndrome on which treatment is based?

Although presumably autoimmune, no specific antigen or well-defined immune abnormality has been detected in Guillain-Barré syndrome. Nevertheless, treatment is still directed towards an immunological cause, and now consists primarily of plasmapheresis. If done early in the disease, this does seem to shorten the overall course. Steroids, once thought to be helpful, are now seldom employed. Because there can be autonomic dysfunction as part of the syndrome, and since respiration is frequently impaired by the weakness, patients usually require management in the intensive care unit. Patient management thus focuses on the day-to-day concerns of respirators, vital signs, nutrition, and other aspects of critical care.

Guillain-Barré Study Group: Plasmapheresis and acute Guillain-Barré syndrome. Neurology 35:1096–1104, 1985.

RADICULOPATHIES

30. What is the most common cause of radiculopathies on the medical ward?

The most common cause of radiculopathy is mechanical compression, such as from spondylosis or a herniated disc. The common manifestations are neck and low back pain.

31. What is the diagnostic evaluation of the patient with a radiculopathy?

The diagnostic evaluation of a patient with a radiculopathy generally begins with an EMG/NCV to identify specifically which root is involved, and hence which muscles are denervated. The next step is often to image the area where the root emerges from the spinal cord, since this is the most common site of disorders causing radiculopathies. This usually requires a myelogram through the level of interest, although noninvasive studies are increasingly used to image the spine and roots, including computed tomography (CT) of the spine and magnetic resonance imaging (MRI). If these studies are negative, showing no root compression, then nonmechanical causes, such as tumor or infection, should be considered (which are similar to those causing peripheral neuropathies).

Deyo RA, Bigos SJ, Maravilla KR: Diagnostic imaging procedures for the lumbar spine. Ann Intern Med III:865–867, 1989.

32. What is the treatment for radiculopathies?

For most mechanical radiculopathies the treatment consists of bedrest, analgesics such as aspirin or other nonsteroidal anti-inflammatory drugs, and heat. There are surprisingly few careful, controlled studies analyzing the amount of bedrest needed or the most useful analgesics. Traction is seldom used for radiculopathies anymore.

33. When is surgery appropriate for a radiculopathy?
One of the most controversial topics arises when radiculopathy due to spondylosis or a herniated nucleus pulposus (slipped disc) requires surgical treatment. Many experts feel that the presence of focal neurological findings is a strong indication for surgery—findings such as weakness, atrophy or fasciculations in the muscles affected, an absent reflex, or dermatome sensory loss. Such hard findings are unlikely to improve and may well progress unless pressure on the nerve is relieved. Much more controversial is surgery for the relief of pain alone, without focal neurologic findings. Even in well-chosen patients with clear lesions and no overlying complications such as litigation or secondary gain, surgery to alleviate pain is effective in only about half the cases. It is therefore often reserved for patients who have "failed medical management," which is a clinical decision and generally implies persistent very severe pain after a 1- to 2-week trial of strict bedrest with analgesics.

34. What are the most common causes of back pain?
Only about 20% of back pain is caused by a slipped disc or root compression. There are many other causes, such as arthritis of the facet joints, but most back pain is felt to be "musculoskeletal," from strain placed on the tendons, ligaments, and muscles of the back. Many experts feel that this pain is largely mechanical, secondary to the inherent instability of the lordotic spine required for the human upright posture and aggravated by the problems of obesity, lack of exercise, and other precipitating factors in the modern lifestyle. For most such pain, conservative therapy and patience are indicated.

Frymoyer JW: Back pain and sciatica. N Engl J Med 318:291–300, 1988.

MYELOPATHIES

35. What are the clinical features of spinal cord compression?
Spinal cord compression will cause the classic cord syndrome of a sensory level, bowel and bladder changes, and upper motor neuron weakness with spasticity, hyperreflexia, and positive Babinski signs. Superficial reflexes may be diminished, such as abdominal reflexes and the anal wink.

36. What are the most common causes of spinal cord compression?
The most common cause of chronic spinal cord compression is **cervical spondylosis.** If there is no history of trauma, the acute syndrome is often due to compression by a neoplasm, usually metastatic. Such compression may develop almost instantaneously and may or may not cause back pain.

37. How is spinal cord compression best managed?
Spinal cord compression is best managed initially by localizing the site of the lesion. Plain x-rays of the spine have a high yield for showing metastatic disease, as evidenced by lytic lesions and erosion of pedicles. Bone scans may be helpful, though the yield is lower. Increasingly, MRI is replacing myelography for the definitive documentation of compression.

Surgical intervention is indicated for compression due to cervical spondylosis or mechanical deformation, such as spondylolisthesis. For neoplastic compression, radiation therapy is increasingly favored over surgical decompression, since results are equally good in many studies. However, this assumes that the tissue type is known and the underlying cancer has been identified. Otherwise surgery may be needed for diagnosis as well as treatment (an excisional biopsy that is therapeutic as well as diagnostic). In either case, high-dose intravenous steroids, such as 100 mg of Decadron daily, may provide additional relief.

Rodichok LD, et al: Early diagnosis of spinal epidural metastases. Am J Med 70:1181–1188, 1981.

Barcena A, et al: Spinal metastatic disease: Analysis of factors determining functional prognosis and the choice of treatment. Neurosurgery 15:820–827, 1989.

BRAINSTEM DISEASE

38. A patient presents with a primary complaint of dizziness. What characteristics of the dizziness should be ascertained during evaluation?

When evaluating a patient with dizziness, the first question should be whether this is true vestibular dizziness (vertigo) or "dizziness" because of near syncope, ataxia, or other etiology. Patients with true vestibular dizziness complain of **vertigo**, which is a sense of spinning or turning of themselves or the environment, much like being on a merry-go-round. In essence, it is an hallucination, the sensation of motion when none is actually present.

The next decision is to determine whether the vertigo is central (due to a brainstem lesion) or peripheral (due to an ear lesion). Although many accompanying signs and symptoms have been promulgated to differentiate central from peripheral vertigo, none has great sensitivity or specificity. The most useful way to diagnose vertigo is by the company it keeps; **brainstem vertigo** is almost always accompanied by other signs of brainstem dysfunction, such as double vision, weakness or numbness of the face, dysarthria, dysphagia, etc. **Vertigo due to an ear lesion** is usually accompanied by tinnitus or hearing loss, but no other neurologic abnormalities.

39. Name the common causes of (1) peripheral vertigo and (2) central vertigo.

Common Causes of Vertigo

Peripheral	Central
Meniere's disease	Stroke
Vestibular neuronitis	Multiple sclerosis
Local trauma	Tumors
Drugs (antibiotics, diuretics)	
Acoustic neuroma	
Benign positional vertigo	

40. Which special procedures are helpful in the diagnostic evaluation of the dizzy patient?

Diagnostic evaluation of the dizzy patient depends heavily upon the history and physical examination. Audiograms are often useful to determine if there is any disease in the ear. Brainstem auditory evoked potentials may also be useful, since they can aid evaluation of both the peripheral eighth nerve in the ear, and also the central nervous system auditory pathways. Structural lesions, such as acoustic neuromas, are uncommon causes of dizziness, but when strongly suspected they may be seen using MRI.

41. What is the best treatment for dizziness?

Vertigo can be treated symptomatically, almost regardless of the cause. Scopolamine has proven to be the best available treatment in head-to-head trials against other drugs and placebos. Amphetamines are also useful, but for obvious reasons are seldom prescribed. Other similar drugs that stimulate the sympathetic autonomic nervous system are helpful, including agents such as ephedrine. Benzodiazepines and antihistamines are of some value, including meclizine (Antivert) and diazepam.

Parker SW: Modern approaches to dizziness and vertigo. Drug Therapy 53–64, 1980.

CEREBELLAR DISEASE

42. What is the most common cause of cerebellar disease?
Alcoholism. Alcohol causes an anterior, midline (vermal) atrophy that leads to leg and truncal instability and thus to gait ataxia. Other metabolic causes of cerebellar disease include hypothyroidism and drugs such as 5-FU and phenytoin (Dilantin). Structural lesions can also cause cerebellar disease. The most common are cerebellar infarcts and hemorrhages, and neoplasms, both primary and metastatic.

43. What is the best treatment for cerebellar dysfunction?
Cerebellar tremor, dysmetria, and ataxia are among the most difficult symptoms to mask or treat effectively. Some studies have shown that high doses of isoniazid (INH), in a range from 900 to 1200 mg a day, are superior to placebo for minimizing cerebellar dysfunction. However the toxic effects on peripheral nerves, requiring pyridoxine supplementation, and on the liver, requiring constant blood monitoring, make it difficult to work with this drug at these high doses. Other medications such as propranolol, primidone, and trihexyphenydil have provided occasional, though sporadic, success.

BRAIN DISEASE

Stroke

44. What is a stroke?
Stroke is focal brain dysfunction due to ischemia. The ischemia may arise from atherosclerotic narrowing of a blood vessel, from an embolus, or from other causes.

45. What are the main kinds of strokes?
Strokes may be divided into four main types: thrombotic, embolic, lacunar, and intracerebral hemorrhagic.

Types of Strokes

TYPE	% OF ALL STROKES	ONSET	PRECEDING TIAs (%)	ALTERED MENTAL STATUS (%)	MRI OR CT SCAN	OTHER FEATURES
Thrombotic	40	May be gradual	50	5	Ischemic infarction	Carotid bruit, stroke during sleep
Embolic	30	Sudden	10	1	Superficial (cortical) infarction	Underlying heart disease, peripheral emboli or strokes in different vascular territories
Lacunar	20	May be gradual	30	0	Small, deep infarction	Pure motor or pure sensory stroke
Hemorrhagic	10	Sudden	5	25	Hyperdense mass	Nausea and vomiting, decreased mental status

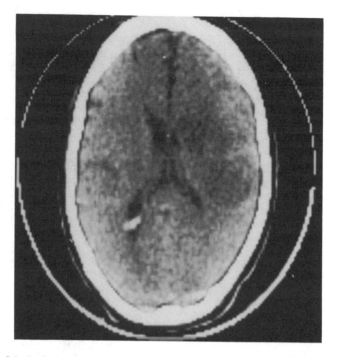

CT scan of the brain showing an ischemic stroke in the right middle cerebral artery territory, which appears as a large hypodense (dark) lesion.

46. What are the clinical features of a thrombotic stroke?

Thrombotic strokes are the most common type and account for approximately 40% of all strokes. They may have a gradual, stuttering, or step-wise onset rather than an abrupt, instantaneous deficit. The cause is generally atherosclerosis, which usually affects large vessels. The large-vessel involvement explains why thrombotic strokes tend to cause considerable neurologic deficit. About one-third to one-half of thrombotic strokes are preceded by transient ischemic attacks (TIAs), which are focal but totally reversible deficits that last from a few minutes to 24 hours.

47. What are the clinical features of an embolic stroke?

Embolic strokes generally arise from the heart and are most often diagnosed in patients with an underlying cardiac disease, such as atrial arrhythmias, valvular heart disease, or mural thrombus. They tend to be abrupt in onset, with more rapid resolution, and tend to cause smaller neurologic deficits than a thrombotic stroke. Because the embolus will travel in the arterial stream until it reaches a blood vessel of sufficiently small caliber to occlude it, it often travels distally all the way to the cortex. Cortical deficits, such as aphasia, are thus characteristic of embolic strokes.

48. What are the clinical features of a lacunar stroke?

Lacunar strokes are very small, discrete infarcts, less than 1 cc in size, occurring deep within the brain or brainstem (lacune means little lake or pond). These strokes are due to occlusion of tiny penetrating or perforating arterioles that supply the deep brain substance, usually in the region of the basal ganglia, thalamus, and internal capsule. The other region of the brain supplied by tiny penetrating arterioles is the brainstem, and this is the other common location for lacunae. Because these strokes are so small, they cause discrete clinical symptoms such as a pure motor stroke (hemiparesis without any sensory loss) or pure sensory stroke.

49. What are the clinical features of a hemorrhagic stroke?

An intracerebral hemorrhage is classified as a stroke because of its abrupt onset with focal neurologic deficits, but it is due to rupture of a blood vessel with subsequent bleeding and intracerebral mass, rather than to ischemia directly. Intracerebral bleeds have an abrupt onset and are usually accompanied by a significant headache and other signs of increased intracranial pressure, such as nausea, vomiting, and a diminished mental status. These are often devastating events with a poor prognosis. Bleeds tend to occur in the same deep locations as lacunae, namely the basal ganglia and brainstem.

50. What are the leading causes of death shortly after a stroke?

The three leading causes of death in the first 30 days after a stroke are not related primarily to the stroke itself or to neurologic deficits. They are listed in the following table:

Leading Causes of Death After a Stroke

1. Pneumonia
2. Pulmonary embolus
3. Ischemic heart disease
4. The stroke itself

51. What is the focus of medical management of the acute stroke patient?

Medical management of the stroke patient should focus on complications that develop after the stroke. Since the leading cause of death is pneumonia, care should be taken that the patient does not aspirate. He should be kept NPO until it is clear that his swallowing is not impaired by his neurologic damage. Fever in the wake of a stroke should always be presumed to be pneumonia until proven otherwise.

Measures to prevent pulmonary embolus should also be instituted, including early mobilization, support hose, and low-dose subcutaneous heparin.

Ischemic heart disease commonly causes death, since many patients who have atherosclerosis affecting the cerebral vasculature also have atherosclerosis of the coronary arteries. It has not yet been demonstrated that admitting stroke patients to an intensive care unit or that constant cardiac monitoring of such patients actually leads to improved survival or outcome. Nevertheless, cardiac assessment should be individualized for each stroke patient.

If there is intracerebral edema and swelling from the stroke itself, hyperosmolar agents to cause diuresis and reduction of the edema, such as mannitol, may be useful.

52. Are steroids useful in treating the acute stroke patient?

Steroids, once a widely popular treatment for massive strokes, have not been shown to be of any value, and may even be contraindicated; they should not be used.

53. Are there any specific treatments for the stroke itself?

Unfortunately, there is no very successful therapy for the stroke itself, other than general supportive measures.

54. What is the role of anti-platelet agents in cerebrovascular diseases?

Anti-platelet agents, specifically aspirin, have been advocated for the *secondary* prevention of stroke. Patients with a TIA or minor stroke are often treated with aspirin, usually in a dose of one tablet (325 mg) per day, to prevent further episodes of cerebrovascular ischemia.

Despite numerous large, multicenter, prospective, randomized, double-blinded trials, and a number of subsequent meta-analyses, the value of aspirin in cerebrovascular disease has never been proven conclusively. It is not clear if aspirin can in fact reduce the risk of stroke. Still, it is a relatively benign therapy for a disease that is otherwise essentially untreatable, so it is given routinely.

Prospective, Randomized, Double-Blind, Controlled Trials of Aspirin For the Prevention of Stroke

STUDY	NUMBER OF PATIENTS	FOLLOW-UP	DAILY ASPIRIN DOSE	STROKES ON ASPIRIN	STROKES NOT ON ASPIRIN	COMMENTS
American: Fields et al.	178	24 mos	1300 mg	11 (12%) n = 88	14 (15%) n = 90	(Stroke 8:301, 1977) No benefit for aspirin.
Canadian: Barnett et al.	585	26 mos	1300 mg	36 (12%) n = 290	48 (16%) n = 295	(N Engl J Med 299:53, 1978) Claimed benefit for aspirin (only in men without heart disease), but controversial.
Italian: Candelise et al.	124	11 mos	1000 mg	2 (4%) n = 63	2 (4%) n = 61	(Stroke 13:175, 1982) No benefit for aspirin.
French: Bousser et al.	604	36 mos	1000 mg	35 (11%) n = 400	31 (18%) n = 204	(Stroke 14:5, 1983) Claimed benefit for aspirin in men and women.
Danish: Sorenson et al.	203	25 mos	1000 mg	17 (17%) n = 101	11 (11%) n = 102	(Stroke 14:15, 1983) No benefit for aspirin; trend favored placebo.
Swedish: Britton et al.	505	24 mos	1500 mg	12 (5%) n = 253	13 (5%) n = 252	(Stroke 17:132, 1986) No benefit for aspirin.
United Kingdom	2,435	48 mos	1200 or 300 mg	158 (10%)	90 (11%)	(Br Med J 296:316, 1988) No benefit for aspirin.

55. Is there any role for aspirin in the primary prevention of stroke?
Aspirin does not seem to be helpful for the *primary* prevention of stroke. In the two large primary prevention trials of aspirin for coronary artery disease, the American and the British physician trials, there was actually an increased incidence of stroke among the subjects taking aspirin compared to those taking placebo.

Steering Committee of the Physicians' Health Study Research Group: Final report on the aspirin component of the ongoing physicians' health study. N Engl J Med 321:129–135, 1989.

56. Is dipyridamole useful in the prevention of stroke?
Dipyridamole (Persantine) has no role in therapy for cerebrovascular disease. A number of large, careful, blinded, multicenter studies have failed to show any benefit from dipyridamole for preventing strokes, or to the combination of dipyridamole and aspirin compared to

aspirin alone. Similarly, sulfinpyrazone (Anturane) and other antiplatelet agents have never been shown to be of value.

57. What is the role of anticoagulation in cerebrovascular disease?
The role of anticoagulation in cerebrovascular disease is very controversial, in part because prospective, randomized, double-blinded, placebo-controlled, multicenter trials, or similar definitive studies, have not been done addressing the most relevant issues. The consensus among most neurologists is that anticoagulation is only of benefit, or possible benefit, in two settings:

1. **Stroke in evolution.** A progressing stroke may benefit from anticoagulation. This is usually due to thrombotic stenosis of a large vessel, such as the internal carotid or middle cerebral artery, leading to progressive deficits that begin gradually and slowly worsen over a period of minutes or hours. Some authorities believe that heparin will prevent the propagating thrombosis and thus the progressive ischemia. In this setting, heparin is generally given without a loading bolus, in a dose of approximately 1000 units/hr continuous IV drip, to maintain the PTT at one and one-half times normal. Some neurologists continue anticoagulation by switching to coumarin for a period of up to several months, whereas others discontinue anticoagulation once the deficit has stabilized, usually in a few days.

2. **Embolic stroke from the heart.** The person with cardiac disease that has caused embolization to the brain will probably benefit from anticoagulation. The usual settings in which this occurs are atrial fibrillation, mural thrombus after myocardial infarction, or thrombosis on abnormal valves (as in rheumatic mitral valve disease). Following an initial brain embolus, the risk of subsequent embolization is high, especially within the first few days and weeks, and evidence suggests that immediate anticoagulation dramatically reduces this risk. Although there is a chance that immediate anticoagulation will worsen a stroke by converting the ischemia into hemorrhage, data suggest that this worsening is minimal and more than outweighed by the benefits in preventing further emboli.

Phillips SJ: An alternative view of heparin anticoagulation in acute focal brain ischemia. Stroke 20:295–298, 1989.

Copenhagen AFASAIC Study: Placebo-controlled randomized trial of warfarin and aspirin for prevention of thromboembolic complications in chronic atrial fibrillation. Lancet i:175–179, 1989.

58. What are the contraindications to anticoagulation in cerebrovascular disease?
In any setting, the contraindications to anticoagulation for ischemic cerebrovascular disease include known hypersensitivity to the drugs, bleeding dyscrasias, active bleeding such as from the GI tract or hematuria, a massive stroke (defined clinically, based on a clinician's judgment that there has been a major amount of brain tissue infarcted), and very frail health (such as an elderly, very sick patient).

59. What is the role of carotid endarterectomy in cerebrovascular disease?
The role of carotid endarterectomy for the treatment of cerebrovascular disease is one of the most hotly debated issues in neurology. Again, the careful prospective studies needed to precisely determine the value of this surgery have not been done, although at the time of this publication a number of trials are underway that will probably clarify this issue more definitively. The preliminary results from one such study, the North American Symptomatic Carotid Endarterectomy Trial (NASCET), suggest that surgery is superior to medical management for patients with a significant stenosis. Certainly, in most communities it is the "standard of practice" to perform carotid endarterectomy on otherwise healthy, good surgical candidates who have experienced a TIA in the carotid distribution, and who have angiographic evidence of a significant appropriate carotid lesion, defined as either a 70% carotid stenosis or deep ulceration.

Cebul RD, Whisnant JP: Carotid endarterectomy. Ann Intern Med 111:660–670, 1989.

AHCPR Health Technology Assessment Reports, 1990, Nos. 5 and 6. Washington, D.C., U.S. Dept. Health and Human Services, 1990, DHHS Pub. Nos. (PHS) 91-3472 and (PHS) 91-3473.

Aphasia

60. How is aphasia defined?

Aphasia is defined as a disturbance in language functions (that is, the ability to manipulate sounds and symbols into concepts or words and phrases). It must not be confused with dysarthria or slurred speech, which is strictly a problem with the motor control of talking. Aphasics not only have difficulty with talking, but also with writing, reading, and all other forms of language production.

61. What are the different types of aphasias?

There are two primary types of aphasias. The many subtypes are of interest primarily only to neurologic specialists.

The two main kinds of aphasia are **fluent aphasia** and **nonfluent aphasia.** Nonfluent aphasias are generally produced by lesions in the cortex, in the anterior part of the dominant hemisphere, around the sylvian fissure, and are often referred to by other expressions such as Broca's aphasia, motor aphasia, expressive aphasia, or anterior aphasia. Such patients have difficulty producing language and either cannot speak or do so only in monosyllables and short "telegraphic" phrases. Naming and repetition are also impaired, but comprehension is relatively preserved.

Fluent aphasias are due to lesions in the cortex in the posterior part of the dominant hemisphere, around the posterior temporal lobe. Such aphasias—also known as Wernicke's aphasia, sensory aphasia, receptive aphasia, or posterior aphasia—result in speech that is fluent and even loquacious, but senseless. These patients can talk but they make no sense. They have many neologisms and paraphasic errors, inventing words and sounds as they go along, and stringing words together in nongrammatical meaningless fashion. Such patients usually have impaired naming, repetition, and severely impaired comprehension as well.

Comparison of the Main Types of Aphasia

TYPE	FLUENT	NAMES	REPEATS	COMPREHENDS
Broca's	No	No	No	Yes
Wernicke's	Yes	No	No	No

Albert M, Helm-Estabrooks N: Diagnosis and treatment of aphasia. JAMA 259:1043–1047, 1205–1210, 1988.

Seizures

62. What is an epileptic seizure?

An epileptic seizure is the abnormal discharge of a neuron or group of neurons that leads to excessive electrical activity in the brain, causing disruption of brain function sufficient to produce clinical symptoms, such as staring spells or jerking of muscles.

63. What are the main kinds of epileptic seizures?

Epileptic seizures are generally divided into four main groups, as shown in the following table:

Classification of Epileptic Seizures

Generalized seizures
    Generalized tonic-clonic (grand-mal)
    Generalized absence (petit-mal)
Partial seizures
    Partial simple (focal)
    Partial complex (psychomotor)

64. What are the clinical features of partial simple seizures?

Most partial simple seizures encountered in a medical setting consist of the focal jerking or twitching of an arm or leg on one side of the body. This is usually due to a structural lesion in the brain (such as a stroke, abscess, or tumor) that leads to local irritation and an epileptic discharge. If this discharge spreads, the focal seizure will also spread, sometimes involving the other side of the brain and causing twitching or jerking of both arms and legs (a generalized tonic-clonic [grand mal] seizure). Occasionally, metabolic lesions, especially hyperglycemia and hyperosmolar states, can cause focal lesions and focal partial seizures.

65. What are the clinical features of partial complex seizures?

Partial complex seizures may be preceded by an aura of abnormal smells or tastes, visual sensations, or mental phenomena, such as déjà-vu. The seizure itself may consist of an episode of staring, lip smacking, and automatic, semi-purposeful movements, such as picking at clothes. Often there is no jerking of muscles, no loss of tone, and no falling down. Patients, however, are in a state of significantly altered mental status and are often completely unresponsive. After a minute or two the seizure passes, leaving a postictal state of confusion and lethargy.

66. What are the clinical features of generalized absence seizures?

Generalized absence seizures, sometimes referred to as petit mal, are seen almost exclusively in children. These seizures usually do not have any significant aura or postictal state, but may consist of just a few seconds of staring and altered mental status. This may be so brief, and clinical manifestations so subtle, as to escape detection by untrained observers. At other times, children are thought to be daydreaming rather than experiencing a seizure.

67. What are the clinical features of generalized tonic-clonic seizures?

Generalized tonic-clonic seizures, the so-called grand mal seizures, consist of the sudden onset, often without any preceding aura, of jerking tonic and clonic activity of both arms and both legs, with a generalized increase in muscle tone and loss of consciousness. There may be tongue biting or incontinence. Seizures usually last a minute or two and then resolve, often with a period of postictal lethargy and confusion.

68. What are the most common causes of seizures in the emergency room or on the medical ward?

The most common cause of seizures in a medical ward or emergency room is anticonvulsant withdrawal (that is, most patients are known epileptics who have been taking medicine, and for one reason or another are noncompliant with their drugs). Alcohol withdrawal is another common cause, as is drug overdose and metabolic derangements such as hyponatremia. Structural brain disease, including stroke and meningitis, is a less common (but still significant) cause of seizures.

69. What are the clinical features of alcohol withdrawal seizures?

Alcohol withdrawal seizures generally occur 12 to 48 hours after cessation or abrupt reduction in the intake of alcohol. These seizures are always generalized tonic-clonic seizures, without focality. They are often single, isolated seizures, but sometimes patients may have two or more. Status epilepticus is rare after alcohol withdrawal but does occasionally happen. Usually the interval between the first seizure and the last seizure is only about 6 hours. Alcohol withdrawal seizures seldom persist and are self-limited.

70. What are the most important principles of seizure management, including patients in status epilepticus?

Most seizures can be controlled completely, or nearly so, by following a few basic principles:

1. Pick the most appropriate anticonvulsant for the type of seizure the patient is experiencing.

2. Steadily increase the dose of that drug, following serum anticonvulsant levels, until seizures are controlled. If the patient becomes toxic on the drug before his seizures stop, then the drug is not the appropriate one. In this case, discontinue the drug and try a different one. Obviously, this should be done by starting the new anticonvulsant and increasing it to therapeutic levels before tapering off the old drug.

3. Monotherapy is preferable. If possible, once the old drug has been eliminated, the new drug should again be increased to the point where seizures are controlled, or the patient becomes toxic. Good therapeutic levels of one drug are preferable to subtherapeutic levels of multiple drugs.

71. Is status epilepticus life-threatening?
Status epilepticus can be life-threatening when generalized tonic-clonic seizures cause hyperpyrexia and acidosis from prolonged muscular activity, as well as occasional hypoxia or other compromise of respiratory function.

72. What is status epilepticus of partial seizures called?
Epilepsia partialis continua. Status epilepticus, defined as prolonged or repetitive seizures without a period of recovery between attacks, may occur with all forms of seizures.

73. What is the treatment of status epilepticus?

Treatment of Status Epilepticus

1. Rapid history and physical examination, including airway, breathing, circulation.
2. Start IV and draw blood for blood count (CBC), electrolytes, and anticonvulsant levels. Administer thiamine and glucose.
3. Infuse phenytoin by slow IV push at 50 mg/min to a dose of approximately 20 mg/kg (1,500 mg). If it is necessary to break a continuous seizure, diazepam up to 20 mg or lorazepam up to 8 mg may be given.
4. Infuse IV phenobarbitol at 100 mg/min up to 600 mg.
5. Institute general anesthesia.

Note: Experts disagree about when to intubate the patient. Some do it in step 2, others wait until step 4. You should always be prepared to immediately intubate any patient in status epilepticus.
Aminoff MJ, Simon RP: Status epilepticus. Am J Med 69:666–697, 1980.
Delgado-Escueta AV, et al: Management of status epilepticus. N Engl J Med 306:1337–1340, 1982.

74. Which drugs are the most useful anticonvulsants?
The most useful anticonvulsants depend upon the type of seizure:
1. Partial simple seizures: phenytoin, carbamazepine, and phenobarbital.
2. Partial complex seizures: carbamazepine, phenytoin, and phenobarbital.
3. Generalized absence seizures: ethosuximide and valproic acid.
4. Generalized tonic-clonic seizures: phenytoin, carbamazepine, and phenobarbital.

Mattson RH, et al: Comparison of carbamazepine, phenobarbital, phenytoin, and primidone in partial and secondarily generalized tonic-clonic seizures. N Engl J Med 313:145–151, 1985.

Parkinson's Disease

75. What are the cardinal features of Parkinson's disease?
Parkinson's disease is a gradual, progressive, degenerative disease of the basal ganglia (extrapyramidal) motor system. It is a very common condition, probably affecting 1% of people over the age of 60.

Cardinal Features of Parkinson's Disease

1. Tremor
2. Rigidity
3. Bradykinesia
4. Postural instability

The tremor is usually a to-and-fro, pronation-supination, resting tremor that diminishes with voluntary movement. It is coarse and slow, and is most prominent in the hands and head. Patients have rigidity, with a diffuse increase in muscular tone, and sometimes a "cog-wheeling" property to their joints when passively moved. Bradykinesia refers to slowness of movement. The patients also have a paucity or lack of movement and tend to show minimal facial expression—they often sit quite immobile, almost like statues.

76. What is the differential diagnosis of Parkinson's disease?
The vast majority of patients with tremor, rigidity, and bradykinesia have Parkinson's disease, but there are a few conditions which can cause parkinsonism, a symptom complex that mimics idiopathic Parkinson's disease. The most common causes are the neuroleptic drugs. Parkinsonian features are frequent side-effects of phenothiazines (such as chlorpromazine, thioridazine, etc.) and butyrophenones (such as haloperidol). Similar symptoms can also be mimicked by multiple strokes, hydrocephalus, and degenerative conditions such as Alzheimer's disease.

77. What is the treatment for Parkinson's disease?
The best treatment for Parkinson's disease is a combination of L-dopa plus carbidopa (Sinemet). The main cause for the symptoms of Parkinson's disease is a deficiency of dopamine within the pathway running from the substantia nigra to the basal ganglia. Since dopamine cannot be given directly (because it does not cross the blood-brain barrier), it is given as L-dopa. To prevent L-dopa from being decarboxylated and metabolized before it can reach the brain, carbidopa is given in combination with it.

Other dopamine agonists are sometimes used to supplement Sinemet. The main one is bromocriptine. Anticholinergic agents, which suppress the overactive cholinergic system and bring it into balance with the diminished dopamine system, can alleviate symptoms of Parkinson's disease. The most commonly used agents are trihexyphenidyl and benztropine.

Antioxidants, which may slow the rate of degeneration in the basal ganglia, are probably of some value in slowing the progression of Parkinson's disease. For this reason, MAO inhibitors such as deprenyl are commonly used.

The Parkinson Study Group: Effect of deprenyl on the progression of disability in early Parkinson's disease. N Engl J Med 321:1364–1371, 1989.

78. What are the other important types of tremors?
Parkinson's disease is the most common form of resting tremor and can usually be recognized by the accompanying rigidity and bradykinesia. However, other important types of tremors include:

1. **Essential tremor.** This is a rapid, fine tremor involving the head and arms especially, which is present at rest but more noticeable with sustained postures or intentional movement. About half the cases have a family history, with an autosomal dominant inheritance.

2. **Cerebellar tremor.** Damage to the cerebellum disturbs motor control by causing a tremor. This is absent at rest and only appears with intentional or voluntary movements. It is a slow, coarse, dyssynergic tremor.

OTHER DISCRETE SYNDROMES NOT ANATOMICALLY LOCALIZED

Headache

79. What are the key principles in evaluating headache?

Headache is an almost universal symptom, at least at some time in life, and is one of the most common reasons for consulting a physician. A few simple principles will aid in the management of headache:

1. The brain is anesthetic. This means that most causes of head pain do not arise from the brain itself but rather from surrounding structures, such as blood vessels, periosteum, etc. Since most headaches are not caused by brain disease, most are benign.

2. The more severe the headache, the more benign the disease. The exception to this is intracranial hemorrhage, but in general, most severe headaches are due to self-limited causes.

3. Eye problems and sinus disease seldom cause headaches. Patients tend to blame their headaches on eye strain or sinusitis, but in fact these are rare etiologies.

Lance JW: Headache. Ann Neurol 10:1–10, 1981.

80. What are the common types of headache?

Common Types of Headaches

Common migraine
Classic migraine
Tension headaches

Other less common or rare types of headaches include cluster headaches and headaches from brain tumor, meningeal irritation, and temporal arteritis.

81. What are the serious disease processes capable of causing permanent neurologic dysfunction that can present as headaches?

Although most processes causing headache are benign, some are serious, as follows:

Serious Causes of Headache

1. Brain tumor, either primary or metastatic
2. Increased intracranial pressure from other mass lesions, such as abscesses, subdural hematomas, etc.
3. Intracranial bleeding, either from subarachnoid hemorrhage or intracerebral hemorrhage
4. Meningitis, either bacterial or viral
5. Temporal arteritis and other vasculitis

82. What are the clinical features of headache due to brain tumor?

Brain tumors generally cause a mild-to-moderate headache, seldom severe, that is rather nonspecific in its symptoms. It is dull, chronic, and throughout the whole head. Often it is not localized to the region of the tumor. The headache is usually worse with maneuvers that cause the tumor to shift around, such as changes in position (as upon getting out of bed in the morning, bending over, etc.). Valsalva maneuvers, which increase intracranial pressure, will also worsen the headache. Most brain tumors produce abnormal findings on physical examination, such as altered mental status, papilledema, or focal weakness or numbness. A headache with a normal neurologic examination is unlikely to be a brain tumor.

83. What are the clinical features of increased intracranial pressure?

Because the brain is completely surrounded by the hard bony skull, any increase in intracranial pressure can impair brain function. The most sensitive indicator of increased intracranial pressure is an altered mental status and it is usually the first symptom to change as the pressure rises. With increased pressure, the brain can herniate downward through the foramen magnum, compressing and destroying the brainstem. Herniation can be recognized by the development of brainstem signs as the top of the brainstem (midbrain) becomes impaired. In addition to altered mental status, these signs include dilatation of one or both pupils ("blown pupil"), hyperventilation, and focal neurologic signs such as hemiparesis. Herniation can progress to coma and death.

84. How can intracranial pressure be lowered?

Lowering intracranial pressure requires reduction of the intracranial contents in order to make room for the mass lesion and increased pressure. The intracranial contents consist essentially of the brain, the cerebral spinal fluid filling the ventricles, and the blood within the blood vessels.

Lowering the blood pressure will of course lower the intracranial pressure, and this can be accomplished with a diuretic such as furosemide. Osmotic diuresis is particularly effective, and therefore mannitol is the mainstay of therapy to lower intracranial pressure. It is given intravenously in a dose of 100 mg, followed, if necessary, by 50 mg boluses every 2 hours. Glycerol and urea are other osmotic diuretics but are employed less frequently than mannitol.

Intubation and hyperventilation will cause vasospasm that reduces the blood volume intracranially. This is temporarily effective in lowering intracranial pressure, but because of compensatory re-equilibration, hyperventilation will provide at most a few hours of relief.

Steroids are useful for reducing swelling secondary to vasogenic edema, such as occurs with neoplasms, but they are not useful for edema that is cytotoxic, such as develops after a stroke or intracerebral hemorrhage. Since they may take hours or even days to work, they have little value acutely.

In emergency situations, intracranial pressure can be lowered by **removal of spinal fluid.** Surgical placement of a shunt in the ventricles to drain off spinal fluid can thus be life-saving.

85. What are the clinical features of headache due to intracerebral hemorrhage?

Intracranial hemorrhage causes the abrupt onset of an extremely severe headache. Patients will report that it is "the worst headache I have ever had in my life." The bleeding may result from the rupture of a vessel outside the brain (subarachnoid hemorrhage) or inside the brain (intracerebral hematoma).

Subarachnoid hemorrhage is usually due to the rupture of a small intracranial aneurysm, called a berry aneurysm, often located on the anterior communicating artery, the middle cerebral artery or their branches. Approximately half of the patients collapse and die at the time of the bleed. The remainder usually present to an emergency room with an altered mental status but may not have significant focal neurologic findings.

An **intracerebral hemorrhage** also causes collapse, coma, and death in a high percentage of patients, but since it occurs within the parenchyma of the brain, there are almost always focal neurologic findings, such as hemiparesis. Most patients also have altered mental status. It is strongly associated with hypertension.

86. What are the clinical features of headache due to meningitis?

The headache of meningitis, as in other severe illnesses, is often mild-to-moderate rather than extremely intense. It, too, is a diffuse pain throughout the head, sometimes accompanied by photophobia, and shows signs of irritation of the brain and meninges, such as a stiff neck. Meningitis is unlikely to be overlooked in the differential diagnosis of headache because of the accompanying signs of fever, elevated white blood count, and other evidence of infection. Meningitis usually presents as an infectious, toxic process rather than as a headache.

87. What are the clinical features of headache due to temporal arteritis?

Temporal arteritis is the confusing term used to describe a giant cell arteritis that may present as headache. It is confusing because the process is not confined to the temporal arteries. This is a systemic illness that usually has generalized symptoms such as fevers, myalgias, arthralgias (polymyalgia rheumatica), anemia, and elevated liver function tests. The erythrocyte sedimentation rate is usually very elevated, generally greater than 100 mm/min. The disease is very rare in people under the age of 55.

The headache of temporal arteritis is a mild-to-moderate, diffuse pain, not necessarily confined to the temples or frontal region of the head. The disease should be suspected in elderly people who develop new headaches, and the sedimentation rate is a good screening test. (Although there are reports of temporal arteritis with normal sedimentation rates, this is uncommon.) The confirmatory test is a temporal artery biopsy showing granulomatous angiitis. This biopsy is a fairly benign procedure, and should be done if the diagnosis is strongly suspected. High-dose steroids for a period of 1 to 2 years are often required, sometimes in doses in the range of 60 mg/day of prednisone or more. This is effective in controlling most symptoms of temporal arteritis, including the most tragic symptom, which is blindness from vasculitic involvement of the ophthalmic blood supply. Approximately 15% of patients with temporal arteritis, if left untreated, will develop significant visual loss.

88. Are migraine headaches a frequent problem in the general population?

Very frequent, with a prevalence of 20–30%. Migraine is much more common in women than men, and usually begins early in life, sometimes even in childhood, diminishing in both frequency and intensity of attacks in later adulthood. About half of all patients with migraine have a family history of the problem.

89. What are the clinical features of migraine headaches?

Migraine headaches are paroxysmal, intermittent headaches occurring on an average of once a month (though the frequency is highly variable) and lasting from 4 to 12 hours or more. About one-third of patients have hemicranial pain, but in two-thirds the headache is actually diffuse over the entire head. Most hemicranial headache is migraine, but most migraine is not hemicranial.

Some patients, with classic migraine (as opposed to common migraine) have a preceding aura for 20 to 40 minutes before the headache. This often consists of visual changes such as flashing lights. Gastrointestinal disturbances are also very common, including nausea and vomiting, and anorexia is almost universal. If you can eat during your headache, it is probably not migraine!

90. What are the most common triggering factors for migraine headaches?

Many patients with migraine have triggering factors that set off their headaches. Hormonal triggers are common, and many women have migraines at the time of their menstrual periods or accompanying ovulation. Alcohol, emotional stress, and some foods such as chocolate can also trigger headaches. A list of triggers includes:

Some Precipitating Factors in Migraine Headaches

1. Head trauma	5. Diet: chocolate, alcohol, etc.
2. Psychological stress	6. Hormonal changes
3. Sleep	7. Physical exertion
4. Changes in weather (barometric pressure)	

91. What is the cause of migraine headaches?

The cause of migraine is not known. A leading theory is that serotonin levels rise in the blood, triggering vasoconstriction. The increased serotonin is responsible for the gastrointestinal symptoms, and the vasoconstriction causes the neurologic deficits, such as visual changes. As the serotonin is metabolized, there is a rebound vasodilatation. It is this dilation and stretching of the blood vessels that causes the actual pain. Migraine is a vascular headache.

Another theory of migraine also involves serotonin, but in this theory low serotonin levels in the brain trigger brainstem neurons to fire, which alters cerebral blood flow. The neurologic deficits and the head pain result from low brain serotonin levels, and the vascular changes are only of secondary importance.

92. What is the best treatment for a migraine headache?

Ergotamines remain the best treatment for migraine headaches. They probably work by promoting vasoconstriction. They are especially useful if the patient has an aura alerting him to the onset of the headache, so that ergotamines can be taken and the vessels constricted, thus preventing the subsequent phase of vascular dilatation that causes the actual head pain.

93. What treatments are useful as prophylactic or preventive therapies in people with migraine?

For patients who have very frequent headaches, or the occasional patient whose headache is complicated by persistent neurologic deficits, prophylactic treatment may be indicated. A variety of drugs from different classes are helpful:

1. **Amitriptyline,** a tricyclic compound, is useful, though doses of 100 mg a day or more may be necessary. Most other tricyclics are not effective.

2. **Propranolol,** a beta adrenergic blocking agent, is also useful, again in doses of 100 mg or more per day. Most other beta adrenergic blockers are not effective.

3. **Calcium channel blockers.** Both nifedipine and verapamil have been shown to be effective in the prevention of migraine.

4. **Cyproheptadine,** in doses of 2 to 8 mg a day, is also useful. This drug is an antihistamine.

5. **Methysergide,** is probably the single most useful prophylactic agent for migraine. It is a serotonin analog but its exact mechanism of action is not clear. Patients who show no response whatsoever to methysergide probably do not truly have migraine.

94. Are there contraindications to the prescription of methysergide for migraine?

Despite the excellent results from this agent, particularly for severe migraine, it is often not prescribed for patients because of fear of side-effects. When the drug was first introduced, patients taking large doses for longer than 6 months occasionally developed fibrotic complications, including retroperitoneal fibrosis with ureteral stricture, and pulmonary fibrosis. Fortunately, in doses less than 8 mg per day this side-effect does not seem to be significant. Nevertheless, it is recommended that patients be given a "drug holiday" and withdrawn from the medication for 1 month out of every 6, since the fibrotic complication is reversible.

95. What are the clinical features of tension headaches?

Tension headaches are diffuse headaches, often described as a band around the head, usually bifrontal but sometimes occipital. Patients with chronic, persistent tension headaches report that the pain is very severe, though it seldom seems so to the physician. Unlike migraine, these headaches are usually not paroxysmal but are constant and chronic. Like migraine, they are most common in women and generally begin early in life, and about half of the patients have a family history. Usually there are no associated neurologic symptoms (such as visual changes) or nausea and vomiting.

Tension and migraine headaches commonly coexist in the same patient.

96. What is the cause of tension headaches?

The cause of tension headache is not known. There is no convincing evidence that they are due to psychological factors or emotional stress, nor are there good data showing they are related to muscle contraction.

97. What is the best treatment for tension headaches?

The best treatment for tension headaches is amitriptyline, sometimes requiring doses of 75 to 150 mg a day. This tricyclic compound works independently of its antidepressant effects. Nonsteroidal anti-inflammatory medications (NSAIDs) are useful for the daily common headache most people experience, but are seldom successful in treating the chronic persistent tension headache seen so often in the patients whose refractory pain spurs them to present to a physician for relief. Muscle relaxant drugs are also not effective (not surprisingly, since muscle contraction is not the cause of the headache).

Dementia

98. What are the clinical features of dementia?

Dementia is a progressive decline in cognitive and intellectual functions in the presence of a clear sensorium. Dementia implies that the person has lost intellectual function from his baseline state—that is, he was not born mentally retarded (this is an acquired process), and he is not delirious, lethargic, or otherwise suffering from an impaired level of consciousness.

99. What are the most common causes of dementia?

The most common cause of dementia is Alzheimer's disease, which probably accounts for at least half of all cases. Second in frequency is multi-infarct dementia, which is a loss of function because of ischemic destruction of significant amounts of brain tissue. The old belief that generalized atherosclerosis and global reduction in blood flow can cause dementia has proven correct in only the rarest of cases. Cerebrovascular disease essentially does not cause dementia except by actual destruction (infarction) of brain tissue.

Other causes of dementia include neurosyphilis, hypothyroidism, HIV infection, neoplasm, subdural hematoma, and head trauma.

100. What is the diagnostic approach to the patient with dementia?

The approach to the patient with dementia is to rule out treatable causes. Most dementias, such as Alzheimer's disease, have no effective treatment, so the best that can be hoped for in evaluating demented patients is that some treatable or reversible cause will be found, and the patient's personality and intellect can be restored. It is often difficult to distinguish the etiologies of dementia on clinical grounds alone, since so many conditions that impair the intellect mimic one another closely. Therefore, this diagnostic philosophy unfortunately requires ordering a variety of tests because of the great similarity in the clinical presentation of the different causes of dementia. Some reversible causes include:

Some Reversible Causes of Dementia

Mass lesions	Hypothyroidism
Meningioma	Drugs
Subdural hematoma	Syphilis
Hydrocephalus	Collagen vascular diseases
Vitamin deficiencies	Alcohol
Uremia	Depression (pseudodementia)

A workup for treatable causes should include CT scan or MRI to image the brain, and an EEG to show metabolic encephalopathies, which will produce diffuse slowing. The EEG helps to identify some specific dementias (such as the periodic sharp waves seen in Creutzfeldt-Jakob disease). Some authorities advocate lumbar puncture to rule out neurosyphilis, cryptococcal meningitis, or other chronic infections. Blood studies detect most other causes of dementia, such as hypothyroidism, B_{12} deficiency, and vasculitis.

Barry PP, Moskowitz MA: The diagnosis of reversible dementia in the elderly. Arch Intern Med 148:1914–1918, 1988.

101. What is Alzheimer's disease?

Alzheimer's disease, first described in 1906–1907 in Germany by Alois Alzheimer, is a degenerative dementing process of unknown etiology. Most elderly patients who were once termed "senile" probably had Alzheimer's disease, which is now felt to be a specific, distinct disease entity rather than the mere loss of intellectual functions with normal aging. Pathologically, Alzheimer's disease is characterized by degenerative changes in the brain, especially senile plaques, neurofibrillary tangles, and granulovacuolar degeneration. These degenerative changes are seen in great concentration in the hippocampus. Unfortunately, there is no biological marker or specific test for Alzheimer's disease, so clinically it is largely a diagnosis of exclusion. The criteria for the diagnosis of Alzheimer's disease, short of a brain biopsy, are summarized in the following table:

The Clinical Diagnosis of Alzheimer's Disease

1. Proof of dementia by neuropsychological testing	4. No disturbance of consciousness
2. Deficits in two or more areas of cognition (i.e., not just memory loss)	5. Onset between ages 40 and 90 (usually after age 65)
3. Progressive worsening	6. Absence of other causes of dementia

Multiple Sclerosis

102. What are the clinical features of multiple sclerosis (MS)?

MS is the most common disabling neurologic disease of young people under the age of 40. It is probably an autoimmune disease, characterized by relapsing and remitting episodes of inflammation in the brain and spinal cord. This inflammation destroys the myelin, which is the insulating sheath around nerve cells, and hence destroys the ability of the nerves to conduct electrical impulses (action potentials).

Clinically, MS may affect almost any part of the brain or spinal cord. Generally symptoms come on fairly abruptly, over a period of hours to days, persist for several weeks, and then resolve over a period of several more weeks, often returning completely to normal. On average, patients have one attack per year, although about 20% of patients with MS have a chronic progressive course of steady worsening deficit, without abrupt attacks.

The highly variable presentation of MS reflects the fact that it may involve the optic nerves, spinal cord, pyramidal tracts, spinothalamic tracts, brainstem, or cerebellum. Common symptoms include:

Most Common Symptoms of Multiple Sclerosis

1. Focal weakness	45%	4. Cerebellar ataxia	30%
2. Optic neuritis	40%	5. Diplopia and nystagmus	25%
3. Focal numbness	35%	6. Bowel and bladder changes	20%

103. How is the diagnosis of MS made?

The diagnosis of MS is primarily clinical, despite the great variability in signs and symptoms. The Schumacher criteria are well-proven guidelines for the diagnosis and include the following:

The Schumacher Criteria for Definite Multiple Sclerosis

1. Two separate CNS lesions	4. Objective deficits on examination
2. Two separate attacks of symptoms	5. Age 10–50 years
3. Symptoms must be consistent with a white matter (myelin) lesion	6. No other diseases with similar symptoms

Generally, young people who have had two separate lesions in the CNS at two separate times have a strong likelihood of having MS. Although these criteria are quite accurate, it is not possible to use them to diagnose MS when the very first symptom appears. A definitive diagnosis requires two separate symptoms. For this reason, patients suspected of having MS often undergo further testing to provide some laboratory confirmation of the diagnosis.

An MRI of the head very accurately shows the white matter lesions of MS. Although it is quite sensitive, it is not very specific, and a diagnosis can seldom be made from the MRI alone. The spinal fluid usually shows immunological abnormalities, specifically the presence of multiple polyclonal concentrations of IgG, which appear on electrophoresis as oligoclonal bands. A third technique for diagnosing MS is the use of evoked potentials, in which visual, auditory, or electrical stimulation is flashed to the brain, whose reactions are recorded using electrodes, similar to an electroencephalogram. A delay in the impulses evoked by the stimuli often indicates an underlying lesion in patients with MS.

104. How are the symptoms of MS best managed?

Because the cause of MS is not known, there is no cure. Steroids often help alleviate attacks, since they can reduce inflammation. However, they do not appear to alter the natural history of the disease.

Symptomatic management consists of medications to improve spasticity, such as baclofen, management of the neurogenic bladder, and braces or other aids to ambulation.

105. What treatments can alter the natural course of MS?

Immunosuppresive therapy is increasingly employed to try to alter the natural course of MS, using such agents as cyclophosphamide, azathioprine, cyclosporine, plasmapheresis, and total lymphoid radiation. At present, it is not clear that any of these therapies work, since no prospective randomized double-blinded trial has confirmed their value. Nevertheless, there are anecdotal data supporting their use and they remain common treatments.

106. What is the average length of survival after the onset of MS?

Although some patients die within a few years after the first attack, most live 30 years or longer. Multiple sclerosis may be disabling but is seldom fatal.

Coma

107. What are the commonest causes of coma?

The Commonest Causes of Coma

1. Drugs (including alcohol, illicit drugs, and accidental or intentional overdose)	4. Other metabolic derangements (sepsis, uremia, hepatic failure, etc.)
2. Hypoxia	5. Structural brain disease (stroke intracranial hemorrhage, etc.)
3. Hypoglycemia	

Most etiologies of coma are medical problems, not primary neurologic diseases.

108. What is the approach to the patient in coma?
Steps in coma management:
1. ABCs = protect the airway, breathing, and circulation.
2. Draw blood to check for metabolic derangements, infection, and drugs.
3. Infuse glucose, thiamine, and naloxone.
4. History and physical exam for clues to the cause of coma. Focus on pupils and extraocular movements for evidence of brainstem dysfunction.
5. Definitive diagnosis (and therapy) may require CT scanning, lumbar puncture, EEG, etc., depending on the situation.

109. What is the prognosis of coma?
Almost 70% of all patients admitted to a hospital in coma die. Brainstem abnormalities carry an especially grim prognosis—absent extraocular movements, absent gag reflex, or spontaneous respirations or unreactive pupils.

OTHER MEDICAL CONDITIONS AND THE NERVOUS SYSTEM

110. How does alcohol affect the nervous system?
Alcohol can affect virtually any part of the nervous system. Alcoholic myopathy may occur in heavy drinkers in a fashion analogous to the alcoholic cardiomyopathy that affects cardiac muscle. Although rare, acute rhabdomyolysis has been reported, associated with heavy alcohol consumption.

Although alcohol does not affect the neuromuscular junction, it commonly causes a peripheral neuropathy, usually a distal, symmetric, stocking-and-glove sensory and motor polyneuropathy. Alcoholics are also more sensitive to nerve compression, such as the classic "Saturday night" palsy, in which the radial nerve is compressed at the humerus, leading to a wrist drop.

There is no alcoholic radiculopathy per se, and myelopathy is very rare except for a few reported cases of a fulminant necrotic myelopathy associated with heavy alcoholic intake.

Alcohol can affect the brainstem, in the classic Wernicke's encephalopathy, which causes a triad of (1) nystagmus with extraocular abnormalities, (2) cerebellar ataxia, and (3) confusion. Wernicke's is really due to a thiamine deficiency rather than to alcohol ingestion itself. Cerebellar ataxia is common because alcohol leads to degeneration of the anterior (vermis) region of the cerebellum, causing a very ataxic gait. Finally, alcohol affects the cerebral hemisphere by causing an alcoholic dementia.

Charness ME, et al: Ethanol and the nervous system. N Engl J Med 321:442–454, 1989.

111. How does the human immunodeficiency virus (HIV) affect the nervous system?
The HIV can cause widespread damage in the nervous system. It probably enters the nervous system through macrophages that cross the blood-brain barrier. Approximately 10% of all AIDS patients present initially with neurologic symptoms.

An inflammatory myopathy has been reported in HIV-infected patients, as has an inflammatory neuropathy, both of which may respond to steroid treatment. The pathogenesis of the inflammation in both these conditions is poorly understood.

The AIDS myelopathy is a vacuolar degeneration that strongly resembles B_{12} deficiency. It is a chronic, progressive spinal cord syndrome.

The virus also affects the brain and cortex diffusely. Acutely, this can take the form of an aseptic meningitis. Chronically, HIV can cause an AIDS dementia complex. This may appear as a personality change, usually apathy and withdrawal, or as an organic dementia with forgetfulness and loss of cognitive functions.

An important consideration in AIDS patients is a CNS mass lesion, causing focal findings, altered mental status, headaches, or seizures. The most common mass lesions are toxoplasmosis and lymphoma.

Gabuzda DH, Hirsch MS: Neurologic manifestations of infection with human immunodeficiency virus. Ann Intern Med 107:383–391, 1987.

112. How does diabetes affect the nervous system?

The primary effect of diabetes on the nervous system is on the peripheral nerves. The most frequent problem is a distal, symmetric, stocking-and-glove sensory and motor polyneuropathy. This usually begins in the feet, generally with numbness, and ascends upwards, appearing in the hands only later. Often there are burning, painful paresthesias. In severe cases, proprioceptive loss may be sufficiently significant to cause Charcot joints. A motor neuropathy frequently accompanies the sensory changes. In addition, mononeuropathy can occur because the small vessel disease that accompanies diabetes frequently leads to infarction of nerves by occlusion of vasa nervorum. Femoral neuropathies and cranial nerve palsies are particularly common.

Another type of neuropathy is the thoracoabdominal neuropathy of diabetes, in which a thoracic root is damaged, again possibly by infarction, leading to severe chest or abdominal pain that is often mistaken for a visceral crisis. Finally, the autonomic peripheral nervous system may be affected, leading to impotence, bowel and bladder dysfunction, gastroparesis, orthostatic hypotension, or arrhythmias. Involvement of the CNS by diabetes is more indirect. Because diabetes is a risk factor for atherosclerosis, there is an increased incidence of stroke. Of course, hypoglycemia from overmedication can lead to focal neurologic findings such as hemiparesis or aphasia, or, if severe, to altered mental status including coma. Hyperglycemia, from diabetic ketoacidosis or from nonketotic hyperosmolar states, also causes altered mental status, sometimes accompanied by seizures.

113. Do drivers with epilepsy or diabetes mellitus have increased risk of traffic accidents compared to unaffected persons?

A recently published study supports earlier studies in concluding that drivers in both groups have slightly increased age-adjusted rates of accidents. However, these rates, especially when compared with other risk groups (e.g., drivers under age 25), do not represent a significant number of accidents or injuries.

Hansotia P, Broste SK: The effects of epilepsy or diabetes mellitus on the risk of automobile accidents. N Engl J Med 324:22–26, 1991.

114. How does renal failure affect the nervous system?

Uremia is one of the most common metabolic abnormalities affecting the nervous system. Again, the main influence is on the peripheral nerves, where there is a stocking-and-glove distal, symmetric, sensorimotor neuropathy. Patients with renal failure are prone to metabolic encephalopathies causing confusion, lethargy, and even coma. This may be aggravated by fluid and electrolyte shifts during dialysis. Also, because of the anticoagulation necessary for dialysis, there is an increased incidence of intracerebral hemorrhage, such as subdural hematomas, in these patients. A special type of mental status change is the syndrome of dialysis encephalopathy, which is a progressive deterioration in mental status, with hyperreflexia and dysarthria, usually accompanied by myoclonus and seizures. This syndrome is often irreversible and progressive until death.

Fraser CL, Arieff AI: Nervous system complications in uremia. Ann Intern Med 109:143–153, 1988.

115. How does cancer affect the nervous system?

Cancer affects the nervous system primarily by direct invasion. Metastases to the brain occur in 10% to 30% of patients with primary neoplasms, the most common being lung and colon cancer in males and breast cancer in females. Metastatic cancer usually presents as a focal neurologic deficit, such as hemiparesis, but may also cause seizures. As the tumor enlarges, it produces increased intracranial pressure, leading to headache, altered mental status, and ultimately herniation and death.

Cancer may metastasize or spread locally to the spinal cord, leading to acute spinal cord compression. Usually this is accompanied by back pain from vertebral body destruction. The onset of symptoms may be sudden with paraparesis, a sensory level, and bowel and bladder disturbances.

Carcinomatous meningitis is most common in lymphomas and leukemias, but can be seen with solid tumors as well. Usually this presents as altered mental status, sometimes with fever, and sometimes with focal neurologic deficits as the cancer invades cranial nerves and roots as they emerge from the CNS.

Involvement of the peripheral nervous system by direct extension is sometimes seen, such as when a Pancoast tumor invades the brachial plexus.

Peripheral neuropathies, however, are uncommon. Paraneoplastic syndromes, or remote effects of cancer, are actually quite rare. They may include myopathy (polymyositis), neuromuscular junction deficit (Lambert-Eaton myasthenic syndrome), or a peripheral neuropathy, predominantly sensory. There is also a condition of diffuse cerebellar ataxia. Most likely these syndromes are caused by circulating immunological proteins or antibodies which cross-react with neurologic tissues.

BIBLIOGRAPHY

1. Adams RD, Victor M: Principles of Neurology, 4th ed. New York, McGraw-Hill, 1989.
2. Asbury AK, McKhann GM, McDonald WI (eds): Diseases of the Nervous System. Philadelphia, W.B. Saunders, 1986.
3. Barnett HJM, Mohr JP, Stein BM, Yatsu FM (eds): Stroke. New York, Churchill Livingstone, 1986.
4. Brooks MH: A Clinician's View of Neuromuscular Diseases, 2nd ed. Baltimore, Williams & Wilkins, 1986.
5. Dalessio DJ (ed): Wolff's Headache and Other Head Pain. New York, Oxford University Press, 1986.
6. Laidlaw J, Richens A, Oxley J (eds): A Textbook of Epilepsy, 3rd ed. New York, Churchill Livingstone, 1988.
7. Matthews WB (ed): McAlpine's Multiple Sclerosis. New York, Churchill Livingstone, 1985.
8. Plum F, Posner JB: The Diagnosis of Stupor and Coma, 3rd ed. Philadelphia, F.A. Davis, 1982.
9. Rowland LP: Merritt's Textbook of Neurology, 8th ed. Philadelphia, Lea & Febiger, 1989.
10. Wilson JD, et al (eds): Harrison's Principles of Internal Medicine, 12th ed. New York, McGraw-Hill, 1991.

15. MEDICAL CONSULTATION SECRETS

Carol M. Ashton, M.D., M.P.H. and Nelda P. Wray, M.D., M.P.H.

When thou arte callde at anye time,
A patient to see:
And dost perceave the cure too grate,
And ponderous for thee:

See that thou laye disdeyne aside,
And pride of thyne owne skyll:
And thinke no shame counsell to take,
But rather wyth good wyll.

Gette one or two of experte men,
To helpe thee in that nede;
And make them partakers wyth thee
In that work to procede. . . .

But one thinge note, when two or moe
Together joygned be;
Aboute the paynfull patient,
See that ye doe agree.

See that no discorde doe arise,
Nor be at no debate;
For that shall sore discomforte hym,
That is in sycke estate. . . .

For noughte can more discomforte him,
That lies in griefe and peyne,
Then heare that one of you dothe beare
To other suche disdeine.

John Halle (1529–1568)
An Historicall Expostulation . . .
with a goodlye Doctrine and Instruction

GENERAL PERIOPERATIVE EVALUATION AND CARE

1. What are the hemodynamic changes that occur with spinal anesthesia?
Spinal anesthesia, the injection of local anesthetic into the subarachnoid space, blocks transmission of the impulses from the sympathetic nervous system as well as those mediating motor and sensory functions. The sympathetic nervous system controls the caliber of the blood vessels. At basal levels of sympathetic tone the vessels are maintained at about half their maximum diameter. Sympathetic stimulation causes vasoconstriction, whereas sympathetic denervation, as in spinal anesthesia, causes vasodilatation. The vasodilatation causes a drop in systemic vascular resistance and consequent pooling of blood in the lower extremities. Arterial blood pressure usually decreases with administration of spinal anesthesia, and the drop is more severe in patients who are volume-depleted prior to the anesthetic. Patients with hypertension (whether controlled or not) also have a tendency to have exaggerated hypotensive responses to spinal anesthesia.

2. What are the four most common causes of hypertension in Recovery Room patients?
Pain, a full bladder, hypothermia with shivering and vasoconstriction, and hypercarbia are the four most common causes of Recovery Room hypertension. Resolving these problems almost always reduces the arterial pressure without the need for specific antihypertensive therapy.

3. What is the correct approach to hypertension in the Recovery Room?
The first task is to assess the immediacy and severity of the situation. This is done not by reliance upon the actual numeric level of blood pressure, but by ascertaining whether acute organ dysfunction is resulting from or worsening because of the elevated pressure. A useful approach is to categorize the situation as a **hypertensive emergency,** in which the blood pressure should be lowered within the hour; a **hypertensive urgency,** in which the blood pressure should be controlled within 24 hours; or **simple hypertension,** in which there is no immediacy to lowering the pressure. A hypertensive emergency is defined by markedly elevated pressures and cerebral dysfunction (malignant hypertension or encephalopathy) or an acute intracranial event, myocardial ischemia, aortic dissection, acute pulmonary edema, pheochromocytoma crisis, or postoperative bleeding. Hypertensive urgencies include

markedly elevated pressures in conjunction with retinal hemorrhages and exudates (but no papilledema), congestive heart failure (CHF), stable angina, transient ischemic attacks (TIA), and renal insufficiency. Simple hypertension is a situation in which the pressure may be quite elevated but there is no acute or worsening chronic organ dysfunction.

Reuler JB, Magarian GJ: Hypertensive emergencies and urgencies: Definition, recognition, and management. J Gen Intern Med 3:64–74, 1988.

4. Intraoperative hemodynamic monitoring using a pulmonary artery catheter is often contemplated in the high-risk surgical patient. What are the potential benefits of such monitoring?

The hemodynamic parameters directly measurable using a pulmonary artery catheter include pulmonary artery systolic, diastolic, and wedge pressures as well as right atrial or central venous pressure. The mixed venous oxygen content, a measure of the adequacy of peripheral perfusion and tissue oxygenation, can be measured from blood obtained via the catheter. Indirect measurement of cardiac output can be performed, and several other parameters such as systemic vascular resistance can be calculated. By far the most clinically relevant use of the pulmonary artery catheter in the perioperative period is the management of intravascular volume. The pulmonary capillary wedge pressure (PCWP) (and also the pulmonary artery diastolic pressure) is an indicator of left ventricular filling pressure (preload); it should be interpreted and manipulated in light of simultaneous measures of the cardiac output. The pulmonary artery catheter is probably a more important tool in the early postoperative period than the intraoperative period.

5. The clinical usefulness of an invasive procedure must be interpreted in light of its risks. What are the risks of hemodynamic monitoring via a pulmonary artery catheter?

Complications associated with catheter insertion include pneumothorax, accidental arterial puncture, and ventricular ectopy and dysrhythmias. Dysrhythmias are a common occurrence but in most cases are self-limited or at least nonfatal. However, insertion of a catheter through the right heart in the patient with a left bundle branch block may interrupt right bundle branch conduction, leading to complete atrioventricular block.

Complications that occur while the catheter is in place include pulmonary infarction and perforation or rupture of the pulmonary artery. The latter is a rare complication but almost always fatal. Catheter-related sepsis and venous thrombosis are complications usually associated with longer-term (days rather than hours) catheterization.

Matthay MA, Chatterjee K: Bedside catheterization of the pulmonary artery: Risks compared with benefits. Ann Intern Med 109:826–834, 1988.

6. What are the general principles governing the use of perioperative antibiotics for prophylaxis of infection?

Perioperative antibiotics are often used to prevent infection from occurring, and the risk of infection varies with the type of surgical procedure. The risk is lowest in **clean procedures,** i.e., those that do not cross a mucous membrane or involve a break in surgical technique. Generally, prophylactic antibiotics are not given for clean procedures unless the operation involves the insertion of some prosthetic material, such as a cardiac valve or artificial joint. In those cases, the drastic consequences of an infection make the use of antibiotics worthwhile, even though the risk is very low. However, recent evidence suggests that prophylactic antibiotics may be cost-effective even in clean procedures not involving prostheses. **Clean-contaminated procedures** are those that cross a mucous membrane such as the urinary tract but do not involve a break in surgical technique. Prophylactic antibiotics reduce endogenous flora and are effective in reducing the rate of postoperative infections. **Contaminated procedures**—those involving traumatic wounds, spillage of gastrointestinal tract contents, or breaks in surgical technique—have a higher rate of infection, and antibiotics are effective in reducing subsequent infection.

Dirty cases, those involving pus or old traumatic wounds, have the highest rate of infection, and antibiotics are always indicated. Because the goal is to attain antimicrobial levels in the tissues by the time bacteria are likely to seed the wound or bloodstream, antibiotics should be given not more than 2 hours before the procedure. Often they are administered with the preoperative sedatives. In general, the duration of therapy need not be longer than 24 hours, and in many cases one preoperative dose will do.

7. What are the pros and cons of substituting spinal anesthesia for general endotracheal anesthesia in patients with lung disease?

Endotracheal intubation breaches the mechanical barriers to lower respiratory tract infection, which is of special concern in the patient with chronic lung disease whose defenses are already impaired and in whom respiratory infection carries a high mortality. Intubation is also associated with increased bronchial secretions, which may be difficult for the chronic lung patient to clear. Intubation may cause bronchospasm in the patient with reactive airways. However, these risks are more than balanced by the fact that intubation and mechanical ventilation allow a measure of control over alveolar ventilation and gas exchange that is not possible in the nonintubated patient.

Spinal anesthesia may cause serious respiratory compromise in the chronic lung patient, depending on the level of the spine to which anesthesia is allowed to extend. Expiration is a passive process during quiet breathing in normal persons, but in patients with obstructive lung disease, expiration is an active process—it requires muscular effort. The most important expiratory muscles are those of the abdominal wall (rectus, internal and external oblique, and transversus) and the internal intercostals. These are innervated by the thoracic nerves (T1–L1). The most important muscle of inspiration is the diaphragm. Because this is innervated by the phrenic nerve (C3, 4, 5), it is very unusual for the diaphragm to be paralyzed by spinal anesthesia. However, during abdominal surgery retractors and packs may interfere with diaphragmatic excursion and compromise the patient with limited respiratory reserve.

8. What are the metabolic-hormonal responses to major surgery?

The most important metabolic-hormonal response to surgery is the stress response. Although anesthesia prevents conscious perception of bodily injury, the body responds to major surgery as it does to any other noxious stimulus, with an outpouring of catecholamines and cortisol. In addition to their multiple hemodynamic effects, the catecholamines epinephrine and norepinephrine stimulate the pituitary gland to produce adrenocorticotropic hormone (ACTH). ACTH stimulates the adrenal gland to secrete glucocorticoids (e.g., cortisol) and mineralocorticoids (e.g., aldosterone). Glucocorticoids promote gluconeogenesis by a variety of mechanisms, most of which are catabolic. Postoperative hyperglycemia, seen even in nondiabetics, often results. Aldosterone acts on renal tubular cells to increase the conservation of sodium (potassium is excreted in exchange). The net effect is to increase the extracellular fluid volume, and ultimately, the intravascular volume. Surgical trauma and postoperative pain also may increase the secretion of antidiuretic hormone (ADH), which decreases free-water excretion by the kidneys. These mechanisms are all devoted to protecting the organism, but at times they overshoot. Starvation, water deprivation, pain, infection, hemorrhage, and drugs often exaggerate their effects.

9. Shifts in blood pressure are most common at what times during the intraoperative course of the patient undergoing general endotracheal anesthesia?

Induction of anesthesia is almost always accompanied by a drop in the mean arterial pressure. The drop can be quite marked in hypertensives (whether or not they are well controlled preoperatively) and in patients with volume depletion. Laryngoscopy and tracheal intubation are often associated with tachycardia and hypertension. Blood pressure usually levels out during the procedure. In uncomplicated surgery, induction is the most dangerous time as far as blood pressure is concerned.

10. In the patient on long-term antianginal or antihypertensive therapy, how should the medications be handled perioperatively?

Antihypertensive and antianginal agents should be continued up until the day of surgery. On the morning of surgery, they should be administered with a sip of water. The patient should resume a normal schedule as soon as possible postoperatively.

One occasional exception to this practice is the patient on chronic diuretic therapy for hypertension. Rarely, such a patient is truly volume depleted as a result of such therapy. Volume status can be assessed by determining whether postural changes occur in the blood pressure and heart rate. If the patient is volume depleted, diuretics should be withheld and the intravascular volume restored prior to surgery.

11. In what surgical populations would it not be cost-effective to obtain a screening preoperative electrocardiogram (ECG)? a screening chest radiograph? screening coagulation studies?

A "screening" test is a test performed on a person who has no clinical evidence of the disease in question. Because of sensitivity and specificity issues, not all tests are good screening tests; furthermore, screening is justifiable only for certain diseases. Preoperative *screening* ECGs, chest radiographs, and coagulation studies have not been shown to be cost-effective because the prevalence of clinically silent but perioperatively important heart, lung, and coagulation disorders is so low in asymptomatic patients. In situations in which the prevalence of those conditions is higher, or there is some indication from history or examination that disease may be present, preoperative tests may be justified. Some believe that all patients over 45 should have an ECG and chest radiograph before elective surgery. Others obtain those tests only in patients suspected of heart or lung disease. It is a common practice to obtain routine screening preoperative coagulation studies, but no studies have shown this to be cost-effective or beneficial. It is recommended that coagulation studies for elective surgery be reserved for patients with a personal or family history of coagulopathy or liver disease.

12. What are the general principles guiding the use of total parenteral nutrition (TPN) in surgical patients?

The hypermetabolic, catabolic state induced by major surgery is compounded by a state of relative starvation in the perioperative period. Though this presents little problem to the well-nourished individual, the incidence of postoperative complications is highly correlated with the severity of malnutrition in less robust patients.

Because of its significant risks and costs, TPN should not be used indiscriminately in surgical patients. Three groups of high-risk patients are almost always benefited from perioperative parenteral nutrition: (1) severely malnourished patients undergoing major intrathoracic or intraabdominal surgery, (2) moderately malnourished or previously well-nourished patients having procedures that result in prolonged (> 1 week) periods of inadequate intake (e.g., pancreaticoduodenectomy), and (3) previously well-nourished patients who develop postoperative complications likely to result in a prolonged period of inadequate oral intake.

American College of Physicians: Perioperative parenteral nutrition. Ann Intern Med 107:252–253, 1987.

13. Induction, maintenance, and reversal are the three phases of general anesthesia. What is induction and what are some of the problems that may occur at induction?

Induction of anesthesia consists of administering medication to the conscious, perceiving patient in order to produce a state of unconsciousness and lack of perception. Though inhalational agents can be used to induce anesthesia, in current practice induction is usually accomplished by the intravenous (IV) route. Though it is advisable to intubate some patients before induction of anesthesia, endotracheal intubation is usually carried out immediately after induction. Problems that may occur include retching, vomiting, aspiration, cough, laryngospasm, hypotension, and cardiac dysrhythmias.

14. What is regional anesthesia?

Any anesthesia that is not general is regional. This includes spinal anesthesia (injection of anesthetic into the subarachnoid space), peridural and caudal nerve blocks, regional nerve blocks (e.g., brachial plexus block), and local anesthesia. In many cases there are great advantages to using regional anesthesia instead of general. However, regional anesthesia demands more technical skill from the anesthetist, modified behavior in the operating room by all members of the surgical team, and considerable psychologic support of the patient during the operation.

SURGERY AND HEART DISEASE

15. What are the components of Goldman's cardiac risk index, and how do the levels of risk as determined by the index correlate with the likelihood of cardiac complications?

Goldman found that nine factors affect the likelihood of a cardiac complication with noncardiac surgery:

Factor	Points
Age > 70	5
Myocardial infarction (MI) in the prior 6 months	10
S_3 gallop	11
Important aortic stenosis	3
A cardiac rhythm other than sinus, or PACs on the ECG	7
>5 PVCs/minute documented at any time prior to operation	7
Poor general medical status	3
Intraperitoneal, intrathoracic, or aortic operation	3
Emergency operation	4

PAC = premature atrial contraction; PVC = premature ventricular contraction; S_3 = third heart sound.

In Goldman's study, the risk of a life-threatening cardiac complication (MI, pulmonary edema, or ventricular tachycardia) increased with the number of points. Patients with ≤ 5 points had a negligible risk. Those with 6 to 12 points had a 5% risk, with 13 to 25 points an 11% risk, and with 26 or more a 22% risk. If possible, it is advisable to delay the surgical procedure in the high-risk patient and correct whatever modifiable problems the patient has, e.g., S_3 or poor medical status.

Goldman L, et al: Multifactorial index of cardiac risk in noncardiac surgical procedures. N Engl J Med 297:845–850, 1977.

16. What are the important issues relating to the perioperative care of the patient with a permanent cardiac pacemaker?

Two issues must be addressed: the cardiac status of the patient, including an assessment of adequacy of pacemaker function, and safety in the operating room. In general, the adequately functioning pacemaker (1) senses the patient's own intracardiac signals and (2) delivers an electric stimulus to depolarize the myocardium, at a time when it is excitable, at an appropriate rate. Pacemaker function should be assessed sometime during the month before elective surgery at the patient's usual source of pacemaker care. Also, the implantation site should be examined for signs of infection.

In the operating room, electromagnetic interference (usually from the electrocautery) may cause the demand pacemaker to fail to pace. This problem can be solved by converting the pacemaker from a demand mode to a fixed-rate mode by placing a high-powered magnet over the generator. The possibility of electromagnetic interference can be minimized by placing the ground plate as far from the generator as possible and by using the electrocautery in short bursts. In the patient with a temporary pacemaker, the pacemaker leads provide a direct pathway by which extraneous external electrical impulses can go directly to the heart. The contact points between the leads and the generator should be covered with a surgical glove, and gloves should be worn when handling the unit.

17. What common postoperative dysrhythmia typically presents with a heart rate of 150?

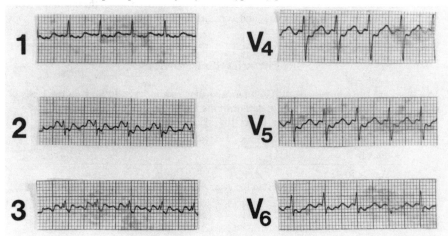

Atrial flutter, a supraventricular tachycardia, is one of the most common dysrhythmias observed in the postoperative period. It may occur in persons with or without heart disease. In atrial flutter the atrial rate is about 300 per minute. Atrial flutter with a 2:1 conduction ratio should be suspected in the patient with a supraventricular dysrhythmia who has a heart rate of 150.

18. Hemodynamically, why do general anesthesia and surgery carry a higher risk for perioperative cardiac complications in the patient who has asymptomatic but significant aortic stenosis (AS)?

The stenotic aortic valve presents a fixed obstruction to the outflow of blood from the left ventricle (LV). In other words, the stenotic orifice limits the maximum cardiac output that can be achieved. In early AS, cardiac output is maintained. The pressure gradient across the stenotic valve during systole increases with increased flow (i.e., increased cardiac output) or as the valve orifice decreases in diameter. The LV hypertrophies in response to the chronic pressure overload. As outflow obstruction worsens, though cardiac output is normal at rest, there is an inability to increase it appropriately with exercise.

In normals, when tissue demands for oxygen go up (such as with exercise), the cardiac output is increased by three mechanisms: (1) arterial dilatation with a drop in LV afterload; (2) enhanced myocardial contractility; and (3) a drop in venous capacitance with increased return to the heart and thus increased preload. In patients with moderately severe AS, arterial dilatation has little effect on improving cardiac output, because the stenotic valve remains the major obstruction to outflow. Because such patients do not have an appropriate response to peripheral dilatation, they are prone to have hypotension with exercise or any other situation in which peripheral dilatation is induced, e.g., anesthesia. Furthermore, because of LV hypertrophy these patients have stiff ventricles, such that for any given intracavitary volume the pressure is higher than normal. When cardiac return is increased in an effort to augment cardiac output, there is the potential for rapid rises in filling pressures and resultant pulmonary edema.

As would be expected in this pathophysiologic state, at the time of surgery, persons with AS are at risk for hypotension, pulmonary edema, and myocardial ischemia. Ischemia can develop in the patient with AS for several reasons. First, atherosclerotic coronary disease frequently coexists with AS. In addition, the pathophysiologic features of AS also affect myocardial oxygen balance unfavorably. Myocardial hypertrophy is associated with an increase in myocardial oxygen demand, and decreases in aortic pressure, especially during diastole, lead to decreases in myocardial oxygen delivery.

19. What is the risk of reinfarction with noncardiac surgery after myocardial infarction (MI)?

In general, the more recent the MI, the higher the chance of reinfarction with noncardiac surgery. Patients operated on within 3 months of an MI may have a reinfarction rate as high as 25%, though intensive intra- and postoperative hemodynamic monitoring and control may reduce that percentage. After 6 months, the reinfarction rate seems to stabilize at about 3–5%. Some recent studies are showing lower rates of perioperative MI with noncardiac surgery. It may be that improved surgical and anesthetic techniques have reduced the incidence of this complication.

Steen PA, et al: Myocardial reinfarction after anesthesia and surgery. JAMA 239:2566–2570, 1978.

20. How is it possible to determine whether myocardial ischemia is occurring intraoperatively?

Continuous ECG monitoring of ST-T wave morphology in lead V5 (one of the "exercise" leads) is the easiest and most reliable way to check for ischemia intraoperatively. Intraoperative transesophageal echocardiography, still an experimental technique, detects transient wall motion abnormalities in the patient having an episode of ischemia. One other possible way is to use changes in pulmonary capillary wedge pressure (PCWP) (data obtained via the pulmonary artery catheter). During ischemia, the diastolic stiffness of the LV increases, leading to an increase in PCWP. This last technique has very little real clinical utility because of the many factors which interfere with the interpretation of the PCWP in the operating room: operative position, blood loss, and fluid and drug administration.

21. What are the risk factors for perioperative MI with noncardiac surgery?

In theory, anything that increases myocardial oxygen demand or decreases oxygen supply to the myocardium, such that irreversible cell injury occurs, is a risk factor for perioperative MI. In practice, however, because of the remarkable range of the autoregulation of perfusion across the coronary bed present in the person with normal coronaries and myocardium, the most important risk factor is some sort of heart disease, such as stenotic coronary arteries, hypertrophied muscle, or dilated chambers. These conditions make the heart less able to compensate for the perturbations of myocardial oxygen demand and supply that may occur with anesthesia and surgery. In other words, they abbreviate cardiac reserve. The occurrence of sustained hypotension intraoperatively seems to be the most important extraneous risk factor. Sustained intraoperative hypertension does not seem to be as important.

22. How do you make the diagnosis of MI in the postoperative patient?

Just as in other settings, the diagnosis of MI rests on the triad of typical symptoms, a typical pattern of change in cardiac enzymes, and ECG changes. However, the postoperative patient presents some diagnostic challenges. Up to half the patients may never have the typical chest pain of MI. Instead they present with unexplained hypotension, dysrhythmias, pulmonary congestion, mental status changes, and restlessness. Though the symptoms are atypical for MI, the truly asymptomatic perioperative MI is an uncommon occurrence. Secondly, of all the so-called cardiac enzymes, only the MB fraction of creatine kinase (CK) is not elevated by the muscle trauma associated with anesthesia and surgery. So although the total CK may be "falsely" elevated in the postoperative patient, CK-MB retains its excellent sensitivity and specificity for acute MI. ECG changes are very common in the postoperative setting, so the ECG by itself is of little utility in diagnosing infarction. Up to 20% of postoperative patients will have new ECG abnormalities, usually minor changes such as T-wave inversion or flattening. In any setting, Q waves pathognomonic for infarction develop in only 60% of patients with documented MIs.

23. What are the principles of evaluation and management of the patient with congestive heart failure (CHF) who must undergo noncardiac surgery?
In the patient with CHF, whether from systolic impairment or diastolic dysfunction, evaluating the state of compensation for CHF is the most important component of the preoperative evaluation, even more important than knowing the ejection fraction. The ejection fraction tells nothing about the state of compensation, and no consistent relationship has been found between ejection fraction and exercise tolerance as determined on a treadmill. Recent declines in exercise tolerance, increasing fatigue, orthopnea, and paroxysmal nocturnal dyspnea are the symptoms of decompensation. The signs of decompensation are weight increase, jugular venous distention, S_3 gallop, hepatomegaly, and edema. It is important to have the patient as well compensated as possible before surgery. CHF seems to be an independent risk factor for perioperative cardiac complications. Monitoring right atrial or pulmonary wedge pressure intraoperatively and even more importantly *post*operatively can help in the management of intravascular volume.

24. How commonly do patients with atherosclerotic peripheral vascular disease and no symptoms or signs of coronary artery disease (CAD) actually have silent, significant ($\geq 70\%$ stenosis of at least one vessel) CAD?
Concomitant coronary atherosclerosis is frequently observed in patients who have atherosclerotic disease in other circulations, such as the cerebral vessels and aorta, and are scheduled to undergo vascular procedures. Usually the CAD is obvious: the patient has a history of MI, angina, or both. However, a significant number (about 30%) of peripheral vascular disease patients who have no historical, clinical, or ECG evidence of CAD will be found to have significant stenosis if coronary angiography is done. This is not to say that all patients should undergo coronary angiography in preparation for vascular surgery. If the goal is to reduce the likelihood that the vascular procedure may precipitate an MI, then the risk of mortality and morbidity from the coronary angiography and subsequent coronary revascularization must be *less than* the chance the patient will have a fatal perioperative MI with the peripheral vascular procedure. This is certainly not the case for most patients.

Hertzer NR, et al: Coronary artery disease in peripheral vascular patients. Ann Surg 199:223–233, 1984.

SURGERY AND LUNG DISEASE

25. What are the changes in respiration that occur postoperatively with upper abdominal surgery?
Vital capacity (VC) is reduced in the early postoperative period after upper abdominal surgery. (VC includes three lung volumes: inspiratory reserve volume, tidal volume, and expiratory reserve volume.) Though pain is an important factor, the reduction in VC is attributable to diaphragmatic dysfunction and not simply to pain. Respirations are

shallower and faster, and sighs occur less frequently. When respiration at lower than normal lung volumes persists, airways at the lung bases are compressed, leading to collapse and atelectasis. Atelectasis causes ventilation/perfusion imbalance, and hypoxemia results. Preoperative and postoperative breathing exercises can minimize the probability of postoperative atelectasis.

26. What are the most common causes of postoperative respiratory failure?

Respiratory failure is defined as a decline in ventilatory performance accompanied by an arterial pO_2 below 50 mmHg and/or a pCO_2 above 50 mmHg. Simply stated, respiratory failure means that the lung is not performing its gas exchange function adequately. By far the most common cause of postoperative respiratory failure is atelectasis due to secretion retention. Aspiration pneumonia (true infection) due to aspiration of oropharyngeal secretions is observed more commonly than pneumonitis due to aspiration of gastric contents (infection is not invariable in this setting). The adult respiratory distress syndrome (ARDS), a noncardiogenic pulmonary edema, frequently occurs in the setting of massive aspiration of gastric contents. However, the overall incidence of postoperative ARDS seems to be decreasing. Other infrequent pulmonary complications associated with respiratory failure include massive pulmonary thromboembolism and fat embolism.

27. What are the symptoms and signs of pulmonary embolism (PE) in the postoperative patient?

Depending on the size of the embolus and the cardiopulmonary reserve of the patient, the clinical signs and symptoms of PE can be dramatic or very subtle, and can range from cardiac arrest to mild or almost no dyspnea. Dyspnea is the most common symptom, and, together with pleuritic pain, occurs in over half of patients. Cough may or may not be present. Hemoptysis is observed in fewer than a third of patients. Syncope occurs infrequently, but PE should be in the differential diagnosis when a patient suffers a syncopal attack on his or her first postoperative ambulation. Tachypnea is observed in most patients, but rales, tachycardia, an increased P_2 on cardiac auscultation, fever, and clinical signs of phlebitis are observed in fewer than half of the patients.

The diagnostic triad of hemoptysis, pleuritic pain, and dyspnea is seen in fewer than 20% of patients, even when massive embolus is present.

28. What are the classic ECG findings in the patient with acute PE? What are the classic arterial blood gas (ABG) findings?

One or more of the "classic" ECG findings of acute cor pulmonale ("$S_1Q_3T_3$," right bundle branch block [RBBB], P pulmonale, or right axis deviation [RAD]) are observed in fewer than 25% of patients. Over 10% of patients will have unchanged ECGs. ECG changes are observed more commonly in patients with preexisting cardiopulmonary disease and in patients with massive emboli. In the majority of patients with PE, the ECG will show only sinus tachycardia and/or ST-segment and T-wave abnormalities.

In most patients with clinically detectable PE, the arterial pO_2 will be less than 90 mmHg. A mild respiratory alkalosis is usually seen. ABGs cannot be relied upon to rule in or rule out the diagnosis of PE, but they are useful in determining the adequacy of the patient's ventilation.

29. What test of pulmonary function is the best predictor of postoperative morbidity in the patient with lung disease?

The single best predictor of postoperative pulmonary complications is an elevated arterial pCO_2. Patients who have chronic CO_2 retention are at high risk for perioperative morbidity and mortality from all causes. Most practitioners believe that there is no place for elective surgery in patients who are chronic CO_2 retainers.

30. What is atelectasis? What effect does it have on gas exchange?

Atelectasis is alveolar collapse. Microatelectasis ("micro" because it is not radiographically apparent) is a prominent feature of the pathophysiology of the adult respiratory distress syndrome (ARDS), whereby defects in the pulmonary surfactant system lead to alveolar instability and collapse. With endobronchial obstruction, radiographically apparent subsegmental, segmental, or lobar atelectasis (some radiologists prefer the term collapse) occurs. Atelectasis is associated with intrapulmonic shunting, i.e., blood courses past poorly ventilated alveoli, with resulting "venous admixture" and arterial hypoxemia.

31. What are the incidence and consequences of aspiration of gastric contents occurring with tracheal intubation in the operating room?

The true incidence is unknown, but aspiration of small amounts of gastric contents may be quite common, occurring in as many as one in four patients. Most times this has no clinically evident consequences. Aspiration of large amounts of gastric contents is uncommon and is immediately apparent to the anesthesiologist. The risk is greatest in nonfasting parturients and patients undergoing emergency operations. Patients with intestinal obstruction or esophageal disorders are also at risk.

Sequelae depend on the amount and type of aspirate. Aspiration of large amounts of acid gastric contents (pH < 2.5) causes a chemical burn of the lung, a pneumonitis. This results in immediate, intense bronchoconstriction, and eventual respiratory distress and insufficiency. Radiographic "white out" of the lungs occurs, and the full-blown ARDS develops. The consequences of aspiration of nonacid gastric contents (pH > 2.5) depend on whether bacteria and/or particulate matter is present in the aspirate. Aspiration of bacteria-containing material leads to development of infection, i.e., aspiration pneumonia. Aspiration of food particles causes obstruction of airways of comparable size.

32. What are the principles of managing the cigarette smoker who must undergo nonpulmonary surgery?

It is important to note that while most smokers do not have chronic obstructive lung disease (COPD), almost all smokers *do* have chronic bronchitis. Chronic bronchitis, a clinical diagnosis, is present if a productive cough has been present for 3 months of the year for 2 consecutive years. The excessive mucus production in smokers/chronic bronchitics is what leads to an increased incidence of postoperative pulmonary complications. Secretion retention and mucus plugging of airways in the postoperative period are associated with microatelectasis or radiographically apparent atelectasis. Atelectasis leads to gas-exchange abnormalities. There is evidence to suggest that smokers who can stop smoking for at least 8 weeks before surgery have a reduced likelihood of postoperative complications. This is probably because the tracheobronchial mucosa can repair itself in that time period and mucus production returns toward normal. Smokers who have a productive cough may benefit from a perioperative pulmonary toilet program, and, in general, the greater the amount of secretions, the more vigorous the program should be. The presence of a productive cough can be best ascertained at the bedside by asking the patient to cough and listening to how much "rattle" is present. Simply asking the patient about productive cough is much less reliable, since most smokers fail to notice their own cough.

33. What are the principles of management of the asthmatic who must undergo nonpulmonary surgery?

The two major principles of managing the asthmatic are **control of bronchospasm** and **control of secretions.** Tracheal intubation can exacerbate bronchospasm and is also associated with increased sputum production. This can be minimized by insuring that bronchospasm is under optimal control before the patient goes to the operating room.

Inhaled bronchodilators should be administered on a regular schedule, and if the patient is receiving theophylline, the serum level should be kept in the therapeutic range. Secretions can be managed by a pulmonary toilet program perioperatively. Such a program usually includes chest physiotherapy in addition to inhaled bronchodilators. Steroid-dependent asthmatics, in whom adrenal function is often suppressed, should receive IV corticosteroids in the perioperative period to cover them for the stress of anesthesia and surgery.

34. What are the principles of management of the patient with severe chronic obstructive pulmonary disease (COPD) who must undergo nonpulmonary surgery?

Postoperative pulmonary complications are most likely with upper abdominal surgery and occur much less commonly with peripheral procedures such as hip replacements. Nevertheless, the principles of management remain the same: **control of secretions** with a program of pulmonary toilet (aerosol bronchodilators, chest physiotherapy, coughing and deep breathing exercises, early ambulation); **avoidance of narcotic analgesics and sedatives,** which suppress respiratory drive and coughing; and **monitoring of gas exchange status** with arterial blood gas (ABG) measurements. In addition, postanesthesia extubation of patients with severe COPD should be postponed until the patient is fully awake, not sedated, and able to cough vigorously.

35. Of what benefit are preoperative basic pulmonary function tests (PFTs—spirometry and lung volume measurement)?

PFTs are an essential part of the workup of the patient who is facing pneumonectomy, lobectomy, or segmentectomy. In that setting, preoperative PFTs can help the clinician estimate the amount of respiratory function the patient will have after lung resection.

In nonthoracic surgery, the place of preoperative PFTs is much less clear. For preoperative PFTs to be of benefit, two conditions must apply:

1. PFTs must provide relevant diagnostic information over and above that which is available from the history and physical examination.

2. PFTs must be able to predict more accurately than the clinician which patients are at risk for postoperative pulmonary complications.

Neither of these conditions has been satisfied. Basic PFTs can diagnose only two conditions: obstructive lung disease and restrictive lung disease. These diagnoses can almost always be made and their severity estimated on clinical grounds, without the need for PFTs. Postoperative pulmonary complications occur most commonly with upper abdominal surgery, and the more severe the respiratory impairment, the more likely it is that complications will occur. The degree of respiratory impairment and the likelihood of postoperative pulmonary complications can be quite accurately assessed by questioning the patient about exercise tolerance (or observing it during a walk around the ward), estimating the amount of tracheobronchial secretions the patient produces, and checking the ABG. These maneuvers cost quite a bit less than the $500 that PFTs cost. The chance of postoperative pulmonary complications can be minimized by a pulmonary toilet program, which is safe, noninvasive, and inexpensive.

Lawrence VA, et al: Preoperative spirometry before abdominal operations: A critical appraisal of its predictive value. Arch Intern Med 149:280–285, 1989.

36. What is the "lesion" in postoperative adult respiratory distress syndrome (ARDS)?

ARDS is a type of **pulmonary edema.** Pulmonary edema is of two types: **cardiogenic,** in which alteration of Starling forces is responsible for increases in water content of the interstitium and alveoli, and **noncardiogenic,** in which the Starling forces are not deranged, but interstitial and alveolar water accumulates because of an increase in capillary permeability. **The "lesion" in ARDS is an injured pulmonary capillary epithelium.** (The Starling forces include the hydrostatic pressure inside the capillary, the hydrostatic forces in the interstitium, the oncotic pressure inside the capillary, and the oncotic pressure in the interstitium.)

It is impossible to distinguish noncardiogenic pulmonary edema (ARDS) from cardiogenic pulmonary edema on the basis of the clinical presentation and radiographic findings. The two conditions can be differentiated by measurement of the pulmonary wedge pressure. The pulmonary capillary wedge pressure (PCWP), which reflects LV filling pressures, is normally 6–12 mmHg. The PCWP is elevated in cardiogenic pulmonary edema, reflecting the elevated LV filling pressures. It is normal in ARDS, because LV filling pressures are normal because the defect is at the alveolocapillary membrane.

37. Who is at special risk for postoperative ARDS?

Factors that seem to predispose the postoperative patient (as well as nonoperative patients) to ARDS include massive aspiration of gastric contents, sepsis, massive transfusion of blood products, fat embolism, and disseminated intravascular coagulation (DIC). Patients with more than one of the above factors are at greatest risk.

38. What is the clinical presentation of fat embolism?

The fat embolism syndrome is a constellation of findings that includes mental status changes, respiratory and sometimes renal insufficiency, and a petechial rash. The syndrome is most commonly observed after fractures of long bones, but occasionally occurs after total hip arthroplasty. Although its delayed appearance lessens its diagnostic usefulness, the petechial rash is very specific for the syndrome. It develops only on the upper torso and in the absence of thrombocytopenia. The mortality rate may be as high as 20%, with respiratory failure accounting for most of the deaths. There is some evidence that corticosteroids may favorably alter the course. An index has been developed that when used in the appropriate clinical setting may lead to earlier diagnosis.

Fat Embolism Index*

FACTOR	SCORE
Petechiae	5
Diffuse alveolar infiltrates	4
Arterial $pO_2 < 70$ mmHg	3
Confusion	1
Fever $\geq 100.4°$ F	1
Heart rate ≥ 120 bpm	1
Respiratory rate $> 30/min$	1

*NOTE: A minimum of 5 points must be present for the diagnosis to be considered highly probable.
Schonfeld SA, et al: Fat embolism prophylaxis with corticosteroids. Ann Intern Med 99:438–443, 1983.

SURGERY AND KIDNEY DISEASE

39. What are the most common causes of postoperative renal insufficiency?

Most cases are due to prerenal causes. Renal parenchymal insults resulting in acute renal failure occur next in frequency. The most common insults are prolonged cross-clamping of the aorta at the time of vascular procedures leading to renal ischemia and nephrotoxic agents. Though contrast agents and aminoglycoside antibiotics are the most frequent nephrotoxins, nonsteroidal anti-inflammatory agents (NSAIDs) can also cause acute renal failure. Postrenal causes of postoperative azotemia are least frequent and include prostatic hypertrophy and the kinked indwelling bladder catheter.

40. How can you minimize the incidence of contrast-related nephropathy in the patient with peripheral vascular disease who must undergo preoperative angiography?

The patients who are at highest risk for the development of dye-induced nephropathy are those who have preexisting renal insufficiency regardless of the cause. Volume depletion at the time of the study is an important additive risk factor. Also, the risk increases with the amount of dye injected. A two-pronged approach should be used:

1. The patient must be adequately hydrated before the procedure.
2. The amount of dye injected should be kept to the minimum.

Normal or half-normal saline should be infused before, during, and after the procedure. Most nephrologists also prescribe a 20% solution of mannitol IV for prophylaxis. If two contrast procedures are necessary, the serum creatinine should be allowed to return to baseline before the second procedure.

41. What is the basic approach to determining the cause of new-onset renal insufficiency in the postoperative patient?

In the postoperative patient, as in other settings, it is useful to classify new-onset renal insufficiency as prerenal, renal, and postrenal. Prerenal azotemia results from decreased renal perfusion. Its causes include **intravascular volume depletion** due to hemorrhage, gastrointestinal losses (as with nasogastric suction or ileostomy), or third-spacing of fluids (as with peritonitis); **decreased cardiac function** due to pump failure, valvular abnormalities, dysrhythmias, or pericardial tamponade; **excessive peripheral vasodilatation** as seen in sepsis or with afterload reducing agents; and **obstruction of blood flow** through renal arteries or veins.

To evaluate for the presence of prerenal causes, a careful history and physical examination should be performed, with special reference to the cardiovascular system. The blood urea nitrogen (BUN):creatinine ratio provides helpful information. In prerenal azotemia, the ratio approaches 20:1 rather than its normal 10:1. Urinary sodium measures are extremely helpful. Because the kidney has only one stereotypical response to what it perceives to be a threat to intravascular volume, namely conservation of sodium (and hence water), in prerenal azotemia the urinary sodium will be very low, less than 10 mEq/L.

Obstruction to urine flow causes postrenal azotemia. In the workup of postoperative renal insufficiency, obstruction at or below the bladder neck should be ruled out by the insertion of a catheter. For obstruction above the bladder to cause renal failure, it must be bilateral. Inadvertent ligation of the ureters during abdominopelvic surgery occasionally occurs. The presence of hydronephrosis/hydroureter can be ascertained by renal ultrasonography.

Renal parenchymal causes of postoperative azotemia include ischemia, as can occur with abdominal aortic aneurysm surgeries, and exposure to nephrotoxins, such as contrast agents and aminoglycosides. The diagnosis is suggested by a BUN:creatinine ratio of > 20:1 and a urine sodium of > 10 mEq/L. The urine sodium is elevated because the injured parenchyma is unable to conserve sodium.

42. Who is at special risk for postoperative renal insufficiency?

Individuals at increased risk for postoperative renal dysfunction can be categorized based on the type of azotemia (prerenal, renal, postrenal) most likely to occur. Patients with cardiac disease are at highest risk for prerenal azotemia. Elderly patients (the glomerular filtration rate [GFR] falls progressively with aging) and patients with preexisting renal insufficiency are at greatest risk for renal azotemia. Patients with structural abnormalities of the lower urinary tract, namely prostatic hypertrophy or urethral stricture, are at greatest risk for postrenal azotemia. Obviously, often several of these risk factors are present in the same patient.

43. What are the principles of managing the patient with chronic renal failure in the perioperative period?

Preoperatively a thorough history, physical examination, and laboratory evaluation should be performed to quantitate the degree of renal dysfunction present. A convenient way to classify renal dysfunction is:

Stage 1: decreased renal reserve
Stage 2: renal insufficiency
Stage 3: moderate renal failure
Stage 4: severe renal failure

Patients in stage 1 are completely asymptomatic but have a glomerular filtration rate (GFR) of only 50–60% normal. BUN is < 20 mg/dl and serum creatinine is < 2 mg/dl. Elderly patients would fall into this stage because of age-related decrements in GFR. In the elderly, BUN and creatinine may be normal in the face of the decline in GFR, because muscle mass is lost with aging. Patients in stage 1 are at increased risk for postoperative renal failure from nephrotoxins. Stages 2–4 are characterized by progressive azotemia accompanied by symptoms and signs of uremia. These patients are unable to excrete volume and salt loads and are at risk for volume overload manifested by pulmonary edema and peripheral edema. In these patients, during the perioperative period, scrupulous attention must be given to intake and output. A pulmonary artery catheter, which allows measurement of pulmonary wedge pressure, is very helpful in managing these patients postoperatively.

Weir PHC, Chung FF: Anaesthesia for patients with chronic renal disease. Can Anaesth Soc J 31:468–480, 1984.

44. What effect do anesthesia and surgery have on ADH? What clinical significance does that effect have?

Anesthesia and surgery seem to provide "non-osmotic" stimuli for the release of ADH (antidiuretic hormone, also called vasopressin) from the posterior pituitary. ADH has a central role in water excretion by the kidney. It increases the permeability of the collecting tubules to water. Without ADH, the collecting tubules are not permeable to water and large volumes of water are excreted in urine. In the presence of ADH, water flows down its concentration gradient from the lumen into the interstitium, and a concentrated urine is excreted. Serum sodium drops. Hyperosmolality is the most potent stimulus for ADH release, though volume depletion is also a potent stimulus.

Depending on the severity of the hyponatremia (and the consequent serum hypo-osmolality) and the rapidity with which it develops, postoperative hyponatremia may cause brain swelling and significant neurologic impairment. The careless administration of high volumes of hypotonic fluids to the postoperative patient can have disastrous consequences.

45. What is the correct diagnostic approach to the patient with postoperative hyponatremia (i.e., serum NA$^+$ of 127)?

The plasma concentration of sodium, the primary determinant of serum osmolality, is maintained within a narrow normal range by means of a balance of water intake, regulated by the thirst mechanism, and water excretion by the kidney. The normal kidney can excrete up to 10 L of water per day. Consequently, hyponatremia is only rarely caused by excessive water intake. The most common cause of hyponatremia is a defect in the renal excretion of water.

Schrier has suggested a very useful approach to the hyponatremic patient. The first step is to assess the patient's volume status by performing a physical examination. Three possibilities exist, each with its own differential. (1) The **volume-depleted patient** is salt- and water-depleted, with the salt deficit exceeding the water deficit. These deficits result from either renal losses (e.g., diuretic excess) or extrarenal losses (e.g., gastrointestinal losses). (2) The **edematous patient** has an excess of total body water and salt, with the water excess greater than the salt excess. The excesses result from the kidney's retention of salt and water in conditions such as cardiac failure and cirrhosis, where it perceives a decrease in the "effective arterial blood volume." Salt and water excess is also seen in nephrosis and advanced renal failure, though the inciting causes are different. (3) The **hyponatremic patient** who appears to be euvolemic is usually modestly volume-expanded and has an excess of total body water, though this is not detectable on examination. The most likely explanation for "euvolemic" hyponatremia is prolonged release of ADH in the face of persistent water intake. Postoperative pain is one stimulus for ADH release. Measurement of the urinary sodium concentration is a useful adjunct in distinguishing among the · diagnostic possibilities in these three categories.

Hyponatremia is very common in postoperative patients. Usually it results from a combination of hypotonic fluid administration and release of ADH. It should be kept in mind that hyperglycemia can cause a "factitious" hyponatremia (called factitious because though sodium is low, plasma osmolality is normal or high). This is an important consideration in the postoperative diabetic with hyponatremia.

Schrier RW, Berl T: Disorders of water metabolism. In Schrier RW (ed): Renal and Electrolyte Disorders. Boston, Little, Brown, 1976, pp 24–36.

SURGERY AND DIABETES AND OTHER ENDOCRINE DISEASES

46. What are the hormonal changes that the patient with insulin-dependent (type I) diabetes mellitus (IDDM) experiences with major surgery?
Just as with the nondiabetic, the diabetic experiences a catabolic state that results from perioperative starvation and the physiologic stress of anesthesia and surgery. However, insulin plays a major role in muting some of the catabolic processes, and the patient with IDDM may develop severe diabetic ketoacidosis (DKA) postoperatively.

Starvation is associated with a drop in plasma glucose and insulin. Lipid metabolites rise as the body switches to alternative fuels. In nondiabetics, basal insulin secretion serves to place a brake on catabolism. In the IDDM patient, lipolysis is uncontrolled. Added to the effects of starvation are the catabolic effects of the "stress response." Surgery causes an outpouring of catecholamines, which in addition to various hemodynamic effects act on the pituitary. ACTH from the pituitary causes release of glucocorticoids from the adrenals. Glucagon and growth hormone are also secreted. By their various pathways, these catabolic hormones lead to gluconeogenesis. In the IDDM patient, severe hyperglycemia develops, lipid mobilization persists unchecked by insulin, and fatty acid and ketone body concentrations rise, causing DKA. It should be clear that insulin administration to type I diabetics is the cornerstone of keeping perioperative catabolic processes under control.

47. How should the oral hypoglycemic agents be handled in the type II diabetic in the perioperative period?
In contrast to type I diabetics, who suffer from insulin deficiency, type II diabetics have three abnormalities contributing to their hyperglycemia:
1. Impaired insulin secretion from pancreatic beta cells.
2. Insulin resistance in peripheral tissues.
3. Increased production of glucose by the liver.
Sulfonylureas are the only oral hypoglycemics used in the U.S. today. Though the precise intracellular events are still unknown, sulfonylureas act on the pancreatic beta cell to increase insulin secretion. The duration of action of these agents is very important in the perioperative patient. The longest-acting drugs are chlorpropamide (duration of action up to 72 hours) and glyburide (16+ hours). Hypoglycemia resulting from sulfonylureas is likely to be prolonged, and its signs and symptoms may be inapparent in the perioperative

patient. Sulfonylureas should be stopped before major surgery, with the timing of discontinuation based on the duration of action of the particular drug. Insulin can be used in the perioperative period. With minor surgery in otherwise healthy patients, who will almost certainly be eating regular meals the day of surgery, the drug need not be interrupted. Frequent measurement of the blood sugar is essential in management, and it should be kept in mind that inaccuracy of glucose monitoring using finger-stick test strips is greatest at low levels of blood glucose.

48. What are the adverse consequences of hyperglycemia (serum glucose > 300 mg/dl) in the postoperative diabetic?

Despite the difficulty of proving the assertion, most believe that **wound healing** is impaired in the poorly controlled diabetic. A second adverse consequence may be a predisposition to **infection.** Although the clinical ramifications are not yet known, several defects in host defense mechanisms have been shown to be present in poorly controlled diabetics. These defects include impaired leukocyte chemotaxis, decreased intracellular bactericidal activity, and an impaired cell-mediated immune response. A third, often forgotten adverse effect is the **osmotic diuresis** hyperglycemia induces. In the renal tubule, the T_m (maximum tubular transport capacity) for glucose is about 375 mg/min. Once the filtered load of glucose exceeds the T_m, no more glucose can be reabsorbed, and glucose appears in the urine. The osmotic presence of glucose in the renal tubular fluid retards water and salt reabsorption. In the postoperative patient (as in other settings), this may lead to volume depletion and prerenal azotemia.

49. What is the approach to managing the insulin regimen in the type I diabetic undergoing major surgery?

One approach to perioperative management is the partial-dose approach, in which the patient is given one-half or two-thirds of his or her usual intermediate-acting insulin on the morning of surgery. Alternatively, a continuous low-dose infusion of insulin can be used perioperatively. In patients whose oral intake is poor in the early postoperative period, use of a sliding-scale approach is warranted.

Alberti K, et al: Insulin delivery during surgery in the diabetic patient. Diabetes Care 5(Suppl 1): 65–77, 1982.

50. Occasionally, a hyperosmolar, hyperglycemic state (HHS) develops in the postoperative period in the previously undiagnosed type II diabetic. What are the symptoms, signs, and management of this syndrome?

The HHS represents an acute decompensation of diabetes mellitus. The syndrome is marked by severe hyperglycemia (blood glucose levels as high as 2400 mg/dl have been observed), a serum osmolarity > 325 mOsm/L, and little or no acidosis. The prodrome, which may last from days to weeks, consists of polyuria, polydipsia, progressive volume depletion as a result of a relentless osmotic diuresis, and mental status changes that progress from lethargy to coma. Occasionally HHS is precipitated by the stress response associated with major surgery. Treatment is directed first at replacement of fluid and electrolyte losses. Fluid losses with HHS may be as much as 20% of body weight. Insulin requirements are much less than with DKA. Mortality, which is still quite high, generally results from thrombotic phenomena.

51. What are the symptoms and signs of postoperative adrenal insufficiency?

Adrenal insufficiency occurring in the perioperative period is rare, and though it is an eminently treatable condition, clinicians often forget to include it in the differential diagnosis of intra- or postoperative deterioration.

Surgery is a physiologically stressful situation that may unmask chronic adrenal insufficiency. The first sign may be persistent intraoperative hypotension. Postoperatively, the patient may be febrile to 103° F, with nausea and vomiting, and severe abdominal pain. These findings are often misdiagnosed as an intraabdominal catastrophe. Hypotension and shock can develop. Whenever the diagnosis is entertained, a serum cortisol level should be drawn and, without waiting for the result, corticosteroids should be administered.

It is the patient with chronic adrenal insufficiency who is at risk for an adrenal crisis precipitated by surgery. The symptoms and signs of chronic adrenal insufficiency are asthenia, fatigue, muscle weakness, postural hypotension, nausea, vomiting, anorexia, weight loss, abdominal pain, hyperkalemia, hyponatremia, anemia, and eosinophilia. Hyperpigmentation may or may not be present. Though very helpful if elicited as part of the preoperative evaluation, in the postoperative patient most of these findings are difficult to interpret, because they can be attributed to iatrogenic causes such as anesthesia, surgery, and fluid and electrolyte administration.

52. What kinds of problems might occur in the perioperative period in the patient with undiagnosed hyperthyroidism undergoing major surgery?
Thyroid hormone has important effects on many organ systems, but in the perioperative patient its effects on heart and lungs are of greatest importance.

Thyroid hormone has direct effects on the cardiovascular system that resemble, but are distinct from, the effects of catecholamines. These effects include an increase in myocardial contractility, an increase in heart rate, and a decrease in peripheral vascular resistance. Stroke volume and cardiac output are increased. High output cardiac failure and consequent pulmonary vascular congestion may occur. The "stress response" evoked by surgery and general anesthesia involves an outpouring of catecholamines. The hemodynamic effects of the catecholamines will be additive to the sympathomimetic effects of excess thyroid hormone. Because of the increase in myocardial oxygen requirements, angina pectoris may occur. Cardiac failure may be precipitated or worsened.

Excess thyroid hormone is associated with increased ventilatory demands (because of increased oxygen demand and increased production of carbon dioxide) and with weakness of the respiratory muscles. This may be a lethal combination in the postoperative patient whose respirations may be further depressed by anesthesia and analgesia, and whose ventilatory capacity is reduced by upper abdominal surgery.

Finally, surgery is known to be one of the precipitating causes of thyrotoxic crisis.

53. What is the approach to perioperative management of the patient on chronic corticosteroid therapy?
Atrophy of the adrenal glands can be induced by exogenous corticosteroids in a matter of weeks. The glands atrophy because the exogenous hormone suppresses pituitary secretion of ACTH. ACTH is trophic for the adrenals, i.e., it is necessary for normal structure and function.

In the preoperative patient on chronic corticosteroids, it is possible to determine whether the hypothalamic-pituitary-adrenal axis is suppressed, and if it is, to administer extra corticosteroids to cover the stress of surgery. However, most clinicians simply assume the axis is suppressed and treat accordingly. A variety of corticosteroid preparations are available, and they differ in potency. For minor surgery, hydrocortisone 100 mg (or its equivalent) should be administered parenterally every 6 hours during the day of surgery. Dosing can begin when the premedication is given. The regular dose and schedule can resume the day after surgery. For major surgery, every-6-hour dosing should begin when the premedication is given and continue for 2 or 3 days postoperatively. If complications occur, this may need to be extended. There is no need to taper the dose to return to usual maintenance doses.

SURGERY IN THE ELDERLY

54. Delirium is a fairly common postoperative problem in the elderly. How do you diagnose it? What causes should be searched for?
The key diagnostic points are:

1. Delirium affects the main aspects of cognition—thinking, perception, memory.

2. Delirium is frequently accompanied by frightening visual (and sometimes auditory) hallucinations.

3. An attention disorder is present, and the level of alertness waxes and wanes throughout the day.

4. The sleep-wake cycle is disturbed, with symptoms typically worse at night.

Delirium is an organic disease. It is a medical emergency, and its cause should be sought immediately. Up to 20% of elderly patients will develop postoperative delirium, and the incidence may be higher in patients with Parkinson's disease. Drugs, especially anticholinergics, are the commonest cause of delirium. However, in the elderly, delirium is often the presenting finding in acute MI, in pneumonia and other infections, and in electrolyte abnormalities. Thus "postoperative" delirium should be considered a diagnosis of exclusion and made only after these other considerations have been ruled out.

Lipowski Z: Current concepts—geriatrics: Delirium in the elderly patient. N Engl J Med 320:578–582, 1989.

55. How do you treat postoperative delirium?
Haloperidol in low doses (0.5 mg twice a day) usually provides good sedation without severe side-effects. However, vigilant supportive nursing and medical care are essential in preventing complications and keeping the period of delirium as brief as possible. Nutritional, fluid, and electrolyte needs must be addressed, and any signs of infection must be investigated promptly. A brightly lit room with a clock and calendar is helpful. Sensory stimuli should be limited. The presence of family members is often calming to the patient.

56. In the healthy elderly (those with no disease), what are the age-related changes that increase the risk of postoperative morbidity due to fluid and electrolyte abnormalities and drug toxicity?

1. Changes in body composition, with loss of lean muscle mass and increase in adipose tissue, such that total body water is decreased

2. Decrease in glomerular filtration rate (GFR)

3. Decrease in the kidney's ability to conserve water

4. Decrease in the kidney's ability to conserve sodium

5. Decrease in perception of thirst

These five factors work together to increase the risk of serious volume depletion, which is likely to be hypertonic in situations where the patient's access to free water is impeded (as in the postoperative period). Changes in body composition change the volume of distribution of drugs. This factor, together with the decline in the kidney's ability to metabolize and excrete certain drugs, increases the risk of drug toxicity.

57. Why would an elderly patient be more likely than a young patient to experience a delay in "waking up" in the Recovery Room after general anesthesia?
Unrecognized hypothermia in the Recovery Room can occasionally be the cause of delayed awakening from general anesthesia. Age-related changes in the autonomic nervous system impair the ability to generate and conserve heat. However, by far the most common cause of delayed awakening in the elderly is delayed metabolism and excretion of drugs used in anesthesia.

Opiates, which can be used as primary or supplementary anesthetics, probably account for most cases of delayed awakening in the elderly. Older people are much more sensitive than younger people to the anesthetic and respiratory depressant effects of opiates. The increased sensitivity is related to greater plasma drug concentrations, which may be due to age-related changes in the drug's volume of distribution and clearance. In older people slow to react in the Recovery Room, CO_2 narcosis resulting from opiate-related respiratory depression should be ruled out by measuring the arterial pCO_2.

MISCELLANEOUS PERIOPERATIVE ISSUES

58. How do you manage the anticoagulants in a patient who has a prosthetic aortic valve and must undergo transurethral prostate resection?
In the anticoagulated patient facing surgery, the task is to balance the risk of bleeding with the risk of thrombosis. It takes 3–5 days for the coagulation cascade to normalize after warfarin is stopped. Many recommend that patients with prosthetic heart valves be admitted 3 days before the planned surgery. At that time the warfarin should be stopped and the patient should be anticoagulated with heparin. Heparin should be stopped 6 hours before the operation. Warfarin should be restarted as soon as the patient can tolerate oral intake, and the prothrombin time will be prolonged within 3 days. The risk of thromboembolism during the period the patient is not anticoagulated seems greatest in patients with a prosthetic valve in the mitral position. In these patients, heparin should be started 6–12 hours postoperatively and continued until warfarin has prolonged the prothrombin time.

59. Is prophylaxis against infective endocarditis necessary in the patient with mitral valve prolapse (MVP)?
MVP, a common valve abnormality estimated to be present in up to 10% of people, is apparently associated with a very low risk of infective endocarditis. Nevertheless, clinical practice varies, with some physicians prescribing prophylactic antibiotics in all patients with MVP, others using prophylaxis only in MVP patients who have associated mitral insufficiency, and still others who believe prophylaxis is simply not necessary in patients with MVP.

60. What are the general principles of prophylaxis against infective endocarditis?
There are three general principles:
    1. Certain types of congenital or acquired structural cardiac lesions place patients at risk for infective endocarditis.
    2. Surgery/invasive procedures that traverse a mucous membrane (oral, genitourinary, gastrointestinal) are more commonly associated with transient bacteremia than incisions across a sterile field.
    3. The presence of circulating antibiotics with appropriate antimicrobial activity during the time of bacteremia reduces the incidence of bacterial seeding and infection of cardiac structures.
    Kaye D: Prophylaxis for infective endocarditis: An update. Ann Intern Med 104:419–423, 1986.

61. What is the risk of transmission of hepatitis C virus (HCV) with transfusion of one unit of packed red cells (RBCs)? What is the risk of human immunodeficiency virus (HIV) transmission?
The risk of infection with HCV (until recently called non-A, non-B hepatitis) is estimated at 1:100 units or greater. HCV accounts for most cases of post-transfusion hepatitis. The risk of infection increases as the number of units transfused increases. A significant proportion of persons with transfusion-associated HCV infection eventually develop chronic liver disease. Currently, screening of donors for HCV is carried out using nonspecific tests (antibody to hepatitis B core antigen, and alanine aminotransferase), but soon a specific test for detection of antibodies to HCV will be available.

The risk of HIV transmission with a transfusion is much less than the risk of HCV and is currently estimated at 1:100,000 units.

62. What is the best way to minimize the possibility of transmission of blood-borne diseases in a patient who will definitely need perioperative transfusions?

The best way to prevent blood-borne diseases associated with homologous transfusion (products from volunteer donors) is to use **autologous blood products** (the donor and the recipient are the same person). Blood can be collected as often as every 4 days up until 72 hours before surgery. Autologous blood can be stored in its liquid form for up to 6 weeks or can be frozen if a longer storage or collection period is necessary. Almost everyone is able to donate blood for autologous use, but blood collection must be performed with extreme caution in patients with severe cardiovascular disease. Iron supplements are necessary for autologous donors.

63. What is malignant hyperthermia? How is it managed?

Malignant hyperthermia is an extremely rare complication of anesthesia with halogenated inhalational agents or the neuromuscular blocking agent succinylcholine. Its incidence is estimated to be 1 in 50,000–100,000 anesthetic episodes.

Many genetic, environmental, and pathophysiologic features of the syndrome are incompletely understood. It is believed to be due to a defect in muscle whereby calcium is handled abnormally by the sarcoplasmic reticulum. An increase in the sarcoplasmic calcium concentration precipitates a generalized hypermetabolic state in muscle. The syndrome is usually heralded by a rise in body temperature, which can get as high as 108° F. Tachycardia is often the first sign noted by the anesthesiologist. Muscle rigidity is a late finding. As soon as malignant hyperthermia is suspected, the operative procedure should be terminated, and respiratory support, circulatory support, body-cooling measures, and fluid and electrolyte therapy should be instituted. Dantrolene sodium, available in all operating suites, is specific therapy.

64. What is the incidence of deep venous thrombosis (DVT) with repair of hip fracture and transurethral prostate resection, two very common operations?

Though the incidence of clinically evident postoperative pulmonary embolism (PE) is low, DVT is a very common occurrence in postoperative patients. It is often inapparent or missed on physical examination.

The control groups of randomized trials concerned with prevention of DVT provide the most accurate data on the incidence of perioperative DVT. Over 40% of patients undergoing hip fracture repair develop DVT postoperatively. In 30% of patients the thrombus is in the proximal veins, which is thought to carry a higher risk of embolization than distal DVT. With transurethral prostate resection, the incidence is lower, about 10%.

65. What prophylaxis against perioperative thromboembolic disease has been found to be successful (i.e., preventing thrombosis without causing significant bleeding) in general, urologic, orthopedic, and gynecologic surgery?

Though many of the clinical trials of measures to prevent postoperative venous thrombo-embolism were too small to detect protective effects, an analysis of the compiled results from multiple studies has provided strong evidence that low-dose heparin given perioperatively confers significant protection against venous thromboembolism without causing significant bleeding. The heparin regimen is 5000 units administered subcutaneously every 8 or 12 hours, beginning before surgery and continuing until the patient is fully ambulatory. Other measures that confer some protection against postoperative thromboembolic disease (at least in some surgical groups) are dextran infusion and mechanical lower-limb compression devices.

Collins R, et al: Reduction in fatal pulmonary embolism and venous thrombosis by perioperative administration of subcutaneous heparin. N Engl J Med 318:1162–1173, 1988.

66. Occasionally, a patient abruptly develops hypertension, tachycardia, diaphoresis, disorientation, hallucinations, and tremor in the postoperative period. What is the most likely diagnosis?

The most likely diagnosis is delirium tremens (DTs), the most serious of the alcohol withdrawal syndromes. Alcoholism is underdiagnosed in general hospitals in the U.S. Its prevalence in adults admitted for general medical problems is estimated to be as high as 30%. The abstinence from alcohol necessitated by hospitalization, anesthesia, and surgery can precipitate DTs, and its development can be quite surprising to the clinician who was unaware that the patient is an alcoholic. The syndrome, which still carries a mortality rate of 10–15%, is associated with marked autonomic hyperactivity manifested by fever, tachycardia, hypertension, diaphoresis, and tremor. The patient is profoundly disoriented and difficult to control. There are massive fluid and electrolyte losses. Treatment is supportive, and benzodiazepines are used for sedation.

PSYCHIATRY: DISTINGUISHING AMONG ABNORMAL MENTAL STATES

67. What is somatization disorder?

According to the *DSM-III-R*, somatization disorder is a psychiatric condition characterized by multiple, recurrent physical complaints for which no organic basis can be found. The disorder begins before the age of 30 and is more common in females. Common physical complaints include vomiting, pain in the extremities, shortness of breath, amnesia, pain in sexual organs or rectum, and dysmenorrhea. The patient with somatization disorder makes frequent visits to physicians because of the physical symptoms, and it is not uncommon for the somaticizing patient to be seeing several physicians concomitantly. Patients undergo extensive, repetitive diagnostic workups for their symptoms, take many prescription drugs, and often undergo surgical procedures. None of these interventions reveals an organic basis for the symptoms. There is no known effective therapy for somatization disorder.

68. What is the most effective way for the internist to approach the patient with somatization disorder?

Because the cycle in somatization disorder (or any somatoform disorder) often is "physical complaint–unrevealing workup–empiric therapy," the danger of iatrogenic disease is very real. The internist or family physician who can establish a long-lasting relationship with a patient who has somatization disorder is occasionally able to break the cycle. To be successful, the physician must be able to have confidence in his or her history-taking and physical examination ability and must be able to exercise diagnostic and therapeutic restraint. Care of the somaticizing patient is extremely difficult in public hospital/clinic settings, because a new physician may see the patient at each visit.

69. Is the patient with a schizophrenic disorder competent to make decisions about his medical care?

The three elements of informed consent (or informed refusal) are:

1. The physician must disclose an adequate amount of information about the risks, benefits and alternatives of the proposed medical intervention.

2. The patient must understand the information provided (i.e., be able to receive, retain, retrieve, and rationally manipulate information).

3. The patient must be able to make a voluntary decision, free from internal and external compulsions.

The natural history of schizophrenia varies. Apparently, fully 20% of patients recover completely, usually after one episode. Obviously such patients are competent to make informed decisions about their medical therapy, except during the active phase of their illness. Another 40% have a waxing and waning course marked by remissions and exacerbations. These patients generally become more impaired with each cycle, and competence may be permanently impaired. The remaining 40% of patients have persistent symptoms and signs of schizophrenia, and they may or may not be capable of making informed decisions about medical care.

Within the individual, the severity of the symptoms and signs of schizophrenia shows marked fluctuation over time. During the active phase of illness, significant disturbances exist in several areas that would almost certainly affect an individual's ability to make informed choices for his care. Areas affected during the active phase include language and communication, thought content, perception, affect, sense of self, volition, and relationship to the environment. With schizophrenics who are not in the active phase of illness, competence to make choices regarding personal medical care must be assessed on a case-by-case, and within the same patient, on an encounter-by-encounter basis. Competence evaluations should be motivated by respect for the patient's autonomy.

70. What is a personality disorder, and how might it interfere in the relationship between patient and internist or family physician?

Personality disorders are very common in medical as well as psychiatric practice. A personality disorder is present when the patient's patterns of relating to, experiencing, and thinking about him/herself, others, and the environment cause internal distress or interfere with the person's social and occupational performance. There are various types of personality disorders, and the manner in which the various types would hinder the relationship between internist and patient is fairly predictable. For example, the medical treatment of the patient with a paranoid personality disorder might be hampered by the patient's suspiciousness about the physician's diagnostic and therapeutic intent. The physician treating the patient with a histrionic personality disorder for a medical problem may have to deal with seductive behavior on the part of the patient. Another problem with this type of patient is that physical complaints are related to the physician in an excessively dramatic way, which can interfere with the physician's ability to assess the severity of the medical illness.

71. What is the difference between delirium and dementia?

In both delirium and dementia, there is impairment of the three main aspects of cognition: thinking, perception, and memory. However, in **dementia,** the cognitive impairment develops insidiously and is enduring, whereas in **delirium** the impairment has an abrupt onset and is short-lived. The table below summarizes the important differences between the two:

Characteristic	Delirium	Dementia
Onset	Sudden	Insidious
Course over 24 h	Fluctuating, worse at night	Stable
Consciousness	Reduced	Clear
Attention	Disordered	Normal except in severe cases
Cognition	Disordered	Disordered
Hallucinations	Visual or auditory	Often absent
Delusions	Poorly systematized	Often absent
Orientation	Usually impaired	Often impaired
Psychomotor activity	Variable	Often normal
Speech	Often incoherent	Difficulty in word-finding, perseveration
Involuntary movements	Asterixis/coarse tremor	Often absent
Physical illness or drug toxicity	One or both present	Often absent

(Adapted from Lipowski ZJ: Delirium in the elderly patient. N Engl J Med 320:578–582, 1989, with permission.)

72. What is the appropriate approach to the delirious patient?

Delirium is a medical, not a psychiatric, emergency. After the diagnosis has been made and the patient's immediate safety assured, the possible causes of delirium should be investigated. In the elderly, delirium is often the herald of serious systemic disease; therefore, the first group of diagnostic possibilities to be explored includes acute MI, pneumonia and other infections, hyper- or hypoglycemia, azotemia, acid-base disorders, and fluid and electrolyte disturbances. The second group of possibilities consists of drug toxicities. Alcohol withdrawal should be considered here. Almost any drug can cause changes in mental status, even when ingested in "therapeutic" doses.

73. What are the somatic signs of depression?

Though nonspecific somatic complaints such as fatigue, headache, and gastrointestinal disorders can accompany depression, by far the most common somatic signs involve sleeping, eating, and sexual function. Sleep disturbances include difficulty in falling asleep and early morning awakening, with the patient sometimes awakening 2 or 3 hours before his or her habitual rising time. On the other hand, hypersomnia occasionally occurs. Often the patient complains that food has lost its taste. Loss of appetite and weight occur more commonly than increases in appetite and weight. Libido may be completely lost.

74. What is the clinical presentation and medical evaluation of the patient with a panic attack?

A panic attack is an episode characterized by intense fear and discomfort. According to the *DSM-III-R,* at least four of the following symptoms must be present to make the diagnosis of a panic attack (typically, nine or ten are present): shortness of breath or a smothering feeling, dizziness, palpitations or tachycardia, trembling, diaphoresis, choking, nausea or abdominal distress, depersonalization, paresthesias, flushes or chills, chest pain, fear of dying, and fear of going crazy or doing something uncontrolled. From the internist's perspective panic attack is a diagnosis that can be made only after organic causes of the above symptoms have been ruled out. The differential diagnosis includes acute MI, cardiac dysrhythmia, pulmonary edema, pulmonary embolism, anaphylaxis, hyperthyroidism, pheochromocytoma, and cocaine intoxication. Panic attacks beginning after age 40 suggest medical illness.

MISCELLANEOUS ISSUES IN MEDICAL CARE
OF THE PSYCHIATRIC PATIENT

75. What is a rational approach to the treatment of chronic hypertension in the patient with depression?

Depression has been reported to occur with (or be exacerbated by) many antihypertensive agents. However, it is important to note that depression is reported by patients in the placebo arms of blinded clinical trials of antihypertensive agents almost as commonly as patients on active therapy. The clinician should therefore be wary of changing medication without substantial indications in the patient complaining of symptoms that may or may not be side-effects of drugs, or an endless cycle of drug changes may be initiated.

Recent evidence has suggested that angiotensin converting enzyme (ACE) inhibitors such as captopril may be a very good choice in the patient with depression. A study comparing the effect of captopril, propranolol, and methyldopa on patient-perceived quality of life found that captopril was associated with an improved performance on the quality-of-life scale. Captopril has also been reported to produce mood elevation in depressed patients. However, selection of antihypertensive agents must be individualized based on the patient's age, race, and coexisting conditions and medications.

76. What is a rational approach to the treatment of chronic hypertension in the patient with psychosis or a major affective disorder?

There are four basic points to remember when treating the hypertensive patient who has psychosis or a major affective disorder:

1. Because of severe agitation and autonomic overactivity, blood pressure will be elevated during a period of acute decompensation. Overzealous use of antihypertensives during this time can be disastrous.

2. Avoid selecting for chronic use agents known to cause rebound hypertension when abruptly discontinued (such as clonidine). Transdermal delivery of antihypertensive medication by means of a skin patch may help in avoiding such a situation in patients with particularly unpredictable behavior.

3. Diuretics should be used as antihypertensives with great caution in patients receiving lithium, and serum lithium levels should be monitored frequently during therapy.

4. Patients are more likely to comply with simple once-a-day regimens.

77. What are the physical signs and symptoms that might be present in the acutely decompensated, severely disturbed schizophrenic?

Acutely decompensated schizophrenics experience intense terror because they perceive that their internal and external milieus are dangerous and uncontrollable. These patients appear terrified and may exhibit signs of strong activation of the sympathetic nervous system (the "fight or flight" reaction). These signs include diaphoresis, increased heart rate, increased arterial pressure, and increased myocardial contractility, among others. Disturbances of motor behavior accompany decompensation; some patients may assume bizarre postures or have almost a total reduction in motor activity (catatonia). Others may engage in repetitive behavior such as head-banging or may pace constantly and rapidly until they are physically exhausted; rhabdomyolysis occasionally results. The internist called to see an acutely disturbed patient should restrict the physical examination to the minimum necessary, because it may be extremely threatening to the patient. Omitted parts may be completed later when the patient is calmer. Therapeutic restraint should be exercised, and it should be kept in mind that adrenergic responses such as tachycardia and hypertension are appropriate to the patient's inner psychiatric experiences and will resolve spontaneously.

78. What are the effects on the cardiovascular system of acute ingestion of cocaine?

Cocaine blocks the presynaptic re-uptake of norepinephrine. Thus acute ingestion has predictable cardiovascular manifestations consistent with sympathetic nervous system overactivity, including vasoconstriction, an acute rise in arterial pressure, tachycardia, and a predisposition to ventricular dysrhythmias. Acute MI occasionally occurs secondary to cocaine ingestion. The increases in heart rate and blood pressure increase myocardial oxygen demand. Though persons with coronary artery disease are at greatest risk for cocaine-induced MI, MI after cocaine use has also been found to occur in persons with normal coronary arteries. Cocaine ingestion predisposes to such cardiac dysrhythmias as sinus tachycardia, ventricular ectopy, ventricular tachycardia and fibrillation, and asystole.

Cregler LL, Mark H: Medical complications of cocaine abuse. N Engl J Med 315:1495–1500, 1986.

79. What policy regarding hepatitis B vaccination should an inpatient drug detoxification/ treatment center have?

IV drug abusers (IVDAs) are at high risk for hepatitis B infection. A safe and effective vaccine against hepatitis B virus (HBV) has been available since 1982. All IVDAs who have not been previously infected with HBV should be offered vaccination. However, since this population has a very high rate of prior infection and a large number of cases are asymptomatic, it may be cost-effective to test for the presence of antibodies in all individuals who deny previous hepatitis and to offer vaccination to those whose tests are negative.

80. What should be included in the medical evaluation of the elderly depressed patient scheduled to begin a course of electroconvulsive therapy (ECT)?

ECT is often more effective than drugs in the treatment of depression. It acts more quickly than drugs, an important consideration when there is a significant risk of suicide. ECT may be of particular value in the depressed elderly because age-related changes, coexisting disease, and the need for concomitant medications often lead to intolerable side-effects with antidepressant drugs. In contrast to the manner in which ECT was provided in the past, in current practice ECT is delivered under controlled conditions, and the patient's cardiovascular and ventilatory status are carefully monitored. The patient receives a short-acting general anesthetic for comfort and a neuromuscular blocking agent to attenuate the seizure. Supplemental oxygen is administered to prevent the development of hypoxia during the seizure, and anticholinergics are given to control secretions and lessen the bradycardia that occurs when the seizure begins.

The most common complications of ECT are cardiac dysrhythmias and exaggerated hypertensive responses. Very rarely, MI occurs. Dysrhythmias are quite common and can involve atrial premature contractions, atrial flutter or fibrillation, AV block, premature ventricular contractions, and rarely ventricular tachycardia. The pretreatment evaluation should be directed at assessing the presence and control of hypertension, the presence and state of compensation of CHF, the presence and severity of angina, and the history of cardiac dysrhythmias. A careful history, physical examination, and ECG are usually the only diagnostic workup indicated.

Elliot DL, et al: Electroconvulsive therapy: Pretreatment medical evaluation. Arch Intern Med 142:979–981, 1982.

MEDICAL DISEASE DUE TO PSYCHIATRIC DRUGS

81. What are the four categories of drugs used to treat psychiatric conditions, and the most common, medically important side-effects of each group?

The four categories are:

1. Antipsychotics (phenothiazines, thioxanthines, butyrophenones, and some miscellaneous compounds).

2. Mood stabilizers (lithium, carbamazepine).

3. Antidepressants (tricyclics, monoamine oxidase inhibitors, and "second generation" antidepressants such as trazodone and amoxapine).

4. Sedative-hypnotics (benzodiazepines, barbiturates, and some miscellaneous compounds).

The most common medically important side-effects of the antipsychotics involve the autonomic nervous system: dry mouth, urinary retention, constipation, and orthostatic hypotension. Lithium, the most widely used mood stabilizer, has important effects on the kidney's handling of water. Of patients taking lithium, 20–70% have polyuria and polydipsia. Nephrogenic diabetes insipidus occurs in more than 5% of patients (some estimates go as high as 25%). In fact, lithium is now the most common cause of nephrogenic diabetes insipidus. Of the antidepressants, tricyclics are in widest use. They have important anticholinergic side-effects and are frequently associated with dry mouth, urinary retention, delirium, tachycardia, and orthostatic hypotension. Benzodiazepines are the most widely used sedative-hypnotics. Their most common medically important side-effects consist of drowsiness and diminished motor skills. The elderly are particularly prone to delirium and falls when using sedative-hypnotics.

82. How does lithium affect salt- and water-handling by the kidney?

When first administered, lithium can cause a brief (1–2 days), transient natriuresis that is usually of no clinical significance. Though there are many similarities in the way the kidney handles lithium and sodium, by far the most important effect of lithium is on the handling of water.

Antidiuretic hormone (ADH, or plasma arginine vasopressin), a hormone secreted by the posterior pituitary, makes the normally water-impermeable collecting tubules in the kidney permeable to water. In the absence of ADH, or with reduced tubular responsiveness to ADH, water is not reabsorbed in the tubules and large amounts of water are excreted in the urine. ADH levels in patients receiving lithium are normal or elevated in the face of impaired free-water conservation. This indicates that lithium interferes with the action of ADH on renal tubular epithelium. The urinary concentrating deficit is usually reversible when lithium is stopped.

83. What are the signs of lithium toxicity?

Early signs of lithium toxicity can be quite subtle. Unrecognized, toxicity gradually worsens over several days to weeks. With serum levels < 1.5 mmol/L, evidence of toxicity consists of a fine intention tremor, lethargy, weakness, and difficulties with concentration and memory. Elderly people can develop lithium toxicity when serum levels are in the so-called therapeutic range. Levels > 1.5 are associated with a coarse resting tremor, muscle fasciculations, increased muscle tone, hyperreflexia, confusion, visual disturbances, ataxia, dysarthria, and extrapyramidal signs. Seizures, coma, flaccid paralysis, and death occur with levels over 3. Dialysis is indicated when levels are above 3 and may be indicated with lower levels, depending on the clinical state.

Simard M, et al: Lithium carbonate intoxication: A case report and review of the literature. Arch Intern Med 149:36–46, 1989.

84. What are "extrapyramidal side-effects"? How are they treated?

Extrapyramidal side-effects (EPS) can be classified into four syndromes, three of which are early and one which is late (tardive dyskinesia). The early syndromes consist of a **parkinsonian complex** indistinguishable from Parkinson's disease, **akathisia,** in which the patient is in constant motion, and **acute dystonia,** which can range from grimacing to oculogyric crisis.

All three of the early syndromes are reversible if the drug is stopped or the dose reduced. The danger is that the EPS syndromes may be misinterpreted as signs of worsening psychiatric disease rather than recognized as drug toxicity, with consequent increase of the dose. Anticholinergics such as benztropine or diphenhydramine relieve the early EPS syndromes promptly.

85. What are the salt and water changes that would occur if a patient on long-term lithium therapy developed gastric outlet obstruction and persistent vomiting, but still took his lithium?

The kidney handles lithium much the same way it handles sodium, and this has important implications for patients taking lithium who, for whatever reason, experience changes in intravascular volume while on the drug. Like sodium, about 75% of filtered lithium is absorbed in the proximal tubule. Thus, in states of volume depletion such as in the patient described, the kidney conserves sodium (in order to protect the intravascular volume), and it also "conserves" lithium. In such a situation, lithium levels will rise and lithium toxicity will develop. Conversely, in volume-expanded states, where the kidney is excreting salt, the kidney also is excreting lithium, and doses may need to be increased to maintain serum levels in the therapeutic range.

86. What is "steroid psychosis"?

Corticosteroid use is frequently associated with changes in mood (euphoria, dysphoria, or emotional lability), changes in sleep pattern (insomnia, weird dreams, nightmares), and changes in appetite (usually increased). Corticosteroids also can have important effects on behavior and thought processes, inducing frank psychosis in persons without a prior history of psychiatric disturbance or causing a decompensation in the known psychotic. The internist and the psychiatrist must work closely in cases in which the drugs used for medical illness worsen psychiatric illness, and vice versa.

87. Chlorpromazine can occasionally cause liver problems. What are the clinical, laboratory, and histologic findings with chlorpromazine-induced liver problems?

Chlorpromazine caused a therapeutic revolution in psychiatry when it was introduced in the early 1950s, but now some psychiatrists consider it obsolete since newer antipsychotics have fewer side-effects. Nevertheless, chlorpromazine is still used quite often. The "liver problem" that chlorpromazine causes is cholestatic jaundice. This occurs in 1–2% of patients, but the incidence may have decreased in the last decade. Previously this problem was thought to be related to hypersensitivity, but evidence now indicates that chlorpromazine is toxic to the liver and that subclinical cholestasis occurs in most patients receiving chlorpromazine. It is not known why some patients develop overt cholestasis. Laboratory findings consistent with biliary obstruction are observed, but fever and right upper quadrant tenderness are minimal. Jaundice becomes apparent during the second through fourth week of therapy. Pathologically, the liver shows bile plugs, portal inflammation, and hepatocellular necrosis. The treatment is discontinuation of the drug. Weeks may elapse before laboratory evidence of cholestasis resolves.

88. What commonly used psychotropic agents cause orthostatic hypotension, a special concern in the elderly?

Orthostatic hypotension is a common occurrence with some of the antipsychotics, particularly chlorpromazine, and the tricyclic antidepressants. Tricyclics are widely used in the elderly, because the prevalence of depression in that age group seems higher than in others. Many elderly have age-related degenerative changes in the autonomic nervous system and/or are taking other medications like diuretics and antihypertensives that exacerbate the postural drop in blood pressure caused by tricyclics. Postural blood pressure changes can cause syncope or near-syncope, with consequent injury from falls. The propensity to cause orthostasis seems to vary somewhat among agents based on affinity for the alpha adrenergic receptor. Lower-affinity agents should, at least in theory, produce fewer postural blood pressure changes. From highest affinity to lowest, the rank is:

Doxepin > amitriptyline > nortriptyline & imipramine > protriptyline > desipramine.

89. What are the cardiovascular effects of therapeutic doses of tricyclic antidepressants?

Tricyclics are commonly associated with orthostatic hypotension (discussed above), with changes in the ECG (see below), and anecdotally, with the development of high-grade heart block in patients with preexisting intraventricular conduction abnormalities. Heart rate increases in some patients. Some of the tricyclics (imipramine) actually seem to decrease ventricular ectopy, and atrial or ventricular ectopy should not automatically preclude the careful use of tricyclics. Early animal studies suggested that tricyclics decrease myocardial contractility, and for a long time these agents were avoided in patients with myocardial dysfunction. However, a study by Veith et al. published in 1982 indicated that LV function in patients with chronic heart disease is not adversely affected by therapeutic doses of imipramine or doxepin.

Veith RC, et al: Cardiovascular effects of tricyclic antidepressants in depressed patients with heart disease. N Engl J Med 306:954, 1982.

90. What changes can lithium produce in the ECG? Tricyclics? Chlorpromazine?

About 20% of patients taking lithium will exhibit flattening or inversion of the T wave. Occasionally, ST-segment depression is found, especially in patients with supratherapeutic levels.

The tricyclic antidepressants produce minor ST-segment changes, but their effect on intramyocardial conduction seems to be more important. In fact, it has been noted in patients taking tricyclic overdoses that the duration of the QRS complex is a good predictor (even better than serum drug levels) of the likelihood that seizures or ventricular arrhythmias will occur.

In patients taking therapeutic amounts of tricyclics, some prolongation of the PR interval, QRS complex, and QT interval may be observed. In patients with preexisting conduction disorders, tricyclics can provoke heart block.

The most common ECG changes observed in patients taking chlorpromazine (and other phenothiazines) consist of T-wave flattening or inversion. ST-segment depression and prolongation of the PR interval and QRS complex are less commonly seen.

91. What is neuroleptic malignant syndrome (NMS)? How often does it occur? What is its clinical presentation and management?

NMS is a rare complication associated with use of antipsychotic agents. The incidence is unknown, but is certainly less than 1% of all episodes of antipsychotic use. A significant proportion of patients who develop NMS have taken antipsychotics in the past without incident. The diagnosis is made clinically. The constellation of signs and symptoms includes delirium, fever (as high as 105° F), tachycardia, blood pressure instability, diaphoresis, and muscle rigidity. The complex develops over 24–72 hours and seems to be occasionally precipitated by or at least associated with volume depletion, physical exhaustion, and use of lithium along with the antipsychotic. The pathophysiology of NMS is unknown. Treatment is supportive. The mortality rate is as high as 30%. Antipsychotics must be stopped when the diagnosis is suspected; continued administration is lethal.

Rosebush P, Stewart T: A prospective analysis of 24 episodes of neuroleptic malignant syndrome. Am J Psychiatry 146:717–725, 1989.

92. Urinary retention is a not uncommon side-effect of which class of drugs used in psychiatry? What is the mechanism? Who is at greatest risk?

Tricyclic antidepressants are frequently associated with urinary retention, and the problem is most frequent, and most severe, in the elderly. Retention in the elderly often develops insidiously and goes unnoticed for several days. Some patients, but not all, complain of difficulty in emptying the bladder and pelvic pain. Nurses or family members may report that the patient has become "incontinent" of urine: this is an overflow type of incontinence. The first sign that something is seriously wrong is often that the patient "takes to his or her bed." This is often interpreted to be a worsening of the depression, when in fact it signifies azotemia or delirium. Delirium commonly accompanies urinary retention. Fever may be present if urinary tract infection has occurred. Physical examination discloses a suprapubic mass that may extend as high as the umbilicus. The mass has a flat percussion note. The diagnosis is confirmed by catheterization of the bladder.

BIBLIOGRAPHY

1. Goldmann DR, et al (eds): Medical Care of the Surgical Patient. Philadelphia, J.B. Lippincott, 1982.
2. Kammerer WS, Gross RJ (eds): Medical Consultation. Baltimore, Williams & Wilkins, 1983.
3. Lubin MF, et al (eds): Medical Management of the Surgical Patient, 2nd ed. Boston, Butterworth, 1988.

16. AMBULATORY CARE SECRETS

Mary P. Harward, M.D.

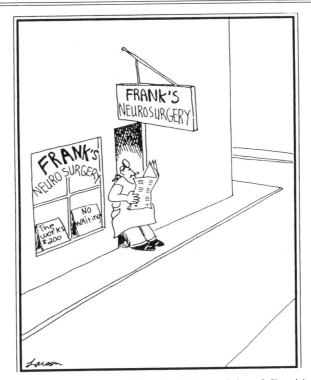

THE FAR SIDE cartoon by Gary Larson is reprinted by permission of Chronicle Features, San Francisco, CA

1. What are Merskey's Rules?

Merskey's Rules

1. Do a silly test, and you get a silly answer.
2. In the hospital, more deaths occur in bed than out of bed, so get the patient out of bed!
3. Any drug can do anything!

(From Matz R: Principles of medicine. NY State J Med 77(1):99–101, 1977, with permission.)

2. What are the most common reasons that patients are seen in ambulatory care internal medicine clinics?

Common Reasons in Rank Order for Ambulatory Visits to Office-based Internists (U.S. Data, 1985)*

REASONS NAMED BY PATIENTS	REASONS NAMED BY PHYSICIANS
General medical examination	Essential hypertension
Hypertension	Diabetes mellitus
Progress visit, no other symptoms	Chronic ischemic heart disease
Chest pain and related symptoms	Acute upper respiratory infection

Table continued on next page.

Common Reasons in Rank Order for Ambulatory Visits to Office-based Internists (U.S. Data, 1985)* (Continued)

REASONS NAMED BY PATIENTS	REASONS NAMED BY PHYSICIANS
Cough	General medical examination
Blood pressure test	Osteoarthritis and allied diseases
Diabetes mellitus	General symptoms
Symptoms referable to throat	Chronic airway obstruction
Abdominal pain, cramps, spasms	Asthma
Headache, pain in head	Bronchitis
Upper respiratory infection, head cold,	Neurotic disorders
coryza	Angina pectoris
Back symptoms	Chronic sinusitis
Vertigo, dizziness	Acute pharyngitis
Shortness of breath	Cardiac dysrhythmias
Tiredness, exhaustion	Catch-all category (diagnosis missing,
Leg symptoms	or illegible)
Shoulder symptoms	Other disorders of soft tissue
Neck symptoms	Other respiratory symptoms
Ischemic heart disease	CHF
	Peripheral enthesopathies

* National Ambulatory Medical Care Survey.
(From Barker LR: Curriculum for ambulatory care training in medical residency: Rationale, attitudes and generic proficiencies. J Gen Intern Med 5(Suppl 1):S3–S14, 1990, with permission.)

3. How should you initially evaluate a 45-year-old black male whose blood pressure (BP), measured on several separate occasions, has been between 140/95 and 155/105 mmHg?
The evaluation of a new patient with hypertension should identify:
1. Treatable causes of secondary hypertension.
2. The extent of end-organ damage due to hypertension.

In this age group, the prevalence of secondary hypertension is small (less than 10%) and does not justify extensive evaluation unless there are suggestive clinical or physical findings. The incidence of secondary hypertension will be increased in patients who experience the onset of hypertension at less than 35 years or greater than 55 years of age.

The evaluation of end-organ damage includes:
1. Funduscopic exam (for retinopathy).
2. Electrocardiogram (ECG) (for left ventricular hypertrophy).
3. Urinalysis (UA) and serum creatinine (for renal function).

4. What are the secondary causes of hypertension and their associated findings?

Findings Associated with Secondary Causes of Hypertension

CAUSE	FINDINGS
Aortic coarctation	Blood pressure difference in arm and leg measurements
Cushing's syndrome	Central obesity, hirsutism, pigmented striae, buffalo hump, moon facies
Primary aldosteronism	Decreased potassium
Renovascular disease	Flank bruit, rapid onset of hypertension, very high BP
Pheochromocytoma	Periodic episodes of headaches, palpitations, and perspiration
Renal parenchymal disease	History of diabetes, elevated creatinine
Hypothyroidism	Fatigue, dry skin, weight loss, cold intolerance, hoarseness, depressed mood
Hyperparathyroidism	Elevated calcium

5. How often should you screen for hypertension in normotensive adults?

Normotensive adults (defined as having a diastolic BP less than 85 mmHg and a systolic BP less than 140 mmHg) should have their BP measured at least every 2 years. Adults with diastolic BPs between 85 and 89 mmHg should be screened annually.

6. Name some of the nonpharmacologic treatments for hypertension.

- Weight loss
- Smoking cessation
- No-added salt diet
- Regular exercise
- Decreased alcohol intake
- Biofeedback/relaxation techniques

7. How would you manage an asymptomatic hypertensive patient with a BP of 170/119 who stopped his medication 1 week ago?

Starting the prescribed maintenance dose of the patient's antihypertensive medications will be sufficient. Oral loading doses or rapid reduction of blood pressure is not needed for the asymptomatic patient without signs of malignant hypertension (papilledema, proteinuria, or confusion).

Zeller KR, Kuhnert LV, Matthews C: Rapid reduction of severe, asymptomatic hypertension: A prospective, controlled trial. Arch Intern Med 149:2186–2189, 1989.

8. When should you begin screening for hyperlipidemia?

Although the optimal frequency of screening for hyperlipidemia has not been determined, a schedule of every 5 years is reasonable. It will be most helpful for middle-aged men, but younger men, women, and the elderly should also be screened.

9. What test(s) should be ordered to screen for hyperlipidemia?

A nonfasting serum cholesterol is sufficient, but several measurements should be done before therapy is initiated due to the wide variation in results. Additional measurements of fasting triglycerides (TG) and high density lipoprotein (HDL) will be helpful if the first cholesterol measurement is elevated (greater than 240 mg/dl) or if the patient has two or more risk factors for coronary artery disease (CAD) *and* a total cholesterol of 200–239 mg/dl. If the TGs are less than 500, the low-density lipoprotein (LDL) value, which can be used to guide therapy, can be calculated from the following equation:

$$LDL = (total\ cholesterol - HDL) - TG/5$$

Report of the National Cholesterol Education Program Expert Panel on Detection, Evaluation, and Treatment of High Blood Cholesterol in Adults. Arch Intern Med 149:505–510, 1989.

10. What are the risk factors for coronary artery disease (CAD)?

The risk factors for CAD include male sex, family history of early myocardial infarction (MI), cigarette smoking, hypertension, diabetes mellitus, and age over 35 years.

11. What advice about sexual activity would you give a patient recovering from an uncomplicated MI?

Sexual intercourse requires about 3 to 5 mets of exertion. (One met is the amount of energy expended at rest.) Most patients recovering from an uncomplicated MI can tolerate this without difficulty. It may be more strenuous for a man to support his weight on his arms in a superior position, and, therefore, other positions for intercourse should be considered.

12. What are the physical examination characteristics of an innocent murmur and of the murmur of mitral valve prolapse (MVP)?

Physical Examination Findings in Innocent and Mitral Valve Prolapse Murmurs

FINDING	INNOCENT	MITRAL VALVE PROLAPSE
Location	Base	Apex (left lateral decubitus position)
Intensity	Less than 3/6	Greater than 3/6
Timing	Early systole	Late systole
Response to maneuvers	Decreases with standing and Valsalva	Begins earlier in systole with standing and Valsalva
Associated signs	Normal S_2	Midsystolic click

13. What are your recommendations for prophylactic antibiotics to a patient with mitral valve prolapse (MVP) scheduled for elective dental procedure? To a patient with a prosthetic aortic valve?

The following recommendations are for patients with previous subacute bacterial endocarditis (SBE), valvular heart disease, prosthetic heart valves, most forms of congenital heart disease (except uncomplicated secundum atrial septal defect), idiopathic hypertrophic subaortic stenosis (IHSS), and MVP with regurgitation. **Viridans streptococci** are the most common cause of endocarditis after dental or upper respiratory procedures; **enterococci** are the most common cause of endocarditis after GI or GU procedures.

Prevention of Bacterial Endocarditis

A. Dental and upper respiratory procedures:
　　Oral
　　Amoxicillin　　　　　　3 grams 1 hour before procedure and 1.5 grams 6 hours later
　　Penicillin allergy:
　　　Erythromycin　　　　1 gram 2 hours before procedure and 500 mg 6 hours later

　　Parenteral
　　Ampicillin　　　　　　2 grams IM or IV 30 minutes before procedure
　　　plus gentamicin　　1.5 mg/kg IM or IV 30 minutes before procedure
　　Penicillin allergy:
　　　Vancomycin　　　　1 gram IV infused slowly over 1 hour before procedure

B. Gastrointestinal (GI) and genitourinary (GU) procedures:
　　Oral
　　Amoxicillin　　　　　　3 grams 1 hour before procedure and 1.5 grams 6 hours later

　　Parenteral
　　Ampicillin　　　　　　2 grams IM or IV 30 minutes before procedure
　　　plus gentamicin　　1.5 mg/kg IM or IV 30 minutes before procedure
　　Penicillin allergy:
　　　Vancomycin　　　　1 gram IV infused slowly over 1 hour before procedure
　　　plus gentamicin　　1.5 mg/kg IM or IV 30 minutes before procedure

Although the risk of SBE after dental procedures has not been clearly defined for patients with MVP, it is probably prudent to administer prophylaxis before the procedure. The risk of SBE may be less in those with only a click and no murmur of MVP.

Oral regimens are more convenient and safer. Parenteral regimens are more likely to be effective, and they are recommended especially for patients with prosthetic heart valves, those who have had SBE previously, or those taking continuous oral penicillin for rheumatic fever prophylaxis.

(Adapted from Prevention of bacterial endocarditis. Medical Letter 31:112, 1989, with permission.)

14. How would you evaluate an asymptomatic patient with new onset of atrial fibrillation?
The evaluation should specifically look for the causes of atrial fibrillation and evidence of cardiac dysfunction.

Evaluation of the Causes of Atrial Fibrillation

CAUSE	HISTORY	PHYSICAL EXAMINATION	LABORATORY
Alcohol use	Daily use, binging	Jaundice, spider angiomata, palmar erythema, hepatomegaly	Liver function tests
Medications	Digoxin		Digoxin level, ECG
Drug use	Stimulant use		Toxin screen
Congestive heart failure	DOE, PND, peripheral edema, nocturia	JVD, rales, edema, S_3	Chest x-ray
Pulmonary embolism	Chest pain, SOB, calf pain, predisposing factors (recent surgery, immobilization)	Calf swelling, pleural rub	ABG, chest x-ray, consider V/Q
Myocardial infarction	Chest pain	S_4	ECG
Cerebrovascular accident	Paresis, paralysis, aphasia, numbness, visual loss	Muscle weakness, sensory loss, dysarthria, reflex changes	Consider head CT scan
Mitral valve disease	Rheumatic fever or valvular disease	Heart murmur	Echocardiogram
Organic heart disease	Hypertension or heart disease	S_3, S_4, elevated BP	Chest x-ray, ECG
Hyperthyroidism	Weight loss, depression	Goiter	Thyroid function tests
Wolff-Parkinson-White syndrome	Palpitations		ECG
Sick sinus syndrome	Syncope		Holter monitor

ECG = electrocardiogram; DOE = dyspnea on exertion; PND = paroxysmal nocturnal dyspnea; JVD = jugular venous distention; SOB = shortness of breath; ABG = arterial blood gas; V/Q = ventilation/perfusion; CT = computerized tomography; BP = blood pressure.

15. What are the LEOPARD and LAMB syndromes?
The acronyms refer to constellations of findings, but both are characterized as hyperpigmentation disorders because of the presence of lentigines.

The **LEOPARD** syndrome consists of the following:
L = lentigines (hundreds covering the body surface, developing in childhood)
E = ECG abnormalities, primarily conduction disorders
O = ocular hypertelorism
P = pulmonary stenosis and subaortic valvular stenosis
A = abnormal genitalia
R = retardation of growth
D = deafness

The **LAMB** syndrome refers to:
L = lentigines
A = atrial myxomas
M = mucocutaneous myxomas
B = blue nevi

16. What should be the therapeutic plan for an adolescent with a moderate case of acne vulgaris?

1. Avoid oily cosmetics.
2. Use mild cleansing soap.
3. Use topical 2.5% benzoyl peroxide gel once or twice daily to cause slight erythema and scaling. If this does not improve the acne, increase the concentration up to 10% benzoyl peroxide or add topical 0.05% retinoic acid.
4. If pustules are present, apply topical clindamycin daily.
5. Use oral tetracycline (500 mg BID) for 6 weeks for severe cases. Stop the antibiotics periodically to assess continued need. Chronic antibiotic use may cause vaginitis in women.
6. Refer to a dermatologist if intralesional steroids or 13-*cis*-retinoic acid is needed.
7. Avoid oral contraceptives for women containing norgestrel or norethidrone.

17. What is hidradenitis suppurativa?

Hidradenitis suppurativa is an infection of the apocrine sweat glands that leads to chronic inflammation and scarring. It occurs in the axilla, groin, buttocks, and under women's breasts. Antibiotic therapy (erythromycin or dicloxacillin) can be useful, but sometimes surgical excision is required.

18. What are the typical locations and appearance of psoriasis?

Psoriasis typically occurs on the extensor surfaces (elbows and knees), waistline, umbilicus, external genitalia, and gluteal fold. The typical lesions are elevated, reddish-brown plaques and papules with silvery scale. Bleeding points occur where the scale is removed (Auspitz's sign). In addition, the nails may be pitted. Some patients will have arthritic involvement of the distal interphalangeal joints.

19. Name some causes of alopecia.

Causes of Alopecia

PATCHY		DIFFUSE
SCARRING	NONSCARRING	DIFFUSE
Tinea capitis with bacterial infection	Alopecia areata	Male-pattern baldness
Discoid lupus erythematosus	Tinea capitis infections	High fever
Third-degree burns	Secondary syphilis	Pregnancy
Trauma	Hair-pulling	Chemotherapy
Herpes infections		Radiation therapy
Neoplasms		Exfoliative dermatitis
Lichen planus		Systemic lupus erythematosus
Scleroderma		Dermatomyositis
		Hypothyroidism
		Cushing's syndrome
		Hypopituitarism
		Anticoagulants
		Oral contraceptives

(From Haynes H, Branch WT Jr: Dermatology in primary care. In Branch WT Jr (ed): Office Practice of Medicine, 2nd ed. Philadelphia, W.B. Saunders, 1987, with permission.)

20. What is the characteristic appearance of tinea versicolor? How do you treat it?

Tinea versicolor, caused by infection with the form-species of fungus *Malassezia furfur*, has various colors (red, pink, brown) and is usually macular with slight scaling. The involved areas of skin do not tan well, and the infection will become particularly obvious in the summer, when the involved areas are hypopigmented. The lesions fluoresce orange and gold under Wood's light. It is treated with 2.5% selenium sulfide suspension applied to the entire body at bedtime and rinsed the following morning. Recurrences are common. Topical antifungal agents (clotrimazole, miconazole) can be used for small areas. Systemic antifungal agents (ketoconazole) can be used in severe cases.

21. How does *Candida albicans* look on a potassium hydroxide (KOH) preparation? How about tinea cruris?

Candida has pseudohyphae and budding spores. Tinea cruris has hyphae and spores with the appearance of "spaghetti and meatballs."

22. What is the proper technique for a KOH preparation?

Moisten the involved skin with water and scrape with a sterile number 10 or number 15 scalpel. Place the scrapings on a glass slide and add one or two drops of 15% KOH. Cover the preparation with a coverslip and heat gently. Examine the slide under low power (10X objective).

23. What is routine follow-up for a patient with diabetes mellitus?

Patients with diabetes mellitus should be seen at least annually if their glucose level is controlled on a stable medication or diet regimen. If insulin or oral hypoglycemic agents require a change, more frequent visits are needed. At the visit, measure the blood pressure; examine the feet for any signs of trauma, blisters, calluses, or improper nail care; test the urine for protein; and examine the eyes for diabetic retinopathy (retinal blood vessel proliferation, microaneurysms, yellow or cotton-wool exudates, and hemorrhages). The latter is probably best accomplished through an annual examination by an ophthalmologist. Check the hemoglobin A1C (glycosylated hemoglobin) as a monitor of glucose control. Review the diet, exercise regimen, home record of blood sugars, and foot-care plan with the patient and ask about symptoms of hypoglycemia, peripheral vascular disease, neuropathy, and sexual function. Administer any needed immunizations. Patients with diabetes require pneumococcal vaccine (once), influenza vaccine (annually), and tetanus/diphtheria toxoid (every 10 years).

24. What are the two most frequent causes of mild, asymptomatic hypercalcemia in the ambulatory population?

Thiazide drugs and hyperparathyroidism are the most frequent causes of hypercalcemia.

25. What are some causes of obesity secondary to excess caloric intake?

Some infrequent or rare secondary causes include hypothyroidism, hypogonadism, Cushing's disease, insulinoma, Froehlich's syndrome, Laurence-Moon-Biedl syndrome, Prader-Willi syndrome, Alström syndrome, and craniopharyngioma.

26. What are some of the adverse consequences of obesity?

Obese patients are more likely to have hypertension, diabetes mellitus, and coronary artery disease than patients who are not overweight. Obesity can complicate chronic obstructive pulmonary disease (COPD) and osteoarthritis. Obese patients will have difficulty following a regular exercise program. They may have a depressed mood and poor self-esteem.

27. What should be included in a treatment regimen for a patient with chronic, idiopathic constipation?

1. Regular bowel habits with attempted bowel movements at the same time each day (15 to 20 minutes after breakfast when the gastrocolic reflex is the strongest).

2. High-fiber diet, including beans (navy, lima, kidney), baked potato with skin, broccoli, peas, corn, apple with peel, oranges, peaches, raspberries, wheat bread, bran cereals.
3. Adequate fluid intake (at least eight 8-oz glasses of water a day).
4. Bulk laxative (psyllium), if needed.
5. Daily exercise.

28. What are the causes of chronic constipation?

Causes of Chronic Constipation

Medications	Calcium channel blockers, antihistamines, opiates, iron, antidepressants, aluminum and calcium antacids, and laxatives (if abused)
Endocrine	Hypothyroidism
Metabolic	Diabetes mellitus, hypokalemia, hypercalcemia
Mechanical obstruction	Tumors, strictures
Neurogenic	Spinal cord disease, multiple sclerosis, scleroderma
Rectal disease	Hemorrhoids, anal fissure
Psychological	Major depression, personality dysfunction
GI disease	Irritable bowel syndrome, diverticular disease
Physical inactivity	

29. Describe the office evaluation of a patient with acute diarrhea for less than 24 hours.

Most causes of acute diarrhea are infectious and many are self-limited. The history and physical examination will help guide further evaluation. In the history, inquire about:
1. Recent travel.
2. Food ingestion (particularly raw meats, poultry and custards).
3. Exposure to animals or to people with similar symptoms.
4. Frequency, volume, and appearance of the stool.
5. Associated symptoms including fever, abdominal pain, tenesmus, blood in the stool, and skin rash.
6. Current medications.

During the physical examination, check the temperature, abdomen, and rectum (including a test for fecal occult blood). The examination should also include a check for the presence of orthostatic changes in blood pressure or a skin rash. A patient with few associated symptoms needs no further evaluation unless the diarrhea does not resolve within a week. In a patient with severe systemic symptoms, a search for and treatment of specific infectious agents will be needed. The stool should be examined for leukocytes by methylene blue or Gram stain. If fecal leukocytes are present, the stool should be cultured. If the patient is severely ill or has bloody diarrhea, sigmoidoscopy may be useful. In the absence of severe symptoms, though, most acute diarrhea in an otherwise healthy patient requires no intervention. Most diarrheas caused by bacteria will be improving by the time the cultures are available.

30. Describe the office evaluation of a patient with diarrhea for 2-3 weeks.

If the diarrhea persists, fecal blood and leukocytes should be rechecked and cultures repeated, with a specific request for ova and parasite examination. Sometimes as many as three specimens are needed for identification of the pathogen. The diagnostic yield can be increased if the examination is done on a fresh stool specimen. Complete blood count (CBC), serum electrolytes, calcium, glucose, liver function tests, and amylase may indicate a systemic illness. Sigmoidoscopy is indicated. In certain patients with evidence of malabsorption (weight loss), a Sudan stain for fat followed by quantitative 72-hour fecal fat collection will be useful. If no etiology is determined, additional evaluations will be needed.

31. What are the symptoms of irritable bowel syndrome (IBS)? How do you treat it?

Because it is the most common gastrointestinal disease seen in clinical practice, most physicians are all too familiar with IBS. However, its management can be frustrating.

Patients with IBS often complain of diarrhea alternating with constipation for months to years. Most patients developed their symptoms before the age of 40. Associated symptoms include depression, anxiety, achy abdominal pain relieved by bowel movements, and excessive flatus. The stool may contain a large amount of mucus. Many patients note increased symptoms with stress.

The treatment of irritable bowel syndrome includes acknowledgment of the symptoms, identification of and counseling for any underlying psychiatric stress or illness, education about the benign nature of the disorder, and therapy for chronic constipation or diarrhea (increased dietary fiber). Short-term limited use of anticholinergic medications is useful in a few patients but should not be the sole therapy.

32. How do you manage an anal fissure?

The patient with an anal fissure usually complains of severe pain with defecation, sometimes associated with bleeding. Most fissures are located in the midline and will be visible. Conservative management with warm baths, stool softeners, and bulk laxatives improves the ease of defecation. Drugs that cause constipation should be avoided. If this therapy fails, the patient should be referred for consideration of surgical repair.

33. What is proctalgia fugax?

Proctalgia fugax is a fleeting, deep pain in the rectum, probably caused by muscle spasm.

34. How should you evaluate and treat a 35-year-old male with dyspeptic symptoms?

For most patients under 50 years of age with vague complaints of dyspepsia ("heartburn," indigestion, "gas"), no evaluation is needed. Symptomatic, empiric therapy can be provided with frequent small meals, smoking cessation, and antacids. Patients who do not respond to 4 weeks of therapy will require endoscopic or radiographic evaluation for possible malignancy. Patients with prior history of peptic ulcer disease or evidence of blood loss should be evaluated when they first complain of the symptoms. Because of the increased prevalence of GI malignancy in those over age 50, earlier diagnostic studies are indicated in this group.

Goodson JD, et al: Empiric antacids and reassurance for acute dyspepsia. J Gen Intern Med 1:90, 1986.

35. What test(s) are most useful in determining if an acute hepatitis is due to viral hepatitis?

If one suspects viral hepatitis based on history, physical examination, and elevated liver transaminases, an HBsAg (hepatitis B surface antigen) can be ordered first. If this is negative, an IgM anti-HBc (hepatitis B core antibody–IgM) will pick up additional cases of acute hepatitis B that are negative for the antigen. Hepatitis A testing includes anti-HAV (total hepatitis A virus antibody) to detect recent or remote infection, followed by IgM anti-HAV for all positive IgG anti-HAV. The IgM anti-HAV is positive only in acute infections. Research is currently under way to develop an easily identifiable marker for hepatitis C.

36. How do you diagnose cervicitis due to *Chlamydia*?

Chlamydiosis is diagnosed by direct immunofluorescent staining or culture of the cervical discharge. Chlamydial cervicitis is suspected in a sexually active woman when a mucopurulent discharge with cervical erythema, ulceration, and friability (easy bleeding) are seen during speculum examination of the vagina. Gram stain of the discharge usually shows greater than 10 leukocytes per high power field.

37. How should you evaluate a 20-year-old sexually active female with the complaint of acute dysuria?

The patient needs to be evaluated for the multiple causes of dysuria, including urethritis, cystitis, vaginitis, and cervicitis. A history of sexual activity (particularly with a new partner) may point toward a vaginitis or cervicitis. The history should focus on the presence of hematuria, vaginal discharge, flank pain, fever and chills. The physical exam should include measurement of the temperature and a bimanual pelvic examination. Any vaginal discharge should be examined microscopically. Cervical discharge needs to be Gram-stained to look for *Neisseria gonorrhoeae* and tested for the presence of *Chlamydia* antigen. A urine sample should be examined in the office for leukocytes and organisms.

38. What are some of the causes of abnormal vaginal bleeding?

Causes of Abnormal Vaginal Bleeding

Anatomic lesions	Uterine fibroids; cervical erosions; cervical polyps; retained gestation products; ectopic pregnancy; endometrial, cervical, or ovarian carcinoma
Dysfunctional bleeding	Immaturity or senescence of the hypothalamic-pituitary-ovarian axis; inadequate luteal phase; ovarian senescence; endometriosis
Inflammation	Pelvic inflammatory disease, intrauterine devices, tampon use
Endocrine disturbances	Hyperthyroidism, hypothyroidism, oral contraceptives
Hematologic disturbances	Bleeding diatheses, iron deficiency, anticoagulation therapy

(Adapted from Goroll AH, et al: Primary Care Medicine: Office Evaluation and Management of the Adult Patient, 2nd ed. Philadelphia, J.B. Lippincott, 1987, p 512, with permission.)

39. How do you manage a woman with postmenopausal vaginal bleeding who has a uterus?

A woman with postmenopausal vaginal bleeding should be referred to a gynecologist for consideration of a dilatation and curettage (D&C) of the uterus.

40. Describe the characteristic vaginal discharges caused by *Candida albicans, Neisseria gonorrhoeae, Gardnerella vaginalis,* and Trichomonas.

Organism	Vaginal Discharge
Candida albicans	White, "cottage-cheese" like, adherent to vaginal wall
Neisseria gonorrhoeae	Purulent with cervical involvement
Gardnerella vaginalis	Foul-smelling, thin, turbid, adherent to vaginal wall
Trichomonas	Foul-smelling (fishy), grayish-green, frothy

41. What are clue cells?

Clue cells are seen in the discharge of vaginal infections caused by *Gardnerella vaginalis.* Microscopically, they appear on a saline wet mount of the discharge as epithelial cells covered with coccobacilli or curved rods.

42. What advice would you give a woman taking combination oral contraceptives who missed a pill?

The patient should take the missed pill as soon as she is aware of the missed dose, then continue the remainder of her pills as scheduled. After a missed pill, it is prudent to use additional barrier contraception until her next menses pill to prevent pregnancy.

43. What are the absolute contraindications to oral contraceptive use?

Absolute Contraindications for Oral Contraceptive Use

1. Pregnancy
2. Severely impaired liver function
3. Undiagnosed vaginal bleeding
4. History of thromboembolic or cardiovascular disease
5. Presence of estrogen-dependent neoplasms

44. How would you evaluate a new breast nodule discovered during a routine physical examination of a woman?

The characteristics of the nodule (size, firmness, mobility) are not predictive of the likelihood of malignancy. If multiple, cystic nodules are present and the woman is menstruating, she should be followed through several menses for any changes in the nodule. Any solitary nodule requires referral for biopsy. A mammogram may be useful for localization of the nodule, but a normal mammogram should not preclude the need for biopsy of a solitary nodule.

45. Is there a proven, validated drug therapy for premenstrual syndrome (PMS)?

Although many agents have been used in the management of PMS (including bromocriptine, diuretics, oral contraceptives, progesterone therapy, prostaglandin synthetase inhibitors, psychotropic agents, and vitamins), there is as yet no scientifically proven therapy.

Clarke-Pearson DL, Dawood MY: Green's Gynecology: Essentials of Clinical Practice, 4th ed. Boston, Little, Brown, 1990, pp 186–193.

Reid Robert L: Premenstrual syndrome (editorial). N Engl J Med 324:1208–1210, 1991.

46. What are the clinical symptoms of influenza?

Influenza typically presents with the sudden onset of high fever, malaise, myalgia, coryza, headache, and sore throat. There may be GI symptoms (nausea, vomiting, and diarrhea). With complications, symptoms of pneumonia, encephalitis, or myositis may develop.

47. How do you differentiate influenza from other acute respiratory illnesses?

It is difficult to distinguish influenza on clinical grounds alone. Although a patient presenting with characteristic symptoms during an outbreak of influenza in the winter months most probably has the disease, laboratory diagnosis is the only way to be certain. Laboratory diagnosis can be made during acute illness from sputum samples, a throat swab, or nasopharyngeal washes.

Streptococcal pharyngitis and early bacterial pneumonia can resemble influenza. Unlike influenza, bacterial pneumonia is generally not self-limited, and a bacterial pathogen can be isolated from purulent sputum by Gram stain.

48. Who should receive the influenza vaccine?

Vaccination with inactivated, trivalent influenza virus vaccine is recommended annually for the following groups:

1. Individuals at increased risk for the complications of influenza virus infection (including death, influenza pneumonia, and secondary bacterial pneumonia):
   a. Adults and children with chronic pulmonary or cardiovascular illnesses (including asthma).
   b. Residents of nursing homes or other chronic care facilities with any chronic medical condition.
   c. Adults 65 years of age or older.
   d. Adults or children with chronic medical conditions requiring regular medical follow-up or hospitalization during the preceding year (including diabetes mellitus, renal dysfunction, hemoglobinopathies, or immunosuppression).

e. Children and teenagers (aged 6 months to 18 years) who are receiving long-term aspirin therapy and are therefore at increased risk for developing Reye's syndrome after an influenza infection.
2. Individuals capable of transmitting influenza to high-risk persons:
  a. Physicians, nurses and other personnel in both inpatient and outpatient settings who have extensive contact with high-risk patients in all age groups.
  b. Providers of home care to high-risk persons.
  c. Household members (including children) of high-risk persons.
3. Other groups:
  a. Anyone, especially those providing essential services, who wishes to reduce his or her chance of acquiring influenza infection.
  b. All HIV-infected persons.
  c. Persons embarking on foreign travel during their destination's influenza season.
Recommendations of the Immunization Practices Advisory Committee (ACIP): Prevention and control of influenza: Part I, Vaccines. MMWR 38:297–298, 303–311, 1989.

49. What are the indications for amantadine in influenza management?

Amantadine, an antiviral agent, is useful in the treatment of and prophylaxis against influenza A infection. It is not useful for influenza B or other viral syndromes.

Although the influenza vaccine is the mainstay of prophylaxis, it is not universally administered. Therefore, in an epidemic amantadine is the drug of choice for chemoprophylaxis. It can be used in patients in whom vaccination was not feasible or was contraindicated. It can also be used for 2 weeks in patients who receive the influenza vaccine during an active influenza season while waiting for the vaccine to produce a protective antibody response. It can also be used in vaccinated patients who are immunocompromised and therefore at greater risk of complications from influenza infection.

As a therapy, it is indicated for uncomplicated upper respiratory tract influenza A infection. It can shorten the duration and decrease the severity of influenza A infections. It should be started within 48 hours of the onset of symptoms and continued for 48 hours after the resolution of symptoms. The dosage is 200 mg on the first day, followed by 100 mg daily. Elderly patients and patients with renal dysfunction or seizure disorder should receive 100 mg each day. Central nervous system side-effects (confusion, hallucinations) can occur and occasionally limit its use.

50. When is combined tetanus-diphtheria toxoid (Td) and tetanus immune globulin (TIG) indicated in wound management?

Tetanus Prophylaxis

History of tetanus immunization	CLEAN, MINOR WOUNDS		ALL OTHER WOUNDS	
	Td	TIG	Td	TIG
Unknown, uncertain, or 0–2 doses	YES	NO	YES	YES[1]
Three or more doses[2]	NO[3]	NO	NO[4]	NO

[1] When Td and TIG are given simultaneously, adsorbed and not fluid tetanus toxoid should be used.
[2] If only three doses of fluid toxoid have been received, a fourth dose of adsorbed toxoid should be given.
[3] Td should be given if more than 10 years since the last dose.
[4] Td should be given if more than 5 years since the last dose. More frequent boosters may increase side effects and are unnecessary.
(From Fedson DA: Adult immunization. In Becker DM, Gardner LB (eds): Prevention in Clinical Practice. New York, Plenum, 1988, p 47, with permission.)

51. What organisms commonly cause nongonococcal urethritis (NGU) in men?

Chlamydia trachomatis and *Ureaplasma* frequently cause NGU. Reiter's syndrome may also cause the symptoms.

52. What is the treatment of epididymitis?

The etiologies of epididymitis include *Chlamydia trachomatis, Neisseria gonorrhoeae*, and gram-negative rods. Appropriate antibiotic therapy will be guided by cultures. For empiric therapy, one should consider treatment for gonorrhea in the young, sexually active male (ceftriaxone followed by 10 days of tetracycline or doxycycline). For the older male, gram-negative rods are more likely. If not systemically ill, therapy can be started with trimethoprim-sulfamethoxazole. If the patient is compromised, hospitalization with intravenous therapy should be considered.

53. How do you differentiate acute epididymitis from testicular torsion?

Differentiation of Epididymitis and Torsion

	EPIDIDYMITIS	TORSION
Age	Older	Prepubertal
Pyuria	+	−
Bacteriuria	+	−
Urethritis symptoms	+	−
Physical exam	Palpable epididymis	Firm, tender mass

54. What are the symptoms of atypical pneumonia? What are its causes?

The cough of atypical pneumonia is usually dry. The chest radiograph has a diffuse infiltrate. Typically, the chest radiograph "looks worse" than the patient. Common causes of the atypical pneumonia syndrome include *Mycoplasma pneumoniae*, viruses (influenza, adenovirus, respiratory syncytial, and parainfluenza), *Chlamydia* (psittacosis), fungi (histoplasmosis, coccidioidomycosis), and *Pneumocystis carinii*.

55. What are the prodromal symptoms of herpes zoster (shingles)?

Before the vesicles appear, infected individuals frequently experience headache and malaise. Pain and paresthesia may be felt in the involved dermatomes. If the involved dermatome is on the anterior chest wall, the pain may be confused with anginal or MI pain.

56. How can the history and physical examination predict if acute pharyngitis in an adult is due to streptococcal infection?

The decision as to whether an adult case of acute pharyngitis is due to group A streptococcal infection or infection with other bacteria or viruses is a commonly encountered clinical problem. Although the history and physical examination cannot conclusively make the etiological diagnosis, several findings are useful. These include:

- Tonsillar exudate (exudate anywhere else in the oropharynx is not helpful)
- Tender anterior cervical lymphadenopathy
- Tonsillar enlargement
- History of a positive throat culture in the preceding year
- Myalgias
- The absence of itchy eyes

When fever, tonsillar exudate, and anterior cervical adenopathy are all present, the probability of streptococcal pharyngitis is about 40%.

  Komaroff AL, et al: The prediction of streptococcal pharyngitis in adults. J Gen Intern Med 1:1–7, 1986.

57. Which adults should receive measles vaccine?

Adults born after 1954 should receive measles vaccine if they:

1. Do not have documentation of immunization with live virus vaccine on or after their first birthday or a record of physician-diagnosed measles.
2. Do not have laboratory documentation of immunity.
3. Have received live virus vaccine before their first birthday.
4. Have received killed virus vaccine alone or followed by live virus vaccine within 3 months.
5. Have received an unknown type of vaccine between 1965 and 1968.

Adults born before 1956 probably have natural immunity. They should be considered for vaccination if they:

1. Are health care workers.
2. Are students entering a college or university.
3. Plan international travel.

ACP Task Force on Adult Immunization: Guide for Adult Immunization, 2nd ed. Philadelphia, American College of Physicians, 1990.

58. What form of polio vaccine should be given to adults?

Adults should receive an injection of inactivated polio vaccine. Adults have a slightly increased risk of developing paralysis from the live-virus polio vaccine (OPV).

59. What are some frequent causes of meralgia paresthetica?

Meralgia paresthetica is caused by localized entrapment of the lateral femoral cutaneous nerve that produces pain over the anterolateral thigh. It may occur with diabetes mellitus and pregnancy (during the final weeks of gestation), or during sudden weight loss or gain. Tight girdles, gun belts, and other accessories have been implicated.

60. What are the typical symptoms of a migraine headache? a tension headache? a cluster headache? (See also pp 442–446.)

Typical Headache Symptoms

SYMPTOM	CLUSTER	MIGRAINE	TENSION
Location	Unilateral	Hemicranial	Entire head or bitemporal
Quality of pain ache, tightness	Burning	Throbbing	Pressure-like
Duration	1–2 hours	2–6 hours	Days
Frequency	1–3 times/day for weeks to months	Flurry of frequent attacks for several weeks	Daily
Associated	Ipsilateral sweating, flushing, lacrimation, and rhinorrhea	Prodrome (scotoma, paresthesia, confusion, or behavioral changes)	Neck and shoulder aching

61. What are the symptoms of a transient ischemic attack (TIA) in the anterior carotid distribution? vertebrobasilar distribution?

Symptoms of Transient Ischemic Attack

ANTERIOR	VERTEBROBASILAR
Transient paresis of face and/or arm	Transient global amnesia
Paresthesia	Ataxia
Aphasia	Dysarthria
Amaurosis fugax (sudden loss of vision in one eye)	Weakness, dizziness
Homonymous hemianopia	Hearing loss

62. What is the triad of symptoms of Meniere's syndrome?
Meniere's triad of symptoms includes paroxysmal vertigo, hearing loss, and tinnitus. It may be accompanied by nausea and vomiting.

63. What are the leading causes of acute impairment or loss of the sense of smell?
Head trauma, especially in children and active young adults, and viral infections, especially in older adults.

64. Describe the typical signs of Parkinson's disease.

Signs of Parkinson's Disease

Pill-rolling tremor	Dementia
Rigidity	Drooling
Bradykinesia (decreased spontaneous movement)	Festinating gait
Immobile facial features	

65. What are the characteristics of bacterial conjunctivitis? viral conjunctivitis? allergic conjunctivitis?

The Red Eye

	CONJUNCTIVITIS			CORNEAL INJURY OR INFECTION	IRITIS	ACUTE GLAUCOMA
	Bacterial	Viral	Allergic			
Vision	–	–	–	↓ or ↓↓	↓	↓↓
Pain	–	–	–	+	+	+++
Foreign body sensation	–	±	±	+	–	–
Itch	±	±	++	–	–	–
Tearing	+	++	+	++	+	–
Discharge	Mucopurulent	Mucoid	–	–	–	–
Preauricular adenopathy	–	+	–	+[1]	–	–
Pupils	–	–	–	NL or small[2]	Small	Mid-dilated and fixed
Conjunctival hyperemia	Diffuse	Diffuse	Diffuse	Diffuse and ciliary flush	Ciliary flush	Diffuse and ciliary flush
Cornea	Clear	Sometimes faint punctuate staining or infiltrates	Clear	Depends on disorder	Clear or lightly cloudy	Cloudy
Intraocular pressure[2]	NL	NL	NL	NL[3]	↓, NL, ↑	↑↑

[1] In herpes keratitis
[2] Indicates secondary iritis
[3] Very low in perforating trauma
NL = normal
(From Steinert RF: Evaluation of the red eye. In Goroll AH, et al (eds): Primary Care Medicine. Office Evaluation and Management of the Adult Patient, 2nd ed. Philadelphia, J.B. Lippincott, 1987, p 835, with permission.)

66. What is a wrist ganglion? How is it treated?

The ganglion is the most common tumor of the hand and wrist, and the most frequent site of origin is the dorsum of the carpus. The cause of ganglia has not been proven, but many patients allude to acute or chronic trauma, sometimes occupational. The ganglia arise from the synovium of a joint or tendon sheath, and occasionally from the tendon itself. They contain a gelatinous fluid and those on the dorsum of the wrist are usually smooth, round, fluctuant, and firm. They are sometimes associated with mild discomfort but ordinarily require no therapy and occasionally resolve spontaneously. They can be treated with rupture, aspiration, or surgery and splinting. Rupture with digital pressure or striking the flexed wrist with an object is sometimes done when a scar is objectionable, but the ganglion can recur when treated by rupture or aspiration.

Milford L: Tumors and tumorous conditions of the hand. In Crenshaw AH: Campbell's Operative Orthopaedics, 7th ed. St. Louis, C.V. Mosby, 1987, p 483.

67. How do you treat a coccygeal fracture?

A coccygeal fracture is treated conservatively with analgesia and use of an inflatable "donut" cushion when sitting. It most often results from a direct blow, usually a fall onto the buttocks.

68. What is Phalen's maneuver? Tinel's sign?

In carpal tunnel syndrome, forced flexion or hyperextension of the wrist (Phalen's maneuver, see figure **A**) reproduces the symptoms of pain and paresthesia as well as numbness in the palm and first three or four fingers. In Tinel's sign (see figure **B**), the symptoms are reproduced when the median nerve is tapped lightly.

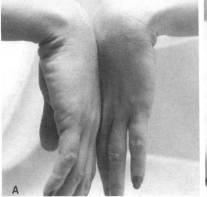 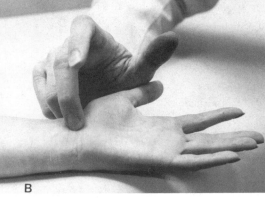

A, Phalen's test.　　　　　　　　　B, Tinel's sign for median nerve at the wrist.

(From Ferlic TP: Hand and wrist injuries. In Mellion MB: The Team Physician's Handbook. Philadelphia, Hanley & Belfus, 1990, pp 357, 358, with permission.)

69. What should be included in the examination of a patient complaining of a "sprained ankle"?

The history should include the details of the injury, particularly whether or not the ankle was inverted or a tearing sensation was felt. Initial exam should check for tenderness along the anterior talofibular ligament (located slightly anterior to the lateral malleolus), fibulocalcaneal ligament (immediately below the lateral malleolus), and the posterior talofibular ligament (posterior to the lateral malleolus). The latter two will be tender usually only in more severe strains. The degree of swelling should be noted. If ecchymosis is present, there is at least a second-degree injury.

Ankle stability is tested by the anterior drawer sign (see figure). The patient should relax. The lower leg is grabbed anteriorly, firmly with one hand. The heel and calcaneus are grasped with the other and the foot is pulled forward. The ankle should be held in 20° flexion. The examiner notes how far the ankle can be moved in comparison to the uninvolved ankle. Foot strength, sensation, and blood flow are noted. An x-ray will be needed in almost all strains to check for a fracture.

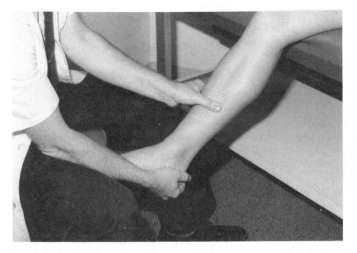

Anterior drawer test. (From Brown DE: Ankle and leg injuries. In Mellion MB: The Team Physician's Handbook. Philadelphia, Hanley & Belfus, 1990, p 441.

70. What is a second-degree ankle sprain? How is it treated?
In a second-degree ankle sprain, a portion of a ligament is torn without complete disruption. On exam, there will be ecchymosis and slight asymmetry between the involved and uninvolved ankle on anterior drawer sign. It is treated with elevation, bulky dressing or elastic bandage, and ice packs for 20 minutes every 3 to 4 hours for 2 to 3 days. The patient should avoid any weight-bearing and use crutches. He or she can begin plantar- and dorsiflexion exercises after 48 hours. Weight-bearing can be allowed after 5 to 10 days if the pain and swelling are decreased.

71. What is the location of muscle weakness, sensory loss, and reflex absence associated with an L4 root compression?

Associated Findings with Root Compressions

ROOT	DISC	MUSCULAR	SENSORY	REFLEX
L4	L3–L4	Leg extensors (quadriceps)	Anterolateral thigh, medial lower leg	Patellar
L5	L4–L5	Large toe dorsiflexion (extensor halluces longus), heel walking (tibialis anterior)	Dorsum of foot	None
S1	L5–S1	Toe walking (gastrocnemius)	Lateral foot and 5th toe	Ankle

72. What toe fractures should be referred to an orthopedist?
Fractures of the proximal phalanx of the 5th toe should be referred to an orthopedist. If a fracture involves the distal phalanx and extends into the interphalangeal joint, this should also be referred.

Birnbaum JS: The Musculoskeletal Manual. New York, Academic Press, 1982.

73. What physical examination findings would you see in a patient with a rotator cuff tendinitis?

With rotator cuff tendinitis, there will be subacromial tenderness and pain on passive elevation (usually to a certain point). Specific findings include:

Positive impingement signs

Rotator cuff and biceps weakness

Positive supraspinatus test

Pain with abduction from 70 degrees to 120 degrees (painful arc)

May be atrophy of shoulder muscles—compare with opposite side

May be tender over coracoacromial ligament

Julin MJ, Mathews M: Shoulder injuries. In Mellion MB: The Team Physician's Handbook. Philadelphia, Hanley & Belfus, 1990, p 326.

74. How do you manage a patient with lumbosacral strain?

Patients with acute back strain should remain at strict bedrest on a firm mattress or a hard floor for at least 3 days. They should not rest in a prone position. If supine, the knees and neck should be supported by small pillows. Lying on one side with hips and knees slightly flexed is also comfortable. Nonsteroidal anti-inflammatory drugs (NSAIDs) and muscle relaxants (diazepam, cyclobenzapine) are helpful, as is local heat.

75. What is Reiter's syndrome?

Reiter's syndrome is common in young, white men and produces arthritis of the lower extremities (knees, ankles, small joints of the feet). Accompanying symptoms include urethritis (dysuria with mucopurulent penile discharge) and mild conjunctivitis. There may also be plantar fascitis (heel pain), diffuse swelling of the toes (sausage digits), shallow painless oral ulcers or penile lesions, and onychodystrophy (crumbling of the nails). The characteristic skin rash is call keratoderma blenorrhagica and appears as discrete papules. The illness may occur after an acute, diarrheal illness. Affected patients frequently have HLA-B27.

76. What conditions may present as chronic fatigue?

Conditions Causing Chronic Fatigue

Psychologic	Depression, anxiety, sleep disorders
Endocrine-metabolic	Hypothyroidism, diabetes mellitus, apathetic hyperthyroidism of the elderly, pituitary insufficiency, hyperparathyroidism or hypercalcemia of any origin, Addison's disease, chronic renal failure, hepatocellular failure
Pharmacologic	Hypnotics, antihypertensives, antidepressants, tranquilizers, drug abuse and withdrawal
Infectious	Endocarditis, tuberculosis, infectious mononucleosis, hepatitis, parasitic disease, chronic Epstein-Barr virus (EBV) infection, cytomegalovirus (CMV), human immunodeficiency virus (HIV) infection
Neoplastic	Occult malignancy
Hematologic	Severe anemia
Cardiopulmonary	Chronic congestive heart failure (CHF), chronic obstructive pulmonary disease (COPD)

(Adapted from Goroll AH, May LA, Mulley HG: Primary Care Medicine: Office Evaluation and Management of the Adult Patient, 2nd ed. Philadelphia, J.B. Lippincott, 1987, p 26, with permission.)

77. To which clinical syndrome does "hay fever" refer?

Hay fever is a quite inexact reference to **seasonal allergic rhinitis**, which is not specifically caused by hay nor associated with fever. This perennial rhinitis has symptoms of sneezing, nasal passage obstruction, rhinorrhea, itching, and lacrimation. It is brought on by airborne pollens being trapped in the nasal folds, with digestion of the outer coat by mucosal enzymes and release of protein allergen. There is usually a family history of similar allergic conditions. **Vasomotor rhinitis** is a kindred symptom complex without a known allergic basis.

Austin KF: Diseases of immediate type hypersensitivity. In Wilson JD, et al (eds): Harrison's Principles of Internal Medicine. New York, McGraw-Hill, 1991, pp 1422–1428.

78. What is Tietze's syndrome?

Tietze's syndrome is mild inflammation of the costochondral junction that produces localized warmth, swelling, erythema, and pain. The symptoms are reproduced by palpation of the involved area.

79. What are the diagnostic criteria for major depression?

Criteria for Major Depression

At least five of the following symptoms have been present nearly every day for 2 weeks:
1. Depressed mood
2. Diminished interest or pleasure in nearly all activities
3. Weight loss or gain (more than 5% of body weight in a month)
4. Insomnia or hypersomnia
5. Psychomotor agitation or retardation
6. Fatigue
7. Feelings of worthlessness or inappropriate guilt
8. Decreased ability to think
9. Recurrent thoughts of death

(Adapted from American Psychiatric Association: Diagnostic and Statistical Manual of Mental Disorders, 3rd ed. Washington, D.C., APA, 1980, pp 213–214, with permission.)

80. What medical illnesses can also cause depression?

Medical Illnesses Causing a Depressed Mood

Endocrine	Hyperthyroidism, hypothyroidism, Cushing's syndrome, Addison's disease, hypercalcemia, hyperparathyroidism
Rheumatic	Rheumatoid arthritis, systemic lupus erythematosus
Neurologic, subdural, cerebrovascular	Temporal lobe epilepsy, chronic hematoma, multiple sclerosis, accident, frontal lobe tumor, senile dementia of the Alzheimer's type
Infectious	Hepatitis, infectious mononucleosis
Nutritional	Vitamin B_{12} deficiency
Toxic	Alcoholism, drug withdrawal

81. Which antidepressants are sedating?

Sedative Potency of Antidepressants

ANTIDEPRESSANT	SEDATIVE POTENCY
Amitriptyline	Marked
Doxepin	Marked
Trazadone (Desyrel)	Marked
Imipramine	Moderate
Desipramine	Mild
Nortriptyline	Mild
Maprotiline (Ludiomil)	None
Fluoxetine (Prozac)	None

82. Which antidepressant causes priapism?
Trazadone (Desyrel) can cause priapism.

83. What is agoraphobia? How is it treated?
Agoraphobia is the fear of being in public places. The patient with agoraphobia may live a reclusive life. It is usually first seen in women in their late teens or early twenties and may be associated with panic attacks. During panic attacks, the patient will have at least four of the following symptoms, in addition to apprehension or fear: dyspnea, palpitations, chest discomfort, choking sensation, dizziness, feelings of unreality, paresthesia, hot and cold flashes, sweating, faintness, trembling, or fear of dying or going crazy.

Severe agoraphobia is best treated in consultation with a therapist skilled in behavioral therapies such as desensitization. If the patient has panic attacks without the avoidant behavior (panic disorder), alprazalom (0.5 mg TID) or imipramine (25 to 250 mg per day) may be useful.

American Psychiatric Association: Diagnostic and Statistical Manual, 3rd ed. Washington, D.C., APA, 1980.

84. What is the hyperkinetic heart syndrome?
This is a syndrome found in asymptomatic young males who present with increased cardiac output of no discernible cause. They usually seek medical attention because of palpitations, tachycardia, and atypical chest pain. The diagnosis is uncertain and has been variously listed as neurasthenia, anxiety neurosis, Da Costa syndrome, effort syndrome, and soldier's heart.

Grossman W, Braunwald E: High-cardiac output states. In Braunwald E: Heart Disease: A Textbook of Cardiovascular Medicine, 2nd ed. Philadelphia, W.B. Saunders, 1984.

85. What are the principles of good sleep hygiene?
1. Set regular bedtime.
2. Set regular wake time.
3. Establish regular exercise program.
4. Establish regular bedtime routine (warm bath, light snack).
5. Avoid caffeine and stimulants within 8 hours of bedtime.
6. Do not read or watch television in bed.
7. Get out of bed if not asleep within 30 minutes.
8. Avoid daytime naps.
9. Do not alter daily activities because of fatigue.

86. How could you improve a patient's compliance with a regimen of multiple medications?
Using as few medications as possible will help the patient to comply. Also, decreasing the number of doses required each day can help. The patient should be instructed to take the medication at the time of some other routine activity (such as meals or bedtime). Asking the patient about side-effects will identify potential problems.

87. What are some of the organic causes of impotence?

Organic Causes of Impotence

Endocrine	Primary testicular failure, hypothalamic disease, diabetes mellitus, acromegaly, adrenal neoplasms, pituitary adenomas, chromophobe adenoma, hypothyroidism, hyperthyroidism
Urologic	Peyronie's disease, prostatitis, phimosis, priapism
Neurologic	Autonomic peripheral neuropathy (including diabetes mellitus), amyotrophic lateral sclerosis, spinal cord tumors or transection, multiple sclerosis, tabes dorsalis

Table continued on next page.

Organic Causes of Impotence (Continued)

Vascular	Athero-obstructive aorto-iliac disease, aneurysm, arteritis
Cardiorespiratory	Cardiomyopathy, coronary insufficiency, chronic obstructive pulmonary disease
Hematologic	Hodgkin's disease, leukemia, chronic sickle cell anemia
Infectious	Genital tuberculosis
Organ failure	Cirrhosis, chronic renal failure, lead, herbicides
Surgical	Aorto-iliac surgery, radical pelvic surgery, postprostatectomy
Medications	Alcohol, benzodiazepine, antidepressants, major tranquilizers, antihypertensive agents

(Adapted from Gottfried LA, Richie JP: Sexual problems. In Branch WT Jr (ed): Office Practice of Medicine, 2nd ed. Philadelphia, W.B. Saunders, 1987, p 1410, with permission.)

88. What are some of the early signs and symptoms of anorexia nervosa?

Anorexia nervosa should be suspected in an adolescent female with amenorrhea, weight loss, and a distorted body image (feeling "fat" in the face of emaciation). It can occur in women in their thirties.

89. What are the risk factors for suicide?

Risk Factors for Suicide

1. Male sex	7. History of impulsive behavior or suicide attempts
2. Single or widowed marital status	8. Presence of chronic pain syndrome, major depression, psychosis, alcoholism, substance abuse, organic brain syndrome, or chronic illness
3. Unemployment	
4. Social isolation	
5. Urban area residence	
6. Recent loss or surgery	9. Family history of suicide

90. How would you evaluate a patient who stated he was considering suicide?

The patient with suicidal thoughts should be questioned about previous suicide attempts, the specific details of the current plan and its feasibility, hopeless feelings, thoughts about the future, presence of significant psychosocial stress, concurrent major depression, and social support. Although suicide risk is difficult to predict, the patient with a well-conceived plan who feels hopeless and depressed should be protected from harming himself. Consultation with a psychiatrist will be helpful.

91. What are the common side-effects of neuroleptic antipsychotic agents?

The neuroleptic medications include haloperidol, chlorpromazine, thioridazine, fluphenazine, perphenazine, trifluoperazine, and thiothixene. They can cause sedation, orthostatic hypotension, and anticholinergic symptoms (dry mouth, constipation, urinary retention, blurred vision, nasal stuffiness). The extrapyramidal symptoms include akathisia (restlessness), parkinsonian symptoms, and acute dystonic reactions (torticollis and oculogyric crisis). Tardive dyskinesia (involuntary tongue, lip, neck, and arm movements) can occur after prolonged use and is usually irreversible.

92. What is an anniversary reaction?

A bereaved patient will frequently experience a depressed mood or somatic symptoms on the anniversary of the death of a close friend or relative. An anniversary reaction can occur after any significant loss such as job loss, amputation of a limb, or divorce.

93. How do you make the diagnosis of alcoholism?

Alcoholism is persistent, heavy drinking that interferes with the person's health, interpersonal relationships, position in society, or means of livelihood. It is the consequences of drinking that define alcoholism. Internists and family physicians often miss, or choose to ignore, the diagnosis of alcoholism in the patients they treat. Unfortunately, this avoidance behavior interferes with the physician's ability to get at the real cause for some common presenting complaints such as insomnia, nonspecific GI symptoms, and depression. It also makes the doctor an unwitting accomplice in the patient's destructive behavior.

One rapid, simple, and reliable screening test for alcoholism is the *CAGE* test, given below with the mnemonic in bold type.

Have you ever felt the need to **C**ut **down** on drinking?

Have you ever felt **A**nnoyed by criticism of your drinking?

Have you ever felt **G**uilty about your drinking?

Have you ever taken a morning **E**ye-opener?

Johnson B, Clark W: Alcoholism: A challenging physician-patient encounter. J Gen Intern Med 4:445–452, 1989.

94. How do you use nicotine gum to aid in smoking cessation?

Nicotine gum should be used by patients who have already stopped smoking to maintain smoking cessation. One piece of gum is chewed slowly and intermittently whenever the urge to smoke is felt. When the patient feels a slight taste or tingling, the gum is held in the cheek until the sensation is over to allow for absorption of the nicotine. Then the patient can resume slow chewing. Most patients need at least ten pieces of gum per day and should not exceed 30 pieces a day. Nicotine gum use should be continued for at least three months.

95. What is the differential diagnosis of chronic cough?

Diagnosis of Chronic Cough

Environmental irritants	Cigarette smoking, pollutants, dusts, lack of humidity
Lower respiratory tract problems	Lung cancer, asthma, COPD, interstitial lung disease, CHF, pneumonitis, bronchiectasis
Upper respiratory tract problems	Chronic rhinitis, chronic sinusitis, disease of the external auditory canal, pharyngitis
Extrinsic compressions	Adenopathy, malignancy, aortic lesions, aneurysm
GI problems	Reflux esophagitis
Psychogenic factors	

(Adapted from Goroll AH, et al: Primary Care Medicine: Office Evaluation and Management of the Adult Patient, 2nd ed. Philadelphia, J.B. Lippincott, 1988, p 185, with permission.)

96. What can an office practitioner do to encourage patients to stop smoking?

1. Ask all patients about smoking.
2. Strongly advise all smokers to stop.
3. Set a quit date and sign a stop smoking contract with the patient.
4. Provide self-help materials on smoking cessation.
5. Provide information about smoking cessation programs in the community.
6. Consider nicotine gum for those who will stop smoking.
7. Arrange follow-up visits or phone calls at 1 to 2 weeks after quit date.
8. Identify "smoker" on the chart and in the problem list.
9. Have a smoke-free office.
10. Set a personal example by not smoking.

U.S. Department of Health and Human Services: Clinical Opportunities for Smoking Interventions. A Guide for the Busy Physician. Washington, D.C., U.S. Government Printing Office, 1986.

Ockene JK, Kristeller J, Goldberg R, et al: Increasing the efficacy of physician-delivered smoking interventions. J Gen Intern Med 6:1–8, 1991.

97. What are the health consequences of smoking?

Smoking is associated with increased morbidity and mortality from COPD, malignancy (including lung cancer), and cardiovascular disease. Smokers also have an increased incidence of recurrent respiratory infections, peptic ulcer disease, cerebrovascular disease, sudden death, death from abdominal aortic aneurysm, and graft occlusion after lower extremity vascular reconstruction. The overall morbidity and mortality among smokers after any type of surgery are also increased.

98. What is the characteristic history of most patients with occupationally related asthma?

The history reveals a cyclical pattern of (1) wellness upon arrival at work, (2) symptoms appearing toward the end of the shift period, (3) symptoms increasing in severity for a period of time after departing from the worksite, and (4) symptoms gradually regressing over time away from the worksite. Holidays and weekends are free from asthma.

99. What are the findings of acute arterial occlusion?

With acute peripheral arterial occlusion, the patient will complain of the sudden onset of severe pain. In some patients there may be a more insidious onset over several hours. The patient may also complain of numbness, paresthesia, and muscle weakness or paralysis. On exam, the involved limb will be pale and cold with no pulses distal to the occlusion.

100. What are the typical symptoms of arterial insufficiency?

The patients are frequently older and have a history of smoking. The typical symptoms are pain or muscle tightness in the calf predictably reproduced after a certain amount of exercise. The pain or tightness is relieved by rest. Other symptoms include numbness and paresthesia. With progressive disease, the patient may develop ulcerations of the feet and pain developing at rest. Patients will also describe pain awakening them from sleep, relieved by dangling the feet over the bed.

101. What should be included in a foot care plan for a patient with arterial insufficiency?

1. Inspect both feet daily, particularly the soles, for trauma.
2. Wash daily with lukewarm water (test the water temperature with the hand or elbow prior to immersing the feet).
3. Avoid prolonged soaking.
4. Use a moisturizing cream daily.
5. Use an antifungal powder as needed.
6. Place lamb's wool between the toes at areas of pressure.
7. Cut toenails straight across.
8. Wear properly fitting shoes at all times.
9. Treat corns and calluses with physician supervision.
10. Avoid trauma.

102. When would you refer a patient with claudication for surgery?

Patients with rest pain, nonhealing distal ulcers, or early gangrene should be referred for surgical evaluation. Patients with disabling symptoms that interfere with their lifestyle should be referred. Counsel all patients with claudication to stop smoking.

103. What are the physical findings of deep venous thrombosis? How sensitive are these findings?

One may find unilateral swelling, warmth, pitting edema, or engorged superficial veins in the involved extremity. The patient may complain of aching pain. The occurrence of deep venous thrombosis, particularly in the postoperative period, may be asymptomatic. The physical findings may be present in as few as 50% of the cases. Although frequently cited as a sign of deep venous thrombosis, Homan's sign (calf pain with forced dorsiflexion) is not useful. There may be a palpable cord.

104. What are the characteristics of an ulcer due to venous stasis disease?
A venous stasis ulcer is usually pigmented with hemosiderin and is located on the medial leg.

BIBLIOGRAPHY

1. Barker LR, Burton JR, Zieve PD: Principles of Ambulatory Medicine, 3rd ed. Baltimore, Williams & Wilkins, 1991.
2. Branch WT Jr: Office Practice of Medicine, 2nd ed. Philadelphia, W.B. Saunders, 1987.
3. Goroll AH, May LA, Mulley AG (eds): Primary Care Medicine: Office Evaluation and Management of the Adult Patient, 2nd ed. Philadelphia, J.B. Lippincott, 1987.
4. Griner PF, Panzer RJ, Greenland P (eds): Clinical Diagnosis and the Laboratory: Logical Strategies for Common Medical Problems. Chicago, Year Book Medical Publishers, 1986.
5. U.S. Preventive Services Task Force: Guide to Clinical Preventive Services. An Assessment of the Effectiveness of 169 Interventions. Baltimore, Williams & Wilkins, 1989.

17. GERIATRIC SECRETS

George E. Taffet, M.D.

> *To be seventy years old . . . is like climbing the Alps. You reach a snow-crowned summit, and see behind you the deep valley stretching miles and miles away, and before you other summits higher and whiter, which you may have the strength to climb, or may not. Then you sit down and meditate and wonder which it will be.*
>
> Henry Wadsworth Longfellow (1807–1882)
> *Letter to George W. Childs, March 13, 1877*

> *When the physician said to him, "You have lived to be an old man," he (Pausanias) said, "That is because I never employed you as my physician."*
>
> Pausanias (479 B.C.)
> *Quoted by Plutarch in: Moralia, "Sayings of Spartans," 231.A.6 (tr. by F.C. Babbitt)*

1. Two things can increase the maximum life span of animals. What are they?

Caloric restriction has been shown to increase the maximum life-span of rodents by over 50%. These animals are fed approximately two-thirds of their ad-lib diet and proper nutrition is insured. On this diet mice will live 4 or more years, longer than animals on a normal diet. The second method of life prolongation will not work for warm-blooded animals. However, in cold-blooded animals, simply decreasing the environmental temperature will increase the maximum life span.

2. Are there any organs in the human body that normally "fold up shop" as we age?

There are a few organs that appear to have programmed death. The ovaries in women seem to have a predetermined rate of follicle production that ends with menopause. The thymus is another such organ that is essentially gone by age 65. The involution of the thymus starts after puberty and is progressive thereafter. The importance of the thymus in maintaining immune function has prompted many to suggest that aging is primarily a loss of immunocompetence.

3. What are the three major theories of aging?

The three major theories of aging are:

1. **Cellular theory:** This theory proposes that genetic instability (such as accumulated errors in DNA replication) and progressive cellular damage (from both internal and environmental factors) cause the aging process.

2. **Autoimmune theory:** This theory proposes that aging is the result of progressive "self-destruction" through autoimmune mechanisms. This process may be mediated by genetic, environmental, endocrine, or other factors.

3. **Neuroendocrine theory:** This theory proposes that changes in the neural and endocrine systems may be the cause of aging. These changes may lead to the development of diseases that limit life span (cancers, atherosclerotic cardiovascular diseases, etc.).

4. What is the rate at which most organ systems age?

Most of the changes seen in organ system function in the aged occur as the result of a gradual loss over the course of a person's life. The "1% rule" expresses the generalized rate of decline. Most organ systems lose approximately 1% of their functional capacity per year after age 30. This generalization is, of course, subject to much individual variation.

5. What overall changes in human morphology are associated with aging?

Overall Changes Associated with Aging

SYSTEM	MORPHOLOGY
Overall	↓ height (stooped posture secondary to ↑ kyphosis) ↓ weight ↑ fat to lean-body-mass ratio ↓total body water

6. Name some organ-specific changes in human morphology and function associated with aging.

Organ-specific Changes Associated with Aging

SYSTEM	MORPHOLOGY	FUNCTION
Skin	↑ wrinkling Atrophy of sweat glands	
Cardiovascular	Elongation and tortuosity of arteries ↑ intimal thickening of arteries ↑ fibrosis of the media of arteries ↓ rate of cardiac hypertrophy Sclerosis of heart valves	↓ maximum cardiac output ↓ heart rate response to stress ↓ compliance of peripheral blood vessels
Kidney	↑ number of abnormal glomeruli	↓ creatinine clearance ↓ renal blood flow ↓ maximum urine osmolarity
Lung	↓ elasticity ↓ cilia activity	↓ vital capacity ↓ maximal oxygen uptake ↓ cough reflex
GI tract	↓ hydrochloric acid ↓ saliva flow ↓ number of taste buds	
Bones	Osteoarthritis Loss of bone substance	
Eyes	Arcus senilis ↓ pupil size Growth of lens	↓ accommodation Hyperopia ↓ visual acuity ↓ color perception ↓ depth perception
Hearing	Degenerative changes of the ossicles ↑ obstruction of the Eustachian tube Atrophy of the external auditory meatus Atrophy of cochlear hair cells Loss of auditory neurons	↓ high frequency perception ↓ pitch discrimination
Immune		↓ T-cell function
Nervous	↓ brain weight ↓ cortical cell count	↑ motor response time Slower psychomotor performance ↓ intellectual performance ↓ complex learning ↓ hours of sleep ↓ hours of REM sleep

Table continued on next page.

Organ-specific Changes Associated with Aging (Continued)

SYSTEM	MORPHOLOGY	FUNCTION
Endocrine	↓ triiodothyronine (T_3)	
	↓ free testosterone	
	↑ insulin	
	↑ norepinephrine	
	↑ parathyroid hormone (PTH)	
	↑ vasopressin	

↑ = increased, ↓ = decreased.
(From Kane RL, et al: Essentials of Clinical Geriatrics, 2nd ed. New York, McGraw-Hill, 1989, p 7, with permission.)

7. What maximum heart rate should be expected for a 75-year-old male wishing to start an exercise program? How about a 75-year-old woman?
Data from men in the Baltimore Longitudinal Study who were vigorously screened for the presence of occult coronary artery disease yielded the following regression equation:

Maximum heart rate = $208.2 - 0.95 \times$ (age in years)

Thus, in a 75-year-old male, the calculation would be:

$208.2 - 0.95 \times 75 = 137$ beats/min maximum heart rate

Women usually only attain 85% of this calculated maximal heart rate. Remember that the target heart rate for training is 50% to 85% of the calculated increase that occurs with exercise. If a patient's resting heart rate is 75, his target range for training should be 106 to 136.

Rodeheffer RJ, et al: Exercise cardiac output is maintained with advancing age in healthy human subjects. Circulation 69:203–213, 1984.

8. THA is an experimental drug with activity in Alzheimer's disease (AD). How does it work? What problems are associated with its use?
THA (tetrahydroaminoacridine) is an anticholinesterase. One of the hallmarks of AD is a decrease in the brain levels of the neurotransmitter, acetylcholine. By blocking the enzyme that metabolizes acetylcholine, more acetylcholine is made available to the receptors.

Two problems are noted with this agent. The first is a dose-related hepatotoxicity that appears to be reversible with decreases in the dose. The second is a hypothetical decrease in cognitive function with further increases in THA. This may be due to excessive acetylcholine at the receptor site. The drug does not appear to change the progression of AD.

9. What is the triad of normal pressure hydrocephalus (NPH)? Why is it important?
The three components of NPH are gait disorders, urinary incontinence, and dementia. This reversible dementia is treated by ventriculoatrial shunting, and a good response is correlated to the presence of all three parts of the triad. The presence of incontinence is unusual early in the course of NPH, as is the presence of gait abnormalities.

Black PM: Idiopathic normal-pressure hydrocephalus. Results of shunting in 62 patients. Neurosurgery 52:371–377, 1980.

10. What are actinic keratoses (AKs)? Can they develop into malignancies?
AKs are premalignant skin changes associated with sun exposure. They may develop into squamous cell carcinoma. They are found in most white people with extensive sun exposure. In some Australian cities they may be found in 95% of elderly men.

Balin AK: Aging of human skin. In Hazzard WR, et al: Principles of Geriatric Medicine and Gerontology, 2nd ed. New York, McGraw-Hill, 1990.

11. What are the types of falls most commonly seen in patients with parkinsonism?

Falls are very common in patients with parkinsonism. The symptoms of bradykinesia, rigidity, gait disturbance, and postural instability contribute to the increased frequency of falls. A festinating gait in parkinsonism, in which patients appear to be accelerating as if to catch up with their center of gravity, may lead to forward falls. At the time of arising, postural instability may lead to falling backwards. Short steps that do not clear the ground adequately will increase the frequency of tripping over objects. To sum up, parkinsonism will lead to many kinds of falls and must be considered in the differential of all patients who fall.

12. Of what significance is jaw pain upon chewing? How about headache with scalp tenderness?

Both of these unusual complaints may be the symptoms of temporal arteritis. Temporal arteritis is associated with polymyalgia rheumatica. Both problems are most common in very elderly women. Temporal arteritis may rapidly produce monocular or binocular blindness and needs to be urgently addressed when suspected. With corticosteroids, blindness can be prevented.

The erythrocyte sedimentation rate (ESR) is usually above 50 mm/hr in these patients. However, the definitive diagnosis requires a temporal artery biopsy. This procedure can be performed shortly after the institution of steroid therapy with prednisone, 60 mg/day, in divided doses.

Grob D. Common muscle disorders. In Reichel W: Clinical Aspects of Aging, 2nd ed. Baltimore, Williams & Wilkins, 1989.

13. What percentage of elderly male patients with congestive heart failure (CHF) have normal ejection fractions (EFs)?

At least 40% of male patients over the age of 75 with CHF have normal EFs as determined by echocardiogram or nuclear ventriculography, a result that is not different from results found in studies that look at all age groups. This group is important to recognize because the elderly are most likely to have problems with digoxin. Unless there is a clear indication for this agent (such as atrial fibrillation with rapid ventricular response), elderly male patients should not receive it.

Luchi RJ: Clinical Geriatric Cardiology. Edinburgh, Churchill Livingstone, 1989.

14. What is the leading cause of death in women aged 55–74? What about women older than 74?

While heart disease is the leading cause of death in men across these age groups, cancer is the number one killer for women aged 55–74. Older women most frequently die of heart disease.

15. From questionnaire data what is the most common "ailment" described in people over 65 years of age and how many reported it?

Responding to a questionnaire, over one-half (53%) of people 65 years of age and over reported the presence of arthritis. Hypertension was reported by 42%, hearing impairments by 40%, heart conditions by 34%, and visual impairments by 23%.

16. The ADL (activities of daily living) are bathing, toileting, dressing, walking, and eating. What percentage of those over 65 are fully independent in ADLs?

Despite the prevalent image of dependent, frail old people, over 90% of people over age 65 do not require any assistance in performing their ADLs.

17. What changes in the eye occur with normal aging other than cataracts?

There are a multitude of changes in the aging eye other than those leading to cataract formation. The periorbital tissues atrophy. The upper lid may droop and the lower lid can turn inward or outward. The pupil will become smaller and adaptation of the eye to changes in lighting is much slower in the older person. The lens will lose elasticity leading to an inability to focus on near items (presbyopia). The ability of the old eye to distinguish objects from background is impaired, and therefore more contrast is needed between objects.

18. What decrease in systolic blood pressure (BP) upon standing is considered normal in patients over 75?

One working definition of orthostatic hypotension requires a decrease of systolic blood pressure of more than 20 mmHg upon arising. However, decreases of greater than 20 mmHg upon arising have been reported in 20–30% of the community-dwelling elderly. The relative contributions of longstanding hypertension, antihypertensive agents, and age have not yet been clarified.

19. What is a positive Osler's maneuver with respect to the diagnosis of hypertension?

Blood pressure measurement, as usually performed today, involves the compression of the brachial artery by pressure applied via the cuff. Patients with heavily calcified arteries will have rigid, hard-to-compress arteries but may not have high intra-arterial pressures. If the cuff is pumped above the systolic blood pressure and the brachial or radial arteries are still palpable, this is a positive Osler's maneuver. Using cuff measurements of BP in patients with a positive Osler's maneuver results in a gross overestimate of the actual intra-arterial pressures.

20. What is the importance of a fourth heart sound (S_4) on cardiac exam in an older person?

Auscultation of an S_4 is very common on exam of an older person and is usually of limited clinical significance. It may be a manifestation of the decreased compliance of the aged heart. However the presence of an S_3 gallop is not normal and is characteristic of CHF.

   Spodick DH, Quarry-Pigot VM: Fourth heart sound as a normal finding in older persons. N Engl J Med 288:140–143, 1973.

21. What changes are seen on a glucose tolerance test in older patients? Why?

Fasting glucose changes very little with increasing age, perhaps 1 mg/dl for each decade over age 30. The impairment in glucose tolerance is much larger. At 1 and 2 hours after the challenge meal (usually 100 grams of glucose), the plasma glucose increases 5–6 mg/dl for each decade above 30. The same impairment is seen with a standard meal. If the normal 30-year-old has a 2-hour postprandial glucose of 140 mg/dl, then the normal 70-year-old might reach 160 or more (diabetic by some criteria). Insulin release is delayed and the maximum serum concentrations of insulin are higher in the older person. Insulin resistance at the tissue level is thought to be a predominant mechanism in the impaired glucose tolerance of the elderly.

22. What percentage of elderly persons with active tuberculosis (TB) have a nonreactive skin test?

In as many as 30% of patients with active TB, the skin test may be negative. The frequency of this situation appears to increase with increasing age. The booster effect (a more powerful reaction seen after a second PPD is applied 7–10 days after the first) reveals that many of the patients who are initially negative have active disease. This is a worthwhile procedure for TB in skin-testing most elderly patients.

23. What is the estimated prevalence of dementia in people over the age of 85?

Severe dementia is present in less than 1% of those over 65 but is seen in more than 15% of those over 85. This group (those over 85) is the fastest growing segment of the population. The incidence of dementia is highest in the ninth decade, and it appears to decline thereafter, so that new onset of dementia due to Alzheimer's disease is less common in patients above 90.

Katzman R: Alzheimer's disease. N Engl J Med 314:964–973, 1986.

24. What percentage of dementia is caused by Alzheimer's disease (AD)?
At least 50–60% of patients with dementia have AD or have a component of AD coexisting with another dementing illness, commonly multi-infarct dementia.

Katzman R: Alzheimer's disease. N Engl J Med 314:964–973, 1986.

25. There are only two ways to make a definite diagnosis of Alzheimer's disease (AD). What are they?
Either autopsy or brain biopsy. The diagnosis of definite AD requires a clinical history consistent with AD and histopathologic confirmation. However, using a reasonable approach to exclude other causes of dementia should allow a practitioner to be 90% correct in using only clinical findings to make the diagnosis of probable AD.

McKhann G, et al: Clinical diagnosis of Alzheimer's disease. Neurology 34:939–944, 1984.

26. What neurologic signs may be present in patients with dementia?
Focal neurologic findings are the clue that the etiology of the dementia may be multiple infarcts and not Alzheimer's disease. Cranial nerve findings should suggest the presence of chronic meningitis and prompt further investigation, including lumbar puncture. There is a set of neurological findings that are seen in dementia, perhaps because of loss of the inhibitory influences. These include the snout reflex, the suck reflex, and the glabellar blink. The sensitivity and specificity of these soft neurological signs in identifying patients with dementia are poor relative to those of a mental status exam.

27. What changes in hearing occur as part of normal aging?
The most representative loss of auditory function that occurs with aging is in the high-frequency range. There is an increase in the loudness of sound that is the minimum appreciated by the older ear. This is sensorineural hearing loss, which is usually noted in middle age and becomes problematic in later life. A parallel finding is the decrease in speech discrimination. When the patient is given words to both ears simultaneously and then asked about information given to one ear, older patients seem to have a large age-related loss in discriminant function. Because this test is performed with sounds above the auditory threshold, it is thought to be due to a central processing deficit independent of the sensorineural problem.

28. How common are macular degeneration and cataracts in those above 75?
The prevalence of these two eye problems is very high. The Framingham study reported macular degeneration in about 6% of patients aged 65–74 and 18% in those 75 or older. Cataracts were noted in 13% of those 65–74 and in approximately 40% of patients 75 and older.

29. What are the ophthalmoscopic findings of senile macular degeneration?
There are two types of senile macular degeneration (SMD). These are the nonexudative (dry) and exudative (wet). The nonexudative type is most common and is characterized by drusen (hyaline excrescences in Bruch's membrane). The underlying changes in the pigmented epithelium can produce geographic atrophy. This disorder produces a slowly progressive central visual loss, though only 10% of patients progress to legal blindness. There is no adequate therapy. The exudative form of SMD is accompanied by neovascularization that weeps and bleeds. Laser photocoagulation can be used to slow the progression of visual loss in the exudative type.

30. What are the complications of nasogastric feeding?

In addition to the displeasure that the patient may express, there are some important complications that may result from enteral feedings. Aspiration pneumonia may be the most important. Trauma to the nasal mucosa or the gastric and esophageal mucosa may produce erosions. Gastric distention may result from feedings in the presence of decreased motility. Diarrhea may result from increased motility or other causes (especially osmotic loading). Fluid overload may result in hyponatremia or CHF. In short, the practice of tube feeding is not benign.

31. What are the risk factors for hip fracture?

Since hip fracture is the most severe complication of osteopenia, many of the risk factors are the same.

Risk Factors for Hip Fracture

Female sex	White race
Thin body habitus	Increasing age
Hemiplegia	Psychotropic drugs
Cigarette smoking	Ethanol use
Chronic corticosteroid use	Previous hip fracture
Prior history of falls	Surgical bilateral oophorectomy (before natural menopause)

32. How frequently do patients with hip fractures have prior falls?

Hip fractures are very common and are one of the most dread sequelae of falling. About 15% of patients with hip fracture report previous falls. Therefore, early intervention in patients who fall may prevent recurrent falls and significantly decrease the number of hip fractures leading to death, disability, or institutionalization.

33. What are premonitory falls and which diseases are associated with them?

About 5% of falls are premonitory, signaling the presence of a serious systemic illness. These typically are pneumonia, urinary tract infections, or CHF. However, a fall can be the presenting complaint in an acute MI in elderly patients.

34. Why do younger women with osteoporosis who fall suffer Colles' fractures, whereas older women suffer hip fractures?

Colles' fracture is a fracture of the distal radius that occurs when persons with osteoporosis try to catch themselves when they fall. With age, the reaction time increases, so that frequently the older person who is falling may not have sufficient time to extend the arm. This leads to trauma absorbed directly by the hip and an increased potential for hip fracture.

35. Besides menopause, what are the other known risk factors for osteoporosis?

There are two types of osteoporosis, postmenopausal and age-related. Risk factors for osteoporosis include female sex, white or Oriental race, thin habitus, increasing age, low calcium intake, surgical bilateral oophorectomy (before natural menopause), hemiplegia, psychotropic drugs, cigarette smoking, ethanol use, chronic corticosteroid use, multiple pregnancies, and sedentary lifestyle.

36. How effective are supplemental estrogens in preventing hip fractures in postmenopausal women?

Supplemental estrogens are very effective, producing a 50% decrease in the incidence of hip fractures. Estrogen replacement will retard bone loss and thereby prevent the development of osteoporosis. The most bone mass is conserved if the estrogen replacement is instituted shortly after menopause; however, the evidence that estrogen is not useful when instituted more than 5 years beyond menopause is hypothetical and has not been rigorously evaluated.

37. What are the potential ill effects of supplemental estrogen?
The most well-known of the adverse effects is the 10-fold increase in the incidence of endometrial cancer in women on supplemental estrogen. This risk can be substantially decreased by the addition of supplemental progestins, which leads to cyclical shedding of the endometrium. The estrogen-replacement therapy does appear to increase the risk of gallstones and may promote the development of breast cancer. The evidence in reference to breast cancer is very controversial.

38. What are contractures? How long do they take to develop?
Contractures are the result of fibrosis of periarticular structures and shortening of muscles and tendons. The process can occur within just 7 days if regular full motion of the joint is not maintained. Any reason for immobility of a joint will produce contractures. Because contractures are so difficult to treat once they are present, preventative measures, such as bedside passive range of motion exercises, may be very beneficial and should be used in all immobilized patients.

39. What risk factors are associated with developing pressure sores (decubitus ulcer)?
The relative contribution of various factors in producing pressure sores is not clear-cut. Some risk factors, in addition to the pressure itself, include hypoalbuminemia, fecal incontinence, immobility, weight loss, hypotension, and fractures. A depressed sensorium will increase the risk of pressure sores, as will any other process that impairs the patient's ability to sense and respond to discomfort.

40. Why do pressure sores heal so much slower than similarly sized skin wounds of other types?
Three factors lead to ischemia of the surrounding tissue and slow healing:

1. **Shear forces:** Many pressure sores involve shearing, which occurs because of body position. In addition to producing ischemia by compressing vessels, the shear forces may disrupt the blood supply to the area.

2. **Thrombosis:** At times of low blood flow (or no blood flow), a clot may form in the vascular supply to the area. There is decreased fibrinolytic activity in the area of the ulcer, which causes the clot to persist.

3. **Transmission of pressure:** There is a tendency to assume that the skin area that is involved projects cylindrically into the deeper tissues. It appears that the projection is more that of a cone, with a narrow skin site of pressure and a much wider, deeper area of ischemia below the surface.

41. How are pressure sores graded? Which grades often require surgery?
All of the popular classification systems to grade pressure sores use maximum depth of penetration to measure the severity of the lesion. Shea's grading system is frequently used and is helpful in deciding on therapy.

Shea's Decubitus Grading System

Grade 1 = decubiti penetrate into the dermis
Grade 2 = decubiti extend into the subcutaneous fat
Grade 3 = decubiti extend into the fascia
Grade 4 = decubiti extend deeper than fascia and are without apparent boundaries

42. Why is the "head-elevated" bed position so likely to produce pressure sores?

The head-elevated position will produce shearing forces at the sacrum. The body is pulled by gravity while friction holds the skin to the sheet, thus producing the shearing force. The patient should not remain in this position for long periods of time.

43. What is the strongest risk factor for adverse drug reactions?

Although there are many risk factors, the strongest is the number of drugs to which the patient is exposed. Other predisposing factors to adverse drug reactions are female sex, small body size, hepatic or renal insufficiency, and previous drug reactions. Additionally, the presence of multiple diseases, altered compliance, and decreased homeostatic mechanisms may also predispose an older person to adverse drug reactions.

44. What characteristics help differentiate depression from dementia?

This differential may be very difficult. Depression has been called pseudodementia. On mental status examination, depressed patients frequently answer questions with "I don't know," whereas demented patients will try to answer even though their answer may be wrong. Depressed patients often have complaints about memory impairments that are out of proportion to the severity of findings on exam. The routine use of a depression questionnaire such as the Hamilton Depression Scale has been suggested, as has neuropsychological testing. If the uncertainty in the diagnosis persists, then a diagnostic/therapeutic trial of a tricyclic antidepressant (with low anticholinergic activity) may be warranted.

Remember, in up to a third of the cases, a demented person will have coexistent depression. These people may improve functionally when their depression is treated, even though the underlying dementia is not affected by the treatment.

Reynolds CF, et al: Bedside differentiation of depressive pseudodementia from dementia. Am J Psychiatry 145:1099–1103, 1988.

45. Why is depression common after a stroke?

Depression is said to affect up to 60% of stroke victims. The reasons are uncertain but appear to be partly due to the physical limitations produced by the stroke. There is a further correlation with the location of the stroke; patients with left frontal infarctions have the highest risk of depression. This area of the brain may play a key role in maintenance of mood.

Collin SJ, et al: Depression after stroke. Clin Rehab 1:27–32, 1987.

46. Why is it important to distinguish patients with cardiovascular syncope from those with syncope of other causes?

The patients with a cardiovascular etiology (anatomic, myocardial, or electrical) for their syncopal episodes have a much higher 1-year mortality (20%) than those with a defined noncardiovascular etiology, or those whose etiology is uncertain after workup. This is thought to be due to the underlying cardiovascular diseases for which the syncope serves as a marker (especially aortic stenosis).

Kapoor A, et al: A prospective evaluation and follow-up of patients with syncope. N Engl J Med 309:197–204, 1983.

47. What percentage of those over age 70 have significant (75% or higher) coronary artery stenoses at autopsy? How about those over age 90?

The prevalence of coronary artery disease (CAD) increases with age, but for men the prevalence appears to level off. Over 50% of all persons over age 70 have at least one arterial site of 75% stenosis at autopsy. By age 90 the prevalence increases to about 70%, women accounting for the increase. By noninvasive testing the prevalence of CAD is somewhat less, but is above 50% in the elderly.

48. What clues point to the possible presence of renovascular hypertension?

Renovascular hypertension is a common secondary cause of hypertension. It should be investigated in the elderly patient with:

1. The sudden development of hypertension (especially systolic and diastolic elevations rather than isolated systolic pressure elevation).
2. A history of well-controlled hypertension, which suddenly becomes difficult to control.
3. Hypertension who develops acute oliguric renal failure when given an angiotensin converting enzyme (ACE) inhibitor.
4. Hypertension who is found to have an abdominal or flank bruit.
5. Known atherosclerotic disease who develops renal insufficiency.

Rosmarin PC: Secondary hypertension. Clin Geriatr Med 5:753–768, 1989.

49. What is the difference between aortic stenosis and aortic sclerosis? How can one make the differentiation on physical examination?

Aortic sclerosis is the source of many benign murmurs in patients over 70 years of age. It is due to sclerosis (hardening and fibrosis) of the aortic cusps and is not hemodynamically significant. Aortic stenosis is not uncommon in the elderly and is usually due to calcification of a bicuspid valve in the younger elderly patient or degenerative calcification in those older than 75. By definition there is impedance to flow in aortic stenosis.

Although many findings on physical examination have been reported to distinguish the murmur of aortic stenosis from that of aortic sclerosis, unless the stenosis is severe (producing a thrill or very prolonged ventricular impulse), they are unreliable. It is most prudent to evaluate the patient with echocardiography. For example, the narrowed pulse-pressure characteristic of aortic stenosis in younger people is not often seen in the elderly with the same degree of aortic stenosis. This is probably due to the age-related increase in stiffness of the arterial tree. For the same reason, the "pulsus parvis et tardus" at the carotids also may not be seen in elderly patients with significant aortic stenosis.

Luchi RJ: Clinical Geriatric Cardiology. Edinburgh, Churchill Livingstone, 1989.

50. What is the natural history of an abdominal aortic aneurysm? If it is more than 6 cm in diameter, what is the chance of it lasting 2 years without rupture?

It appears that all abdominal aneurysms enlarge progressively but do so at varying rates. The likelihood of a 6-cm aneurysm lasting 2 years without rupture is less than 50%. It is this threshold (6 cm in diameter) in which elective surgery is most appropriate and probably should be recommended.

51. Are the symptoms of abdominal or low back pain important in patients known to have an abdominal aortic aneurysm?

Abdominal aortic aneurysms (AAAs) tend to rupture, not dissect. Elective aneurysmectomy can be performed with acceptable operative mortality; however, emergent surgery is very risky (50% mortality). Hypogastric pain or low back pain in a person known to have an AAA is often due to rapid expansion and may suggest that rupture is occurring or is imminent.

52. What is the importance of a positive antinuclear antibody test (ANA) in an older patient?

The increase in erythrocyte sedimentation rate in the normal elderly is well known; additionally, there is a 15% frequency of a positive ANA in normal older people. These are usually of low titer (1:16 or less) and, in isolation, are of little clinical significance.

53. What joints are most commonly involved in osteoarthritis?

The joints most frequently involved in osteoarthritis are the distal interphalangeal and proximal interphalangeal joints of the hands, the knees, the first carpometacarpal joint of the feet, and less frequently the hips. The distribution presented here is from radiologic survey data and does not reveal whether or not there was any limitation of function or other symptomatology associated with the radiologic changes.

54. What neurologic examination findings are abnormal in a young patient and normal in an older one?

The passage of time has many effects on the normal nervous system, and a multitude of changes occur with aging alone. On cranial nerve exam, a marked limitation of upward gaze is seen in most elderly persons as well as relatively constricted pupils. There is a slowing of rapid alternations of movement, which is termed dysdiadochokinesia. In the distal extremity there may be sensory impairments, and ankle jerks may frequently be absent. Abdominal reflexes may also be absent.

55. What can handwriting tell you about the differential diagnosis of tremor? What can a glass of wine do in this regard?

Essential tremor will worsen with intention and will usually improve with ethanol. Parkinsonism patients characteristically have micrographia, a condition in which the handwriting is very small. The administration of ethanol does not significantly alter the tremor of Parkinson's disease.

56. Who gets tardive dyskinesia? How is it treated?

Tardive dyskinesia usually follows prolonged exposure to neuroleptic agents. Although older patients seem to be more likely to get tardive dyskinesia, it is not clear that duration of exposure, the specific agent, or the total dose has any relation to the appearance of the involuntary movements. There is little evidence that tardive dyskinesia can be treated with drugs, although in a certain percentage of patients the movements may disappear, even with the continuation of the neuroleptic agent.

57. What are the long-term complications of cascara or senna laxatives?

The most important side-effect of long-term use of these laxatives is degeneration of myoneural chains in the colon. This impairs peristalsis and may set up a vicious cycle in which decreased colonic motility leads to worsened constipation and increased use of laxatives.

58. What group of elderly patients is at risk for osteogenic sarcoma? Is there a marker for malignant conversion?

Although osteogenic sarcoma is usually found in growing adolescents and is quite rare in the elderly, it occurs in one subgroup of elderly patients. Patients who have active Paget's disease of the bone also have a marked increase in their risk of developing osteogenic sarcoma. In these patients there usually is a significant increase in serum alkaline phosphatase heralding the malignancy. Although these tumors develop in less than 1% of elderly patients with Paget's disease, their prognosis and response to treatment are very poor.

59. What percentage of men over age 80 are still having intercourse?

A recent survey of healthy men aged 80–102 revealed that 63% were having sexual intercourse at least several times a year. For women, the percentage was only 30%. This may be a reflection of the much higher numbers of women alive in these age groups (six women for each man). The point is that the male climacteric (age-related hypogonadal state) is an unusual phenomenon.

60. What differences are seen between breast cancers in younger women and those in older women?

The overall prognosis for breast cancer is probably unchanged with age. This is due to a number of factors, some positive and some detrimental. At the time of diagnosis of breast cancer, elderly women are more likely to have distant metastases and therefore a poor prognosis. However, elderly women are much more likely to have estrogen-receptor-positive breast cancer, implying a well differentiated malignancy that will be more responsive to hormonal manipulation and will possibly be slower growing. The less aggressive nature of these malignancies has been confirmed using thymidine labeling to determine what percentage of cells are actively making DNA. This percentage goes down linearly with increasing patient age.

Cox EC: Breast cancer in the elderly. Clin Geriatr Med 3:695–713, 1987.

61. What percentage of prostate cancers is confined to the prostate or local pelvis at time of diagnosis?

Only about 30% of prostate cancers are local at time of diagnosis. This means that two-thirds are widespread and incurable at diagnosis. Fortunately the malignancy is usually responsive to hormonal manipulation, which controls the disease and alleviates symptoms.

62. When an older person is found to a have a monoclonal gammopathy of undetermined significance (MGUS), what are the chances of developing a related malignancy in the next 10 years?

A monoclonal gammopathy is a monoclonal protein noted on serum protein electrophoresis of less than 3 g/dl and without associated signs or symptoms of hematological abnormalities. At 10 years of follow-up, 40% of elderly patients with MGUS are stable, 40% are dead from other causes, and 10–20% have myeloma, macroglobulinemia, amyloidosis, or non-Hodgkin's lymphoma.

63. What age-related changes make the older person more likely to develop pneumonia?

There are multiple changes that occur with aging that make the older person more likely to develop pneumonia. The most common way for an older person to introduce pathogens into the lungs is aspiration. Older people appear to aspirate more frequently while swallowing and to have a poorer cough reflex, thus incompletely clearing the aspirate. The organisms that inhabit the oropharynx are usually nonpathogenic in the younger person (with some exceptions). However there appears to be an increase in the amount of gram-negative organisms in the flora in up to 20% of community-dwelling elderly individuals, as well as almost all nursing home residents.

Changes in the immune system, especially T-cell changes and antibody affinity changes, may also increase the risk of pneumonia. Drugs that sedate the patient and allow aspiration to occur are more frequently administered to the elderly. Finally, the increased frequency of influenza leads to an increased frequency of pneumonias.

64. What are acceptable reasons for a chronic Foley catheter?

There are only a few indications for a chronic indwelling Foley catheter. Urinary retention should be treated with chronic catheterization if it produces renal dysfunction, infections, or overflow incontinence, and if it is not treatable with surgery, medications, and intermittent catheterization. If incontinent urine is soiling skin wounds, decubitus ulcers, or skin irritations, then the catheter is appropriate. There is a small group of patients with terminal illnesses or severe debility (a person with severe rheumatoid arthritis where any movement is very painful) that may require the catheter and an even smaller group that wants the catheter for patient or caregiver convenience.

65. What can be done to decrease the rate of colonization of indwelling urinary catheters?

Almost all patients with indwelling Foley catheters become colonized with bacteria. Irrigation or antibiotic therapy does not eradicate colonization but does produce changes in the flora. For suspected urinary tract infection, it is important to remove the old catheter and get urine for cultures from the new catheter. Condom catheters, when they get twisted, kinked, or clogged, have a frequency of infection that is as bad as the indwelling catheter. Perhaps the most important point is to evaluate the absolute indication for the catheter and be certain that it is not just for nursing convenience.

66. What is the role of antiviral therapy in the treatment of herpes zoster in the immunocompetent elderly?

In general, neither acyclovir nor vidarabine is recommended for immunocompetent elderly patients with uncomplicated shingles because of the expense and potential side-effects. For ophthalmic zoster infection, immunocompetent patients should be treated with oral acyclovir. Prednisone is given to many immunocompetent elderly with shingles to prevent post-herpetic neuralgia, but the effectiveness of this therapy is uncertain. Post-herpetic neuralgia is 3–5 times more frequent in patients over 60 years of age.

67. Are patients with shingles very likely to have an underlying malignancy?

No. Although there probably is a small increase in the chance of cancer in patients with herpes zoster recurrence, it is not large enough to merit evaluation for malignancy in every patient who presents with shingles.

Raggazino MW, et al: Risk of cancer after herpes zoster: A population-based study. N Engl J Med 307:393–397, 1982.

68. What are seborrheic keratoses? What treatments are effective for them?

Seborrheic keratoses are benign epidermal lesions frequently seen in the elderly. These hyperpigmented, hyperkeratotic lesions have distinct borders and an irregular, scaly surface. They are light or dark brown, wart-like papules of varying size, generally described as having a "stuck-on" appearance. They are usually multiple and are most commonly found on the trunk. As they enlarge, they darken and develop a greasy scale.

Although they have no malignant potential, because of their dark color they can sometimes be confused with malignant melanoma. These lesions can be treated with curettage, electrodesiccation, liquid nitrogen, and topical glycolic acid.

Kleinsmith DM, Perricone NV: Common skin problems in the elderly. Clin Geriatr Med 5:189–211, 1989.

69. What age-related skin changes produce xerosis?

Rough, dry skin (xerosis) is the reflection of a number of age-related skin changes. There are a decrease in sebum secretion and a decrease in eccrine sweat glands. There are also changes in the stratum corneum and epidermal atrophy. All these changes facilitate drying of the skin.

70. Hepatic metabolism of drugs has three components that determine handling. What are they and how are they affected by aging?

There are three important determinants of hepatic metabolism of drugs: (1) hepatic blood flow, (2) phase I reactions, and (3) phase II reactions. Hepatic blood flow decreases with age in both the arterial and portal systems. This decreased delivery will make an important contribution to increasing the half-life of certain agents and narrowing the oral dose/parenteral dose discrepancies for drugs that are heavily metabolized during the "first pass" through the liver. The liver handles drugs in two general ways: phase I reactions are oxidations and reductions, and phase II reactions are acetylations and glucuronidations. Phase I reactions decrease significantly with age, whereas phase II reactions are well preserved. All these are important issues in choosing an agent with which prolonged half-life might have serious adverse effects.

71. Why are older people more prone to accidental hypothermia?

More than half of patients hospitalized with accidental hypothermia are over age 65. This is due in part to the impairment in temperature regulation that is seen in normal elderly people. The "thermostat" is within the hypothalamus, and it is less responsive to changes in both skin temperature and core temperature in the elderly. Therefore, the hypothalamus will signal shivering to begin at a lower temperature. However, shivering in the elderly appears to generate normal amounts of heat. The loss of subcutaneous tissue with aging produces a loss of insulation, so the older person will lose or gain heat more rapidly. The basal metabolic rate of the older person is lower than in the young, so there is less heat to conserve in the first place. Finally, the older person has a reduced drive to micro-acclimatize (put on warm clothing) when the surroundings are cold. All of these small changes (especially in the presence of impaired cognition or sedative medications) add up to a large risk of accidental hypothermia.

72. What significant changes in body composition occur as we age from 25–75? Does gender make a difference?

Displayed graphically in the figure below are the marked increase in fat mass and corresponding decrease in lean body mass that accompany normal aging in men. For women, the changes are less dramatic, since they have significantly more fat mass throughout life.

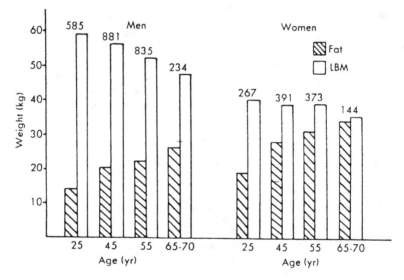

Changes in lean body mass (LBM) and fat content as a function of average age in men and women. Number of subjects at each age is shown above bar graphs. (Data from Forbes GB, Reina, JC: Metabolism 19:653, 1970. From Conrad KA, Bressler R: Drug Therapy for the Elderly. St. Louis, C.V. Mosby, 1982, p 44, with permission.)

73. Why are old people more likely to become dehydrated?

Water and salt homeostasis are well maintained in the healthy elderly in the absence of stress. With stress, however, this may not be the case. The elderly have a decreased thirst drive, and it takes a larger change in plasma osmolarity to stimulate water intake. Even then, the amount of water ingested is less than in the young and is often less than necessary. The amount of sweat produced is decreased, the threshold temperature for sweating is increased, and the renal losses seem to be more significant. The renal changes with aging are multiple, but most relevant to this question is the impairment of the maximum concentrating ability of the kidneys (1200 mOsm in the young and less than 800 mOsm in the elderly). Furthermore, the elderly are slower to respond to a water deficit. It takes 24 more hours of water deprivation for the older person to reach maximum urine concentrations.

74. Why is it that in men, lung cancer peaks in incidence at age 70 and declines afterwards?
The development of lung cancer is very strongly associated with cigarette abuse. Above age 70, many of the smokers are dead or have stopped smoking for other reasons. Therefore, the population as a whole has a lower risk of developing lung cancer. For smokers, the risk of lung cancer appears to continue to increase with increasing age.

75. Which groups of patients are at increased risk of untoward reactions when vitamin D supplementation is used for prophylaxis against osteoporosis?
Vitamin D supplementation has an unclear role in prevention of osteoporosis; however, some physicians do administer this agent for prophylaxis. The groups at risk for untoward reactions to this therapy are those with kidney stones, patients with sarcoidosis, and, if the active form of vitamin D (1,25 di-hydroxy vitamin D) is administered, anyone with decreased creatinine clearance.

76. Does sweating change with aging?
Yes. The temperature required to produce sweating in a healthy elderly person sitting in a sauna is 1-2 degrees higher than in a young person (the threshold temperature is increased). The maximum sweating rate is lower due to either a decrease in the number of glands and/ or a decrease in the maximum production by each gland. The sweat glands of older patients are less responsive to exogenous or endogenous acetylcholine. The decreased function is seen in both eccrine and apocrine sweat glands.

77. How frequent is urinary incontinence in community-dwelling elderly? How about those in nursing homes?
The frequency of insignificant loss of urine is quite common in women of all ages. However, the frequency of urine loss of sufficient magnitude to produce social compromise or health problems is found in 10-30% of community-dwelling elderly, with a lower frequency in men. Surveys of elderly nursing home residents have reported urinary incontinence in 50% of inhabitants. The very high frequency in institutionalized populations is primarily due to their underlying diseases, but it is sometimes the product of physical restraints and medications.

78. What are the four different types of urinary incontinence? What are their distinguishing features and causes?
Urinary incontinence is not a part of normal aging, nor is it caused by aging. However, many of the physiologic consequences of aging can contribute to urinary incontinence. The four types of urinary incontinence are:
    1. **Stress incontinence:**
    Definition: The involuntary loss of small volumes of urine related to events that cause increased intraabdominal pressure (coughing, laughing, exercise). It is more common in females (present with laughing in 50% of young females) and increases with aging.
    Causes: Weakness or laxity of pelvic floor muscles, bladder outlet, or urethral sphincter.
    2. **Urge incontinence:**
    Definition: The involuntary loss of larger volumes of urine due to the inability to delay voiding when the sensation of bladder fullness (urge) is perceived.

Causes: Detrusor motor and/or sensory instability, either alone or in combination with one of the following:

- Local genitourinary conditions such as cystitis, urethritis, tumors, stones, diverticula, and outflow obstruction.
- CNS disorders such as stroke, dementia, parkinsonism, suprasacral spinal cord injury, or disease.*

3. **Overflow incontinence:**

Definition: Involuntary loss of small amounts of urine resulting from mechanical forces on an over-distended bladder or from other effects of urinary retention on bladder and sphincter function.

Causes: Anatomic obstruction by prostate, stricture, or cystocele; acontractile bladder associated with diabetes mellitus or spinal cord injury; neurogenic (detrusor-sphincter dyssynergy), associated with multiple sclerosis and other suprasacral spinal cord injury.

4. **Functional incontinence:**

Definition: Leakage of urine associated with inability to toilet because of impairment of cognitive and/or physical functioning, psychological unwillingness, or environmental barriers.

Causes: Severe dementia and other neurological disorders. Psychological factors such as depression, regression, anger, and hostility.

*When detrusor motor instability is associated with a neurological disorder, it is termed "detrusor hyperreflexia."

(From Kane RL, et al: Essentials of Clinical Geriatrics, 2nd ed. New York, McGraw-Hill, 1989, p 151, with permission.)

79. What are the primary treatment modalities for the four types of urinary incontinence?

1. **Stress incontinence:** Pelvic floor (Kegel) exercises, alpha-adrenergic agonists, estrogen, biofeedback, behavioral training, surgical bladder neck suspension.

2. **Urge incontinence:** Bladder relaxants, estrogen (if vaginal atrophy is present), training procedures (e.g., biofeedback, behavioral therapy), surgical removal of obstructing or other irritating pathological lesions.

3. **Overflow incontinence:** Surgical removal of obstruction, intermittent catheterization (if practical), indwelling catheterization.

4. **Functional incontinence:** Behavioral therapies (e.g., habit training, scheduled toileting), environmental manipulations, incontinence undergarments and pads, external collection devices, bladder relaxants (selected patients), indwelling catheters (selected patients).

(From Kane RL, et al: Essentials of Clinical Geriatrics, 2nd ed. New York, McGraw-Hill, 1989, p 168, with permission.)

80. What are the important causes of acute and reversible urinary incontinence?

Because of the severe physical, psychological, social, and economic costs of urinary incontinence, it is important to identify reversible cases and render the needed treatment. The causes of acute and reversible forms of urinary incontinence can be remembered by the "DRIP" acronym:

D = delirium

R = restricted mobility, retention

I = infection,[1] inflammation,[1] impaction (fecal)

P = polyuria,[2] pharmaceuticals

[1]Acute symptomatic urinary tract infection, atrophic vaginitis or urethritis.

[2]Hyperglycemia, volume-expanded states causing excessive nocturia (e.g., CHF, venous insufficiency).

(From Kane RL, et al: Essentials of Clinical Geriatrics, 2nd ed. New York, McGraw-Hill, 1989, p 149, with permission.)

81. What are the complications and adverse effects of urinary incontinence?

Potential Adverse Effects of Urinary Incontinence

Physical health:	**Social:**
Skin breakdown	Stress on family, friends, and caregivers
Recurrent urinary tract infections	Predisposition to institutionalization
Psychological:	**Economic:**
Isolation and dependency	Supplies (padding, catheters, etc.) and laundry
Depression	Labor (nurses, housekeepers)
	Management of complications

(From Kane RL, et al: Essentials of Clinical Geriatrics, 2nd ed. New York, McGraw-Hill, 1989, p 140, with permission.)

82. How do the age-associated changes in body composition affect drug pharmacokinetics?
There is more fat and less muscle (water volume) in which the drug can distribute. Water-soluble drugs may have higher concentrations due to this decreased volume of distribution. Highly fat-soluble drugs may have lower concentrations at effector sites in the elderly. Furthermore, these drugs are stored in body fat, which then acts like a depot when therapy is discontinued and may take a very long time to "wash out."

83. Does an asymptomatic carotid bruit imply impending stroke?
NO. The risk of a cerebrovascular accident (CVA) without warning transient ischemic attacks (TIAs) is only about 1% in the year following the discovery of a bruit. However, the bruit is a marker of widespread atherosclerosis and the risk of CVA is elevated. The scenario becomes quite different once the bruit becomes symptomatic with ipsilateral TIAs. At this point, therapy is indicated.

84. How large is the age-associated decrease in hemoglobin seen in healthy men and women?
Trick question! There is no decrease in hemoglobin in healthy elderly men or women.

85. Are vaccinations useful in preventing illness in the elderly? If so, which illnesses and in which elderly patients?
Influenza, pneumococcal, and tetanus-diphtheria vaccinations are all recommended for older patients. The flu vaccine is about 70% effective in elderly patients and should be given yearly, in the fall, to all people over 65, especially those who live in nursing homes. The newest pneumococcal vaccine includes antigen from 23 serotypes that probably cause 85% of pneumococcal pneumonias. The current recommendations suggest that patients over 65 have one lifetime pneumococcal vaccination and that those who received the earlier (14 serotype) vaccine do not need to be immunized again. Although tetanus is still a fairly uncommon disease, the percentage of patients over the age of 50 has been increasing. These people often have been immunized in the remote past but not recently. The same is true for diphtheria. Booster immunizations with ADULT diphtheria-tetanus should be done every 10 years throughout adult life.

86. Are there any types of hearing loss that do not respond to hearing aids?
Though there are still some who do not believe that sensorineural hearing loss will respond to amplification, it appears that both of the common types of age-associated hearing loss, conductive and sensorineural, will respond to amplification provided by hearing aids. The third type of communication defect is a central processing problem in which the words are heard but not properly understood. This problem may be made worse by a hearing aid that also amplifies the background sound. These patients need to have extraneous sound reduced for optimal function.

87. Is there any benefit to smoking cessation for smokers above age 65?

Yes. The most immediate benefit is to the heart and circulation where the benefits may be seen almost immediately.

FEV$_1$ decreases at a much faster rate in smokers than in nonsmokers. Although the absolute level of FEV$_1$ does not improve with cessation of smoking, the rate of decline does. The rate of decrease that occurs in smokers (about 75–100 cc/year) will quickly return to the rate of decrease seen in nonsmokers (about 25–30 cc/yr). The elderly smoker is difficult to change, and successful cessation rates for those over 65 are not good. Nevertheless, the elderly smoker has much to gain by stopping.

88. Is single-dose therapy for cystitis as successful in older women as it is in younger women? How long should treatment be continued?

No. Even with the lower bacterial load seen in asymptomatic bacteriuria, single-dose therapy was effective in less than two-thirds of elderly women. It is anticipated that symptomatic UTI would be even less responsive to this treatment regimen. Most experts are currently recommending 7 to 10 days of antibiotic therapy for uncomplicated urinary tract infections.

89. Many old people complain about difficulties sleeping. How many hours of sleep does the average 75-year-old require and will the requirement change with further aging?

There is considerable controversy in this area, but it is now thought that the number of hours of sleep per 24-hour period changes very little throughout adult life. Older persons seem to increase their daytime sleeping (naps) and decrease their nocturnal sleeping, so the number of hours of sleep at night goes down. There is a large change in the amounts of sleep time spent in the various stages of sleep. Older persons spend more time in stage I (light sleep/sleep-awake transition). There is also an age-associated decrease in stage-IV sleep.

90. What are the common causes of lower GI bleeding in an elderly person?

Bleeding from diverticula is the most common cause of bleeding in the elderly, followed by bleeding from angiodysplasia. These two conditions make up 75% of lower GI bleeding. Other causes of blood loss in the elderly are colonic polyps, colon carcinoma, ischemic colitis, and inflammatory bowel disease. Old people can also have hemorrhoids as a cause of bleeding. One study has shown that 30% of the elderly known to have diverticula were bleeding because of another reason. It is therefore unwise to empirically attribute lower GI blood loss to diverticula.

91. What treatments are used for early chronic lymphocytic leukemia (CLL)?

None. At the present time, patients with a normal hemoglobin and a normal platelet count should be monitored frequently for any progression of the disease. Therapy can be useful for more advanced stage CLL; however, most elderly die *with* CLL, not *from* it.

92. Sjögren's syndrome is more common than previously thought in older patients. What findings are seen in this syndrome? (See also pp 349–350.)

Sjögren's syndrome has recently been reported in up to 2% of nursing home residents (predominantly women). This chronic inflammatory disease of unknown etiology primarily involves the lacrimal, salivary, and excretory glands. The symptoms are dry mouth, dry eyes, recurrent salivary pain or swelling, dyspareunia, cough, and dysphagia. In most patients the erythrocyte sedimentation rate (ESR) is elevated, but since the ESR may be elevated in the healthy elderly, this is nondiagnostic. Antibodies to the Lane SSB antigen are diagnostic. In the elderly population the extraglandular involvement is less frequent than in younger patients with Sjögren's syndrome.

93. How much money was spent in 1985 on health care costs for each person over 65? How much of this was their own money?

Incredibly, about $4000 was spent on health care for each elderly person. Even though many of these expenses were covered by private insurance or Medicare, out-of-pocket expenses totaled $1000 for each person over 65 that year. One can expect that the total figure per person over 65 in 1991 has almost doubled since 1985.

94. How is Paget's disease of the bone most often diagnosed in the elderly?

Paget's disease of bone is frequently recognized in the elderly via multichannel screening of blood. The elevation of alkaline phosphatase in the absence of liver disease is often found to be a marker of the increased bone turnover that is part of Paget's disease. Confirmation is made radiographically. Paget's disease is present in over 10% of those over age 80 and is more common in the northern U.S. than in the southern U.S.

95. What are the clinical manifestations of Paget's disease of bone?

Although most patients are asymptomatic at the time of diagnosis, in 90% of cases it has a variety of manifestations. These include:

Bone manifestations (commonest):
1. Bone pain in the pelvis, hips, and back
2. Bone deformities due to the remodeling process. This is most commonly seen as bowing of the femur and tibia, skull enlargement, and loss of height due to scoliosis and vertebral collapse.
3. Pathologic fractures due to bone remodeling
4. Increased warmth over the affected areas of bone due to an increase in vascularity

Cardiovascular manifestations (rare):
1. High cardiac output state with or without CHF
2. Hypertension
3. Exacerbation of ischemic heart disease
4. Cardiomegaly
5. Arterial and valvular calcifications

Neurological manifestations (rare):
1. Compression of cranial nerves (all can be involved, but Paget's disease most often involves the eighth cranial nerve, causing a variety of symptoms) or blood vessels (causing stroke).
2. Middle ear deafness due to ossification of the stapedius tendon
3. Hydrocephalus due to compression of the foramina of Luschka or Magendie
4. Spinal compression syndromes

Other manifestations:
1. Hypercalcemia and hypercalciuria (with or without renal calculi)
2. Osteogenic sarcoma

96. What are the indications for specific treatment of Paget's disease of bone?

Criteria for Specific Treatment of Paget's Disease

1. Disabling pain not relieved by analgesics or anti-inflammatory medications.	3. Neurologic complications
	4. Increasing deafness
2. Progression of skeletal aspects of the disease, as indicated by increasing deformity, head or appendicular bone enlargement, frequent fracture, nonunion of fractures, vertebral compression, or acetabular protrusion.	5. High-output congestive heart failure
	6. Immobilization hypercalcemia, before and after major orthopedic surgery

(From Lifschitz ML, Harmon CE: Musculoskeletal problems in the elderly. In Schrier RW (ed): Clinical Internal Medicine in the Aged. Philadelphia, W.B. Saunders, 1982, p 193, with permission.)

97. What are the treatment modalities available for Paget's disease of bone?

Treatment Modalities for Paget's Disease of Bone

1. **Nonsteroidal anti-inflammatory/analgesic agents:** for relief of symptoms.
2. **Calcitonin:** Inhibits osteoclast production and activity, which may decrease and improve manifestations of the disease, reverse some of the pathological changes, and lead to partial normalization of the biochemical markers of the disease. The initial effects are seen in approximately 2 weeks, and therapy reaches maximal effectiveness in 6 to 12 months. Side-effects (which are usually not significant) include nausea, vomiting, facial flushing, and polyuria. Development of resistance due to antibodies against salmon calcitonin may require the use of human calcitonin.
3. **Diphosphonates:** Causes a slowdown in bone growth and turnover by binding to hydroxyapatite crystals in the bone; blocking their growth and dissolution, and inhibiting osteoclast activity. Diphosphonates have the advantage of oral administration and are usually given in 6-month courses. Side-effects are usually not significant.
4. **Mithramycin:** Although not approved for use in Paget's disease, mithramycin, a cytotoxic antibiotic, has been used to suppress the manifestations of the disease in some patients. Remissions of many years' duration have been reported after a single course of therapy. Side-effects can be severe, and include hepatic, renal, and bone marrow toxicities.
5. **Surgery:** Can be used to increase mobility and joint motion, as well as to relieve nerve compression syndromes. Should be performed after several months of medical therapy to decrease postoperative bleeding and hypercalcemia.

98. How frequently is amyloid protein seen on autopsy in atria of hearts from patients aged more than 90? What is its significance?

Small amounts of amyloid protein, limited to the atria of the heart, may be seen in 80–90% of autopsy specimens when the hearts are from the very elderly. This protein has not been shown to have pathological importance, and it is considered a benign age-associated marker. Some researchers consider this amyloid to be similar to the atrial natriuretic peptide.

99. How is the antibody response to an antigen different in an old person as compared to a younger one?

The total amount of antibody produced in response to a challenge (perhaps an immunization) is essentially unchanged with increasing age. The quality of the antibody produced is poorer because the affinity of the antibody for its intended antigen may be less than that produced by a young person. The specificity of the antibody is a function of the T cell that is directing the B-cell response. Many of the functions of the T cell, especially those dependent on interleukin-II, are significantly impaired with increasing age.

100. What are the causes of fecal incontinence?

Causes of Fecal Incontinence

1. Fecal impaction with overflow diarrhea
2. Laxative overuse or abuse
3. Neurological disorders:
    Dementia
    Stroke
    Spinal cord injury
4. Colorectal disorders:
    Diarrheal illnesses
    Rectal sphincter damage
    Neoplastic or inflammatory processes

101. Is there any evidence that supports the idea that our life span is programmed in our genes?

Yes, there is substantial evidence that our maximum life span is primarily genetic:

1. There are large differences in maturation and maximum life span among species, from days to more than a century.

2. In some short-lived species, breeding has been very successful in lengthening maximum life span about 50% (fruit flies).

3. In almost all species the female will outlive the male.

4. The similarities in aging and life expectancy between monozygotic twins are remarkable and are closer than dizygotic twins.

102. How can John Adelbert Kelley still run the Boston Marathon at age 83?

Kelley claims he now trains harder to compensate for age decrements. At this writing Mr. Kelley is about to run his 60th Boston Marathon and he is the oldest person actually to run this marathon (26 miles, 385 yards). He is a medical wonder, with a resting pulse of 60 bpm versus the normal of 72 bpm. His goal is to run until he is 100, at least.

BIBLIOGRAPHY

The primary references and sources for many of the answers that are not referenced are listed below. The *Syllabus* is a highly readable resident- or intelligent-student-level text. *Principles* is an encyclopedic reference work.

1. Beck JC: Geriatrics Review Syllabus: A Core Curriculum in Geriatric Medicine. New York, American Geriatrics Society, 1989.
2. Hazzard WR, Andres R, Bierman EL, Blass JP: Principles of Geriatric Medicine and Gerontology, 2nd ed. New York, McGraw-Hill, 1990.

Other reference sources:

3. Kane RL, et al: Essentials of Clinical Geriatrics, 2nd ed. New York, McGraw-Hill, 1989.
4. Schrier RW (ed): Clinical Internal Medicine in the Aged. Philadelphia, W.B. Saunders, 1982.

INDEX

Entries in **boldface** type indicate complete chapters.